# BSAVA Manual of Canine and Feline Behavioural Medicine

## Second edition

Editors:

## Debra F. Horwitz
**DVM DipACVB**

Veterinary Behavior Consultations, 11469 Olive Boulevard #254,
St Louis, MO 63141-7108, USA

**and**

## Daniel S. Mills
**BVSc PhD CBiol FIBiol FHEA CCAB DipECVBM-CA MRCVS**

Department of Biological Sciences, University of Lincoln,
Riseholme Park, Lincoln LN2 2LG, UK

Published by:

**British Small Animal Veterinary Association**
Woodrow House, 1 Telford Way, Waterwells
Business Park, Quedgeley, Gloucester GL2 2AB

A Company Limited by Guarantee in England.
Registered Company No. 2837793.
Registered as a Charity.

Copyright © 2023 BSAVA
First edition published 2002
Second edition published 2009
Reprinted 2012, 2015, 2017, 2018, 2020, 2021, 2023

A catalogue record for this book is available from the British Library.

ISBN 978 1 905319 15 2

The publishers, editors and contributors cannot take responsibility for information
provided on dosages and methods of application of drugs mentioned or referred to
in this publication. Details of this kind must be verified in each case by individual
users from up to date literature published by the manufacturers or suppliers of those
drugs. Veterinary surgeons are reminded that in each case they must follow all
appropriate national legislation and regulations (for example, in the United Kingdom,
the prescribing cascade) from time to time in force.

Printed in the UK by Severn, Gloucester GL2 5EU – a carbon neutral printer
Printed on ECF paper made from sustainable forests

18597PUBS23

# Other titles in the BSAVA Manuals series:

*Manual of Avian Practice: A Foundation Manual*
*Manual of Backyard Poultry Medicine and Surgery*
*Manual of Canine & Feline Abdominal Imaging*
*Manual of Canine & Feline Abdominal Surgery*
*Manual of Canine & Feline Advanced Veterinary Nursing*
*Manual of Canine & Feline Anaesthesia and Analgesia*
*Manual of Canine & Feline Behavioural Medicine*
*Manual of Canine & Feline Cardiorespiratory Medicine*
*Manual of Canine & Feline Clinical Pathology*
*Manual of Canine & Feline Dentistry and Oral Surgery*
*Manual of Canine & Feline Dermatology*
*Manual of Canine & Feline Emergency and Critical Care*
*Manual of Canine & Feline Endocrinology*
*Manual of Canine & Feline Endoscopy and Endosurgery*
*Manual of Canine & Feline Fracture Repair and Management*
*Manual of Canine & Feline Gastroenterology*
*Manual of Canine & Feline Haematology and Transfusion Medicine*
*Manual of Canine & Feline Head, Neck and Thoracic Surgery*
*Manual of Canine & Feline Musculoskeletal Disorders*
*Manual of Canine & Feline Musculoskeletal Imaging*
*Manual of Canine & Feline Nephrology and Urology*
*Manual of Canine & Feline Neurology*
*Manual of Canine & Feline Oncology*
*Manual of Canine & Feline Ophthalmology*
*Manual of Canine & Feline Radiography and Radiology: A Foundation Manual*
*Manual of Canine & Feline Rehabilitation, Supportive and Palliative Care: Case Studies in Patient Management*
*Manual of Canine & Feline Reproduction and Neonatology*
*Manual of Canine & Feline Shelter Medicine: Principles of Health and Welfare in a Multi-animal Environment*
*Manual of Canine & Feline Surgical Principles: A Foundation Manual*
*Manual of Canine & Feline Thoracic Imaging*
*Manual of Canine & Feline Ultrasonography*
*Manual of Canine & Feline Wound Management and Reconstruction*
*Manual of Canine Practice: A Foundation Manual*
*Manual of Exotic Pet and Wildlife Nursing*
*Manual of Exotic Pets: A Foundation Manual*
*Manual of Feline Practice: A Foundation Manual*
*Manual of Practical Animal Care*
*Manual of Practical Veterinary Nursing*
*Manual of Practical Veterinary Welfare*
*Manual of Psittacine Birds*
*Manual of Rabbit Medicine*
*Manual of Rabbit Surgery, Dentistry and Imaging*
*Manual of Raptors, Pigeons and Passerine Birds*
*Manual of Reptiles*
*Manual of Rodents and Ferrets*
*Manual of Small Animal Practice Management and Development*
*Manual of Wildlife Casualties*

For further information on these and all BSAVA publications, please visit our website: **www.bsava.com/store**

# Contents

# Client handouts

## Client handouts

### Behaviour problems

#### Aggression
Avoiding aggression in cats
Handling exercises for an aggressive cat
Ladder of Aggression
Redirected aggression in dogs

#### Fear and stress
Taking your cat in the car
Treating a fear of car journeys using desensitization and counter-conditioning
Treating a fear of the veterinary clinic using desensitization and counter-conditioning
Treating a noise fear using desensitization and counter-conditioning

#### House soiling and marking
Avoiding house soiling by cats
Avoiding house soiling by dogs
Avoiding urine marking by cats

#### Senior pets
Cognitive dysfunction syndrome

#### Separation anxiety
Treating separation anxiety in dogs

### New pets
Adopting a rescue dog: the pros and cons
Introducing a new cat into the household
The newly adopted rescue dog: preventing problems

#### Puppies and kittens
Handling exercises for puppies and kittens
Litterbox training
Playing with your kitten
Puppy socialization: getting used to new people
Your puppy's first year

## Owner aids for training
Down–stay mat exercises
Headcollar training
How to find a good trainer
'Leave it' exercises
Muzzle training
'Nothing in Life is Free'
Recall exercises
Sit–stay exercises
Teaching your dog to go to a place on command

### Welfare
Environmental enrichment for cats in animal shelters
Environmental enrichment for dogs in animal shelters
Playing with your dog – toys
What your cat needs
What your cat needs: multi-cat households
What your dog needs

### Miscellaneous
Complementary therapies in behaviour problems

## Client questionnaires

Canine behaviour profile
Canine behaviour questionnaire
Feline behaviour questionnaire
Noise fear score sheet
Pet selection questionnaire
Questionnaire to assess separation anxiety
Request for information on problem behaviours

## Referral form

The Companion Animal Behaviour Therapy Study Group Referral Form

## Client handouts

To access the client handouts and other leaflets that accompany this manual, visit bsavalibrary.com/behaviour_leaflets or scan the QR code on your mobile device.

# Contributors

**Melissa Bain** DVM DipACVB MS
University of California, School of Veterinary Medicine, Clinical Animal Behavior Service, 1 Shields Avenue, Davis, CA 95616, USA

**Jon Bowen** BVetMed DipAS(CABC) MRCVS
Behavioural Medicine Referral Service, Queen Mother Hospital for Animals, The Royal Veterinary College, Hawkshead Lane, North Mymms, Hatfield, Hertfordshire AL9 7TA, UK

**Rachel Casey** BVMS PhD DipECVBM-CA Dip(AS)CABC CCAB ILTM MRCVS
Department of Clinical Veterinary Science, University of Bristol, Langford House, Langford, Bristol BS40 5DU, UK

**Claire Corridan** BVMS MRCVS
Animal Behaviour, Cognition and Welfare Group, Department of Biological Sciences, University of Lincoln, Riseholme Park, Lincoln LN2 2LG, UK

**Sharon L. Crowell-Davies** DVM PhD DipACVB
College of Veterinary Medicine, University of Georgia, Athens, GA 30602, USA

**Sagi Denenberg** DVM
North Toronto Animal Clinic, 99 Henderson Avenue, Thornhill, Ontario L3T 2K9, Canada

**Jaume Fatjó** DVM PhD DipECVBM-CA
The Society for the Protection of Animals of the City of Mataró, C/Galicia s/n, 08303 Mataró, Spain

**Sarah Heath** BVSc DipECVBM-CA CCAB MRCVS
Behavioural Referrals Veterinary Practice, 10 Rushton Drive, Upton, Chester CH2 1RE, UK

**Debra F. Horwitz** DVM DipACVB
Veterinary Behavior Consultations, 11469 Olive Boulevard #254, St Louis, MO 63141-7108, USA

**Katherine A. Houpt** VMD PhD DipACVB
Department of Clinical Sciences, College of Veterinary Medicine, Cornell University, Ithaca, NY 14853-6401, USA

**Wayne Hunthausen** DVM
Animal Behavior Consultations, 4820 Rainbow Boulevard, Westwood, KS 66205, USA

**Hildegard Jung** DVM Zusatzbezeichnung Verhaltenstherapie
Veterinary Behaviour Consultations, Stengelstrasse, 6a D-80805, München, Germany

**Tiny De Keuster** DVM DipECVBM-CA
Veterinary Behaviour Consultations, Oostveldkouter 222, 9920 Lovendegem, Belgium

**Gary M. Landsberg** BSc DVM DipACVB DipECVBM-CA MRCVS
North Toronto Animal Clinic, 99 Henderson Avenue, Thornhill, Ontario L3T 2K9, Canada

**Emily D. Levine** DVM DipACVB MRCVS
Animal Emergency & Referral Associates, 1237 Bloomfield Avenue, Fairfield, NJ 07004, USA

**Ellen Lindell** VMD DipACVB
Veterinary Behavior Consultations, 6 Brenner Ridge Road, Pleasant Valley, NY 12569, USA

**Samantha Lindley** BVSc MRCVS
Glasgow University Veterinary School, 461 Bearsden Road, Bearsden, Glasgow G61 1QH, UK

**Andrew U. Luescher** Drmedvet PhD DipACVB ECVBM-CA
Purdue University, Veterinary Clinical Sciences, 625 Harrison Street, West Lafayette, IN 47907-2026, USA

**Daniel S. Mills** BVSc PhD CBiol FIBiol FHEA CCAB DipECVBM-CA MRCVS
Department of Biological Sciences, University of Lincoln, Riseholme Park, Lincoln LN2 2LG, UK

**Jacqueline C. Neilson** DVM DipACVB
Animal Behavior Clinic, 809 SE Powell Boulevard, Portland, OR 97202, USA

**Lorella Notari** DVM MSc
Veterinary Behaviour Clinic, Via Donatello, 6 21100 Varese, Italy

**Clara Palestrini** DVM PhD Dip ECVBM-CA
Sez. di Zootecnica Veterinaria, Dipartimento di Scienze Animali, Facoltà di Medicina Veterinaria, Università degli Studi di Milano, Via Celoria, 10 20133 Milano, Italy

**Irene Rochlitz** BVSc MSc PhD MRCVS
Department of Veterinary Medicine, University of Cambridge, Madingley Road, Cambridge CB3 0ES, UK

**Kersti Seksel** BVSc(Hons) MA(Hons) FACVSc DipACVB CMAVA DipECVBM-CA MRCVS
Sydney Animal Behaviour Service, 55 Ethel Street, Seaforth, New South Wales 2092, Australia

**Sheila Segurson** DVM DipACVB
Animal Rescue League of Boston, 10 Chandler Street, Boston, MA 02116, USA

**Kendal Shepherd** BVSc CCAB MRCVS
16 Church Street, Finedon, Wellingborough, Northants NN9 5NA, UK

# Foreword

The *BSAVA Manual of Canine and Feline Behavioural Medicine, second edition*, is an updated source of information which provides new ideas and concepts about a subject that fascinates and frustrates pet owners. The first edition of the *BSAVA Manual of Canine and Feline Behavioural Medicine* was a big success because it proved to be an excellent resource for veterinarians wanting to incorporate animal behavior into their companion animal practices. It was written by experts in the field of behavior in a concise but thorough way.

Companion animals have become significantly more important to their owners over the past 25 years, but with this increased closeness has come less understanding of what animals do and how to prevent unacceptable behaviors developing. In fact, owners often have a tendency to reward the very behaviors they do not want. At the same time, research is providing a greater respect for the interconnections between mind and body. From the simplest concept – that stress to an individual affects cortisol levels – we have progressed. As an example, for years a cat that urinated in the house had a behavior problem. Well, it is still a behavior problem, but we now recognize that a certain percent of these cats may have interstitial cystitis with bladder wall pathology. Feline hyperesthesia is now a condition with identifiable microscopic changes at the cellular level, and not just a neurotic cat on which to try a variety of drugs, hoping that one will be helpful. In addition, we are appreciating that psychopharmacologic agents not only alter behavior, they also alter the chemistry of the brain in many more subtle ways.

Behavioral medicine continues to advance at a rapid rate, so it is important for veterinarians to have excellent sources of information in order to be able to stay current. Because this subject is often not taught in the veterinary curricula of many universities, it becomes even more important to have up-to-date information available to practitioners. It is also important that this material be easy to understand. The *BSAVA Manual of Canine and Feline Behavioural Medicine, second edition* provides just that type of material. The Editors have again tapped global experts in animal behavior to provide the reader with the 'latest and greatest' for helping their clients. The Manual is practical in scope and broad in subject matter. It is an outstanding book that should find its way on to the shelves of progressive practitioners everywhere.

**Bonnie V. Beaver BS DVM MS DPNAP DipACVB**
Executive Director, American College of Veterinary Behaviorists

# Preface

In the seven years since the first edition of this Manual was published much has changed in veterinary behaviour. More specialists have entered the field, and an increase in information and research has moved us forward in our understanding of canine and feline behaviour and its management. Although veterinary surgeons are as busy as ever, they are increasingly aware of the impact of behaviour on all facets of veterinary medicine. This updated Manual is our effort to share that new knowledge with our colleagues.

This new edition attempts to help both the general and aspiring specialist practitioner continue to expand their knowledge and provide them with useful information that can be readily applied to the daily practice of veterinary medicine. The Manual begins with a highly informative discussion of the impact of medical issues on behaviour and what the veterinary surgeon should know to make sure an animal receives appropriate care. Only the veterinary profession has the unique responsibility for the medical aspects of any case. The next chapters cover the area of behavioural husbandry and will enable the veterinary surgeon to create a behaviour-friendly practice and increase the welfare and satisfaction of both their patients and clients. The following chapters are designed to give valuable information on how to optimize the welfare of our canine and feline patients, and to educate and teach our clients about this most important issue.

The remainder of the chapters cover various areas of behaviour problems in dogs and cats. We have also added a special chapter on shelter animals as they deserve special attention, and this is an area where veterinary support is increasingly sought in both health and husbandry. This new Manual places the emphasis on diagnosis, understanding the behavioural biology of the condition, and detailed treatment plans. At the end of each chapter there is a listing of accompanying handouts to enable the veterinary surgeon to create detailed and functional treatment plans for their patients. These handouts, along with a detailed behavioural questionnaire for each species, are available from **bsavalibrary.com/behaviour_leaflets**.

Our goal is to optimize the welfare and health of our companion animals, and toward that end new information on communication and learning helps readers shed old myths about canine and feline behaviour. We hope through an understanding of our patients we can improve their behavioural health, strengthen the human–animal bond and keep pets happy, safe and in their homes.

**Debra F. Horwitz**
**Daniel S. Mills**
**August 2009**

# Medical and metabolic influences on behavioural disorders

## Jaume Fatjó and Jon Bowen

## Introduction

There is general agreement in the field of veterinary medicine that canine and feline behaviour problems referred to veterinary surgeons may often be related to the existence of an underlying medical condition.

This statement has two important practical consequences:

- A veterinary surgeon should be the first professional to evaluate a dog or a cat presented for a behaviour problem
- A diagnostic protocol for a behaviour problem should always include a medical examination; and a diagnostic protocol for a medical problem should always consider the possibility of a behaviour problem.

In fact, the idea that medical conditions can alter behaviour is probably the most important and genuine contribution of veterinary medicine to the field of applied ethology.

Medical disorders may have 'deficit' and 'productive' effects on behaviour:

- *Deficit effects* are characterized by a decrease in certain behaviours, such as alertness, exploratory behaviour, eating, drinking and social interaction
- *Productive effects* facilitate the expression of certain behaviours that were previously less intense, less frequent or not present at all, for example aggression, inappropriate elimination, vocalization, eating, drinking or self-mutilation.

Some reviews offer extensive lists of medical disorders that may be considered to be differentials for, or contributory factors to, behavioural disorders. Whilst these appeal to common sense and may be supported by evidence from human medicine, there is a lack of specific evidence to support many of these associations in the veterinary context. This chapter will therefore avoid this area of contention and rather discuss a systematic approach that allows veterinary surgeons to apply their existing knowledge within a framework that incorporates behavioural information.

## How medical conditions may affect behaviour

One of the most important features of biological systems is that they are adaptive. Within the animal, adaptation can occur in a number of ways, including alterations in gene expression, the regulation of biochemical pathways and the production of specialized proteins or cells (e.g. immunoglobulins, T cells). Behaviour is the adaptive output of the central nervous system (CNS), enabling the animal to respond to environmental changes, motivational states (such as hunger or thirst) and pathological states (such as pain). Through its behaviour the animal maintains its bodily integrity by protecting itself and gaining the resources it needs. Medical conditions can affect behaviour in a number of different ways, which include: alterations in motivation; a general response to illness; and direct impairment of brain function.

### Altered motivation

An individual's time and energy need to be divided efficiently between a range of activities. At any given moment, behaviour is the product of the balance between numerous motivational states that arise out of an animal's need to maintain itself, protect itself and reproduce.

Motivational states have subtle effects on an individual's behaviour. For example, as hunger increases, an animal's priorities gradually shift away from other activities towards obtaining food.

Medical conditions that alter motivation have subtle and general effects on an animal's behaviour. For example, the superficial effect of diabetes is that the animal eats and drinks more. Since this animal may experience an almost permanently raised level of hunger and thirst, the priority to maintain access to valuable food and water resources may cause it to engage in aggressive behaviour that is to the detriment of social relationships with the owner and other animals in the household. Due to the constant need to find opportunities to get food the animal may be active at times when it might otherwise choose to rest, causing fatigue and irritability.

Any adaptive behavioural change, such as lameness, polyphagia, polydipsia, or increased grooming due to pruritus, should be seen as evidence that the animal's priorities and motivations are also altered.

### Examples of pain

Pain alters motivation in favour of avoidance and defensive behaviours. In a study to validate an owner questionnaire to evaluate quality of life in dogs experiencing pain, Wiseman-Orr *et al.* (2006) produced a consistent 12-factor model that included dimensions such as 'listless–reluctant', 'panicky–nervous', 'aggressive–unresponsive', 'confused–complaining', 'attention-seeking–comfort-seeking', and 'whining–crying'. This model forms a reliable basis for assessing quality of life in patients with pain and provides direct evidence that the behaviour of animals is altered by pain.

Pain also causes subtle adaptive changes in normal behaviours, such as altered gait in arthritic patients. The lameness that these animals display is an adaptation that allows the animal to continue to move whilst experiencing reduced discomfort. This type of adaptation can persist long after the pain has subsided.

A relevant behavioural example is persistent house soiling by cats that have previously experienced tenesmus and pain on defecation. It is suspected that these cats may shift the site of their elimination away from familiar places where pain has previously been experienced, causing them to defecate in places undesirable to the owner.

## General response to illness

When animals suffer from illness they tend to become withdrawn, reduce their energy expenditure by resting more often and disengage from social contact. Previously it was assumed that this was merely a product of debilitation or dysphoria resulting from the disease state. Current evidence indicates that, in the same way that fever is part of an immune defence strategy to combat infectious disease, 'sickness behaviour' (Figure 1.1) is, in fact, a highly motivated adaptive response that enables the animal to recover and prevents disease transmission. In preference tests, for example, animals will work harder to gain access to opportunities to rest and withdraw than to gain access to water (Johnson, 2002). This change of priorities is mediated by the effect of inflammatory interleukins on the CNS (Dantzer, 2001). The characteristic 'sickness behaviour' appears similar to that of behavioural inhibition seen in animals under psychological stress, but may be differentiated on the basis of signs of illness such as pyrexia or an inflammatory leucogram.

| Behaviour | Change |
|---|---|
| General activity | Reduced |
| Exploratory behaviour | Reduced |
| Food and water intake | Reduced |
| Play | Reduced |
| Wakefulness | Reduced (sleep increased) |
| Social interaction | Reduced |

**1.1** Characteristic 'sickness behaviour'.

## Conditions arising out of brain dysfunction

Any medical condition that directly or indirectly affects the normal functioning of the CNS has the potential to alter behaviour. Primary CNS dysfunctions that could alter behaviour include brain tumours, hydrocephalus, cerebral trauma and partial psychogenic seizures.

The effects on behaviour of a particular lesion depend on the structure or neural pathway that is affected, regardless of the exact aetiology. For instance, the amygdala is a part of the limbic system involved in the regulation of many aspects of behaviour, including emotional responses, such as fear and rage. Thus, any lesion affecting the amygdala could facilitate aggression, no matter whether it results from neoplasia, trauma or a vascular disorder.

Neurological function can be compromised by conditions that arise within the CNS and other organ systems. It is important to remember that nervous tissue is specialized and is highly sensitive to any systemic metabolic or hormonal disturbance. Systemic diseases with behavioural manifestations include: canine hypothyroidism, feline hyperthyroidism and other hormonal disorders; hepatic encephalopathy; uraemic encephalopathy; and exposure to toxic materials or infectious agents (Overall, 2003; Bagley, 2004a).

### Brain tumours

Tumours located in the brain are often slow growing and lead to behavioural changes, with or without accompanying physical signs such as circling, ataxia, cranial nerve deficits and seizures. Neurological dysfunction results from local compression of the surrounding parenchyma, ischaemia due to vascular damage and oedema, inflammation and increased intracranial pressure. Behavioural clinical signs are usually focal and specifically related to the affected area or neural pathway (Figure 1.2). A pattern of altered behaviour may also result indirectly from the induction of partial psychomotor seizures that affect the function of structures of the limbic system, which is primarily involved in the regulation of emotional reactions.

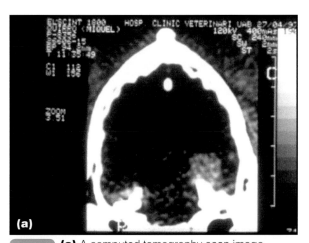

(a)

**1.2** **(a)** A computed tomography scan image showing a homogenously enhanced, well defined, round, broad-based lesion located in the region of the left piriform lobe. The patient was presented for aggression in the absence of other obvious clinical signs. Physical and neurological examination did not reveal any abnormality and the results of routine blood tests were within the normal range. (continues) ▶

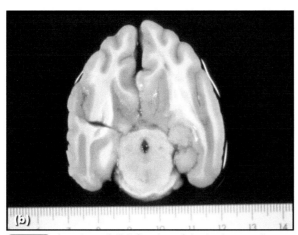

**1.2** (continued) **(b)** Section of the brain revealing a nodular, well demarcated, unencapsulated mass (1 × 1 × 0.7 cm) between the mesencephalon and the left temporal lobe.

## Clinical approach

### Problem presentation

In the presentation of any behavioural or medical problem there is often a difference of perspective between the client and the veterinary surgeon. A pathological process may produce behavioural and physical signs, but of differing importance and relevance to the veterinary surgeon and the client. The same condition, and pathological process, may present as a different balance of behavioural and physical signs in each patient, so that no two cases will be identical. This presents a challenge to the veterinary surgeon, who must appreciate all dimensions of the presentation.

Signs of illness recognized by the owner will include many items that are behavioural, but the veterinary surgeon will tend to focus on physical signs, as these are the most observable in the clinic. This difference in perspective might result in one of the following situations.

- The owner's and veterinary surgeon's perceptions might agree, though they may each be unaware that they are seeing the same underlying disease process from completely different points of view. This situation is achieved by a combination of good history taking and an appreciation of the owner's observations of the animal's behaviour within the context of a pathological process.
- If behavioural signs are very apparent to the owner but the physical signs are subtle or not readily observed, or are complex, or inconsistent with an obvious disease process, then the veterinary surgeon may label the problem as 'behavioural', without considering medical aspects. However, there is a real possibility that the behavioural changes are actually the first indication of a disease process that has not yet resulted in readily observable physical signs. It is important to regard this situation as a justification for medical testing, rather than a reason to overlook the involvement of disease and falsely underestimate the current pathological state.

- Physical signs may be of such prominence that both the veterinary surgeon and the owner overlook the behavioural signs and fail to appreciate the full consequences of the illness. For example, a dog with a painful paw shows facial and body postural signs that indicate its emotional response to the situation (Figure 1.3). This should suggest that its reaction to normal contact, such as handling, may be uncharacteristically aggressive and defensive because of its altered motivations and priorities.

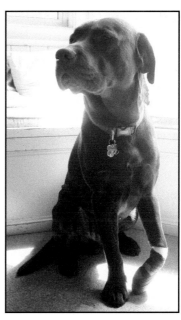

**1.3** A dog with a painful paw may react in an uncharacteristically defensive manner. The veterinary surgeon should be aware of behavioural changes that may be linked to physical signs.

In all of these situations there is a physical pathology or pathological process that is the common factor between the behavioural and physical signs, with behavioural signs often being observed well in advance of physical changes.

The aims of the clinical evaluation of a patient presented for a change in behaviour are to answer four fundamental questions:

- What are the biological meaning and motivation underlying the reported behaviour problem?
- Could the change in behaviour be related to an underlying medical condition?
- What disease processes could explain the change in behaviour?
- Is the medical condition the primary cause or just a contributing factor in the expression of the problem behaviour?

In order to answer these questions the veterinary surgeon should take the following steps:

1. Obtain a complete behavioural history.
2. Perform a thorough medical examination.

### Behavioural history

From a diagnostic perspective behaviour must be understood as a complex sign that should be carefully evaluated. In most cases the problem behaviour cannot be directly observed by the veterinary surgeon,

3

who must depend on information provided by the owner. This situation is not unique to behavioural problems; the owner's recollection of the dog's behaviour is considered to be the fundamental source of information required to characterize neurological conditions such as epileptic seizures.

Sample behavioural history forms for dogs and cats are provided in the Appendix. Information gathering includes the following key steps:

- Record and detail *all* changes in behaviour
- Describe and evaluate the level of consistency of the behavioural pattern
- Collect details of the origin and evolution of the behaviour.

### Record and detail all changes in behaviour
The chief complaint is the reason for the owner to seek advice, but a complete description of the dog's overall behaviour is fundamental.

- Problem behaviour: is this a new behaviour or a change in an existing but previously tolerated behaviour?
- Changes in other behaviour (e.g. eating, drinking, social interaction, play).

### Describe and evaluate level of consistency of behavioural pattern
There needs to be a clear description of the problem

behaviour, including:

- Motor sequence
- Body posture
- Stimuli that may trigger the behaviour
- Contexts within which the behaviour occurs, including early presentations and present occurrences.

It is important to judge whether the pattern of the patient's behaviour is well organized and consistent. This applies not only to the specific problem behaviour, but also to the individual's general behaviour. For example, patterns of behaviour that are the product of learning and refinement through experience should be responsive to specific stimuli and contexts, but if there is a reduction in performance this may indicate ill health.

Sequences of behaviour should possess a narrative quality, with an initiating event followed by a flexible set of behavioural responses and finishing when an outcome is achieved or when there is some terminating event. If these conditions are met, the implication is that the behaviour is normally organized and less likely to be the result of CNS pathology. Figure 1.4 can be used as a practical visual scale to estimate the consistency between the problem behaviour, any external stimuli that it relates to, and the contexts in which it appears.

---

Answer each question by placing a mark at some point along the line beneath it. This provides a visual analogue scale.

Does the problem behaviour occur in response to an external event?
ALWAYS _____ NEVER

Does the problem behaviour occur in response to the same range of stimuli?
ALWAYS _____ NEVER

Does the problem behaviour occur in a well defined set of contexts?
ALWAYS _____ NEVER

Does the animal easily respond to environmental cues while performing the problem behaviour? (Is the behaviour easily interrupted by the opportunity to engage in other activities?)
ALWAYS _____ NEVER

Does the behaviour stop spontaneously?
ALWAYS _____ NEVER

Does the behaviour last longer than expected?
NO _____ YES

Is this individual's behaviour typical of that which would be expected for its age and developmental circumstances?
YES _____ NO

Is the current behaviour characteristic of the individual's previous adult pattern of behaviour?
YES _____ NO

Can the change in behaviour be linked to an identifiable change in the environment or a significant experience?
YES _____ NO

Is this a normal but unwanted behavioural response (for example, food-guarding behaviour)?
YES _____ NO

**What is the likelihood that an organic lesion is responsible for the change in behaviour?**
LOW _____ HIGH

**1.4** Evaluation of behaviour. When answering the following questions a trend to mostly left-sided marks suggests a consistent behavioural pattern, whereas a trend to the right indicates less consistency and a greater probability that there is an underlying medical condition. This should be taken only as a guide, but a strong bias to the right should prompt an increased depth of medical investigation even in the relative absence of conventional physical indicators of disease.

### Collect details of origin and evolution of the behaviour

Answers to the following questions will help to reveal the precise nature and underlying motivation of the problem behaviour.

- How did the behaviour first become apparent?
- How has the behaviour developed and changed over time?

In the absence of underlying medical factors, behavioural problems often follow a trajectory through the animal's life, with signs becoming more severe or evolving in character and frequency over time. For example, a dog that is presented with fear-related aggression towards people may have exhibited early signs of fear and avoidance of people when younger, as a result of a lack of socialization or a series of aversive experiences. Thus a consistent narrative exists within the patient's history. Barring specific negative experiences or changes in environment, an individual's personality and style of response to situations is relatively stable from maturity onward.

## Medical examination

Medical examination is a key step in evaluating behavioural problem cases. The current evidence is that the combination of a routine medical examination with a thorough behavioural examination is sufficient to detect the majority of behaviour problems where a medical condition is implicated (Luescher, 1998). Consequently, veterinary surgeons should be familiar with the basic patterns of problem behaviour in dogs and cats, since diagnosis in behavioural medicine should not be restricted to specialists.

### Physical examination

The routine physical examination should encompass all body systems and should include:

- Abdominal palpation
- Auscultation of the chest (heart and lungs)
- Flexion and extension of all limbs and neck
- Assessment of muscular development and symmetry
- Palpation of the spine
- Examination of sensory systems
- Surface examination (skin and mucocutaneous junctions)
- Measurement of blood pressure (where possible).

### Pain evaluation

It is important to discover sources of pain and to rule out painful illness during the initial assessment of behaviour cases. This is critical for welfare, especially when behavioural therapy may involve a demanding programme of training. The American Animal Hospital Association (AAHA) and American Association of Feline Practitioners (AAFP) Pain Management Guidelines for Dogs and Cats (Hellyer *et al.*, 2007) list signs of pain (Figure 1.5), identify a number of commonly overlooked causes of pain (including cardiopulmonary, dermatological, dental and ocular) and suggest methods of managing pain.

| Loss of normal behaviour |
|---|
| Reduced locomotor activity<br>Reduced general activity<br>Lethargy<br>Reduced appetite<br>Reduced grooming (cats) |

| Expression of 'abnormal' behaviours |
|---|
| Inappropriate elimination<br>Vocalization<br>Aggression<br>Decreased interaction with other pets or family members<br>Facial and body posture<br>Restlessness<br>Hiding (especially cats) |

| Reaction to touch |
|---|
| Increased body tension or flinching in response to gentle palpation of injured area and palpation of regions likely to be painful, e.g. neck, back, hips, elbows (cats) |

| Physiological parameters |
|---|
| Raised heart rate<br>Raised respiratory rate<br>Increased body temperature<br>Increased pulse rate<br>Pupil dilatation |

**1.5** Signs of pain (after Hellyer *et al.*, 2007)

They place pain into two broad categories:

- 'Adaptive' pain (inflammatory or nociceptive)
- 'Maladaptive' pain (neuropathic or functional).

Adaptive pain is the normal response to damage to tissues and will resolve with proper treatment. However, inappropriately treated chronic adaptive pain leads to physical changes in the brain and spinal cord, so that the pain becomes maladaptive. Pain is therefore not only an immediate welfare issue for the animal, but can also have a long-term impact unless properly treated.

Many different classes of drug may be used, singly or in combination, in the management of pain, including alpha-2 agonists, corticosteroids, local anaesthetics, $N$-methyl-D-aspartate (NMDA) receptor antagonists, non-steroidal anti-inflammatory drugs (NSAIDs), opioids, topical anaesthetics, tricyclic antidepressants and antiepileptic drugs.

Non-analgesic anxiolytic drugs may be used to reduce anxiety (which increases perception of pain). As the nature of pain changes over time, pain management must also involve regular re-evaluation and modification. The response to NSAIDs, or other analgesic drugs, should not be used as a diagnostic tool to identify the presence of pain: failure to respond to such drugs does not mean that the animal is not in pain. The full AAHA/AAFP Guidelines are available online at www.aahanet.org/PublicDocuments/PainManagementGuidelines.pdf.

For patients that are known to suffer from painful conditions, such as osteoarthritis, it is important to monitor pain regularly, not only so that treatments can be modified to reduce suffering but also so that self-defensive motivational effects of pain are minimized.

No single scale has been agreed for pain assessment and management, but a questionnaire-based approach that uses owner observation to evaluate quality of life (Wiseman-Orr *et al.*, 2006) has been validated. The information from this questionnaire is in accordance with the expectation that pain is associated with emotional and motivational changes.

### Routine laboratory tests
Disease processes may produce behavioural change without strongly evident physical signs. A physical examination, while essential, may be insufficient for the evaluation of many behavioural problems. It is therefore recommended that routine urinalysis, haematology and biochemistry examinations be performed as a health screen for behaviour cases. Additional tests, such as those for thyroid disease or adrenocortical function, should be added in line with physical and behavioural indications. Nevertheless, there is still a lack of consensus between authors regarding the minimum set of laboratory tests that should be included in a routine examination of a behaviour problem or what the contribution of abnormal results may be to an observed behavioural pathology.

### Neurological examination
Neurological disorders, such as epilepsy or a traumatic brain injury, may have profound effects on behaviour without signs that may be observed in a physical examination or routine laboratory tests. It is important to perform a neurological examination to identify any abnormalities and, where possible, to localize any lesion. A definitive neurological examination may require specialist referral if the general practitioner finds subtle or multiple signs that are difficult to interpret. Additional tests, including conduction tests and imaging, may be required.

### Medical investigation prior to referral
The level of medical investigation required prior to referral depends on the professional training and competence of the individual to whom cases are referred. If that person is a veterinary surgeon working within a referral centre such as a university, it may be acceptable for the referring veterinary surgeon to perform only basic preliminary investigations before referral on the basis that expert investigation is available within the referral practice. The demands on the referring veterinary surgeon are much greater if the case is to be referred to a non-veterinary behaviourist and such cases should be investigated more thoroughly. If a patient is known to suffer from concurrent disease, it is generally recommended that it should be referred only to a veterinary behaviourist, especially if the referring veterinary surgeon is unsure about the potential interaction between the disease, its treatment and the animal's behaviour.

### Medical investigation prior to prescribing of psychoactive medication
Before prescribing a licensed preparation it is important to consult a current product monograph in order to identify drug interactions and contraindications. It is advisable that a baseline blood workup be carried out (unless one has been performed very recently), as many psychoactive medications have metabolic and haematological effects that may need to be monitored. A blood workup is even more important if a preparation is to be used 'off-label', or a non-licensed preparation is to be used. Non-licensed preparations should only be used where evidence of efficacy and safety is available, from either reference texts (see Chapter 21), peer-reviewed publications or expert or specialist sources. They should not be used simply on the advice of a non-veterinary behaviourist. Ultimately the dispensing veterinary surgeon is responsible for all treatments administered.

## An integrative approach
Investigation of behavioural problems must integrate information about the animal's development, environment, diet, behaviour and health status.

In terms of health, a common approach is to assume that a problem can only be considered to be purely behavioural once all potential medical disorders have been ruled out. Unfortunately, this 'diagnosis of exclusion' approach faces a fundamental problem: certain medical conditions that affect behaviour can be excluded only by using advanced, and costly, diagnostic techniques such as computed tomography or magnetic resonance imaging (e.g. brain tumours, see Figure 1.2).

The challenge is to determine the sensible limit of the clinical investigation (Figure 1.6). Once basic medical data have been obtained, the level of consistency between a particular pattern of behaviour and the environment within which it is expressed may help to decide whether there is likely to be an underlying medical condition, and whether it may be necessary to perform additional medical tests (Figure 1.7).

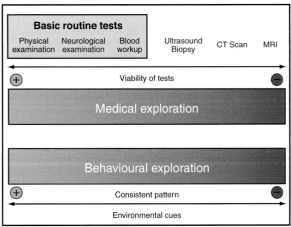

**1.6** How far to investigate? The clinical evaluation of a patient presented for a change in behaviour should simultaneously include a behavioural and a medical examination. Once basic medical data have been obtained, behavioural assessment may help to decide whether additional medical tests should be performed. As a general rule, the more directly and consistently linked the behaviour and the external cues are, the more likely it is that an organic condition is not involved.

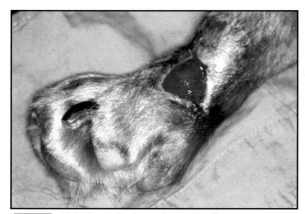

**1.7** Lick dermatitis/granuloma in a German Shepherd Dog, a condition that could result from medical and non-medical factors (i.e. a type of stereotypic or compulsive behaviour). The behavioural history did not reveal any environmental cues that could explain the occurrence of this self-mutilating behaviour. Additional neurological examination including electrophysiological techniques confirmed a sensory neuropathy.

Further evidence of the potential for an underlying medical factor comes from the behavioural history. If the current behaviour of a previously emotionally normal adult animal represents a significant departure from what is characteristic for that animal, and no influential experience or environmental change can be identified, this indicates the possibility of an internal cause. Likewise, if the individual's pattern of development is at odds with what would be expected, given its rearing conditions and current environment, this is a signal that a medical issue may be important.

However, some conditions clearly demonstrate that disease may also lead to well organized and consistent patterns of behaviour that are impossible to differentiate from the non-medical. The explanation could be related not only to the practical limitations of history taking and owner observation (a truly complete picture of the animal's behaviour is not available), but also to the way in which medical conditions affect behaviour. There is increasing evidence that in some instances medical factors could add to other causes in the expression of many behaviour problems, as has been well established in the field of human psychiatry (Cummings and Mega, 2003; Fatjó et al., 2003). In veterinary medicine, some case reports suggest that certain pathological conditions, such as hypothyroidism, could lower the threshold for specifically motivated forms of aggression, such as that relating to fear or resource competition (Fatjó et al., 2003). The resulting behavioural pattern could be very similar to that observed when no medical factors are involved. At least in some cases a careful behavioural history could help to reveal certain inconsistencies in the pattern of aggression, thus stressing the necessity to recover additional information from more specific diagnostic procedures.

**Hypothyroidism**

Canine hypothyroidism has been linked to different behaviour problems and could be present in 1.7% of all canine aggression cases (Reinhard, 1978; Beaver, 1999).

Dogs affected by hypothyroidism and aggression show aggression in contexts similar to those involving social conflict or fear aggression. Common signs of thyroid deficiency in these dogs are very mild or not present at all (Dodman et al., 1995; Beaver, 1999).

The pattern of behaviour shown by these patients may be characterized by different levels of consistency. Although in some cases affected dogs show relatively out-of-context aggression, in others the behaviour could be very difficult to distinguish from aggressive cases where no medical factors are involved. In fact, some recent reports suggest a more complex relationship between hypothyroidism and aggression, where the former will reduce the threshold for the latter. This point of view suggests that hypothyroidism will be not necessarily the primary cause of aggression but one of the many factors that could contribute to its manifestation (Fatjó et al., 2003; Overall, 2003). Thus, thyroid supplementation for hypothyroidism-related aggression should only be considered in conjunction with other therapeutic measures, such as behaviour modification techniques, and only after a functional diagnosis has been established through a complete behavioural history.

The biochemical processes that explain the relationship between hypothyroidism and aggression have still to be clarified. One hypothesis is that thyroid deficiency alters the turnover of serotonin, which is one of the main neurotransmitters involved in the regulation of aggressive behaviour (Aronson, 1998; Kulikov and Zubkov, 2007).

The medical diagnosis of hypothyroidism-related aggression must be done with extreme care, since it almost exclusively relies on laboratory results. A combination of measurements of total or free T4 plus endogenous TSH is usually recommended (Kemppainen and Behrend, 2001). Hypothyroidism can only be suspected when both parameters are outside their normal range and nothing else could account for the lower T4 concentration. In any case, some endocrinologists and behaviourists recommend a more complex diagnostic panel, including total and fractional T3 and T4, as well as anti-T4 and anti-T3 autoantibodies and TSH (Ferguson, 2007).

## How behaviour influences health status

As has already been discussed, medical conditions may have a profound effect on behaviour. However, it is also true that management practices and the level of adaptation to the environment could affect the animal's health. From a practical perspective, the effects of diet and environmental stress in behaviour deserve a more detailed discussion.

### Diet

A properly balanced diet is the basis of good health and development. Prepared diets are generally balanced with respect to protein, carbohydrate, fat, vitamins and minerals, but there is variation in protein source or quality and micronutrient content. Specialist diets have therefore been developed for the treatment of medical conditions such as renal disease, osteoarthritis and cognitive disorder. In addition, many nutraceutical products are available in the form of food supplements. Homemade diets may be seriously nutritionally unbalanced, for example when clients attempt to feed a 'natural diet' that is 100% meat from raw chicken carcasses. Diet and behaviour are discussed further in Chapter 22.

Two areas where there has been some interest are: the use of dietary modification to enhance CNS availability of the serotonin precursor amino acid tryptophan; and supplementation with polyunsaturated fatty acids (PUFAs) such as docosahexanoic acid.

### Tryptophan

Low-protein, high-carbohydrate diets have been advocated for the treatment of behavioural problems in dogs. Dietary amino acids, including tryptophan, have been shown to have an effect on serotonin function and behaviour and tryptophan uptake can be increased by elevating dietary carbohydrate levels (Markus, 2008). In humans, a diet rich in protein-source tryptophan has been shown to have a positive effect on social anxiety disorder (Hudson *et al.*, 2007). Dietary modification of this kind may be routinely prescribed by some behaviourists, but evidence is lacking regarding cases in which it may be of benefit.

### Polyunsaturated fatty acids

PUFAs such as the *n*-3 fatty acids eicosapentanoic acid (EPA) and docosahexanoic acid (DHA) have been proposed as dietary supplements for behavioural disorders and also to promote proper brain development. There is some evidence that PUFA supplementation can produce beneficial effects on cognitive function, attention and mood, but not anxiety, in humans (McCann & Ames, 2005; Ross *et al.*, 2007). PUFA supplementation has also been shown to have positive effects on attentiveness, hyperactivity and impulsiveness in children with attention deficit hyperactivity disorder (Sinn *et al.*, 2008).

There are few studies of the effect of PUFA supplementation in companion animals, other than in dogs with cognitive disorder.

Kelley *et al.* (2004) found that the fatty acid status of puppies, based on red blood cell membrane fatty acid profiles, was significantly affected by fish oil supplement, and puppies given 1.1% fish oil showed significant increase in performance in a discrimination learning task. Heinemann *et al.* (2005) found that bitches fed a diet rich in alpha-lipoic acid (ALA) produced milk with high ALA but not DHA. Puppies fed with this milk had higher plasma DHA, but not as high as those fed a preformed *n*-3 (DHA)-rich diet. Puppies fed the preformed *n*-3 diet showed an improved electroretinogram (ERG) at 12 weeks, with increased light sensitivity and dynamic responses to stimulation. These findings are consistent with those from the human and animal literature and it seems appropriate to recommend that the diet of bitches and puppies be properly balanced with respect to PUFAs.

### Environmental stress

Stress, which may be the product of an inappropriate environment or husbandry, not only alters the individual's sense of dysphoria and pain that make the experience of being ill more difficult to tolerate, but can also play a role in the presentation and severity of certain conditions such as feline interstitial cystitis (Buffington *et al.*, 2006) (see below). In particular, animals expressing 'sickness behaviour' (see Figure 1.1) have a very specific need for opportunities to perform the sickness behaviour, such as having access to places in which to hide or withdraw from contact. Without these opportunities their welfare may be impaired and they may become highly stressed and even aggressive. There is further discussion on the effect of stress on problem behaviour in Chapter 13.

### Feline interstitial/idiopathic cystitis

Feline interstitial cystitis (FIC) is a commonly occurring condition that underlines the potential complexity of pain management. The aetiology of this condition is unclear, but affected individuals may have spinal cord changes and/or altered bladder wall function that could result from a constellation of risk factors, including diet and environmental stress (Figure 1.8). Management may involve the use of analgesic drugs, tricyclic antidepressant drugs and antispasmodic drugs, together with environmental modification and pheromone therapy to reduce stress in a multimodal strategy (Buffington *et al.*, 2006).

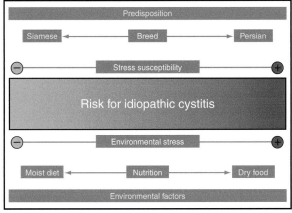

**1.8** A number of different factors combine to contribute to overall risk for feline idiopathic cystitis.

### Feline hyperaesthesia syndrome

In the field of veterinary medicine, feline hyperaesthesia syndrome (rolling skin syndrome, feline neurodermatitis) is an excellent example of a condition in which neurological as well as behavioural factors seem to be involved and provides an opportunity to apply a multidisciplinary approach in the diagnosis and treatment of a behaviour problem.

Affected cats show short episodes of thoracolumbar skin rolling or rippling and epaxial muscle spasms. During episodes patients act in a very anxious manner, with paroxysmal agitation, exaggerated tail movements, dilated pupils, vocalization, running and biting of their flanks and tail (Landsberg *et al.*, 2003).

Feline hyperaesthesia syndrome is referred to as 'idiopathic' in both neurology and behavioural medicine textbooks. Many causal factors have been hypothesized, including focal seizures, a neurological disorder similar to Tourette's syndrome in humans, sensory neuropathies, a vacuolar myopathy, food allergies and environmental stress (Landsberg *et al.*, 2003; Bagley, 2004b). Suggested treatments reflect the wide range of putative aetiological factors and include antiepileptics, amitriptyline, fluoxetine, NSAIDs and hypoallergenic diets. It is possible that many of these factors could operate concurrently in the onset of the problem, with environmental stress and other external stimuli triggering the condition in an otherwise predisposed individual. Thus, the diagnosis should include medical and behavioural assessment and the treatment must be multimodal, combining medical as well as behavioural intervention.

## Conclusion

The border between medically and non-medically related behaviour problems is becoming less well defined as more information is available on the mechanistic aspects of behaviour. The identification of such medical factors in the expression of behaviour depends heavily on the accuracy of the behavioural and medical analysis.

The use of advanced ancillary diagnostic techniques such as electroencephalography (EEG) and positron emission tomography have revealed brain dysfunctions at the deepest level of analysis, i.e. in the turnover of certain neurotransmitters and even in the expression of certain genes, not only in human beings but also in domestic animals (Reisner *et al.*, 1996; Peremans *et al.*, 2003).

Nevertheless it should be remembered that many behaviour problems presented to the veterinary surgeon are just an expression of normal species-specific behaviour that may be appropriate but unwanted. Further, brain functioning and behaviour has proved to be a bidirectional process, where the former affects the latter and *vice versa*. Thus, simple statements on cause-and-effect relationships between behaviour and its neurophysiological correlates should be considered with care.

## References and further reading

Aronson LP (1998) Systemic causes of aggression and their treatment. In: *Psychopharmacology of Animal Behavior Disorders*, ed. NH Dodman and L Shuster, pp. 64–102. Blackwell Sciences, Malden, MA

Bagley RS (2004a) Coma, stupor and behavioural change. In: *BSAVA Manual of Canine and Feline Neurology, 3rd edn*, ed. SR Platt and NJ Olby, pp. 113–132. BSAVA Publications, Gloucester

Bagley RS (2004b) Tremor and involuntary movements. In: *BSAVA Manual of Canine and Feline Neurology, 3rd edn*, ed. SR Platt and NJ Olby, pp. 189–201. BSAVA Publications, Gloucester

Beaver B (1999) *Canine Behavior: A Guide for Veterinarians*. WB Saunders, St Louis

Berendt M, Gredal H and Alving J (2004) Characteristics and phenomenology of epileptic partial seizures in dogs: similarities with human seizure semiology. *Epilepsy Research* 61, 167–173

Buffington CAT, Westropp JL, Chew DJ and Bolus RR (2006) Clinical evaluation of multimodal environmental modification (MEMO) in the management of cats with idiopathic cystitis. *Journal of Feline Medicine and Surgery* 8, 261–268

Cummings JL and Mega MS (2003) *Neuropsychiatry and Behavioral Neuroscience*. Oxford University Press, New York

Dantzer R (2001) Cytokine-induced sickness behavior: where do we stand? *Brain, Behavior and Immunity* 15, 7–24

Dodman NH, Mertens PA and Aronson LP (1995) Animal behavior case of the month. *Journal of the American Veterinary Medical Association* 207, 1168–1170

Fatjó J, Amat M and Manteca X (2003) Aggression and hypothyroidism. *Journal of the American Veterinary Medical Association* 223, 623–626

Fatjó J, Martín S, Manteca X, Añor S, Pumarola M and Palacio J (1999) Animal behavior case of the month. Dominance aggression and pathologic aggression secondary to a brain tumor. *Journal of the American Veterinary Medical Association* 215, 1254–1256

Ferguson, D (2007) Testing for hypothyroidism in dogs. *Veterinary Clinics of North America: Small Animal Practice* 37, 647–670

Heinemann KM, Waldron MK, Bigley KE, Lees GE and Bauer JE (2005) Long chain (*n*-3) polyunsaturated fatty acids are more efficient than alpha-linolenic acid in improving electroretinogram responses of puppies exposed during gestation, lactation and weaning. *The Journal of Nutrition* 135, 1960–1966

Hellyer P, Rodan I, Brunt J *et al.* (2007) AAHA/AAFP Pain Management Guidelines for Dogs & Cats. *Journal of the American Animal Hospital Association* 43, 235–248

Hudson C, Hudson S and MacKenzie J (2007) Protein-source tryptophan as an efficacious treatment for social anxiety disorder: a pilot study. *Canadian Journal of Physiology and Pharmacology* 85, 928–932

Johnson RW (2002) The concept of sickness behaviour: a brief chronological account of four key discoveries. *Veterinary Immunology and Immunopathology* 87, 443–450

Kelley RL, Lepine AJ and Burr JR (2004) Effect of dietary fish oil on puppy trainability. In: *Proceedings, Preconference Workshop, 6th International Society for the Study of Fatty Acids and Lipids Congress*, p. 51

Kemppainen RJ and Behrend EN (2001) Diagnosis of canine hypothyroidism. Perspectives from a testing laboratory. *Veterinary Clinics of North America: Small Animal Practice* 31, 951–962

Kulikov AV and Zubkov EA (2007) Chronic thyroxine treatment activates the 5-HT serotonin receptor in the rat brain. *Neuroscience Letters* 416, 307–309

Landsberg G, Hunthausen W and Ackerman L (2003) Stereotypic and compulsive disorders. In: *Handbook of Behavior Problems of the Dog and Cat*, pp. 195–225. Saunders-Elsevier, Philadelphia

Luescher UA (1998) Pharmacologic treatment of compulsive disorder. In: *Psychopharmacology of Animal Behavior Disorders*, ed. NH Dodman and L Shuster, pp. 203–221. Blackwell Science, Oxford

Markus CR (2008) Dietary amino acids and brain serotonin function; implications for stress-related affective changes. *NeuroMolecular Medicine* 10, 247–258

McCann JC and Ames BN (2005) Is docosahexaenoic acid, an *n*-3 long-chain polyunsaturated fatty acid, required for development of normal brain function? An overview of evidence from cognitive and behavioral tests in humans and animals. *American Journal of Clinical Nutrition* 82, 281–295

Mills DS (2003) Medical paradigms for the study of problem behaviour: a critical review. *Applied Animal Behaviour Science* 81, 265–277

Overall K (2003) Medical differentials with potential behavioral manifestations. *Veterinary Clinics of North America: Small Animal Practice* 33, 213–229

Peremans K, Audenaert K, Coopman F *et al.* (2003) Estimates of regional cerebral blood flow and 5-HT2A receptor density in impulsive, aggressive dogs with 99mTc-ECD and 123I-5-I-R91150. *European Journal of Nuclear Medicine and Molecular Imaging* 30, 1538–1546

Reinhard DW (1978) Aggressive behavior with hypothyroidism. *Canine Practice* 5, 69

Reisner IR, Mann JJ, Stanley M, Huang YY and Houpt KA (1996) Comparison of cerebrospinal fluid monoamine metabolite levels in dominant-aggressive and non-aggressive dogs. *Brain Research* 714, 57–64

Ross BM, Segin J and Sieswerda LE (2007) Omega-3 fatty acids as treatments for mental illness: which disorder and which fatty acid? *Lipids in Health and Disease* 6, 21

Sinn N, Bryan J and Wilson C (2008) Cognitive effects of polyunsaturated fatty acids in children with attention deficit hyperactivity disorder symptoms: a randomised controlled trial. *Prostaglandins, Leukotrienes and Essential Fatty Acids* 78, 311–326

Wiseman-Orr ML, Scott EM, Reid J and Nolan AM (2006) Validation of a structured questionnaire as an instrument to measure chronic pain in dogs on the basis of effects on health-related quality of life. *American Journal of Veterinary Research* 67, 1826–1836

## Client handouts (bsavalibrary.com/behaviour_leaflets)

- **Canine behaviour questionnaire**
- **Cognitive dysfunction syndrome**
- **Feline behaviour questionnaire**
- **Request for information on problem behaviours**

# 2

# Behavioural medicine as an integral part of veterinary practice

## Kendal Shepherd

## The behaviourally sensitive practice

**The veterinary surgeon's role in the human–animal bond is to maximize the potential of this relationship between people and animals.**

*American Veterinary Medical Association mission statement regarding the human–animal bond*

To fulfil this aim and implicit obligations, as well as enhancing the welfare of both the client and their pet, it is impossible to ignore the emotional and behavioural aspects of the human–animal bond and focus on purely physiological illness and disease. Not only may behavioural clinical signs be indications of underlying physical disease, but problem behaviour and associated stress can frequently result in physical malaise and illness. For the complete needs of any cat or dog to be met by their attending veterinary surgeon, it is therefore essential that the mental health of the patient is taken as seriously as its physical health. Management systems, and their impact upon behavioural as well as physical health, should be as routinely considered for the cat and dog as for the cow, pig or chicken. Not least of the environmental factors that impact upon behaviour and wellbeing is the relationship an animal has with its owner and family and other people it may come into contact with, including its attending veterinary surgeon. Behavioural awareness and concern must therefore be integrated into every aspect of veterinary intervention, rather than being reserved only for the patient who is already presented by their owner as needing behavioural help.

The concept of **behavioural husbandry** involves:

- Creating an appropriate management system by giving guidance at the start of a pet–human relationship. Opportunities can be created during vaccinations, puppy parties and classes. The veterinary consulting room and clinic should be presented as a role model for the rest of an animal's life
- Sustaining the relationship by identifying and optimizing the home management system. This includes the communication system between pet and owner, the relationship between pet and environment and awareness of the impact of veterinary intervention upon both.

Any form of veterinary intervention should, at the very least, aim for limitation of behavioural damage and at best ('best practice') should achieve an improvement in the relationship between the pet and the veterinary clinic and between the pet and its owner and environment.

## Awareness of a patient's behavioural needs

Just as the physical nature of a patient can become immediately apparent in the waiting and consulting rooms, so can its temperament and behavioural nature. Boisterous, vocal, timid, fearful and potentially aggressive animals are all readily identifiable from the moment they enter the waiting room, as are calmer, more convenient patients. Although a visit to the veterinary clinic can bring out the very worst in a pet, how an animal behaves when under duress is frequently a reflection of behavioural tendencies in the rest of its life. A client's embarrassment at the way their pet behaves in the clinic may preclude their asking for vital help with behavioural issues in other contexts, with serious implications for the routine welfare and mental wellbeing of that animal. These clients urgently need advice, which should be offered in an informed, non-judgmental and empathetic manner. Most clients do not automatically know how best to manage their pet at the clinic, any more than they should be aware of which diseases a dog or cat should be vaccinated against and when. Dispensing advice about both will help to ensure that the pet's entire needs are properly fulfilled.

The day-to-day behaviour of an animal, and how it may deviate from an accepted norm, should be considered as reflections of its inner mental state in the same way that clinical signs, such as vomiting or a cough, reflect bodily dysfunction or disease. To evaluate behavioural abnormalities fully, a normal behavioural state (for dogs and cats in general, as well as for an individual pet) should first be identified. Baseline behavioural values for cats and dogs can be recorded for future reference to help with later evaluation of any deviations from baseline behaviours. The 'C-BarQ' (Canine Behavioural Assessment and Research Questionnaire) is a reliable standardized method for evaluating and screening dogs for the presence and severity of behavioural problems (Hsu and Serpell, 2003) and can also be used to monitor changes over time. But what may be presented as a reflection of an acute behavioural problem by one owner may be considered entirely normal behaviour by another. Variations in perception of the behaviour of a pet provide valuable insights into the relationship between a pet and their owner or family – insights that are relevant to the care and treatment of both physical and mental conditions. Despite appearances, the behaviour exhibited in the veterinary clinical setting may or may not reflect behaviour in the home environment.

Information regarding both perceived behaviour and home management systems can be gleaned by use of routine questionnaires, either for the clients to be asked to fill in or the questions routinely incorporated into the history taking on a pet's first visit to the clinic. The answers may prompt early behavioural intervention for emergent behavioural problems as well as provide the impetus for giving preventive advice. The same checklist can later be used to update a patient's progress. Sample behaviour questionnaires for dogs and cats are provided in the Appendix.

## Building design and specifications
Behavioural awareness should be evident in the practical design and use of veterinary premises, whether the clinic is custom-built or a conversion from an existing building. A patient's view of the clinic will be formed immediately it enters the premises according to the environmental information presented to it. Cats are often less dependent upon individual relationships with people and more upon the relationship they have with their environment. The opposite is true for dogs: regardless of where they are, their relationship and communication with human beings is paramount. A vital source of information is therefore their owner and most relevant companion, so it is equally important to make the clients feel at home. Do the facilities on offer enable the attendant human to relax and behave as they would elsewhere? Do clients have enough room to allow their pet to maintain a degree of personal space from other people or animals? Or do they feel under pressure to ensure that their pet 'behaves' itself, regardless of the facilities on offer, thus creating context-specific tension in both themselves and their pet?

### The waiting room
Simple provisions can make it easier for dogs to behave appropriately. Having separate entrance and exit points and, if at all possible, a one-way system in and out of the reception area avoids dogs meeting each other going in opposite directions through one doorway. Dogs will be put under less social pressure, feel less threatened and therefore behave better if they are following other dogs rather than being forced to come face to face with them. As much space as possible should be provided around the reception desk and wherever possible the reception desk should not be placed in front of the main front door, to reduce overcrowding of both clients and their pets.

Even if a dog is relatively obedient, it can be extremely difficult for it to sit upon request on a slippery waiting room floor. Although non-slip abrasive surfaces in the form of riven tiles or vinyl textured finishes have

been used, the frequent specialist cleaning required may outweigh behavioural concerns and advantages. Instead, the provision of non-slip washable mats, particularly for larger canine patients, can make sitting or lying down a more comfortable and therefore feasible option in the waiting room. Clients can also be encouraged to bring in their own mats, as they may well have done in puppy class at the clinic or elsewhere (Figure 2.1).

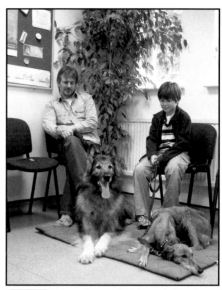

**2.1**   Non-slip washable mats for dogs to sit or lie on can be supplied, or the owners may bring in their own mat.

The waiting area should be large enough to ensure that, even at busy times, dogs are not forced to invade each other's personal space. If the waiting area has to be communal, a separate area should be partitioned off for cats. Cats may feel less vulnerable if flat surfaces at a height are provided on which clients can place their cat carriers. A separate cat clinic with its own waiting area away from hustle and bustle is an even better option.

All parts of the waiting area should be easily visible from the reception desk to enable pre-emptive action to be taken for animals that are obviously distressed by the veterinary experience. To minimize arousal prior to veterinary consultation, particularly anxious, distressed pets or dogs that are aggressive toward other dogs may be left in the client's car (if weather allows) until a consulting room becomes available or led immediately from the waiting room into another empty room. Making special provisions for such animals is a necessary part of consideration for their mental welfare and future treatment.

### Consulting room
Consulting rooms should be as large as possible to allow any animal a sense of freedom in which to explore its surroundings. Dogs should always be allowed the opportunity to settle on the floor on a relaxed or trailing lead before being lifted on to the table. Much information, both physical and behavioural, can be gleaned from a few moments of surreptitious observation of the patient while the history is being

taken from the client and recorded. By the same token, as far as possible cats should be allowed to emerge from their carriers voluntarily rather than being dragged out; alternatively a modular carrier can be disassembled and the cat lifted out with a towel. Top-loading wire carriers often allow for easier and stress-free handling. The installation of feline and canine pheromone diffusers in the consulting room as well as elsewhere in the practice may help cats and dogs, respectively, to feel more immediately at home (Mills *et al.*, 2006).

The decision whether to lift a dog on to an examination table is often made purely on the basis of size rather than what the individual dog might prefer and where it will feel less threatened. A smaller dog may feel uncomfortable being leant over and handled from above and happier if raised at a height for handling. When safety allows after an initial assessment, crouching down and even sitting on the floor to examine certain dogs and cats may alleviate the threat that veterinary examination inevitably entails. A hydraulic-lift table on to which dogs can voluntarily walk or be lifted without intrusive handling is beneficial (Figure 2.2).

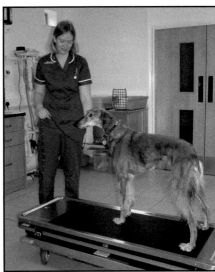

**2.2**

Hydraulic lift-table.

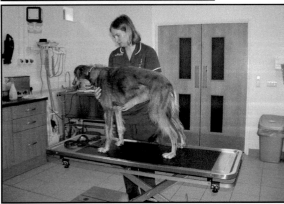

### Kennelling

Kennelling is most frequently installed with the ease of staff access and cleaning in mind rather than the needs of individual animals. Reducing the inherent threat that both cats and dogs perceive in confinement will in turn improve their emotional welfare. Cats

should be kennelled separately from dogs to reduce all-round stress. Although stainless steel is easy to clean, laminate surfaces for cats or ceramic tiles for dogs provide both insulation and noise reduction. Rehoming centres have found glass doors very beneficial in reducing noise stress and these can equally be considered in the clinic context (Figure 2.3a). A combination of glass and more standard cage door is ideal, enabling dogs that are able to eat to be rewarded with treats by passing staff members for

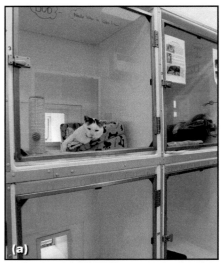

(a)

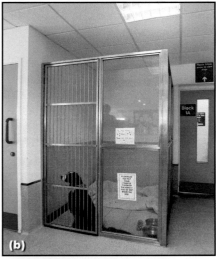

(b)

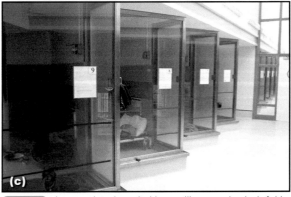

(c)

**2.3** Appropriate hospital kennelling can be helpful in reducing stress. **(a)** Glass doors are useful to cut out noise. **(b)** A combination of glass and caging allows calm dogs to be rewarded with treats. **(c)** Setting kennels at an angle avoids animals facing each other directly.

sitting calmly in the clinic (Figure 2.3b). Acoustic ceiling tiles can be used to reduce noise impact and improve quality of life for both patients and staff (Coppola *et al.*, 2006). Kennels or pens set at an angle avoid forcing animals to face each other directly, thus reducing social pressure (Figure 2.3c).

The provision of vertical space is an essential part of the cat's environment, as is a covered bed in which to hide. Although an installed shelf is ideal, on which a soft igloo bed can provide both warmth and privacy at a height (Figure 2.4), the 'hide and perch' box has been shown to reduce stress in cats awaiting rehoming and is equally suited to clinic confinement (see Chapter 23).

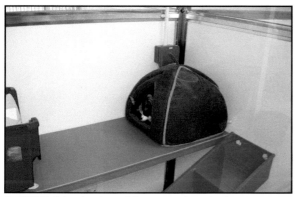

**2.4** Igloo bed providing warmth and privacy at a height.

## The practice of behavioural medicine on a daily basis

Behavioural husbandry involves the incorporation of awareness of, and care for, behaviour into all aspects of an animal's life, including during any necessary veterinary intervention. While at the clinic, any interaction with a pet should be considered as an opportunity to create positive associations, both with the practice and with any particular member of staff, as well as to guide behaviour in a calm and convenient direction. Using basic behavioural principles, iatrogenic behavioural damage may be limited or avoided altogether and a patient amenable to future handling and treatment is both created and maintained, to all-round benefit. Ideally, all staff should become familiar with the theory and practice of reward-based training, if only to be able to teach a dog to sit on command. Demonstrating such humane training methods to clients and leading by example, whether in the waiting room or during consultation, will have huge educational and welfare benefits in all areas of a pet's life.

### Application of behavioural principles

All staff should be well informed regarding the basis upon which behavioural decisions are made by an animal. In general terms, decisions are motivated by the need either to gain something that is desired or to avoid something unpleasant. Any behaviour that proves successful in either direction is likely to be repeated later in a similar context. In addition to

learning which behaviours 'work' best in achieving such goals, positive and negative associations are made by an animal with features of the environment which will subsequently trigger both emotional and behavioural change, for better or worse (see Chapter 5). Staff should also develop an awareness of the behavioural choices available to a cat or dog at any time and of the potentially damaging effect that the restriction of choice, by confinement or restraint, may have. In any situation where an animal is likely to be apprehensive and in a negative emotional state, every effort must be made to avoid undue threat or coercion in view of the very real risk of triggering an aggressive response. Once thus aroused, pets will find it difficult to follow any behavioural guidance that may be offered, instead focusing only on perceived threat.

Many dogs can be calmed simply by demonstrating to their owners, with the use of readily available and tasty food rewards, how to teach a dog to sit. To this end, all staff (including receptionists) should carry food titbits on their person. Whether a dog learns to sit or not, and a titbit is simply taken from the hand, veterinary staff will begin to be seen as 'good news' by their patients. With cats, exactly the same principles can be used to create pleasant associations with their visit to the clinic, thus reducing the likelihood of defensive scratching or biting. In the waiting room, receptionists and veterinary nurses can demonstrate calm, non-threatening intervention to prevent owners from reprimanding their pet, either physically or verbally, for its 'bad' behaviour, to the benefit of all concerned. Owner anger and anxiety coinciding with a veterinary visit can only make a pet's emotional state, and its reflected behaviour, worse.

It is frequently assumed that the more a dog or cat is restrained, by enlisting the help of however many people seem to be necessary at the time, the better controlled it is. Although in the short term such an approach may get the job done, in the long term severe behavioural damage may be caused and result in a worsening of behaviour over every subsequent visit to the clinic. By associative learning, restraint becomes a reliable predictor of discomfort for the pet. In addition to the inevitable association with unpleasantness, restraint simply denies an animal the 'flight' option when faced with a threat and makes a 'fight' response far more likely. Apparent passivity does not necessarily reflect willing compliance.

### The Ladder of Aggression
The Ladder of Aggression (Figure 2.5) is a depiction of the gestures that any dog will give in response to an escalation of perceived stress and threat, from very mild social interaction and pressure, to which blinking and nose licking are appropriate responses, to severe, when overt aggression may well be selected. The purpose of such behaviour is to deflect threat and restore harmony and the presence of appeasing and threat-averting behaviour in the domestic dog's repertoire is essential to avoid the need for potentially damaging aggression. The dog is a social animal for whom successful appeasement behaviour is highly adaptive and it is used continually and routinely in everyday life.

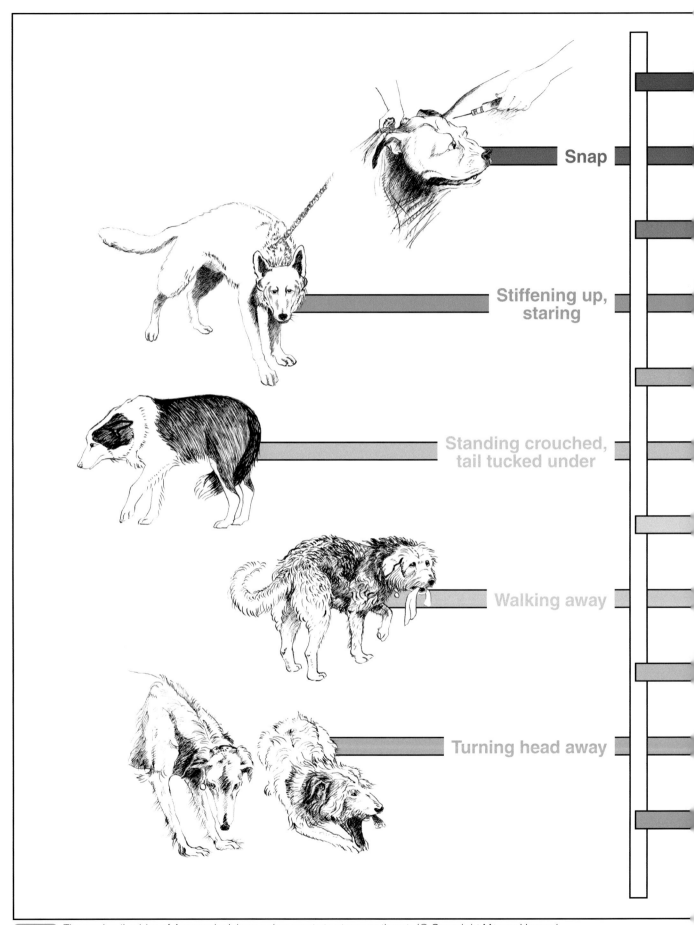

Snap

Stiffening up, staring

Standing crouched, tail tucked under

Walking away

Turning head away

**2.5** The canine 'Ladder of Aggression': how a dog reacts to stress or threat. (© Copyright Maggy Howard and Kendal Shepherd) The Canine Ladder of Aggression concept was developed by Kendal Shepherd.

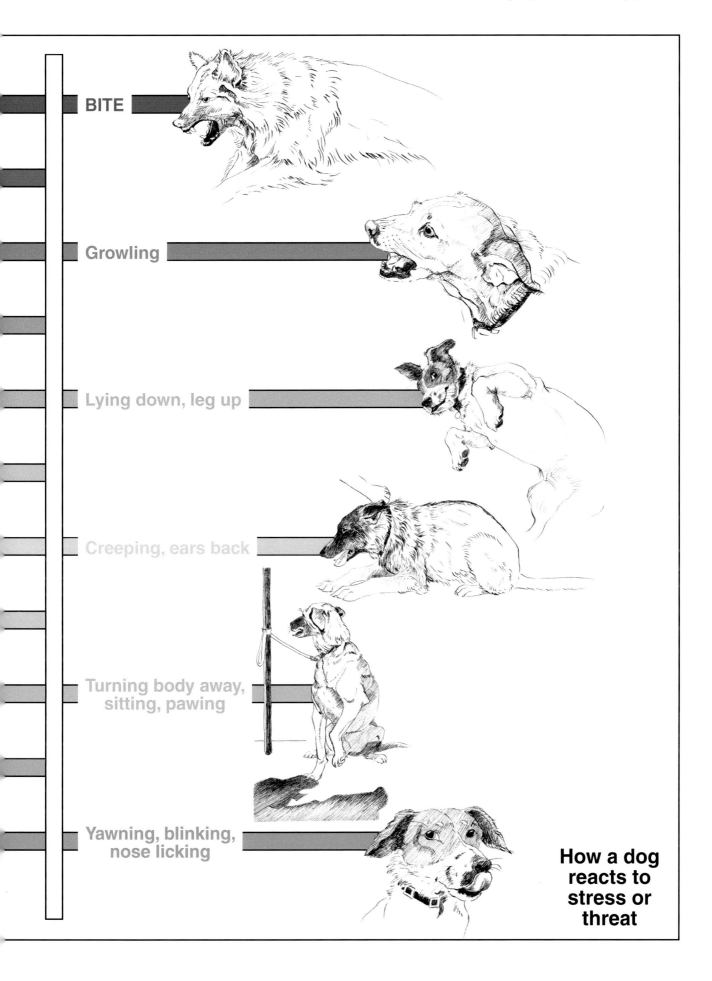

BITE

Growling

Lying down, leg up

Creeping, ears back

Turning body away,
sitting, pawing

Yawning, blinking,
nose licking

**How a dog
reacts to
stress or
threat**

It is most important to realize that these gestures are simply a context and response-dependent sequence that will only culminate in threatened or overt aggression if all else fails. Contrary to persistent misinformation, the gestures identified are nothing to do with a purported dominant or submissive state (see Chapter 17). In all dogs, inappropriate social responses to appeasement behaviour will result in its devaluing and the necessity, from a dog's perspective, to move up the ladder. Aggression is therefore created in any situation where appeasement behaviour is chronically misunderstood and not effective in obtaining the socially expected outcome. Dogs may progress to overt aggression within seconds during a single episode if the perceived threat occurs quickly and at close quarters, or learn to dispense with lower rungs on the ladder over time, if repeated efforts to appease are misunderstood and responded to inappropriately. As a consequence, a so-called 'unpredictable' aggressive response, without any obvious preamble, may occur in any context that predicts inescapable threat to the dog, when in reality it was entirely predictable.

Unfortunately, appeasement behaviour is often ignored, misunderstood and devalued during dog–human communication in the veterinary clinic. The dog sitting in the corner of the consulting room with laid-back ears, turned head and raised paw is communicating a visual plea to be left alone, yet is still approached to be given an injection. Increased understanding and recognition of early signs of unease will do much to obviate the risk of aggression. Simply taking steps to encourage a dog to walk voluntarily towards veterinary staff on a loose lead, for example, rather than being dragged in their direction, may help to ensure that the dog remains below the 'walk away' behavioural option on the ladder. A dog should never be dragged into the consulting room or out of a kennel if at all possible. If such action appears to be necessary from the point of view of either the client or the attending veterinary staff, an emotional problem exists in that animal associated with the circumstances. This must be addressed, rather than exacerbated, if future aggression is to be prevented and the demeanour of the patient at subsequent visits improved.

### The puppy and kitten vaccination

The young animal's first visit to the clinic is the most crucial and attitude-forming that it will ever experience. It is essential that this visit is made as pleasant and as educational as possible, however long it takes, as lessons learned at this time will form the point of reference for all future experiences in this environment. If handled well, the dog or cat when adult may forgive a multitude of sins because previous pleasant memories help to protect against future unpleasantness (see Chapter 5). If handled badly, the experience may create a pet readily prepared to use aggression when threatened, at any time in the future and in any similar context. The single human action that is most likely to create such a context in a pet's mind is that of forceful restraint by either owner or veterinary staff.

The majority of the vaccination consultation must therefore be spent ensuring that the puppy or kitten not only enjoys itself but begins to learn the behaviours that will be the most convenient all round for the rest of its life. There are very few puppies that will not eat in the consulting room at this stage of their lives, if tasty food is both offered 'for free' and given as rewards for suitable behaviour, *before* anything unpleasant has happened to them.

It is arguable that discussions regarding worming, diet and neutering should be left to a competent veterinary nurse or technician while the veterinary surgeon's time is better spent teaching the puppy to sit on the consulting room table, using food as a lure (Figure 2.6). By contrast, the most important lesson to avoid any puppy learning is that being held firmly predicts pain and discomfort. At the moment an injection is given, the puppy must be let go and allowed to eat the offered food. Evidence of success includes smiling owners and a puppy who sits willingly on the table when presented for its second vaccination.

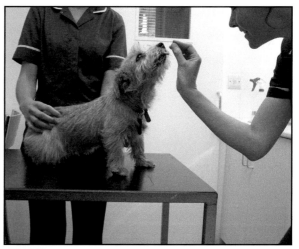

**2.6** Food can be used as a lure to teach a puppy to sit on the examination table.

### Food used to guide behaviour

The use of food is to be encouraged throughout the veterinary clinic, not only as a behaviour manipulator but also as a rough guide to a dog's emotional state. Although it is a not uncommon finding that dogs who are emotionally aroused will not want to eat and will therefore not be motivated by food alone to behave as might be required, this must not be used as an excuse for not offering food to all dogs who walk through the clinic door. The earlier this pleasant association is made in a pet's veterinary career, the more useful it will be at subsequent visits. For those animals who cannot be given food prior to a general anaesthetic, it is absolutely essential that the body gestures and instructions of the handler maintain previously taught associations with the imminent arrival of food. A closed hand moved upwards while a dog is asked to sit in a jolly tone of voice maintains the belief that food might arrive. By contrast, common practices such as collar corrections, shouting, or pointing a finger downwards and a stern 'No' do not.

An owner's frequent response that 'he doesn't take food from strangers' should be more accurately reinterpreted as 'he is rather worried by strangers and, if circumstances dictate, may try to bite them'. In other words, if food is refused, there is something worrying the dog and, in a veterinary context, it is most likely to be the attendant veterinary surgeon or nurse, or their handling. Concerns arising from the proximity of other animals may also result in 'redirected aggression' toward those nearby. However, once a certain response has been linked with both a reward and command, a conditioned emotional response is generated as well as a conditioned behaviour. Such an emotional response will frequently allow sufficient positive emotional change as to enable a dog to feel like eating. In practical terms, if a dog is asked to sit, a food titbit will frequently be taken *after* completing this task, which would have been refused if simply offered from the hand. A window of opportunity to begin to alter an anxious dog's view of the clinic is thereby created (Figure 2.7).

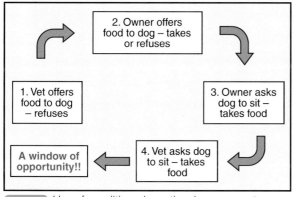

**2.7**  Use of conditioned emotional responses to environmental information, including obedience commands.

### Behaviour management during a routine consultation

What any puppy or older dog learns in a 'party' or class must extend beyond the remit of the veterinary nurse or dog trainer and into every aspect of the veterinary consulting room. Particular attention must be paid to those behaviours that best allow veterinary handling and examination; namely the sit, the stand, the down and the roll over (Figure 2.8). Although taught as 'tricks' in class and a client's sitting-room, they are generally very ill-rehearsed, if at all, in the veterinary consulting room. It is therefore imperative that veterinary surgeons are also involved in the 'puppy training' process. For a task or trick to be deemed worth doing, there must always be both anticipated and tangible rewarding payback for the pet. Conflicting messages are received when a food treat is earned for an obedient 'hands off' sit in a puppy party, but a 'sit' in the consulting room results in restraint and a painful injection. In the case of cats teaching them to 'high five' is usually simpler than a sit, but just as effective, since they will often focus and paw at a treat held close to the raised hand in front of them (Figure 2.9).

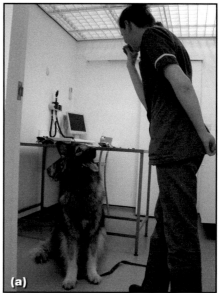

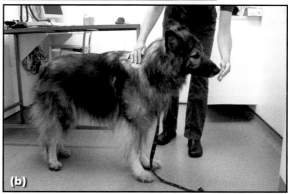

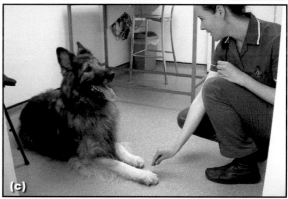

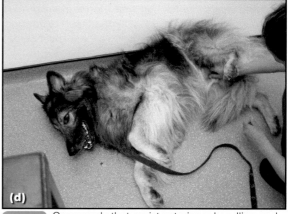

**2.8**  Commands that assist veterinary handling and examination: **(a)** 'sit'; **(b)** 'stand'; **(c)** 'down'; and **(d)** 'roll over'.

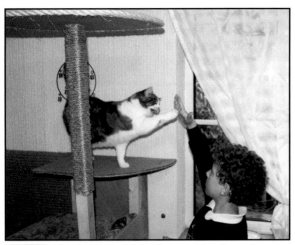

**2.9** Teaching a cat to 'high five'. (Courtesy of D. Mills.)

### Involving the owner in behavioural management

Training and resultant behaviour are dependent upon the information the environment presents to the animal at any given time. An owner, if properly instructed, can become a significant source of information to their pet, but the way owners are often asked to behave in the clinical context is at odds with how they transmit information and communicate with their pet in training class or at home. The question therefore arises: should any owner be used merely to restrain their pet or also to inform it in an appropriate manner?

The typical way in which an owner may be asked to restrain their dog for the administration of an intranasal vaccine is illustrated in Figure 2.10a. In this situation, all the environmental information presented to the patient is threatening and predicts the lack of 'flight' as a behavioural option. It has already been stressed how the inability to use this option is frequently instrumental in engendering a 'fight' response. The dog is restrained on a lead, is being held tightly by the owner as well as a veterinary nurse, and has its eyes covered. By contrast, Figure 2.10b illustrates how to give multiple non-threatening and informative signals to a patient. The owner now presents herself to the dog in 'training mode' by removing her shoulder bag and the restraining lead and not holding on to her dog. Instead, she is wearing a 'treat' bag predicting food, giving a clear hand signal for the required behaviour, giving a verbal 'sit' command and smiling. To her dog, the 'flight' option is also still available, making an aggressive response far less likely. Such control does not come without practice on the part of the owner and the attending veterinary surgeon. But it is often surprising how, when an owner uses only commands known to their pet, they can immediately alter its behaviour for the better, even if not specifically rehearsed in the clinic context.

For the already more difficult dog, there are various forms of head restraint available, the most useful of which are those with an effective muzzling action. With the lead loose, the dog may pant and feel unrestrained but the mouth can be shut as a

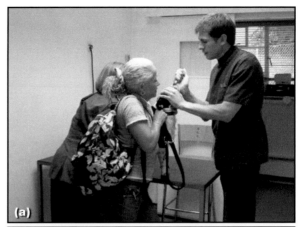

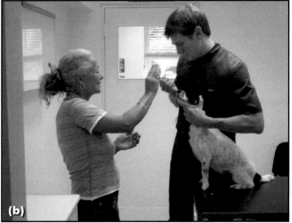

**2.10** Involving the owner. **(a)** Holding a dog for intranasal vaccination. **(b)** The owner in 'training mode'.

precautionary measure when necessary (Figure 2.11). A wary dog, already accustomed to and presented wearing such a device, is immediately easier to control in a less threatening manner than one who has to be manoeuvred into a muzzle after threatening to bite (see Chapters 8 and 17).

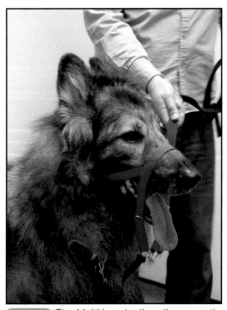

**2.11** The Halti headcollar allows panting. (continues) ▶

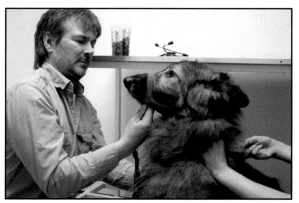

**2.11** (continued) The Halti headcollar also allows head control and closing of the mouth if necessary.

## Pre-admission information

According to the principles of behavioural husbandry, any interaction with any dog and client is an opportunity to inform both the veterinary surgeon and the owner regarding the most humane way to promote appropriate behaviour. Although it is essential to identify any organic disease that may be contributing to a behaviour problem, it is when an animal is ill, injured or in recovery following routine surgery that consistent behavioural guidance may most be needed. Questions asked upon admission and advice given upon discharge may be of great importance in generating a successful outcome.

In addition to the information regarding behaviour already recorded (see Appendix), certain questions may have increased relevance for the behavioural care of dogs being admitted into the veterinary hospital. Such questions and the practical reasons for asking them are summarized in Figure 2.12. Once admitted into the veterinary hospital and without an owner present, the patient is entirely reliant upon information given by veterinary staff as to what to do. The significance of the information gathered is to allow as much cross-context consistency in the handling and management of a dog between home and the clinic as possible. The answers may also reveal deficiencies in management as well as owner concerns regarding inappropriate behaviour, which may well impact upon the prognosis for clinical success. If a dog is extremely difficult to walk on a lead, for example, how might this affect client compliance with a postoperative requirement of six weeks' lead exercise following orthopaedic surgery? How might enforced cage rest impact upon a dog that is unable to be left in a room alone, let alone 'home alone'?

## Blood sampling, intravenous injection and other procedures

A fairly common practice in veterinary medicine has become the use of routine blood screening prior to surgical procedures. Veterinary surgeons should be aware of the potential behavioural consequences for some animals who may perceive these procedures as intrusive, painful or anxiety-provoking. It is imperative to understand the welfare implications of taking blood from a patient and to take appropriate steps to ameliorate the stress and distress possibly associated with this procedure.

These steps might include ensuring that the person responsible for the procedure is proficient in the technique as well as aware of behaviourally friendly means of obtaining a blood sample. These may include using a butterfly catheter in smaller animals to minimize pain, using a syringe rather than a vacutainer, obtaining only necessary amounts of blood, avoiding rushed encounters, giving the animal time to adjust to each step and delaying drawing blood if the animal is profoundly distressed and waiting does not compromise their medical condition. The value of

| Question | Reasons for question | Action |
|---|---|---|
| 1. How has your dog been trained? | How are the dog's decisions made? What emotional responses have been conditioned and why? | More awareness of emotional change associated with human words and gestures |
| 2. What words or hand signals does the dog know? | What information does the dog need to make decisions? Is it reliant on collar and lead? | Maintain consistency for patient – use the same signals |
| 3. Any concerns regarding reactivity to noises? | Noise fears underdiagnosed in the pet dog | Protect dog in hospital. Facilitate early intervention for treatment |
| 4. Where and when does the dog usually eliminate? | Is there a substrate preference? Who initiates elimination? On command or 'asks' to go out? On a lead or off? Loss of 'training' if owner not present | Provide same substrate choice (gravel, grass, earth, concrete) Give same command |
| 5. What is the dog's reaction to other dogs? | May affect kennelling choice | Avoid contact between dogs. Early intervention for dog–dog aggression |
| 6. What is usual lead restraint? | How does the dog behave on the lead? Is communication lead-dependent? | Pre-prepare with Halti or Gentle Leader. Long-line training – educational freedom |
| 7. How does the dog react to grooming? | Is there a difference between home and groomers? Are there handling issues with familiar people? How does this impact upon veterinary care? | Consider whether better to have owner present or absent. Early intervention for relationship dysfunction |

**2.12** Useful questions to ask on admission.

blood samples from highly stressed animals is itself questionable from a clinical perspective, regardless of the behavioural impact.

When done without regard to behavioural input, venepuncture may be quite intolerable to the veterinary patient. Some restraint, however minimal, is always necessary and is usually from humans unknown to the animal. Significant and possibly threatening eye contact may occur and the patient may receive no meaningful guidance as to what it is expected do in order to get the job done efficiently. Vocal exhortations to 'behave' tend to increase in volume and inherent threat and may make matters worse.

To help the patient to cope, meaningful guidance by both verbal and visual means is essential. A dog's name followed by known commands only (e.g. 'sit', 'down', 'stay') should be used rather than conversation. Only the behaviour the dog is performing at the time should be praised; for example, 'Good stay!'. This is far more effective than the universal 'Good boy!' and identifies the behaviour that the dog is required to repeat. The patient should be approached from the side rather than from directly in front; eye contact should be avoided by turning the head and blinking; and the handler should maintain a relaxed body posture and try to smile when approaching the dog. For many dogs the use of a headcollar will facilitate control in a friendlier and less intimidating way, allowing for control while perhaps minimizing distress.

To maintain appropriate behaviour in any animal at the clinic, 'good' behaviour must be routinely and meaningfully rewarded. All dogs, regardless of reputation, should be treated in the same way, and tolerant appropriate behaviour should be encouraged and rewarded at every opportunity. It must never be assumed that any dog is 'fine' and therefore needs no inducement to continue to behave well. Unless positive emotions are deliberately generated and appropriate behaviour is regularly rehearsed, as with any other task, they will be lost from a dog's repertoire in a veterinary context.

## Incorporating behaviour into the practice

### Attitude of the practice
The first step towards successful treatment of any behavioural condition is for the initial contact within the practice (be it receptionist, veterinary nurse or veterinary surgeon) to be as concerned and informative as they would be over any physical sign. Ideally, neither the veterinary practice nor its clients should consider the course of action regarding a pet's behaviour to be in a different category from any other of the animal's needs. Explaining the potentially life-saving nature of a behavioural workup, diagnosis and therapy should be just as normal as for any other injury or disease state. After all, the suddenly noticed 'lump' described on the telephone that so concerns the client may be either a benign mass, easily excised, or a malignancy that will eventually prove fatal. But what of the social ramifications of a dog growling at its owner or next-door-neighbour's child and the implications for the patient's own life?

### Dog trainers and behaviourists
The impression created by advertisements on the practice notice board and the products offered for sale in the waiting room reflect and reveal the practice's attitude towards behaviour. Any individual dog trainer or behaviourist wishing to be associated with the practice must be as professional and reliable as any other member of staff. Unless an individual's experience and qualifications have been scrutinized and accepted by the practice, their details should not be displayed.

Visiting and personally ratifying dog training classes is essential. What training methods are employed? Do dogs and attendant owners look happy? Would the veterinary surgeon want the same methods used on their own dog? Does the trainer have public liability insurance? Figure 2.13 is a checklist for assessing training classes.

| Question | Comments |
| --- | --- |
| Are instructors qualified? | e.g. APDT Association of Pet Dog Trainers, APBC members |
| Do they have public liability insurance? | Accidents do happen! |
| How many instructors are there per student/dog? | Suggested minimum requirement of 1 trainer per 6 student/dog pairs |
| Is there an invitation to observe one free class? | No obligation if not happy |
| How noisy is the class? | Calm with no shouting to be recommended |
| What training methods are being used: positive reward or 'do it or else'? | Threat-based training methods may create aggression |
| What types of training tool are utilized? | e.g. headcollars, pinch collars, choke collars, flat collars, body harnesses |
| Are there indoor and outdoor facilities? | Year-round and all-context training |
| Can methods recommended be used in the sitting room or by a small child? | If not, irrelevant for real life |
| Is further specialized help available for 'difficult' dogs? | Appreciation of individual dogs' needs essential |
| Is a training class what the dog needs? | Where will it find learning the easiest? |

**2.13** Checklist for assessing training classes.

Moves are afoot to regulate and monitor those setting themselves up as 'behaviourists'. For example, in the UK, accreditation as a certificated clinical animal behaviourist, regulated by the Association for the Study of Animal Behaviour (ASAB), has set a 'gold standard' in the burgeoning field of animal behaviour, to which it is hoped other organizations will aspire. The criterion for full membership of the Association of Pet Behaviour Counsellors (APBC) from 2011 will be accreditation by ASAB as a certificated clinical animal behaviourist.

### Products for sale
The behavioural implications of products offered for sale (Figure 2.14) and their suitability for purpose

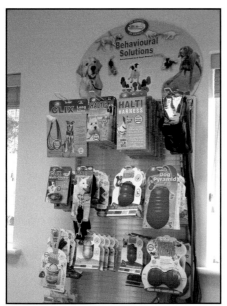

**2.14** Behaviour products offered for sale may require specialist guidance.

should be as carefully considered as any medication that might be prescribed. Any products that require fitting to an individual animal, such as harnesses or headcollars, should not be sold unless a fully informed member of staff has ensured their suitability. The response to requests for any aversive and punishing device should trigger an enquiry by a practice member of staff as to why such measures are thought to be necessary. What is it that the client does not like about their pet's behaviour and how are they trying to address it? How might their attempts impact upon their pet's emotions and is punishment the appropriate and humane course of action? To fulfil their 'constant endeavour to ensure the welfare of animals committed to (their) care' (RCVS Guide to Professional Conduct) the attending veterinary surgeon should be fully informed regarding training devices and methods used at home, and the emotional impact they may have upon the animal's life.

## Advice given during routine consultations

It is widely assumed that working with behaviour is far too time-consuming to be fitted into the busy day of a general veterinary practice. This assumption may have its roots in the historical nature of the field of behaviour management. As few veterinary surgeons receive thorough training in behavioural medicine at veterinary school, treating animal behaviour problems has become a 'specialty' with concurrent need for referral, without recognizing that such problems may feasibly be tackled in general practice. Although veterinary surgeons in general practice may well feel out of their depth when presented with an apparently complex behavioural issue, they can address many problems on a daily basis. First principles and the adage that 'common things occur commonly' can be used to address clinical signs of diarrhoea or pruritus; therefore, certain simple rules based on the assumption that 'common mistakes occur commonly' can transform the relationship between an owner and

their pet. In this way, valuable behavioural advice can be incorporated into everyday consultations in a time-efficient fashion.

Any routine 'do as I do' demonstrations that can be inserted into any veterinary activity will have the beneficial effect of encouraging clients to think about how they themselves deal and communicate with their pet in everyday life, especially if the veterinary surgeon, nurse or technician explains to the client why they do things a certain way (i.e. to reduce the stress on their pet). Such welfare-oriented promotion of behaviour will also favourably impress clients and is more likely to result in positive publicity. Instructing an owner to ask their dog to sit and to deliver food treats while an ear is examined (whether or not the dog seems to 'need' them) can also be used to demonstrate how a dog may be rewarded for sitting instead of barking or jumping up at passers-by, for example. Many episodes of threatened or actual aggression toward family members at home can be prevented by the thorough explanation of the 'Ladder of Aggression' (see Figure 2.5) and the nature and purpose of appeasement behaviour (Shepherd, 2007). Simply emphasizing how sufficient rehearsal and succinct use of obedience commands in all contexts enhances the relationship between dog and owner will go a long way towards creating a more secure and balanced pet.

Above all, the routine consultation should provide a sufficiently empathetic atmosphere for an owner to begin to talk about problematic behaviours, regardless of the reason for the initial consultation. Any admitted difficulties in administering topical or oral medication are of clinical importance. This should therefore prompt the offer of behavioural help and be seen as an opportunity to help clients to learn appropriate interactions with their pet. If a surgical procedure is being proposed, in order for a client to be in a position to give thoroughly informed consent to the procedure the discussion must include a pet's less than desirable behaviour, its potentially adverse effect upon prognosis and what helpful steps might immediately be taken to address it.

## Organizing behavioural referrals

The referral of a behaviour case must be with the full involvement of a referring veterinary surgeon, in the same way as for any other discipline or specialty. It is not acceptable for the receptionist simply to hand out the contact number of a purported 'behaviourist' in response to a behavioural enquiry: it may result in a great number of dogs being denied potentially life-saving advice and could leave the practice open to litigation under its duty of care.

Many clients still expect advice to be given over the telephone and that such 'quick-fix' advice will be both cheap and easy to implement. The referring veterinary surgeon must make them fully aware of what is involved in the diagnosis and treatment of behavioural problems in terms of commitment, family involvement, expectations of outcome and, not least, cost, in much the same way as for any other clinical referral. The uptake of a behavioural service and consequent client compliance, leading to a much improved prognosis, is far greater if a veterinary surgeon has been intrinsically involved in the entire referral process.

An obligatory pre-referral veterinary consultation emphasizes the importance that the practice attributes to their client's concerns and, according to the terms of certain insurance companies, is a prerequisite for a client's claim for behavioural treatment to be honoured. When the referral is to a non-veterinary specialist, it is essential that any underlying health issues and treatment requirements are identified, so that such considerations may be taken into account during both the diagnostic process and any subsequent behaviour modification plan. This does not imply that behavioural advice must be denied to a patient until other health issues are completely resolved (see Chapter 1). As already stated, it is at times of ill health that behavioural guidance may be the most needed by both client and patient.

To this end, a working relationship should be established with a suitably qualified individual into whose behavioural care a client's pet can be reliably entrusted. This person may be already employed by the practice or they may visit on a regular basis to conduct a behaviour clinic. It may, on the other hand, be a behaviourist who has their own clinic elsewhere or who conducts their consultations during a home visit. In all cases, a post-consultation written report should be expected in which a summary of history, the contribution that any underlying medical conditions may be making to expressed behaviour, and the treatment protocol with rationale are all detailed. It is particularly important that any cases that may require further clinical investigation or medication are verbally discussed with the referring veterinary surgeon and that a timescale is set for feedback between veterinary surgeon and behaviourist regarding results and progress.

### In-practice or clinic referral

Prior to behavioural referral, all issues should be identified and addressed and the client made aware of the attending charges of a behaviour consultation, whether carried out in-house or referred elsewhere, if necessary in a separate consultation. If conducted in a clinic, the facilities must be sufficient to allow both owner and animal to behave in as 'normal' a manner as possible. This requires a room of sufficient size and furnished in as home-like a manner as possible. Although it is not necessary for problem behaviours to be seen or deliberately replicated during a consultation in order for relevant advice to be given (a dog growling at a child, for example), owner-absent or compulsive behaviour, which cannot be adequately described, is best recorded and reviewed during the consultation. A video recording also gives the clinician a 'virtual' impression of home circumstances, which may well be essential to the provision of a relevant management protocol.

Part of the consultation must entail a practical demonstration of training methods and their relevance, both to the patient in its home situation and in the context of the problem behaviour. Although much

problematic behaviour occurs in a home context only, behaviour and control outside the home also frequently prompt the need for behaviour advice, if only owing to public liability concerns. An open but enclosed space in which a dog may be given freedom and in which problem scenarios may be played out for training purposes with stooge people or other dogs is highly recommended if it can be safely provided.

### Home visit referral

There are many advantages to the home visit. A client is as relaxed as they can be in their own home; the pet is seen *in situ* and the behavioural effects of its routine environment can be identified at first hand; relevant behavioural modification and training techniques can be demonstrated in the context in which they are required; the whole family can be involved in the consultation process and the relationship between them and their pet, for good or bad, ascertained. This is particularly important when dealing with a very common reason for behavioural referral, namely aggression shown toward family members or visitors.

The advantages and disadvantages of clinic and home-based behavioural consultations are summarized in Figure 2.15.

| Clinic | Home visit |
|---|---|
| Support staff available if needed for handling and stooge exercises | No help available if needed for handling |
| Some animals may be safer in the clinic | Some animals may be more dangerous at home |
| Some animals may be more dangerous in the clinic | Some animals may be safer at home |
| Efficient use of time as no travelling | Travelling time must be added |
| Appointment times must be adhered to | Consultation may overrun |
| No unnecessary interruptions | May be interruptions |
| Behavioural equipment to hand and products readily available for sale | All equipment and products must be transported |
| Suitable home-like room required | Normal living accommodation available |
| Suitable outdoor facility required | Garden, normal exercise areas available |
| Behaviour of animal changed by novel environment | Behaviour of animal seen in routine environment |
| Consultation more formal and clients may be less relaxed | Consultation more informal and relaxed |
| Whole family may not be able to attend | Easier for whole family to attend |
| Context not relevant to real life | Context relevant to real life |
| No first-hand information regarding home life | First-hand experience of home life |

**2.15** Advantages and disadvantages of clinic consultations *versus* home visits.

## Follow-on use of dog trainers

Although canine behaviour management of necessity involves training dogs, the two fields of behaviour modification and dog training are often perceived as different by many behaviour consultants and referring veterinary surgeons. The differences, however, are not in the underlying learning principles and training methods used, but in the context in which they are performed and their relevance to the real life of the dog concerned. Dog training tends to happen at a specific time and place in the company of other like-minded owners and their dogs. Behaviour management, on the other hand, must happen in all contexts of a dog's life in which it is expected to behave appropriately. Very beneficial use can be made of dog trainers, either in class or on a one-to-one basis, but only if the techniques recommended, demonstrated and learned can be practically transferred to the client's kitchen, sitting room, garden, local park and their veterinary clinic. Some behaviour problems, such as aggression, reflect underlying anxieties and fears that must be addressed. It is therefore important to recognize that obedience training alone is not sufficient, and the involvement of a veterinary surgeon is essential.

Ideally the attending veterinary surgeon, behaviour counsellor and dog trainer should all work hand-in-hand to the benefit of the patient. Although a behaviour problem may be viewed simply as a 'training issue' (poor recall, for example), addressing the problem in a highly distracting and socially pressured dog-training class may not be the best initial step. Poor recall and other apparent 'disobedience' are often underpinned by other relationship deficiencies which are best identified by a behaviour counsellor and addressed and rehearsed initially at home. A dog trainer may be best utilized to help clients to rehearse recommended training techniques and goals regularly, either on a one-to-one or in-class basis, depending upon progress at home. In all contexts, however, the welfare and behavioural benefit of sufficient mental exercise in preventing and treating behaviour problems cannot be underestimated.

## References and further reading

Coppola CL, Enns MR and Grandin T (2006) Noise in the animal shelter environment: building design and the effect of daily noise exposure. *Journal of Applied Animal Welfare Science* **9**, 1–7

Griffith CA, Steigerwald ES and Buffington T (2000) Effects of a synthetic facial pheromone on the behavior of cats. *Journal of the American Veterinary Medical Association* **217**, 1154–1156

Hsu Y and Serpell JA (2003) Development and validation of a questionnaire for measuring behaviour and temperaments traits in pet dogs. *Journal of the American Veterinary Medical Association* **223**, 1293–1300

Mills DS, Ramos D, Estelles MG and Hargrave C (2006) A triple blind placebo-controlled investigation into the assessment of the effect of Dog Appeasing Pheromone (DAP) on anxiety related behaviour of problem dogs in the veterinary clinic. *Applied Animal Behaviour Science* **98**,114–126

Moffat K (2008) Addressing canine and feline aggression in the veterinary clinic. *Veterinary Clinics of North America: Small Animal Practice* **38**, 983–1003

Shepherd K (2007) *The Canine Commandments*. Broadcast Books, Bristol

Tod E, Brander D and Waran N (2005) Efficacy of dog appeasing pheromone in reducing stress and fear related behaviour in shelter dogs. *Applied Animal Behaviour Science* **93**, 295–308

## Useful resources

The Association for the Study of Animal Behaviour Accreditation Scheme (www.asab.nottingham.ac.uk)
The Association of Pet Behaviour Counsellors (www.apbc.org.uk)
Feline Advisory Bureau Cat-friendly Practice Scheme (www.fabcats.org)
British Columbia Society for Prevention of Cruelty to Animals (www.spca.bc.ca)
Canine Behavioural Assessment and Research Questionnaire (www.cbarq.org)
Animal Behavior Resources Institute (abrionline.org)
American Veterinary Society of Animal Behavior (www.avsabonline.org)
American College of Veterinary Behaviorists (www.dacvb.org)
Association of Pet Dog Trainers (www.apdt.com)

## Acknowledgments

With many thanks to Alex Darville and Agora Management (www.agoramanagement.com) for advice and reference photographs. Thanks also to the Oundle Veterinary Surgery for photo opportunities.

---

## Client handouts (bsavalibrary.com/behaviour_leaflets)

- Adopting a rescue dog: the pros and cons
- Avoiding aggression in cats
- Avoiding house soiling by cats
- Avoiding house soiling by dogs
- Avoiding urine marking by cats
- Canine behaviour questionnaire
- Cognitive dysfunction syndrome
- Feline behaviour questionnaire
- Handling exercises for an aggressive cat
- Handling exercises for puppies and kittens
- Headcollar training
- How to find a good trainer
- Introducing a new cat into the household
- Ladder of Aggression
- Litterbox training
- Muzzle training
- 'Nothing in Life is Free'

- Pet selection questionnaire
- Puppy socialization: getting used to new people
- Redirected aggression in dogs
- Request for information on problem behaviours
- Sit–stay exercises
- Taking your cat in the car
- Teaching your dog to go to a place on command
- Treating a fear of car journeys using desensitization and counter-conditioning
- Treating a fear of the veterinary clinic using desensitization and counter-conditioning
- What your cat needs
- What your dog needs
- Your puppy's first year

# 3

# Basic requirements for good behavioural health and welfare in dogs

## Claire Corridan

## Introduction

Scientific interest in canine ethology has grown rapidly over the past two decades and expansion of knowledge in this field should enable validation of the information that is used when advising dog owners on the management of their pets. It is crucial that veterinary personnel have a thorough knowledge and understanding of normal canine behaviours and husbandry practices so that they can advise dog owners appropriately. Behavioural problem prophylaxis should be just as important as advising on diet and vaccination protocols for new dog owners. Without understanding the functional importance of normal canine behaviours, solutions for getting rid of behavioural problems will not be easy to find. Before veterinary surgeons can hope to tackle the abnormal, they must ensure that they fully comprehend the normal.

There have been numerous studies that have contributed to the understanding of the normal canine ethogram. When consideration is given to the ways in which species-related, and particularly breed-related, traits are expressed in dogs living in domestic environments, it is easy to identify the source of many of the 'undesirable behaviours' for which dog owners seek help.

Fear and anxiety are normal responses to real or perceived threats; aggression signals can be used to evade further social or physical conflict or protect a particular resource or individual; barking is an effective way for dogs to communicate with people. Each of these 'normal behaviours' has the potential to be misinterpreted or become exaggerated to the point where it becomes problematic for either the dog, the owner or both.

Throughout this chapter the daily requirements of the dog in order to achieve optimal physical and psychological health are discussed. The particular requirements of puppies and juvenile dogs will be highlighted, but it is important to remember that dogs continue to require stimulation, behavioural reinforcement and training throughout life. Too often new dog owners make a concerted effort to ensure that their new puppy is socialized and trained, receiving lavish attention, but unfortunately allow these efforts to wane as their dog reaches adulthood. The over-representation of dogs aged 5–24 months in rescue shelters in the USA (Salman et al., 1998) highlights the potential weakening of the human–dog bond as 'puppy novelty' wears off. Some behavioural problems

may be over-represented in juvenile dogs, and studies have identified that hyperactivity, elimination behaviours, aggression, destructive chewing, fearfulness and barking (Miller et al., 1996) all increased the risk of relinquishment to shelters. Patronek et al. (1996) identified the following potential risk factors, in order of decreasing importance:

- Lack of veterinary care
- Lack of participation in dog obedience classes after acquisition
- Inappropriate elimination behaviours
- Ownership of a sexually intact dog.

This again highlights the vital role of veterinary practices in ensuring that they are perceived as the primary and most reliable source of information for new dog owners on how best to care for their dogs, in every regard (Figure 3.1).

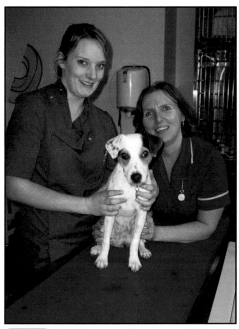

**3.1** Veterinary practices pay a vital role in canine welfare.

A word of caution: sometimes, despite having the ideal building blocks in place (selecting the right puppy from the right source, obtaining and implementing appropriate veterinary behavioural advice and training), some owners still experience behavioural difficulties with their dogs further down the line. The genetic components of an animal's behaviour should not be underestimated. Breed, parental temperament, prenatal stress (Serpell and Jagoe, 1995) and early postnatal experience (Scott and Fuller, 1965) will significantly influence the behavioural phenotype of the dog. The added complications of any congenital or acquired disease process can also hinder behavioural development and, again, necessitate veterinary intervention as early as is feasible.

The relevance of a number of normal canine activities will be covered in the following sections, with recommendations and discussion of the potential behavioural and welfare implications of each activity. Each dog is an individual and it is important to remember that, although generalizations for advice can be helpful, ultimately the advice may need to be tailored to the individual needs of the dog and the lifestyle and requirements of its owner. Client handouts on the basic requirements for good behavioural health and welfare and a checklist for the first year of life are provided online.

## Meeting basic nutritional needs

### Water

Provision of water should be on an *ad libitum* basis, unless there are specific medical reasons why this is contraindicated. Whilst out on long walks or during long car journeys, dog owners must always consider the dog's requirement for access to water. Various bowls, bottles and gadgets have been developed to provide novel solutions for both the carrying and delivery of water away from home.

If water is withdrawn for any reason (e.g. an owner attempts to control urination in the home) the dog's motivation to drink may result in drinking from inappropriate sources (e.g. the toilet) or hyperactivity and attempts by the dog to find its own source of water, resulting in destructive behaviours or escape attempts. If chronic, this problem can lead to medical complications, whether urogenital, gastrointestinal or neurological (effects of hyperosmolarity, electrolyte imbalances and metabolic acidosis).

### Food

Adult dogs vary in terms of their nutritional requirements, depending on breed, activity levels, health and reproductive status, and the nutritional aspects of feeding a dog will not be discussed here. Commercially produced dog foods may ensure the appropriate nutritive content of the canine diet.

The subject of how dogs should be fed is a huge source of debate for those working with them. Dogs evolved as hunters (searching for, stalking, catching and eating prey) and scavengers (seeking out nutritional waste in the environment). These activities, which would form a substantial percentage of their daily time budget, are largely unavailable for pet dogs that are simply handed a bowl of food. However, dry kibbles and canned food provide the potential for using the dog's daily food allowance for both training and stimulation: the owner can ask the dog to 'work' for its food.

- Programmes such as 'Learn to Earn' (Campbell, 1999) and 'Nothing in Life is Free' (Voith and Borchelt, 1996; see client handout) require the dog to follow a command or complete a task in return for food rewards.
- Food trails or 'treasure hunts' provide mental stimulation and keep the dog occupied, particularly in the absence of the owner. Care must be taken to ensure that hidden food is indeed consumed and that the dog has an adequate intake to provide for its daily requirements. In a multi-dog household this technique could result in fighting or unequal division of food rations; this can be minimized by supervising the dogs carefully and, in the absence of owner supervision, dividing access to the areas of the home or garden where trails are set. If resources are abundant there is less risk of provoking conflict.
- Commercially produced or home-improvised toys and objects can be filled with kibbles, so that the dog has to work to release the food, offering both stimulation and novelty.

Most animals will actually prefer to work for food than be provided with it *ad libitum* – a phenomenon known as contra-freeloading. Making the dog work for its food and ensuring that the food has stimulating sensory qualities may therefore be enriching.

Often dog owners like to have a set routine for the care of their dog (though this may vary between weekdays and weekends). Having a routine for meal times has advantages and disadvantages: the dog will expect its meal and should therefore avoid the stresses associated with sourcing food for itself (raiding waste containers and eating inappropriate items), but can experience a stressful response to any changes in that routine (for example, if its owner is late home or if someone unfamiliar is caring for the dog). Set feeding times allow the owner to determine how much a dog consumes in a day and food consumption is one marker of good health and welfare.

Other considerations may be needed in households with more than one dog. Because dogs might fight about food or guard their food bowl, in certain situations separating dogs at meal times will improve safety, increase consumption and be more relaxing for an individual dog.

Some dogs develop habits designed to solicit feeding of meals, treats or table scraps. It is up to the owners to set a precedent for this situation from the outset, when they first acquire their dog. If they reward the dog by providing the food or treat in response to begging, barking or pestering, the dog will learn that this is an effective strategy for eliciting the desired response from its owner, and potentially from any other humans that it comes across. This situation can soon become a problem for owners, if not during their day-to-day routine, certainly when visitors come to the house. The best means of preventing this situation is to prevent the habit from forming in the first place and only allow eating to occur at a designated time and place.

## Elimination and toileting behaviours

Age, neutering status, health, diet and individual variation will all influence the frequency with which dogs need to eliminate.

### Puppies

In newborn puppies, urination and defecation only occur if stimulated by maternal licking of the perineal area (or artificial substitution of the stimulation of the anogenital reflex in orphaned puppies). Urination and defecation come under voluntary control during the transitional period (14–21 days; see Figure 3.6). Tightening of the urethral sphincter muscles takes a variable amount of time in puppies and stimulation or excitement from play, feeding, activity or fear can lead to involuntary urination.

It is important that puppies are directed to appropriate substrates for elimination purposes from as young an age as is feasible. Most dog owners will not want to have an adult dog eliminating on newspaper in the kitchen and so it is vital that owners have access to an area where they can safely take their puppy (without risk of exposure to canine pathogens or parasites) to eliminate after elimination triggers such as waking up after rest, feeding and play. Ignoring mishaps but rewarding the puppy with praise for eliminating in the right place will soon teach it how best to achieve desirable responses from its owner, though the duration of the 'toilet training' period can be hugely variable (see Chapter 6). Owners should be informed that the reward is for eliminating at that moment and in that location, so it is essential that they go outdoors with their puppy to help it to learn the correct tasks.

### Adult dogs

Adult dogs may have superior urethral and anal sphincter tone compared with puppies but the triggers for elimination will remain the same. This must be a consideration for dogs left indoors for lengthy periods in the absence of their owners: another means of accessing appropriate areas for elimination should be provided. The psychological stress associated with any mishaps can easily be imagined:

- Stress from the impulse to eliminate but absence of appropriate area or substrate
- Possible anticipation of admonishment on the return of their owner.

Illness, exposure to fearful stimuli or any changes in diet, activity or routine could increase the risk of indoor elimination. Owners often misunderstand a dog's anticipation of reprimand and perceive it as a demonstration of 'guilty behaviour' instead of the appeasement (conflict-deflecting) behaviour that it represents.

After training their puppies, owners often take it for granted that their dog will remain toilet-trained. Episodes of illness (e.g. cystitis, diabetes or gastroenteritis), stress (e.g. moving house or bringing a new dog into the home) or the natural ageing process (e.g. senility or urinary/faecal incontinence) can result in loss of toilet training or lead to problem elimination behaviours. It is important that good behaviours are rewarded continually throughout the dog's life and this may necessitate a repetition of puppy toilet training in geriatric dogs that may have difficulty retaining their previous training (see Chapter 10).

## Shelter and resting areas

Within some countries there is legislation that enforces specific responsibilities for dog owners; for example, in the UK the Animal Welfare Act (2006) states that the owners of companion animals must provide them with a suitable environment that protects them from the elements and affords them a safe and comfortable place to sleep. Dog owners must consider the implications of providing a secure environment for their dog (for example: fencing the garden to ensure that the dog is contained; or ensuring that it is not left unsupervised off-lead whilst away from home). Within the home, dogs should have an easily identifiable bed or lying area to which they can retire when they need to rest or be left uninterrupted. This becomes particularly important when dogs seek a refuge (or 'den') during stressful situations, such as if they experience fearful responses to fireworks, or in an attempt to escape the curiosity and probing fingers of small children or even punishment from the owner.

Several studies have investigated the effect of positioning the dog's bed in relation to its owner; for example, in one study (Atkinson et al., 2005) one-third of dogs were allowed to sleep in their owners' bedroom. A recent study investigating risk factors for return of rehomed dogs to a rescue shelter found that owners who allowed the dog to sleep in a family member's bed were less likely to return the dog (Diesel et al., 2008).

There has been much debate amongst dog trainers and behaviourists as to the implications of allowing dogs to spend the night in close proximity to their owners but to date there have not been any conclusive scientific studies. Ultimately, if neither owner nor dog has a problem with their chosen sleeping arrangements, it is difficult to argue that they should be behaving otherwise, as long as the owner does not potentially provoke conflict by changing the arrangements. Consistency is the key. On acquisition of a new puppy, owners often either underestimate or overestimate the developmental maturity of their new ward. If they allow their new puppy to sleep on the bed or on the sofa, it will soon consider this to be the accepted routine. If the owner changes their mind when the 'puppy' is 6 months of age or when it can no longer be described as 'lightweight', they may have difficulty changing the rules. Owners must be encouraged to think ahead and start as they mean to go on. They must also consider any lifestyle changes in the future that may influence the accepted living conditions for their dog. For example, if they currently live alone with their dog, would any future partner tolerate their current sleeping arrangements? Any changes in routine or inconsistencies in implementation of the rules can be potential sources of stress and conflict between dogs and their owners.

## Physical activities

### Exercise

As crepuscular animals it could be expected that dogs would be most active in the early morning and evening. In the absence of the necessity to forage for food, they may spend substantial periods of time resting. If the nutritional input of the dog is in excess of its activity levels, this can lead to obesity and its resultant effects on the welfare of the dog: circulatory and articular or locomotor problems, as well as exacerbation of reduced activity levels and reduction of mental stimulation (Figure 3.2).

The exercise requirements of dogs will vary depending on their age, breed, health status and motivation. Provision of exercise away from the dog's home environment should be dependent on the owner, who should be encouraged to consider the exercise requirements of their chosen dog before acquisition in order to ensure that their lifestyle, home environment and available time are suitable. When acquiring a puppy or young dog, owners need to think about the lifestyle changes they might expect to happen over the next 10–15 years that their dog is likely to live (e.g. moving house, changing jobs, having children). They must also consider planning for any contingencies, such as who will care for the dog if they become ill or go on holiday. Owners may decide that their dog has sufficient exercise in their own garden and so they need not worry about desensitizing them or socializing them to other people or dogs; but a change of circumstances necessitating a change in the dog's routine could be a substantial stressor for the dog. It is advisable to provide exposure to novel environments from an early age and throughout the first year of life, irrespective of an owner's expectations about the life their dog is likely to lead. Priorities and circumstances change and a dog that has been restricted in its early socialization is more likely to develop an agonistic attitude towards novelty in later life (Serpell and Jagoe, 1995).

Routine is an important factor when considering exercise. Predictability may lead to a reduction in general stress responses but changes in routine may result in more acute stress responses. A dog that expects the same walk every day, or that it will be let off-lead at a certain point on its walk, or that its owner will throw a ball for it in the same location every time, has the potential to become stressed when this expectation is not met. Routines may become interrupted for a variety of reasons, such as ill health of either the dog or the owner restricting exercise, changes in work routines for the owner, or identification of potential hazards on the usual walking route that

| Category | Potential consequence | Comments |
|---|---|---|
| Physical | Obesity | If nutritional input exceeds daily requirements |
| | Overgrown nails, thin pads | |
| | Articular/locomotor problems | E.g. degenerative joint disease |
| | Cardiovascular and respiratory problems | Associated with obesity |
| | Lethargy | Motivation to be active reduced |
| Psychological | Reduced stimulation or frustration | Can cause variable effects in different dogs: some become hyperactive, others appear apathetic |
| Behavioural | Increase in inappropriate use of aggressive behaviours | Due to frustration, lack of interaction with unfamiliar dogs or people |
| | Increase in fears/anxieties | Reduced exposure to novelty may result in dishabituation to previously accepted stimuli and general reduction in acceptance of novelty |
| | Overactivity | Response to frustration |
| | Problematic sexual behaviours | Response to frustration or reduced interaction with other dogs, or attention-seeking behaviours |
| | Increase in owner control or training problems | Exercise outdoors inevitably results in increased interaction and reinforcement of training, so lack of exercise will reduce this effect |
| | Repetitive-type behaviours increased | Result of frustration, attention-seeking behaviours, learned helplessness |
| Human–dog bond | Effect on owner is variable | Owners may experience guilt from reduced interaction with dog but may not have time or physical ability to be able to commit to activity |
| | Effect on dog more likely to be negative | As result of potential consequences listed, more likely that dog will be affected negatively by lack of exercise |
| | Dependence on owner may be variable | Dog may spend less time actively engaging with owner whilst sharing outdoor activities, but this may increase risk of attention-seeking behaviours in the home |

**3.2**   Welfare implications of lack of exercise for dogs.

restrict off-lead exercise. There may be resultant attention-seeking behaviours from the dog: pestering, barking or jumping up, which can become a source of annoyance for owners. Variety may well provide a solution to some of these potential problems. Providing the dog with adequate exercise and stimulation, with variation in the time, duration and location of its walks as well as any specific interactions with its owner during the walk (being let off-lead or playing games) may help to improve the adaptability of the dog, thereby reducing the potential for acute stressful episodes and the development of attention-seeking or obsessive behaviours.

Locations that are safe for walking dogs off-lead and where it is legally permitted are becoming increasingly difficult to find. The ability to run, sniff and explore without restriction is pleasing and a desired activity for the majority of dogs. Bekoff and Meaney (1997) found that, in general, off-lead dogs induced a manageable amount of problems to 'off-leash' humans: 81% of dog–dog contacts were friendly and 85% of dog–human contacts were friendly or neutral. These figures obviously indicate a considerable number of unfriendly dog–dog and dog–human interactions which, this study concludes, should be tackled through education of people about canine behaviour and matters of etiquette and responsibility (see also Dumont, 1996; Beck, 2000).

The high incidence of aggressive episodes reported by dog owners whilst their dogs are on the lead highlights the importance of teaching dogs during the socialization and juvenile stages of life to walk on-lead and practise encounters with new people and dogs in a controlled manner with appropriate use of rewards for good behaviour.

Certain types of off-lead situations may create anxiety and welfare problems for both dogs and owners. Unpublished studies by the author have found an association between high frequency of on-lead exercise and an increase in behavioural problems and a decrease in dog owner satisfaction. Causation of this effect requires further investigation as it may be influenced by many secondary factors. In simplistic terms, dogs with a history of misbehaving off-lead may be less likely to be trusted off-lead on a regular basis. Dog owners who can enjoy walking their dog off-lead, reassured that it will behave appropriately, may receive more pleasure from the experience and less anxiety than those whose dogs misbehave.

Regulations relating to walking dogs off-lead, or banning access for dogs completely (for example, on beaches during the summer) have meant that it can be difficult to find safe areas to exercise dogs off-lead. In some countries dog parks have been established to facilitate exercising and socializing of dogs in designated areas without the risk of upsetting cyclists and runners or straying too close to children's playgrounds. Users of this valuable resource have the opportunity to socialize and share dog experiences whilst exercising. The success of these parks very much depends on responsible dog ownership, where owners maintain adequate control of their dogs, dispose of dog faeces appropriately and treat other park users with respect.

## Play

### Puppies

Dogs refine their methods of play to enable them to engage with playmates without the risk of inflicting any injury. This skill, referred to as bite inhibition, requires practice in order to ascertain the pressure and vigour with which another individual can be 'mouthed' without causing harm. Beaver (1999) showed that 87% of interactions between puppies involved biting: they will bite their littermates and dam as well as any humans they come into contact with. This is a normal and essential part of their social education, which if denied (due to either isolation or ill-timed human interference) can result in inappropriate use of mouthing and biting during future interactions. Such mishaps can sometimes be misinterpreted by owners as expressions of 'aggression' or 'dominance' and can, at best, result in the puppy or adult dog having limited access to play and interactions with humans or other dogs; at worst the dog, unable to gauge its own bite strength, may inflict significant damage when this was not its intention, or the owner's use of harsh techniques to curb this behaviour results in fear and anxiety associated with owner handling.

Learning social signals when interacting with littermates (play bows, paw raising, tail wags and the use of barking to elicit play) are vital if the dog is to interact safely with conspecifics in the future. Growling, biting and scruffing are also normal behaviours during play and it should be vocal responses or withdrawal by the playmate, rather than intervention by humans, that serve to educate the puppy when it has 'gone too far'. Puppies and juvenile dogs benefit hugely from interacting with adult dogs that are well socialized themselves (Figure 3.3). They can be taught the subtleties of vocal and physical gesturing that will enable them to assess future encounters with unfamiliar dogs appropriately and safely.

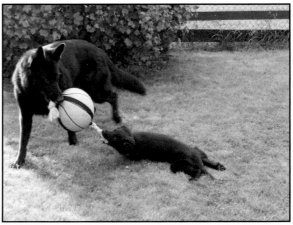

**3.3** Puppies benefit hugely from engaging in play with well socialized adult dogs.

### Adult dogs

Despite the fact that dogs reach sexual maturity between 9 and 18 months of age, depending on breed variation, they do not display fully adult behaviour until 2–3 years of age. Dogs often continue to display play behaviours well into adulthood (Figure 3.4) – an

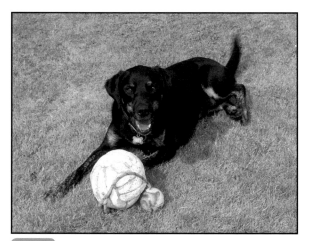

**3.4** Play behaviour lasts into adulthood.

example of paedomorphism (the retention of juvenile characteristics into adulthood), which is a feature of the domestication of the dog.

In social mammals with complex behavioural patterns, play can facilitate the establishment of behavioural routines, provide physical and mental exercise and strengthen individual relations (Bekoff and Byers, 1981). Play rarely occurs if the dog is on its own, which would infer that it should primarily be considered as a social exercise. This may limit the benefits of using toys to stimulate dogs experiencing separation-anxiety signs.

There will be breed variation in the amount and type of play exhibited: Beagles play more than wolves (Beckoff, 1974), who play more than poodles (Fedderson-Pederson, 1991). The differences between play behaviours in differing breeds may be due to restrictions on their ability to display play signals (as a result of selection for different conformations) but comparative studies are lacking. It is important that, during play, both individuals (human–dog or dog–dog) continually signal playful intent.

Rooney & Bradshaw (2003) surmised that dog–human play might influence the relationship between the partners. The input of time spent together and mutually shared positive experiences can only be beneficial to the development of a successful bond (Figure 3.5).

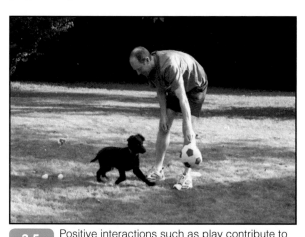

**3.5** Positive interactions such as play contribute to development of the human–dog bond.

## Chewing

Neonatal puppies will suck on any smooth warm object, presumably in an attempt to elicit milk letdown. Oral exploration of the environment continues through transitional, socialization and juvenile periods (Figure 3.6) and it is important that puppies and adult dogs are directed to appropriate chew material in order to satisfy this behaviour safely and without causing annoyance to their owners (see Chapter 6). Provision of chews and appropriate chewable toys will help to maintain the dog's dental health and also avoid misdirection of this behaviour to less suitable items (e.g. sticks, stones, socks, slippers, furniture), which might result in damaged teeth or gums, gastrointestinal foreign bodies, damage to property and irate owners, or any combination of the above.

| Sensitive period | Approximate time frames | Comment |
|---|---|---|
| Prenatal | –63 to 0 days | *In utero* stress or exposure to teratogens may have permanent effects on canine development |
| Neonatal | 0–14 days of age | Period of rapid sensory and locomotor development. Chemical learning well established |
| Transitional | 14–21 days of age | Development of coordination, motor skills and voluntary control of urination and defecation, auditory and visual sensory learning and adaptation to environment |
| Socialization | 3–12 weeks of age | Neural development and maturation facilitates puppy's ability to respond fully to environmental stimuli |
| Juvenile | 3–9 months of age | Exploration of environment increases and behavioural responses refined |
| Social maturation | 12–18 months of age | Learning continues but formation of stable dominance relationships, defence of territory and emergence of aggression demonstrate social maturity |

**3.6** Sensitive phases in dog development and maturation.

Possessiveness may become important where access to chew items is limited and may become a source of conflict if the dog is not trained to leave or release chew items reliably. Ideally it should have *ad libitum* access to appropriate chew items so that this natural urge can be satisfied as and when the dog requires. When there is more than one dog within the home, care may need to be exercised to avoid conflicts over extremely desirable chew items.

## Treats and rewards

Food treats have become the 'gold standard' for dog training and they are used effectively for rewarding good behaviour and successful training. Most dogs are food-motivated (particularly if the rewards constitute their daily food allowance) but for those that are not, praise (physical or vocal) or favoured toys can be used instead. However, excessive use of food rewards can devalue the reward and in extreme cases contribute towards obesity if total food intake is not carefully regulated. Care should be exercised to utilize treats properly for good behaviour, i.e. all treats and rewards must be earned (see Chapter 5).

## Tactile affection

Predisposition towards affinity for humans is another consequence of the domestication of the dog. With wolves, human stimuli in the neonatal period are effective in bonding only if exclusive, and exposure to conspecifics has the potential to override this effect. In contrast, dogs socialized in a similar way show a preference for the human if they are given the choice of another dog instead (Miklósi *et al.*, 2007). This factor may become important where owners are considering acquisition of a second dog to provide 'company' for their first dog.

The calming effects of human presence during petting and grooming have been identified in a number of studies (Kostraczyk and Fonberg, 1982; McGreevey *et al.*, 2005), as have the reciprocal effects on dog owners (Odendaal and Meintjes, 2003). Results indicate that, during positive interaction, concentrations of beta-endorphin, oxytocin, prolactin, beta-phenyl-ethylamine and dopamine increase in both species, whilst levels of cortisol decrease in the humans only. Ultimately these studies confirm the beneficial effects of tactile affection and positive interactions for both the human and the dog. Where these effects are enjoyed over a lengthy period, as in the dog–owner relationship, they must contribute towards strengthening the resultant bond (Figure 3.7).

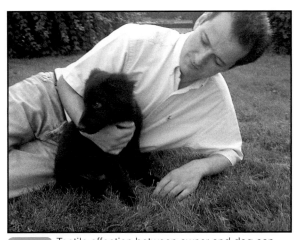

**3.7** Tactile affection between owner and dog can have emotional and physiological benefits for both.

It is recommended (and in some countries, legally required) that dog owners check their dog regularly for any abnormalities or signs of ill health. This activity should be introduced during puppyhood and may constitute part of grooming or petting activities.

Cooperation by the dog can be rewarded with praise or food treats and it is important that owners respond with consideration if their dog responds with aversion, as this may indicate a source of pain or irritation and will inevitably require further intervention (seeking veterinary advice or becoming a focus for further desensitization training).

## Independence from owner

In the course of an average day, dogs may spend a substantial amount of time in the company of their owner without direct interaction. Examples include the dog lying under the desk while the owner is working, or beside the sofa while they are watching television, or under the dining table while the owner is eating. It is important that puppies learn some independence so that proximity to their owner does not always equate with attention (petting, play or feeding). They should be encouraged to explore and work for rewards on their own, either indoors or outdoors (Figure 3.8), and owners can facilitate this by setting up treasure hunts or scent trails, using stimulation toys and appropriate chew items as discussed previously. Simply teaching a puppy or dog how to settle and relax in its own space is also a useful strategy for encouraging independence and calm behaviours.

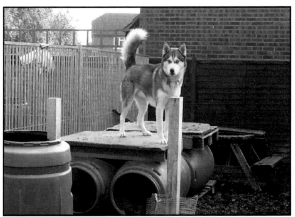

**3.8** Owners can create an enriched environment for their dogs at home using simple garden furniture, plastic drums and pallets.

It is important that a precedent is set from the outset with puppies and juvenile dogs, so that they become accustomed to spending time on their own and do not successfully use pestering tactics to seek attention from their owners, as this habit is much harder to break in adult dogs.

Entertaining themselves in this fashion (exploring, sniffing, digging and chewing) will help to provide exercise, mental stimulation and a reduction in frustration-type behaviours. It will also enable them to cope with spending time in the absence of their owner, perhaps reducing the occurrence of separation behaviours. Figure 3.9 gives a summary of welfare implications for dogs of spending long periods at home in the absence of their owner. Unpublished studies by the author have shown that when dogs are left at home alone in a confined space (single room,

| Category | Potential consequence | Comments |
|---|---|---|
| Physical | Obesity | Long periods of inactivity may increase risk of obesity unless sufficient exercise provided on daily basis |
| | Over-grooming | Hair loss, pyoderma, acral lick granulomas |
| | Self-induced injuries from inappropriate behaviours or attempts to escape | Damaged nails, paws, limbs, or mouth/tooth lesions |
| Psychological | Frustration | |
| | Hyperactivity or inactivity | Variable depending on dog's personality and experience |
| | Loneliness | |
| Behavioural | Inappropriate use of aggression | May be result of frustration or reduced socialization and training |
| | Increase in separation-type behaviours | |
| | Increase in fears or phobias | |
| | Problematic sexual behaviours | Motivated by frustration or attention-seeking behaviours |
| | Increase in owner control or training problems | |
| | Increase in inappropriate elimination problems | May be related to separation distress, or due to prolonged period *per se* |
| | Increase in repetitive-type behaviours | Self-mutilation or attention-seeking behaviours |
| Human–dog bond | Effect on owner variable | Increase in behavioural problems likely to be detrimental, as are feelings of guilt associated with leaving dog for lengthy periods<br>Increased flexibility in freedom of movement could be perceived by owners as beneficial, depending on their work, family and social commitments |
| | Effect on dog more likely to be negative | |
| | Dependence on owner could increase or decrease | Depending on dog's personality, increased chance of over-attachment or aloofness |

**3.9**   Welfare implications of dogs spending too much time at home alone.

training crate or kennel) where options for stimulation are minimal, there is a significantly increased risk of development of behavioural problems and ultimately relinquishment of the dog.

## Obtaining another dog

The companionship provided by multi-dog households may depend on a number of factors (age, breed, neutering status, health status, motivation and sociability of the dogs) and will vary considerably for every dog–dog dyad. When this situation goes wrong, inter-dog aggression within the household can be one of the most difficult problems for dog owners to come to terms with, particularly if the solutions offered include rehoming or euthanasia of one of the dogs.

It is a popular but erroneous belief amongst dog owners that owning more than one dog is less work in that the dogs provide a source of play, companionship and stimulation for each other. Dog–dog stimulation may not be a sufficient substitute to replace lack of interaction with human household members (Tuber *et al.*, 1996; Coppola *et al.*, 2006). Human (but not dog) companions have been shown to be effective at reducing the elevation in cortisol associated with social isolation. The social support effect of multi-dog households is an area that warrants further scientific exploration before there can be confidence about recommending it to dog owners, particularly those who own dogs that are already experiencing problems.

## Training and structured activities

Lack of training has been identified as a contributing factor for relinquishment, and learning the basics of canine behaviour and the etiquette and responsibility associated with dog ownership should be compulsory for all dog owners (see Chapters 5 and 6). Dogs, like children, need to understand the rules if they are to have any hope of obeying them and receiving the praise and acceptance of their owners. The rules must be clearly explained to the dog, using verbal and/or visual cues so that the dog understands what is being asked of it; they must be reinforced consistently, by all members of the household and visitors where possible, irrespective of time of day, owner mood and occasion; success or compliance should be rewarded, throughout the dog's life. It is important that children within the household (perhaps with parental supervision) are involved as much as possible in reinforcing the training of the dog (Figure 3.10) so that appropriate boundaries are set.

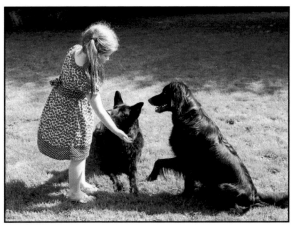

**3.10** Children should be encouraged to participate in reinforcement of the dog's training.

Punishment is a very difficult tactic to get right and is often used whilst the owner is experiencing anger, impatience, embarrassment or other stresses, which further reduce their ability to use it appropriately. The resultant stresses for the dog experiencing the punishment can include confusion, fear and aversion toward their owner and can increase the risk of future anxieties and the likelihood of an aggressive response. In most cases dog owners should be actively discouraged from engaging in this approach or reactionary stance, as the detrimental effects are likely to outweigh the positives (see Chapter 5).

Attendance at structured activities (puppy parties, obedience classes, agility, fly ball, hunting and shooting events or dog shows) provides an ideal opportunity for dogs and owners to engage in shared pleasurable experiences whilst spending time together. However, not all dogs respond well to all aspects of these activities (for example: travelling in the car; loud noises; proximity to other dogs without the opportunity to interact; the pitfalls associated with poor performance and disappointing the owner) and any detrimental effects must be weighed against potential benefits. Owners must consider the temperament and specific likes and dislikes of their dog as an individual and can be encouraged to try out a variety of activities, possibly in the absence of their dog initially, so that they can judge exactly what is entailed and make a reasoned choice about whether they and their dog can benefit from the particular activity.

## Routine activities

### Travel
Dogs often travel by car, train or ferry with their owners and it is important that the dog learns positive associations with this experience early on. If a car journey is always followed by a visit to the groomer, veterinary clinic or boarding kennels, the dog may develop a negative association that can result in travel sickness or other signs of anxiety (e.g. hyperaesthesia, vocalizing, trembling, elimination problems). Ideally, travel should be associated with positive experiences too, such as novel or familiar walks, or visiting human or canine friends. Journeys should be kept short

initially and owners must ensure that the dog's accommodation is safe and comfortable, minimizing the pet's ability to fall or be thrown around. Dog guards, car cages (Figure 3.11) and harnesses are available to provide this stability, but it is important that there is a contingency plan so that the dog can be removed safely in the case of an emergency.

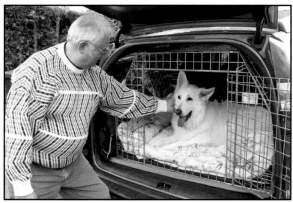

**3.11** Cars should be equipped to carry dogs safely and in comfort, providing access to water where feasible.

## Dog walkers, dog sitters and boarding kennels
Dog owners are not expected to be with their dogs all the time and work, family or social commitments may mean that the dog is left in the care of other people. Puppies and young dogs should be trained to accept this experience early on, so that they can develop coping strategies in the absence of their owner. Dogs can benefit from the novelty of this experience – new people, perhaps exposure to unfamiliar dogs or other animals, visiting novel places and participating in new activities and games – but this has the potential to become an overwhelmingly stressful experience if the dog has not learned appropriate adjustment tactics. Weight loss, reduced disease tolerance, acral lick lesions and signs of anxiety or 'depression' are often associated with prolonged absence from the owner. This can be dismissed as 'missing their owner' but the psychological impact of these stressful experiences is not, as yet, fully known.

Desensitizing puppies and young dogs to going for walks with other people, short stays in boarding kennels or with friends or family and visits to the hospitalization kennels of their veterinary practice can help to minimize future problems. Where the dog's life is based on a specific routine (for sleep, walks, meal times) it is important that the dog sitter or kennel is briefed and as far is feasible that they try to continue the normal routine. They must also be fully briefed if unusual words or commands have been used for training (to take food, or urinate on command, for example).

## Visiting the veterinary practice and grooming salon
Dog owners should be encouraged to find a veterinary practice that fulfils their needs (e.g. proximity, parking, opening hours, level of expertise, facilities) and those

of their dog (friendly staff, quiet well arranged waiting area, use of treats, capable veterinary personnel and 'dog friendly' hospitalization facilities) (Figure 3.12). Frequent visits should be encouraged early on, not necessarily associated with a clinical appointment: to collect food, to be weighed, or just to visit staff and receive a fuss or treat reward, so that the dog becomes familiar with the practice (smells, noise, people). This will help to reduce the stress associated with future visits when the dog is unwell or injured and receiving treatment there (see Chapter 2).

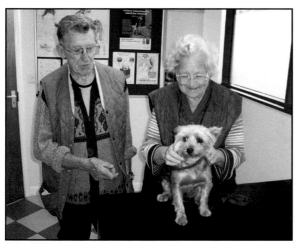

**3.12** Once clients have found a veterinary practice where they and their dog both feel comfortable, they are more likely to remain bonded with that practice.

Selection of a grooming salon should be based on similar criteria. Owners can often judge the response of their dog to a particular boarding kennel or grooming salon based on the willingness or reluctance of the dog to approach the staff and its overt behavioural signs: trembling, attempts to escape or go in the other direction, lowered tail and body postures.

## Conclusion

Although dog ownership may be affected by the increase in popularity of perceived 'low-maintenance' pets such as rabbits, human coevolution with dogs gives them a unique advantage in fulfilling the role of 'man's best friend'. Their sensitivity and responsiveness to human emotional states as well as their ability to enjoy shared activities, walks, play and tactility further endear them to their owners.

If dog owners are to be encouraged to maximize these benefits and minimize problematic behaviours, whilst ensuring the physical and mental wellbeing of the dog, a holistic approach to their care must be employed that encompasses the dog's physical, mental and behavioural wellbeing. Veterinary practices should offer adequate pre-purchase counselling and prophylactic behavioural advice, early response to potential problems identified by owners or by veterinary personnel during routine treatments and consultations, and sensitive and comprehensive management of problem behaviour cases either in-house or through veterinary behavioural referral.

A healthy, happy dog is largely dependent on having an owner who is sensitive to its needs and willing to invest the time and commitment to ensure that these are provided for. The role of veterinary surgeons is to provide the education, support and encouragement that enables dogs and their owners to enjoy a successful human–dog bond.

## References and further reading

Aloff B (2009) *Canine Body Language: a photographic guide: interpreting the native language of the domestic dog.* Dogwise, Wenatchee, Washington

Atkinson TL, Casey R and Bradshaw JWS (2005) Are the amount and type of exercise taken, and proximity to owners at night, related to the incidence of behaviour problems in the domestic dog? In: *Proceedings of the 2005 Companion Animal Behaviour Therapy Study Group Study day.* pp. 35–36

Beaver B (1999) *Canine Behaviour: A Guide for Veterinarians.* WB Saunders, Philadelphia

Beck AM (1996) Ecological aspects of urban stray dogs, In: *Readings in Companion Animal Behavior,* ed. VL Voith and PL Borchelt, pp. 185–191. Veterinary Learning Systems, Trenton, New Jersey

Beck AM (2000) The human–dog relationship: a tale of two species: In: *Dogs, Zoonoses, and Public Health,* ed. CN Macpherson *et al.,* pp. 1–17. CABI, Wallingford

Bekoff M (1974) Social play and soliciting by infant canids. *American Zoologist* **14**, 323–340

Bekoff M and Byers JA (1981) A critical reanalysis of the ontogeny of mammalian social and locomotor play. An ethological hornet's nest. In: *Behavioural Development, The Bielefeld Interdisciplinary Project,* ed. K Immelman *et al.,* pp. 296–337. Cambridge University Press, New York

Bekoff M and Meaney CA (1997) Interactions among dogs, people, and the environment in Boulder, Colorado: a case study. *Anthrozoös* **10**, 23–29

Bradshaw JWS and Nott HMR (1995) Social communication and behaviour of companion dogs. In: *The Domestic Dog,* ed. J Serpell, pp. 116–130. Cambridge University Press, Cambridge

Campbell WE (1999) *Behavior Problems in Dogs, 3rd edn.* Dogwise Publishing, Wenatchee, Washington

Coppola CL, Grandin T and Enns RM (2006) Human interaction and cortisol: can human contact reduce stress for shelter dogs? *Physiology and Behavior* **87**, 537–541

Diesel G, Pfeiffer DU and Brodbelt D (2008) Factors affecting the success of rehoming dogs in the UK during 2005. *Preventive Veterinary Medicine* **84**, 228–241

Dumont G (1996) A telephone survey on attitudes of pet owners and non-owners to dogs and cats in Belgian cities. *Anthrozoös* **9**, 19–24

Edney AT and Smith PM (1986) Study of obesity in dogs visiting veterinary practices in the United Kingdom. *The Veterinary Record* **118**, 391–396

Feddersen-Petersen D (1991) The ontogeny of social play and agonistic behaviour in selected canid species. *Bonner Zoologische Beiträge* **42**, 97–114

Feddersen-Petersen D (2001) Zür Biologie der aggression des Hündes. *Deutsche Tierärztliche Wochenschrift* **108**, 94–101

Fox MW (1970) A comparative study of the development of facial expressions in canids; wolf, coyote and foxes. *Behaviour* **36**, 49–73

Goodwin D, Bradshaw JWS and Wickens SM (1997) Paedomorphosis affects visual signals of domestic dogs. *Animal Behavior* **53**, 297–304

Kostraczyk E and Fonberg E (1982) Heart rate mechanisms in instrumental conditioning reinforced by petting dogs. *Physiology and Behavior* **28**, 27–30

McGreevey PD, Righetti J and Thomson C (2005) The reinforcing value of physical contact and the effect of grooming in different anatomic areas. *Anthrozoös* **18**, 236–244

Miklósi Á, Topál J and Csányi V (2007) Big thoughts in small brains? Dogs as model for understanding human social cognition. *NeuroReport* **18**, 467–471

Miller DD, Staats SR, Partlo C and Rada K (1996) Factors associated with the decision to surrender a pet to an animal shelter. *Journal of the American Veterinary Medical Association* **209**, 738–742

Mineka S and Henderson R (1985) Controllability and predictability in acquired motivation. *Annual Review of Psychology* **36**, 495–529

Odendaal JSJ and Meintjes RA (2003) Neurophysiological correlates of affiliative behaviour between humans and dogs. *The Veterinary Journal* **165**, 296–301

Packard JM (2003) Wolf behaviour: reproductive, social and intelligent. In: *Wolves: Behaviour, Ecology and Conservation,* ed. D Mech and L Boitani, pp. 35–65. University of Chicago Press, Chicago

Patronek GJ, Glickman LT, Beck AM, McCabe GP and Ecker C (1996)

Risk factors for relinquishment of dogs to an animal shelter. *Journal of the American Veterinary Medical Association* **209**, 572–581

Pongrácz P, Miklósi Á, Molnár Cs and Csányi V (2005) Human listeners are able to classify dog barks recorded in different situations. *Journal of Comparative Psychology* **119**, 136–144

Rooney NJ and Bradshaw JWS (2003) Links between play and dominance and attachment dimensions of dog–human relationships. *Journal of Applied Animal Welfare Science* **6**, 67–94

Salman MD, New JG, Scarlett JM *et al.* (1998) Human and animal factors related to relinquishment of dogs and cats in 12 selected animal shelters in the United States. *Journal of Applied Animal Welfare Science* **1**, 207–226

Schenkel R (1967) Submission: its features and function in the wolf and the dog. *American Zoologist* **7**, 319–329

Scott JP and Fuller JL (1965) *Genetics and Social Behaviours of the Dog.* University of Chicago Press, Chicago

Serpell J and Jagoe JA (1995) Early experience and the development of behaviour. In: *The Domestic Dog: Its Evolution, Behaviour and Interactions with People*, ed. J Serpell, pp. 79–102. Cambridge University Press, Cambridge

Tuber DS, Henessay MB, Sanders S and Miller JA (1996) Behavioral and glucocorticoid responses of adult domestic dogs (*Canis familiaris*) to companionship and social separation. *Journal of Comparative Psychology* **110**, 103–108

Voith VL and Borchelt PL (1996) *Readings in Companion Animal Behaviour.* Veterinary Learning Systems, Trenton, New Jersey

Yin S (2002) A new perspective on barking in dogs (*Canis familiaris*). *Journal of Comparative Psychology* **116**, 189–193

## Client handouts (bsavalibrary.com/behaviour_leaflets)

- Adopting a rescue dog: the pros and cons
- Avoiding house soiling by dogs
- Down–stay mat exercises
- Environmental enrichment for dogs in animal shelters
- Handling exercises for puppies and kittens
- Headcollar training
- How to find a good trainer
- Ladder of Aggression
- 'Leave it' exercises
- Muzzle training
- 'Nothing in Life is Free'
- Pet selection questionnaire
- Playing with your dog – toys
- Puppy socialization: getting used to new people

- Recall exercises
- Redirected aggression in dogs
- Request for information on problem behaviours
- Sit–stay exercises
- Teaching your dog to go to a place on command
- The newly adopted rescue dog: preventing problems
- Treating a fear of car journeys using desensitization and counter-conditioning
- Treating a fear of the veterinary clinic using desensitization and counter-conditioning
- Treating separation anxiety in dogs
- What your dog needs
- Your puppy's first year

# Basic requirements for good behavioural health and welfare in cats

### Irene Rochlitz

## Introduction

In recent years the popularity of the cat has increased: in 2008 the UK cat population was 7.2 million and 18% of households owned at least one cat. Despite this, many cats are relinquished to shelters, abandoned, or presented for euthanasia. Behaviour problems, as reported by owners, are one of the most important causes for this failure of the cat–human relationship. Very often the behaviour is normal for cats but problematic for the owner, or is abnormal behaviour that has developed because of a failure of the owner to meet the cat's needs. A better understanding of the normal repertoire of feline behaviour and how to meet the cat's requirements should lead to a reduction in the number of abandoned, relinquished and euthanized cats, an improvement in the cat's welfare and a strengthening of the bond between the cat and its owner.

## Feeding behaviour

Cats are obligate carnivores, with specific nutritional requirements and a much narrower range of tolerance for various dietary components than dogs and humans. Providing proper guidance about cat nutrition requires not only an understanding of the unique nutritional needs of cats, but also of their feeding behaviour.

- Feral domestic cats typically eat 10 to 20 small (prey-sized) meals throughout the day and night, with most of the diet comprising mainly rodents and other small mammals, as well as some birds, reptiles and insects (Fitzgerald and Turner, 2000).
- Repeated cycles of hunting throughout the day and night are required to provide sufficient food, as there is less than a 50% chance of success with every hunting cycle.
- While pet cats share many feeding behaviours with their wild counterparts, they generally have little control over their food supply and are usually offered two or three meals a day. Some cats adapt well to this feeding regime and will not eat all the food immediately, thereby increasing the number of meals eaten throughout the day and mimicking feral feeding behaviour. However, many cats will consume all the food rapidly (more so in a multi-cat household where there is competition, or where the food is very palatable) and then prompt the owner for more food.
- When food is offered *ad libitum*, cats may take many small meals throughout the day and night. However, because of the palatability of the food, as well as competition from other cats in the case of multi-cat households, many cats will overeat.
- In the domestic situation, feeding is not preceded by hunting activity.

The lifestyle of the domestic cat has changed: rather than spending most of the day and night as a predator hunting small, single-meal prey, it now expends very little, if any, energy and time on hunting. Instead, the pet cat receives highly palatable food throughout the day, or in several large meals, from its owner. This resulting overconsumption of food and lack of activity, most evident in indoor-only cats, has led to an obesity epidemic in pet cats in the Western world. Obesity predisposes them to a range of conditions such as insulin resistance and diabetes mellitus, lower urinary tract disease and respiratory difficulties.

Stimulating normal feeding behaviour will increase activity, reduce boredom, help with weight management and prevent obesity, and also strengthen the bond between cat and owner (who will enjoy interacting with their cat). This can be achieved by:

- Hiding dry food (kibble) around the house, or putting food on a high shelf for the cat to discover
- Using puzzle feeding cubes and other puzzle feeders
- Tossing dry food so that cats can chase after their food as they would prey; cat treat dispensers that do this are available commercially
- Using plastic drink bottles or yoghurt pots perforated with dry food-sized holes and part-filled with dried food, which falls out when the item is rolled (Figure 4.1)
- Using food as a reward, possibly with a clicker, for performing tricks and obeying commands
- Using timed automatic feeders for feeding small meals more frequently during the day even when the owner is absent (Figure 4.1)
- Using toy-like objects that are destructible and have nutritional value (few such items are available commercially).

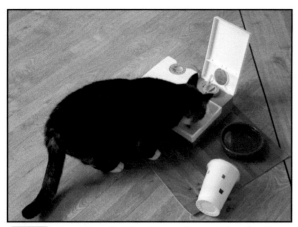

**4.1**   An automated feeder can be used to offer the cat small meals during the day when the owner is absent. When rolled, the white plastic container delivers the daily dry-food ration through cut-out holes.

Because neutering reduces the energy requirements of cats by 24–33%, owners should be advised about the cat's caloric requirements at the time of neutering and also as the cat ages and becomes more sedentary.

Having at least one food bowl per cat in the household will avoid food guarding and agonistic interactions. Multiple feeding stations and individual food dishes, especially if put at multiple levels and in quiet hiding spots, offer timid cats a secure place to eat away from more assertive cats. Assertive cats also benefit, by having more time to eat quietly in a social environment that they do not have to control.

Cats may develop a learned aversion to certain foods if the feeding of the food is paired with a negative experience. For example, cats can develop a food aversion to a food they were eating when they developed an illness, as they associate the food with feeling unwell. Food aversion may also develop as the result of stressful experiences such as hospitalization and force-feeding, or when medication is administered to the cat at the time of feeding.

When introducing a new food, it is best to increase the amount of new food over a period of several days while gradually decreasing the amount of the old food over the same period. The addition of small amounts of another food that the cat likes can help the cat adjust to its new food.

## Drinking behaviour

- Cats often prefer to drink away from the feeding area and at times not connected with feeding, so there should be bowls of water in a number of locations (both indoors and outdoors) away from the feed bowls.
- Some cats like to be in a slightly downward position when drinking; and some like drinking running water, such as from a dripping tap or small water fountain.
- Some cats do not like water straight from the tap (whether it is hard or soft) and may prefer bottled or filtered water; the reverse is true for other cats and many cats like to drink rainwater outdoors.

- Ice-cubes of frozen tuna-flavoured liquid (taken from a can of tuna in spring water and separated from the tuna flesh itself) can be used to encourage water intake; the ice-cube is allowed to melt in a saucer before being offered to the cat.

## Elimination behaviour

One of the reasons why cats are popular as indoor pets is that they can be trained to use toilet facilities indoors. House soiling is the most common feline behavioural problem presented to behaviourists, so client education about normal elimination behaviour and litter tray requirements is crucial (the terms box and tray are used interchangeably). To avoid things going wrong, the conditions of the toilet facilities must meet the cat's needs.

The main function of urination and defecation in cats is to eliminate waste products; these behaviours are not usually used for marking. Cats eliminate waste products in three ways: by squat urination, defecation and, much less commonly, urine spraying. Most house cats squat urinate twice or three times and defecate once daily, but this will vary depending on diet, water intake and other factors. For urination, the cat will usually dig in the substrate, squat urinate, then turn and sniff at the voided urine before covering it with litter (some cats may not cover their urine). After defecation, the cat may or may not cover its faeces.

A cat should never be trapped or cornered in its litterbox to give it medication or administer any aversive procedure, as this is likely to cause the cat to develop a strong aversion to the litterbox that will be very difficult to resolve (see Chapter 11).

## Litterbox provision

- The ideal number of litterboxes is thought to be one per cat in a unique location, plus one.
- Boxes should be placed in quiet private locations, away from traffic areas in the home and noisy appliances.
- As a minimum, litterboxes should be placed in at least two different locations and preferably more in a multi-cat household (feral cats usually deposit urine and faeces in separate locations). Several boxes next to each other really make one larger area, which can be blocked by one cat.
- There should be easy access to, and exit from, the box, to avoid blockage to the litterbox exit or entry of another cat.
- Boxes should be at least one and a half times the length of the cat, but many commercially available boxes are too small. For this reason, other containers such as shallow storage boxes (without the lid), trays used in gardening, and dog litter trays may be preferable.
- Some cats prefer open boxes and others prefer covered ones.
- Arthritic cats and small kittens may benefit from more shallow litter trays that are easier to climb in and out of.

- Most cats prefer a fine-grained, unscented litter (e.g. clumping litter), but an individual cat's preferences for litter substrate should be explored and met.
- Many cats prefer a litter depth of approximately 4 cm (1.5 inches), but preferences vary. Deep litter may be difficult for some cats to manipulate.
- Plastic liners may be aversive to some cats, as may scented litter.
- Some cats with outdoor access will nevertheless prefer to use a covered litterbox provided outdoors (for example, if the ground is hard or in bad weather).

## Litterbox maintenance

- Boxes should be scooped at least twice daily, or as often as is required to keep the box clean and free from odour.
- Clumping litter should be completely changed at least weekly and more often if more than one cat uses the box or if this is necessary to keep the box clean and free from odour.
- Clay litter should be changed at least every other day and more often if more than one cat uses the box or if this is necessary to keep the box clean and free from odour.
- The litterbox should be washed with warm soapy (using a mild kitchen soap) water, rinsed and dried well before adding new litter. Only soaps safe for cats should be used and strong-smelling products should be avoided.
- Boxes should be replaced annually, as plastic absorbs and retains odour over time.

## Social behaviour and organization

Many households now have more than one cat, so understanding cats' basic social organization and structure can help families better provide for their needs. Cats were once thought to be asocial solitary animals, only coming together for breeding. It is now known that the feline social system is flexible, with a complex range of social behaviours that allow cats to live alone or in groups of varying size, depending on resource availability (Macdonald *et al.*, 2000).

- Feral cats form complex matrilineal societies whenever resources (such as food and shelter) allow.
- Within these colonies there is extensive cooperation between adult females in the care and rearing of kittens, including communal nesting, grooming and guarding.
- Some males may remain with a group of females, while others have large home ranges that overlap the ranges of a number of different female groups.
- Cats have a polygamous mating system: females mate with multiple males and males mate with multiple females.
- There is resistance to the introduction of newcomers into the social group, and unfamiliar cats are usually driven away.

- Affiliative behaviours, such as touching noses (usually used as a greeting behaviour), allogrooming (when one cats licks another, often on the head or neck) and allorubbing (when two cats rub their heads, bodies or tails on one another) (Figure 4.2), play and resting together, probably serve to strengthen bonds within a social group.
- As cats become more familiar with each other, they are more likely to remain close and allogroom and less likely to be aggressive.
- Related cats are more likely to be close and allogroom than unrelated cats of equal familiarity.

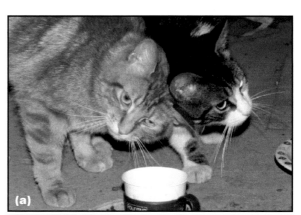

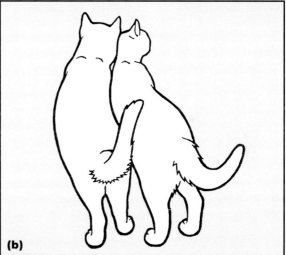

**4.2** Allorubbing probably serves to strengthen bonds within a group. **(a)** Head rub: one cat rubs its head on another. (Courtesy of T. De Keuster.) **(b)** Body rub: one cat rubs its body on another cat. (Illustration reproduced by permission of the UK Cat Behaviour Working Group, 1995.)

The existence of hierarchies, where there is a fairly well defined social ranking with dominant and subordinate cats, is still being debated among those studying cat social behaviour.

- Some describe hierarchical relationships within a group where there are higher-ranking, or dominant, and lower-ranking, or subordinate, cats and a range of dominance and submission signals (Crowell-Davis, 2005). The higher-ranking cats control access to the important resources such as food.

- The alternative view, which will be adopted in this chapter, is that a specific hierarchy with a definite ranking of status does not form, or does not have social significance, in an established group of cats (Heath, 2005).
- Unlike social species such as the dog, cats do not have obvious signals for diffusing conflict, or post-conflict mechanisms such as reconciliation.
- Overt physical aggression is mild and infrequent; much of feline communication within social groups enables individuals to avoid physical conflict wherever possible by ensuring that they maintain their distance from other cats or are able to run away or hide.

## Creating harmony in multi-cat households

Recent data show that the increase in the UK cat population is due to an increase in the number of cats per household rather than an increase in the number of cat-owning households, and this probably holds true for other industrialized countries where there is an increase. Based on knowledge of feline social behaviour and organization, this trend may not be in the best interest of the cat, as the keeping of several unrelated cats together, or introducing newcomers into an established social group, often leads to chronic stress and social disruption in the home (see Chapters 9, 11 and 19). Chronic stress in the multi-cat household has been associated with behavioural problems such as intercat aggression and urine spraying, and medical conditions such as idiopathic cystitis.

Some owners think that getting another cat will be beneficial for their existing single cat, but this is rarely the case. Provided that the single cat has a secure territory, a regular supply of good quality food and water, shelter and privacy, and rewarding interactions with its owner, it is likely to lead a happy life on its own (Bowen and Heath, 2005). For particularly sociable cats, social contact can occur with other cats in the neighbourhood where cats are allowed to go outdoors.

Ensuring harmony within a multi-cat household may be difficult. A number of strategies can be adopted in order to help to prevent problems arising (see **client handouts**).

- Create social groups of related or familiar cats:
  - If the intention is to have a multi-cat household, it is best to start with two or more kittens or adults that are littermates
  - If this is not possible, kittens of a similar age, even if of different litters, are likely to bond well provided that they are still young (less than 2 months)
  - Nevertheless, it is not unusual to find pairs (sometimes called 'preferred associates' (Crowell-Davis, 2005)), or larger groups of cats, that form stable and harmonious groups despite not being related.

- Choose carefully the additional cats to be introduced:
  - Many multi-cat households develop in a haphazard way, with the intermittent addition of stray or rescued cats
  - Resident adults are more likely to be tolerant of younger cats than of same-aged or older cats, and of cats of the opposite rather than the same sex
  - In cases of same sex pairs, two males are more likely to be compatible than two females
  - An older cat may not be able to cope with the play demands of a young kitten, in which case getting two kittens may be the solution
  - A new cat should be introduced following a carefully planned protocol (see below).
- Provide a sufficient number, and distribution, of resources, and sufficient space:
  - Important resources for cats are litterboxes, food and water stations, surfaces for scratching (such as scratch posts), and places for resting and sleeping (some of which also serve as hiding places)
  - Cats should have free and easy access to the resource; for example, the resource should not be placed at the end of a narrow corridor where access can be controlled by one cat
  - These resources should be plentiful for the number of cats, and distributed throughout the home; for example, there should be at least two separate feeding stations for three or four cats
  - Food bowls can be placed on high shelves where more timid cats often choose to go, rather than on the floor where timid cats feel more vulnerable
  - Ideally, the number of litterboxes in a multi-cat household should be one per cat plus one (see Elimination behaviour, above); however, this number may be reduced if the cats have access to the outdoors and there are good outdoor toileting areas, but this number should not be reduced for indoor-only cats
  - In multi-storey houses, there should be at least one litterbox on each storey
  - Sufficient space is crucial, as cats avoid conflict largely by avoiding each other
  - The vertical dimension should be exploited as much as possible, using structures such as activity centres (Figure 4.3), shelving, tops of wardrobes and cupboards and other similar structures
  - Having most of the resting and hiding places big enough for just one cat may help to reduce confrontation and fights
  - Resting and hiding places on the floor, preferably in a corner, may be necessary for kittens, elderly or infirm cats
  - Cardboard boxes, baskets and other similar structures are suitable hiding places.

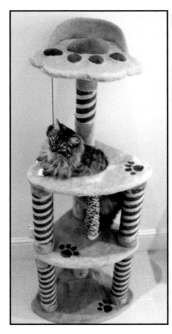

**4.3**

This cat activity centre has several platforms and a rest area covered in soft material, with scratching posts and toys.

Additional techniques can be used to reduce tension.

- If a neighbouring cat enters the home and threatens the resident(s), an electronic cat flap that only recognizes and allows the residents entry can be installed.
- The feline F4 pheromone (available as Felifriend®) is recommended for the introduction of unfamiliar cats.
- The feline F3 pheromone (available as Feliway®) is said to make a cat feel more secure in its home environment, and may help to reduce overall tension where there is no overt aggression and cats are known to each other.
- Food supplements are available that are said to have a calming effect in stressful conditions.
- If a particular cat in the group tends to intimidate other cats, it can be fitted with a quick-release collar with noisy bells to provide an advance warning system for the intimidated cats (Horwitz and Neilson, 2007).

More confident cats (sometimes known as 'despots') are able to choose where they want to go and when, and often try to control the floor of the home and access paths to resources. More timid cats (sometimes called 'pariahs') tend to look for elevated places in a corner, from where they can survey their surroundings and avoid being attacked. For these cats, unhindered access to resources may be difficult unless the resources are well distributed and access to them does not involve crossing large floor areas.

### Introduction of a new cat into the household

Introducing a new cat without careful planning and sufficient control can lead to severe disruption that may be difficult to rectify. The introduction of a new cat may take several weeks to several months. A **client handout** on this topic is provided. The following protocol should be used.

- An F3 pheromone product such as Feliway® should be placed in both the new and the resident cats' areas 2 weeks before the introduction, while an F4 fraction such as Felifriend® should be used at the time of introduction.
- The new cat is kept in a separate room, with food, toys, a litter tray, scratch post, rest and hide areas and perches off the floor, and allowed to adapt to its new environment.
- Limited interaction with the resident cat(s) is allowed under the separating door, as the cats get used to each other's scents and sounds.
- Bedding and other objects are exchanged between cats to intermingle their scents.
- Scent is also exchanged by rubbing a facecloth on the face and body (especially the cheeks and base of tail) of residents and newcomer. The facecloth should be rubbed against door and furniture corners, to spread the cats' group scent in the core territory.
- The newcomer is allowed to explore other areas of the house and become familiar with its layout and potential hiding and escape areas while the resident cat is kept away.
- Initial short visual introductions are made, with either the newcomer or resident(s) contained in a cage, or across a glass door, window or mesh screen. This should be done several times a day, and treats should be given to reward friendly or calm behaviour. If aggressive responses are noted, the visual introductions should be stopped and specialist help obtained.
- Once the cats appear to tolerate each other's presence and there is no aggressive posturing, cats are given short periods of supervised physical contact by being allowed to interact freely in one room.
- Owners should be prepared to intervene if there is any escalation in aggression, chasing or fighting, by using distraction methods (noise, water from bottle) or a heavy blanket to restrain a cat, but an aggressive aroused cat should not be handled directly as it may redirect its aggression to the handler.
- Cats should not be allowed together without supervision until several supervised interactions without aggression have occurred and the cats are calm in each other's presence.
- Newcomer and resident cats should continue to have their own feeding bowls and they should not be placed close together, as this can cause chronic stress in both new and resident cats.

### Kittens

The sensitive phase is the time during which an animal is most susceptible to learning from certain types of experience; these experiences will have a profound influence on the cat's behaviour throughout its life (see Chapter 7). The sensitive phase for the socialization of kittens to humans lasts from approximately 2 or 3 to 7 or 8 weeks of age. Because of this early sensitive phase, the responsibility for adequate socialization rests largely with the breeder of the kitten. It is likely that the phase for socialization to other cats also occurs during this time, though it may continue until 12–14 weeks of age (Hunthausen and Seksel, 2002). Social play peaks at approximately 3–4 months, and object play at 5 months of age (Crowell-Davis, 2005).

Genetic effects on social behaviour are recognized; for example, kittens sired by fathers that are friendly or bold towards humans are more likely to be friendly or bold towards humans themselves than kittens sired by unfriendly or timid fathers (McCune, 1995).

- Kittens should receive high-quality kitten food and fresh water daily, to meet their nutritional requirements.
- While weaning can start as early as 4 weeks, kittens should not be separated from their mother for rehoming before 6–8 weeks of age.
- Kittens learn about appropriate elimination behaviour from their mother, and are also naturally interested in materials that can be dug and raked. Kittens should experience a range of litterboxes and litter substrates before rehoming, particularly during the sensitive phase, to ensure some flexibility in their acceptance of toilet facilities later on.
- A kitten can be trained to use a scratching post or other scratching surface. This can be achieved by enticing the kitten to the post upon wakening with a food treat, by rubbing treats on the post, and by holding treats or toys some way up the post, to encourage the kitten to stretch and to scratch it.
- Play in kittens is thought to provide practice in motor, cognitive, predatory and social skills; kittens also learn skills by watching their mother.
- Kittens should experience frequent handling and play sessions with a variety of people, including men, women and children. They can be habituated to other species such as dogs.
- They should be exposed to a variety of experiences, such as being placed and carried in a cat carrier, being groomed and having their ears, teeth and nails examined.
- Some owners may be prepared to brush their kitten's teeth as part of a preventive health programme.
- Provided that there are no health risks, singleton kittens benefit from interacting with other kittens of a similar age.
- The hand rearing of kittens may be associated with the development of frustration-related aggression towards humans (see Chapter 19).

## Territory and home range

Cats are described as having core and peripheral territories as well as home ranges.

- The core territory of the neutered pet cat is usually its indoor home, and the periphery its garden or immediate surroundings.
- Cats will mark their territory with behaviours such as facial and body rubbing against objects, claw scratching and urine spraying.
- Urine spraying (and sometimes the deposition of faeces) and scratching are more likely to be performed at the periphery of the territory, and the deposition of body odours by rubbing within the core territory.
- In the right conditions, cats within a social group peacefully cohabit by sharing territories.
- Problems arise when the integrity of the core territory is disrupted (for example, due to building work in the home) or when unfamiliar cats invade the peripheral territory (for example, when a new cat moves in next door).

Territories are found within larger home ranges, which usually overlap with those of other cats. Much of feline communication with marking behaviours appears to be designed to enable cats to avoid each other while crossing these home ranges but actual data for this are lacking. Neutered cats have a smaller home range than entire cats.

## Communication

Cats communicate with each other and with humans in many ways, using visual signals, vocalization, tactile behaviours and olfactory signals. The importance and function of olfactory communication in cats is inadequately understood, partly because of the poor sense of smell in humans and our reliance on visual and verbal communication.

### Visual communication

Visual signals are mainly used in regulating aggressive behaviour, whether offensive or defensive (Bradshaw and Cameron-Beaumont, 2000) and it is important for humans to be able to recognize them. Visual signals are also important for indicating friendly intentions, both within a feline social group and from cats to humans.

- An offensive aggressive cat will piloerect, prick its ears forward and stand at its full height with a puffed-up tail (to look bigger).
- A defensive cat that wants to withdraw will crouch on the ground, flatten its ears to the sides of its head, wrap its tail closely to its body and withdraw its head into its shoulders (to look smaller) (Figure 4.4).

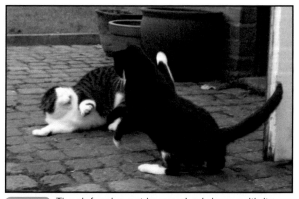

**4.4** The defensive cat is crouched down, with its ears flattened and its head drawn into its shoulders. The offensive cat is rearing up with its ears pricked forwards. (Courtesy of A. Lummerzheim.)

- Other positions observed in offensive encounters include the tail being carried low, held out stiffly behind the body or held out stiffly for a few inches and then forming a 90 degree bend as the tail turns downwards.
- Lashing the tail from side to side is often seen when the cat is very aroused or during aggressive encounters.
- At the beginning of agonistic encounters cats tend to avoid looking at one another simultaneously, thereby trying to avoid confrontation, as direct eye contact (mutual gaze) is interpreted as a threat signal.
- In non-agonistic encounters the amount of mutual gaze does not appear to be used as a signal.
- Direct eye contact between humans and cats does not seem to elicit aggression in cats in the way it can in dogs; usually cats avert their gaze or move away.
- Rolling on the ground is a component of female sexual behaviour and is usually accompanied by purring, stretching and rhythmic opening and closing of the claws and bouts of object rubbing, while male-to-male rolling appears to be a form of appeasement.
- Rolling behaviour directed towards humans is thought by some behaviourists to be a solicitation to play or to another kind of friendly interaction.
- The normal, relaxed tail carriage for most cats is the horizontal or half-lowered position.
- The 'tail-up' position, where the cat approaches another cat (Figure 4.5a), human (Figure 4.5b) or other animal with the tail sticking up in the air,

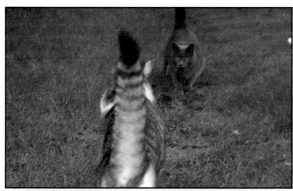
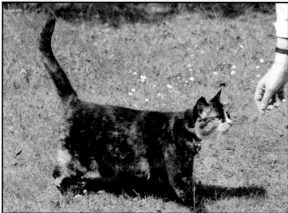

**4.5** The cat's tail is held almost perpendicular to the ground in the 'tail-up' position, indicating its friendly intentions towards another cat or person.

perpendicular to the ground, is a visual signal that indicates friendly intentions. The tail-up position has probably developed as an affiliative signal during domestication, perhaps consecutively with increased sociality which necessitated an additional visual signal in order to avoid unnecessary conflict as cats adapted to living in higher densities with humans.
- Cats also create long-term visual signals by scratching on surfaces, such as vertical and horizontal tree trunks, posts, logs and similar objects.

## Vocal communication

Vocalizations in cats are restricted to four major types of interaction: agonistic, sexual, mother–young and cat–human (Bradshaw and Cameron-Beaumont, 2000).

- Most of the offensive and defensive sounds (for example: growling, yowling, snarling, hissing and spitting) are strained intensity calls where the cat is tensing its body in preparation for a fight or in reaction to threatening predators or humans.
- Queens use the trill or chirrup to call to their kittens. As these calls are also heard between adult cats and between cats and people, they are probably greeting calls.
- The purr is also a friendly greeting call and occurs between cats during a variety of amicable social interactions.
- While it is usually interpreted as indicating pleasurable circumstances, cats may purr when they are seriously ill or in severe pain and so purring may also function as a contact- and care-soliciting signal, possibly derived from its presumed function in the neonate (kittens are able to purr almost from birth).
- The miaow is commonest in human–cat interactions and not often heard during cat–cat interactions.
- Humans are very responsive to the miaow and so, by reinforcement, it often becomes the signal that a cat uses to get attention.
- Some cats can learn to produce different miaows for different purposes and some breeds, such as the Siamese and other Orientals, are known for their 'talkativeness'.

## Tactile communication

Cats that are members of the same colony are often in tactile contact through such behaviours as allorubbing, allogrooming, touching noses and resting together.

- Allogrooming and allorubbing may be signals to redirect or avert aggression or may serve to strengthen social bonds within a group.
- Allorubbing occurs most frequently if one or both cats approach each other in the tail-up position; they may rub their heads and bodies together (see Figure 4.2) and intertwine their tails.
- Resting or sleeping together in close physical contact is a common phenomenon among both

feral and house cats and may be a measure of social bonding.
- Cats will also rub themselves against humans, often in the friendly tail-up position (Figure 4.6), and against objects in their core territory.

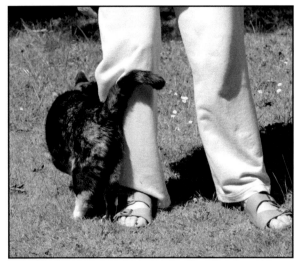

4.6   This cat is communicating by touch, as well as depositing scent by rubbing its body and tail against the person's legs.

## Olfactory communication

Olfactory signals, which last over a period of time and give messages to other cats remotely, enable cats to learn about each other without having to meet physically. It is possible that scent communication in domestic cats, who usually live at a higher density than their ancestors, has been modified during domestication.

Cats have an excellent sense of smell; in addition to a nasal epithelium that is dense with olfactory receptors, they have vomeronasal organs located behind the upper incisors that are used in the '*flehmen*' response. Since flehmen is only performed in response to odours from other cats, it is presumed to gather social information. Olfactory communication consists of the deposition of scent (scent marking), primarily by urine spraying and by claw scratching, and also by urination, defecation and tactile rubbing.

## Marking behaviours

### Urine spraying

Spraying consists of deliberate scent marking with urine: the cat backs up to a vertical surface and urinates backwards, often while quivering its tail (Figure 4.7). The tail is raised vertically and then lowered, and usually only a small amount of urine is voided. In addition to olfactory cues, the marks of sprayed urine leave visual signals. Sprayed urine may contain other secretions, such as those from the preputial or anal glands. Urine spraying is a poorly understood behaviour; it probably has multiple meanings depending upon the context and the exact molecules within a given spray of urine.

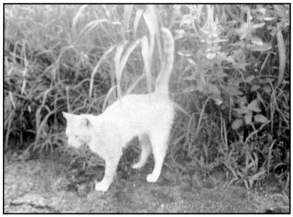

4.7   A free-living entire male spraying urine backwards on to grass at the ege of a field in which he hunts. (Courtesy of S. Crowell-Davis.)

- Spraying is most frequent in mature entire males, but queens also spray, as do neutered cats (urine spraying is a component of sexual behaviour and is greatly reduced after neutering).
- While all cats investigate spray marks intently, usually by sniffing and often followed by flehmen, spray marks are rarely observed to act as a deterrent in their own right (Bradshaw and Cameron-Beaumont, 2000) and are not necessarily deposited at the edges of territories.
- Cats do not attempt to cover urine marks with their own, but may urine spray to add their own scent.
- Urine spraying probably gives identifying information, particularly about reproductive status (when performed by entire cats), about which cat was at a given location at a given time, as well as about emotional state.
- In neutered cats urine marking within the home is often associated with the presence of other cats, both inside and outside the home, or with environmental changes or other causes of stress (see Chapters 11 and 19).
- Synthetic analogues of the feline facial pheromones, such as Feliway®, are widely used for the treatment of spraying behaviour (see Chapter 21).

### Claw scratching

The action of scratching on trees, fence posts or sofas has a marking function for domestic cats, through the formation of a visual mark as well as a scent mark that is deposited from the scent glands in the paws. Scratching also enables cats to condition their claws, stretch their body and exercise the muscles and tendons involved in claw protraction and retraction (Figure 4.8). The location that the cat chooses to scratch on will vary depending on whether it is motivated by the need to leave a mark or to condition the claws.

- Scratching sites are more common along regularly used routes, rather than at the periphery of the territory or home range, and may serve as landmarks that the cat uses in navigation.

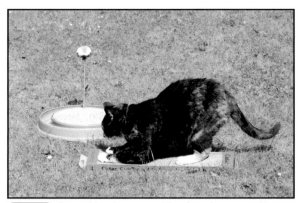

**4.8** Scratching has a marking function, as well as enabling the cat to condition its claws and stretch. This cardboard scratching post is impregnated with catnip; behind it is a toy on a spring with a cardboard centre.

- When scratching as a marking behaviour occurs within the home, which should normally be regarded as a safe and secure core territory, the behaviour is thought to indicate that the cat is feeling insecure (Heath, 2005).
- The cat may scratch at sites of exit and entry (such as by doors and windows) where it feels most threatened.
- Cats may also scratch on objects in the home to condition their claws, without necessarily intending to scent mark.
- After resting or sleeping, cats will often scratch to help stretch their muscles.

## Other forms of olfactory communication

Cats usually bury their faeces, especially when they are in their core territory, and are generally not thought to use faeces as scent markers. However, the deposition of unburied faeces in prominent places ('middening') has been described as a form of territorial scent marking. Cats may also leave scent by squat marking with urine and by rubbing their body against objects and against other cats and humans (see Tactile communication, above).

- Sebaceous glands are located throughout the body, especially on the head (base of ears, chin and around the sides of the mouth), in the perianal area, and between the digits.
- The frequency with which cats rub and sniff each other supports the idea that olfactory cues from these areas are important.
- Cats frequently rub their heads on each other and rub their bodies together (see Figure 4.2) and rub on humans (see Figure 4.6) and objects in their home environment, often purring as they do so.
- The cat's behaviour suggests that it is depositing scent on conspecifics and humans with which it has a friendly relationship, and depositing scent within the core territory; this exchange of scent may lead to the establishment of a 'group odour'.
- This scent exchange can be done artificially, by using a cloth to transfer body scent between cats, and will help with group stability and the acceptance of newcomers.

## Activity and play

Cats are often described as being naturally crepuscular, i.e. most active at dawn and dusk, as this coincides with the peak activity of small mammals that they hunt. However, some studies suggest that the cat has developed a more diurnal pattern of activity as a result of domestication and an adaptation to life with diurnal humans. Nevertheless, high levels of activity at dawn or dusk (and sometimes during the night) are often reported by owners and occasionally considered to be problematic (see Chapter 9).

- In most situations the performance of play, a 'luxury' activity, is driven by a positive emotional state and is inhibited by acute or chronic stress.
- Playfulness, essentially practice for predatory behaviour, is an attractive attribute of cats that is often sought after by owners.
- Some cats prefer to be groomed and petted, while others want to interact through play.
- Most cats play alone or with their owner, though some cats will 'play-fight' with other cats (see Chapter 19).

## Predation

Cats are specialized carnivores, finely attuned to respond to the acoustic and visual cues of their prey (Figure 4.9). Feeding a cat does not necessarily reduce its motivation to hunt. Capture of prey, killing and consumption are relatively independent of each other, and the former two activities are independent of hunger (Fitzgerald and Turner, 2000). Hunger can serve to intensify the effort put into the hunting sequence, but even if a cat has just eaten a full meal

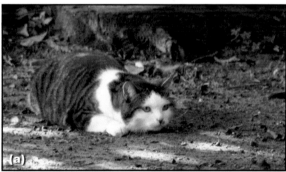

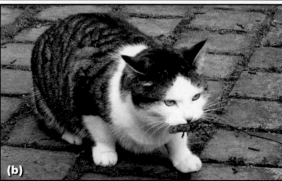

**4.9** Cats are finely attuned to respond to the acoustic and visual cues of their prey. **(a)** Crouching low while watching prey. **(b)** With prey in mouth. (Courtesy of A. Lummerzheim.)

it will not ignore the signals of high-pitched sound, rustling and rapid movement of its prey. In consequence, cats will capture and even kill prey that they have no intention of consuming. This behaviour can sometimes be problematic for humans, and they may try to prevent cats from catching prey by attaching bells or a bib to the cat's collar or by restricting the cat's access to the outdoors during times when their prey is most active.

## Environmental enrichment

Understanding of a cat's needs arises mainly from examining, and extrapolating from, the cat's evolutionary history and from observational studies of the cat's behaviour in different situations. Goals of environmental enrichment for cats include:

- The presence of a wide range of normal behaviour patterns
- The absence of abnormal behaviour
- Positive interaction with the environment (for example, through stimulation of the senses, exploration and play)
- The ability to cope with and adapt to challenges
- A strong bond between the animal and its owner.

Among the major reasons for the development of behavioural problems, such as fearful or avoidance-related behaviours, are environmental stressors and a high proportion of these relate to social factors, such as relationships with other cats or with humans. It follows that the environment in which the cat is housed will affect the development and maintenance of these behavioural problems.

The following aspects (summarized in Figure 4.10) should be considered when attempting to meet a cat's needs by enriching its environment.

### Quantity and quality of space

The home range of the pet cat confined indoors is inevitably very small compared with that of cats allowed to roam freely. Nevertheless, having outdoor access does not compensate for poor conditions in the home that may cause the cat to leave and join the stray cat population.

- Ideally, a cat should have access to at least two rooms.
- Beyond a certain minimum size, it is the quality rather than the quantity of space that counts.
- The cat can be regarded as a semi-arboreal animal that spends some of its time off the floor, on elevated surfaces. Cats use elevated areas as secure vantage points from which to survey what is going on around them. Structures within the home that enable cats to use the vertical dimension include shelves, climbing posts, windowsills and platforms.
- Timid cats and those less well integrated into the social group often occupy the higher positions, particularly those in corners, as they provide the best vantage points and protect the cat from being approached from behind.
- Cat activity centres (see Figure 4.3) can be obtained from good pet shops and plastic children's furniture can also be used.

### Resting and sleeping behaviours

Cats spend a large portion of their day either resting or sleeping, so it is important that there are plenty of rest areas with comfortable surfaces.

- As cats are more likely to rest alone than with others, there should be a sufficient number of comfortable resting areas for all cats in the home.
- Some of the rest areas should be off the floor (cats often indicate their preference for this by sleeping on the chair, bed or the top of the refrigerator, cupboard or wardrobe).

### Hiding behaviour

Hiding is a coping behaviour that cats often show in response to stimuli or changes in their environment. It is seen when cats want to avoid interactions with other cats or people, and in response to other potentially stressful situations.

- In addition to open resting areas, there should be resting areas where cats can retreat to and be concealed, such as high-sided cat beds and boxes (see Chapter 2).
- Some of the hiding places should be off the floor, such as on a shelf or on top of or inside a cupboard or wardrobe.

| Form of enrichment | Components of enrichment |
|---|---|
| Space quantity and quality | Sufficient space (at least two rooms). Use of the vertical dimension |
| Sleeping and resting behaviours | Comfortable resting and sleeping places, some on raised surfaces, throughout the home |
| Hiding behaviour | Comfortable hiding places, some on raised surfaces, throughout the home |
| Claw scratching behaviour | Vertical and horizontal surfaces suitable for claw scratching, placed in strategic locations |
| Social contact | Contact with other cats (related or familiar). Distribution of resources to prevent competition |
| Contact with humans, activity and play | Offer opportunities to explore, to exercise and to play. Short (10–15 minutes) frequent daily interactions with owner via play with toys, petting and grooming. Stimulate feeding behaviour to encourage activity |
| Stimulation of the senses | Olfactory stimuli (e.g. catnip). Visual and auditory stimuli (views from windowsill, audiovisual programmes). Tactile stimuli (e.g. soft bedding, scratch posts). Access to the outdoors |
| Control and choice | Offer predictability and routine, opportunities to have control and make choices |

**4.10**    Approaches to enrichment of the home environment for cats.

• Visual barriers, such as vertical panels, curtains and other room divisions, also enable cats to get out of sight of others and hide.

### Claw scratching behaviour

As well as a marking behaviour, claw scratching is used to stretch the muscles and maintain the claws in good condition. Occasionally, cats may scratch furniture in order to attract human attention.

• Preferred surfaces for the deposition of olfactory and visual signals by claw abrasion include scratch posts, sisal rope, rush matting, cardboard and pieces of carpet and wood.
• Scratching surfaces should be positioned at places of entry and exit in the home where new smells are brought in, and also next to the resting or sleeping area (as cats often stretch and sharpen their claws after waking).
• Prominent surfaces such as corners of furniture can be covered with a suitable material for scratching, or scratch posts can be placed next to them.
• Cats often prefer vertical scratching surfaces that are high enough for them to stretch fully, stable enough so that they can exert some pressure on the surface, and with a vertical thread to pull the claws through.
• Scratching surfaces that are horizontal may also be used (see Figure 4.8).
• Outdoor scratching places, such as softwood posts and logs, in the garden, especially on its borders, will help the cat to control access to its territory.

### Social contact

Cats are semi-social carnivores that regularly interact with others. Their environment may be enriched by having contact with other cats, provided that they are well socialized; ideally the cats should be related. Owners should be aware of the social dynamics between their cats and the particular requirements necessary for cats to live peacefully together. Strategies to help to ensure harmony in multi-cat households have been described in detail above and include:

• Sufficient space (particularly the vertical dimension)
• A sufficient number of resources, distributed in a number of different sites (to prevent monopoly and confrontation)
• Easy access to, and exit from, the resources
• Resting or hiding places big enough for just one cat, or in some cases two (e.g. related cats)
• Use of the F3 feline pheromone to reduce overall tension.

### Contact with humans, activity and play

As well as routine care such as feeding, owners need to spend time with their cats in order to enjoy the benefits of cat ownership.

• Owners should have regular, short but frequent daily play sessions with their cat, which serve to strengthen the cat–owner bond and provide the cat with some stimulation and exercise (especially for indoor-only cats).
• Cats differ in their preference for the type of toy they enjoy playing with.
  – Objects that are mobile, have complex surface textures and mimic prey characteristics (such as sudden jerky movements and squeaks) are often the most successful at promoting play.
  – Toys such as lengths of string, moving furry objects that need winding-up, laser pointers and 'fishing' toys are best for interactive play between the cat and its owner (Figure 4.11).
  – Toys with which the cat can also play on its own include ping-pong balls, artificial feathers and other lightweight objects, soft furry artificial mice and self-propelling or springy toys.
• Cats habituate to toys rapidly and so a variety should be provided and they should be replaced regularly.
• Some toys are made to look attractive to humans, but they may not be very effective at eliciting play or predatory behaviour in the cat.
• Some cats may not be playful but will still enjoy being groomed, petted and interacting with their owner.
• Using techniques to stimulate feeding behaviour will also encourage activity and play.
• Cats benefit from opportunities to explore and suitable novel objects such as boxes, large paper bags and other structures can be introduced into the home environment intermittently.
• Access to the outdoors provides the cat, in most instances, with a wide range of stimuli and opportunities for exercise but may be associated with certain hazards.

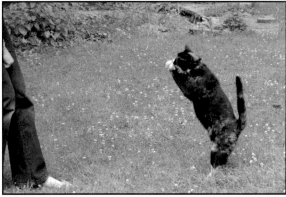

**4.11** Toys on a string are suitable for interactive play between a cat and its owner.

### Stimulation of the senses

Cats have highly developed senses and benefit from being able to use them. Their senses can be stimulated in a number of ways.

• Access should be given to outdoor stimuli (sounds, sights and smells) even if cats are confined indoors (using windowsills, viewing platforms near windows, secure balconies or other enclosures).

- Audiovisual products are available for cats and usually contain images and sounds of nature that are thought to be stimulating for them.
- Catnip is a well known stimulant for cats, though it can cause some cats to become quite aroused and aggressive, and others may not be affected by it.
- Some cats like to chew certain types of grass that can be grown in containers; it is thought that this can help with the elimination of furballs (trichobezoars).
- In order to maintain some olfactory continuity within the home, surfaces that cats have used for olfactory marking (such as corners of tables and doors that they have rubbed against) should not be cleaned too often.
- Household sprays containing citrus scents should be avoided as these scents are aversive to cats.

## Control and choice

An important objective of good housing is to improve welfare by giving the animal a degree of control and choice in its environment.

- While housing in a barren environment leads to apathy and boredom, cats do not like excessive novelty such as contact with unfamiliar cats or humans, or an unfamiliar and unpredictable routine.
- How the cat responds to the level of stimuli, and predictability, in the environment will depend on many factors, including the cat's temperament or personality and previous experiences.
- If the cat has a variety of behavioural choices and is able to exert some control over its physical and social environment, it will develop more flexible and effective strategies for coping with stimuli (provided that extremes are avoided). For example, if a careful protocol is followed when introducing an unfamiliar cat into the household (see above), this enables both resident and new cats to develop effective strategies to cope with the change.

## Assessment of welfare in cats

Some of the measures indicating poor and good welfare are summarized in Figure 4.12 (the list is not exhaustive). The emphasis in research has been biased towards measures of poor rather than of good welfare. Which measures are used will depend on how appropriate they are to the individual cat being assessed. Clearly, the animal's physical condition will have an impact on the behaviours the cat shows and on its psychological health. Physical health can be ascertained by a full veterinary clinical examination together with input from the owner.

## Personality and breed differences

Most studies consist of descriptive aspects of a cat's behaviours towards people and towards novelty, as these are the measures most often used to describe a cat's personality. Factors influencing the response of kittens to humans and to novelty include early social

| Behaviour | Good welfare | Poor welfare |
|---|---|---|
| Maintenance behaviours [a] | Normal levels | Inhibited or absent |
| Activity | Normal levels | Reduced |
| Exploration and investigation of surroundings | Normal levels | Absent or reduced |
| Social interactions with other cats in household | Present and positive | Absent, reduced or hostile |
| Positive interactions with humans | Initiates | Fails to initiate |
| Friendly behaviours | Displays tail-up position, rubbing, vocalization | Persistent signs of timidity, anxiety, fear or aggression |
| Play behaviour (on own, with objects, other cats or humans) | Present | Absent or inhibited |
| Other behaviours | | Hiding or attempting to hide for long periods Over-grooming and other forms of self-mutilation Excessive vocalization Excessive vigilance, feigned sleep [b], scanning behaviour |

**4.12**   Some behavioural measures of good and poor welfare in cats. [a] Maintenance behaviours: sleeping, resting, eating, drinking, elimination (urination and defecation), grooming, claw scratching. [b] Feigned sleep: cat appears to be asleep or resting (body in sleep posture, eyes closed or partly closed) but is awake and vigilant.

experience with mother and siblings, paternity, breed, coat colour, maternal care, aspects of kitten curiosity and fear, duration and quality of interaction with humans, and environmental complexity (Bernstein, 2005). While handling by humans during early development can help kittens to be less fearful and friendlier towards people, some kittens seem resistant to change in their original types. Some friendly kittens remain friendly whether handled or not, and some fearful kittens remain so despite handling. Some behaviours are stable within an individual over time and others may change.

- From observing the behaviours of a group of cats in a laboratory, a number of personality types were identified and categorized as active/aggressive, timid/nervous, and confident/easygoing (Feaver et al., 1986).
- In cats entering a shelter, Casey (2007) identified two coping styles: active and passive.
- Relatively little is known about the origins of other aspects of cat personality, such as friendliness towards other cats or playfulness, and the factors that influence them, despite many owners perceiving their pet cat as a unique individual with its own distinct personality.

Although breed societies and many popular cat books describe physical and behavioural characteristics, few studies have examined behaviour differences among breeds.

## Travel and visits to the veterinary surgery

Cats should be habituated to short trips in the car from a young age, while safely contained in a carrier (see **client handout**). Trips should be slowly increased in duration provided that the cat remains calm.

- The cat should be habituated to its carrier in its home environment, so that the carrier is not only associated with journeys to the veterinary surgery when the cat is sick.
- Treats, toys and familiar bedding should be left in the carrier, and the carrier should be left out in the home so that it is regarded as a safe and familiar area.
- Struggles while getting the cat in and out of the carrier are all too common, but should be avoided as the cat will rapidly become fearful and difficult to handle, both at home and at the veterinary surgery. Carriers with top and front openings are best, as this greatly facilitates getting the cat in and out of the carrier.
- Unless cats are well socialized to each other, each cat should be transported in its own carrier.
- The F3 pheromone fraction, such as Feliway® spray, is recommended for having a calming effect on cats during travel by making them feel more secure in their environment. The product is sprayed in the carrier about half an hour before the journey.
- Cats should not be fed immediately before travel, though cat treats can be given while the cat is in its carrier.

Attention to the cat's welfare while at the veterinary surgery will help to ensure that the visit is not an unpleasant experience (see www.fabcats.org on 'Creating a cat friendly practice'). Attention should also be paid to the cat's experience while hospitalized (see Chapter 2).

- Ideally, there should be a separate waiting area for cats, and waiting times should be short.
- Fractious cats can sometimes be examined safely while still in the lower part of the carrier, if the top can be lifted off.
- The pheromone F4 fraction (Felifriend®) may help to reduce the cat's aggression towards the vet during the consultation.
- If a cat is very frightened, it may become aggressive and dangerous to handle. It is preferable to sedate the cat effectively prior to examination rather than to continue struggling with it, as this will only make the cat even more difficult to handle the next time.

- Ideally, there should be a separate ward for the hospitalization of cats.
- A pheromone diffuser (Feliway®) should be used continuously in the cat ward.
- Cats benefit from having their own familiar bedding, but it may be difficult to keep track of the bedding during hospitalization and ensure that it is returned to the owner.
- Many cats will benefit from having a hiding box, basket or high-sided bed within their cage; being able to hide will enable the cat to cope better with stress.

A cat returning to the home environment after a period of hospitalization may elicit anxious or aggressive reactions from the resident cat, as its familiar group odour will have been replaced with strange unfamiliar odours at the veterinary surgery. In some instances, using a facecloth rubbed over the resident cat and then applied to the returning cat is sufficient to restore harmony, but in extreme cases, a 'new cat introduction' protocol, or parts of it, may have to be followed.

## Indoor *versus* outdoor housing

In Europe the majority of cats are allowed access to the outdoors; it is generally considered that this is the natural thing for cats to do. In the United States, 50–60% of pet cats are housed indoors, and many humane organizations and veterinary associations advise this. In some areas of Australia, concerns about the effects of cat predation on wildlife have led to the adoption of regulations restricting access by pet cats to the outdoors. The risks and benefits associated with confining a cat indoors or allowing it outdoors are summarized in Figure 4.13. There are a number of websites that give advice to owners on how to enrich the indoor environment for their cats.

- The main concern with an indoor environment is that, compared with the outdoors, it can be relatively impoverished, predictable and monotonous, and does not allow the cat to express many of its normal behaviours.
- It is generally assumed that indoor cats are less stimulated and less active, and that this leads to frustration, boredom, obesity and other problems.
- Certain behaviours, such as scratching items and spraying urine, may be considered normal when performed by a cat outdoors but become problematic when performed indoors.
- In urban areas where there is a high density of cats living in homes set closely together, some cats may be fearful of going outdoors because of the challenge from neighbouring cats.
- Scratching places (such as wooden posts or logs), hiding places (such as a dense plant area) and raised vantage points (such as a platform fixed to a tree or fence) in the garden will help the cat feel more secure in its outdoor territory.

| Cat confined indoors |
| --- |
| **Risks** |
| Feline lower urinary tract disease (e.g. feline idiopathic cystitis) <br> Odontoclastic resorptive lesions <br> Hyperthyroidism (may occur also in outdoor cats) <br> Obesity and associated conditions (e.g. diabetes) <br> Household hazards <br> Undesirable behaviours (e.g. scratching) and behavioural problems (e.g. elimination out of litterbox) <br> Boredom and inactivity |
| **Benefits** |
| Protection from some infectious diseases <br> Protection from road traffic accidents <br> Protection from theft or going astray <br> Protection from injury by other animals <br> Protection from extremes of weather <br> More opportunities to interact with owner <br> May live longer |
| **Cat allowed outdoors** |
| **Risks** |
| Infectious diseases (viral, parasitic, etc.) <br> Road traffic accidents <br> Other accidents (e.g. falling from tree) <br> Fights with other cats <br> Attacks by dogs and other animals <br> Poisoning <br> Theft or straying |
| **Benefits** |
| Access to stimulating and changing environment <br> Opportunities for social contact <br> Opportunities for predation <br> Opportunities to perform behaviours that are undesirable if performed indoors (e.g. scratching) <br> Opportunities for exercise (e.g. climbing) |

**4.13** Risks and benefits associated with confining a cat indoors or allowing it outdoors. (Data from Buffington (2002) and Rochlitz (2005).)

Road accidents are a major threat to cats allowed outdoors. They are more common in younger cats, and in males (whether neutered or not). Keeping cats indoors when it is dark or the light is failing (dawn, dusk and at night) and using reflective collars may help to reduce incidence. Controlled and safe access to the outdoors can be achieved using purpose-built outdoor enclosures or specialist fencing, or by training the cat to accept being taken out on a harness and lead.

## Conclusion

A sound understanding of normal behaviour is a prerequisite for ensuring good behavioural health and welfare in cats. Based on this sound knowledge, inventive and effective ways of enriching a cat's environment can be devised so as to minimize stress, promote good behavioural health and welfare and strengthen the relationship between owners and their cats.

## References and further reading

American Association of Feline Practitioners (2004) *Feline Behaviour Guidelines* (see www.aafponline.org/index.htm)

Bernstein P (2005) The human–cat relationship. In: *The Welfare of Cats*, ed. I Rochlitz, pp. 47–9. Springer, Dordrecht, Netherlands

Bowen J and Heath S (2005) *Behaviour Problems in Small Animals: Practical Advice for the Veterinary Team.* Elsevier Saunders, Edinburgh

Bradshaw JWS and Cameron-Beaumont C (2000) The signaling repertoire of the domestic cat and its undomesticated relatives. In: *The Domestic Cat: the Biology of its Behaviour, 2nd edn*, ed. D Turner and P Bateson, pp. 68–93. Cambridge University Press, Cambridge

Buffington CAT (2002) External and internal influences on disease risk in cats. *Journal of the American Veterinary Medical Association* **220**, 994–1002

Casey R (2007) Do I look like I'm bothered! Recognition of stress in cats. In: *Scientific Proceedings of the ESFM Feline Congress 2007*, pp. 95–97. European Society of Feline Medicine, Tisbury, Wiltshire

Crowell-Davis SL (2005) Cat behaviour: social organization, communication and development. In: *The Welfare of Cats*, ed. I Rochlitz, pp. 1–22. Springer, Dordrecht, Netherlands

Feaver J, Mendl M and Bateson P (1986) A method for rating the individual distinctiveness of domestic cats. *Animal Behaviour* **34**, 1016–1025

Fitzgerald BM and Turner DC (2000) Hunting behaviour of domestic cats and their impact on prey populations In: *The Domestic Cat: the Biology of its Behaviour, 2nd edn*, ed. D Turner and P Bateson, pp. 152–175. Cambridge University Press, Cambridge

Heath S (2005) Behaviour problems and welfare. In: *The Welfare of Cats*, ed. I Rochlitz, pp. 91–118. Springer, Dordrecht, Netherlands

Horwitz DF and Neilson JC (2007) *Blackwell's Five Minute Veterinary Consult: Canine and Feline Behavior.* Blackwell Publishing, Ames, Iowa

Hunthausen W and Seksel K (2002) Preventive behavioural medicine. In: *BSAVA Manual of Canine and Feline Behavioural Medicine*, ed. D Horwitz *et al.*, pp. 49–60. BSAVA Publications, Gloucester

McCune S (1995) The impact of paternity and early socialization on the development of cats' behaviour to people and novel objects. *Applied Animal Behaviour Science* **45**, 109–124

Macdonald DW, Yamaguchi N and Kerby G (2000) Group-living in the domestic cat: its sociobiology and epidemiology. In: *The Domestic Cat: the Biology of its Behaviour, 2nd edn*, ed. D Turner and P Bateson, pp. 95–118. Cambridge University Press, Cambridge

Rochlitz I (2005) Housing and Welfare. In: *The Welfare of Cats*, ed. I Rochlitz, pp. 177–203. Springer, Dordrecht, Netherlands

UK Cat Behaviour Working Group (1995) *An Ethogram for Behavioural Studies of the Domestic Cat (Felis silvestris catus L.).* UFAW Animal Welfare Research Report No 8. Universities Federation for Animal Welfare, Wheathampstead

Wooding B and Mills DS (2007) Drinking water preferences in the cat. *Proceedings, 6th International Veterinary Behaviour Meeting and European College of Veterinary Behavioural Medicine – Companion Animals and European Society of Veterinary Clinical Ethology*, p. 120.

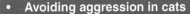

**Client handouts (bsavalibrary.com/behaviour_leaflets)**

- Avoiding aggression in cats
- Avoiding house soiling by cats
- Avoiding urine marking by cats
- Environmental enrichment for cats in animal shelters
- Feline behaviour questionnaire
- Handling exercises for an aggressive cat
- Handling exercises for puppies and kittens
- Introducing a new cat into the household
- Litterbox training

- Playing with your kitten
- Request for information on problem behaviours
- Taking your cat in the car
- Treating a fear of car journeys using desensitization and counter-conditioning
- Treating a fear of the veterinary clinic using desensitization and counter-conditioning
- What your cat needs
- What your cat needs: multi-cat households

# Training and learning protocols

## Daniel S. Mills

## Introduction

Although learning, training and behaviour modification are often thought of as the foundation of veterinary behavioural medicine, it is important to recognize that the practice of veterinary behavioural medicine begins with the recognition and adoption of good general veterinary procedures, such as:

- Good clinical skills to evaluate to what extent the problem may be affected by ill health (see Chapter 1). The importance of this role should not be underestimated as only the veterinary surgeon has the qualification to make a medical diagnosis
- Good behavioural management of the patient, to avoid problems developing as a result of interaction with the clinic. In much the same way that an owner can expect that their pet will not pick up an infection from the clinic or slip and damage itself somehow, they should also be able to expect that their pet will not develop some behavioural problem as a result of its visit to the clinic (see Chapter 2)
- Good knowledge of the species and, if relevant, breed of the patient and its husbandry requirements for good physical and psychological health, in order to undertake an assessment of the care of the animal in its home environment (see Chapters 3 and 4).

Only with these foundations in place do the more specific knowledge and skills associated with behaviour modification become relevant in order to aid the direct management of the behaviour that has become problematic for an animal's owner.

Although every interaction with a conscious patient represents a learning experience for that animal, this chapter will focus on developing an understanding of learning as it applies to the development of training protocols. While it is not reasonable to expect the general veterinary surgeon in practice to be an expert trainer, it is reasonable to expect them to have a working knowledge of the subject, if only so that they can evaluate the advice being given by others concerning the husbandry of a client's animals and offer informed advice on how to find a good trainer (Brammeier *et al.*, 2006) perhaps by way of a suitable **client handout.**

## Learning and training: starting from the basics

'Learning' is about how an animal's potential for a behaviour changes with experience; by contrast, 'training' describes the techniques used to ensure that learning comes about in a predictable way in response to human intervention. Thus learning is about the laws governing how the effects of the environment can change behaviour; training is about how this can be brought about in practice. This involves not only the application of learning theory, but also an understanding of interspecific communication (i.e. how to communicate what you want to the animal you want to change). There is an enormous literature on learning theory and so this chapter will inevitably be a précis of the most important elements that the general practitioner needs to and should know. Further information is provided in the reading list at the end of the chapter.

Relevant to behaviour modification there are three important learning processes. The first two (operant and classical conditioning) are forms of associative learning and the last (habituation and its reverse, sensitization) is an example of non-associative learning.

### Associative learning

#### Operant conditioning

Operant conditioning, also known as **trial-and-error learning** or **instrumental conditioning**, is learning as a result of one's actions. Operant conditioning is a form of associative learning because the animal learns to associate its behaviour with a particular outcome. In the long run, behaviours that are rewarded (reinforced) are more likely to recur and those that are punished are less likely to recur in similar situations.

*Example 1:* **A cat learns that when it miaows its owner feeds it and so it becomes a more vocal cat around the owner.**

Note that the definitions of reinforcement and punishment are both dependent on their long-term effects and not on their immediate effects.

*Example 2:* **A dog that whines and whose owner tells it to 'shut up' may go quiet in the short term because the action of the owner may have** been rewarding or punishing. It would be rewarding if the animal were attention-seeking, because the action of the owner gave it what it wanted – some acknowledgement; alternatively, the animal may have been punished (as the owner thought) and so was put off doing the behaviour. Which of these two explanations is correct can only be determined by looking at the situation over a longer time frame. The reality in this situation, more often than not, is that the behaviour is actually inadvertently rewarded by this sort of action by the owner, and the dog becomes more likely to repeat the behaviour the next time it is ignored for a prolonged period of time.

### Classical conditioning

Classical conditioning, also known as **Pavlovian learning** or **respondent conditioning**, is learning that one event predicts another that causes an instinctive response.

*Example 3:* A dog's new headcollar means nothing to it initially, but the dog does enjoy going for a walk. If the owner makes sure that the dog wears the headcollar whenever it is taken out for a walk, it soon learns that the headcollar predicts going for a walk and so starts to get excited when it sees the owner get the headcollar out. This is a form of associative learning because the animal learns to associate one event with another (the headcollar with the walk), so both now trigger a similar response (excitement).

Classical conditioning can be used to create conditioned rewards or conditioned punishments by pairing them with a reward or punishment. The conditioned stimulus then becomes a signal that certain events will follow and so is sometimes referred to as a **bridging stimulus**.

*Example 4:* The sound of a click may be followed by a treat. Eventually the sound of the click comes to predict the treat and so it can be used in place of the treat some of the time (especially when it would be difficult to deliver food) as a *conditioned reinforcer* (conditioned reward) or simply to predict the later arrival of a treat. However, if primary reinforcement is not maintained for very long, it will soon lose efficacy as a secondary reinforcer.

*Example 5:* A sound (e.g. a disapproving sound, the sound of a kazoo or some deep tone that has a naturally more inhibitory effect) is followed by a form of punishment such as the removal of food, or cessation of social contact and associated activities ('time out'). This sound comes to predict such punishment and can be used in its place as a *conditioned punisher.*

Note that the difference between the two forms of associative learning (operant and classical) is that in the first it is a *behaviour* that is associated with an event (its outcome), and in the second it is two *stimuli* that are associated, one of which already produces the behaviour. In reality, a given training exercise may employ both types of learning, e.g. when a classically conditioned reinforcer (such as the clicker) is used to reinforce appropriate operant behaviour (such as the response to an obedience command).

### Non-associative learning

#### Habituation
Habituation is learning *not* to respond to a stimulus that triggers an instinctive response.

*Example 6:* It is natural for a dog to bark when it is first startled by a sudden noise, such as a bang on the door, but if this noise is not associated with anything significant the dog will learn to ignore it.

Since the animal is simply learning not to respond, no association is being made and so this process is sometimes referred to as a form of non-associative learning.

#### Sensitization
This is a fourth form of learning which is basically the reverse of habituation, i.e. the animal becomes *more* reactive each time a harmless stimulus is presented. It is not used therapeutically in behaviour modification plans, but it is important to be aware of this process as it can give rise to problematic responses, such as hyperexcitability and fear responses. There are several features of a stimulus that increase the chance that an animal will become sensitized rather than habituated, including the form of the stimulus and its intensity, but another important factor concerns the time between repeat presentations. If the animal is still aroused physiologically when a harmless stimulus is re-presented, or already negatively aroused when it is first presented, then the animal may be more likely to become sensitized. It is important to note in this regard that physiological de-arousal often takes longer than behavioural de-arousal and so the animal may look calm from the outside even when it is still at risk. Sensitization is thought to explain how some firework and thunderstorm fears are established, because the sounds, while possibly harmless in themselves, occur at irregular intervals when the animal is still aroused.

### Contingency *versus* contiguity
These are two related but importantly distinct concepts.

- **Contingency** describes the way two events co-vary, or the extent to which one event predicts another.
- **Contiguity** describes the closeness of two events in either time (temporal contiguity) or space (spatial contiguity).

Training is most effective when both contingency and contiguity are high. Historically most training texts place an emphasis on the importance of contiguity, i.e. the importance of delivering rewards in close association with a behaviour in order to reinforce it (operant conditioning), or the importance of initially pairing a click sound with the rapid delivery of a food reward to develop the clicker as a means of providing conditioned reinforcement (clicker training). However, when the two are in conflict, contingency tends to be more important than contiguity. A common example concerns the cueing of treat delivery. Many owners give a treat and say 'good boy' or 'good girl' to their pet. The timing of the two events (treat and speech) is critical to what the animal will learn.

- If the owner speaks first and then gives the treat, both the contingency and contiguity are high for the words predicting the treat and so the animal learns that the words indicate that something good is coming (i.e. the words become a form of praise).
- If the owner speaks at the same time as or after giving the treat, the contingency for the words predicting the treat is low (the treat has already arrived and so the words at best predict nothing and at worst predict no more treat), but the contiguity remains high. In this case, at best the words are meaningless and at worst the words now come to predict no more treat and so become a conditioned punisher – the exact opposite of what the owner thinks they are communicating. It is attention to the relationship between events (especially those that predict reward and punishment) that helps to explain the failure of training and also the development of anxiety and confusion in pets.

## Latent inhibition

Latent inhibition describes how the initial pairing of two events may result in the formation of an association, which means that when a third event is introduced into the relationship with one of these factors, its association is not learned as efficiently as might have been predicted if it had not been previously associated with something else. In other words, the learned prior association between two events interferes with learning about a third event that is introduced concurrently with one or both of the first two.

An understanding of the application of latent inhibition is therefore quite important in behaviour therapy. By training responses with rewards away from the problem situation, their association can be maintained in the presence of aversives, when the animal may otherwise be prone to seeing them as predictors of this unpleasant situation. Thus, latent inhibition helps to explain a number of phenomena. For example:

- If a car ride usually predicts a trip to the park, an occasional trip to the veterinary clinic will not make car rides aversive; conversely, if the car ride always predicts a visit to the veterinary clinic, one trip to the park may not be as joyful until the animal is out of the car

- If a stimulus is initially conditioned in association with a reward, then when it is subsequently encountered in a more aversive context an avoidance reaction is not established. This is one of the principles underpinning socialization and acceptance of novelty in puppies and kittens (see Chapters 6 and 7)
- If a dog is trained to perform a specific response, such as lying down on a particular mat, should this mat then be presented to the dog in a situation that it finds unpleasant (e.g. just before its owner is about to leave, in the case of an animal with a separation-related problem) the dog does not start to avoid the mat, nor respond to it as a predictor of the owner's imminent departure
- If a cat is trained with treats to accept being handled as if being given a pill, then if it is uncomfortable for the cat to be dosed at a later date (perhaps because it is in some pain) it does not learn to resent handling at other times. This also helps to explain why some animals are very forgiving of owners who can at times treat them very harshly.

## A closer look at reinforcement and punishment

It is important to appreciate that reinforcement and punishment are defined by their effect, not by the intent of anyone who may be delivering them. If the recipient of either does not perceive them the same as the deliverer, it does not matter what the person delivering them meant them to mean.

Both reinforcement and punishment may be delivered by applying something or taking something away from the animal. This element of the process is described as being positive when something is added and negative when something is taken away. It has nothing to do with whether the stimulus is pleasant or unpleasant.

- **Positive reinforcement** is achieved by *adding something* to *increase* the likelihood of the desired behaviour recurring in similar circumstances. This will inevitably be something pleasant, such as a treat.
- **Negative reinforcement** is achieved by *taking something away* to *increase* the likelihood of the desired behaviour recurring in similar circumstances. This will inevitably be something unpleasant, such as pressure from a headcollar when the dog turns its head in the desired direction.
- **Positive punishment** is achieved by *adding something* to *decrease* the likelihood of undesired behaviour recurring in similar circumstances. This will inevitably be something unpleasant, such as a loud noise that scares the animal.
- **Negative punishment** is achieved by *taking something away* to *decrease* the likelihood of the undesired behaviour recurring in similar circumstances. This will inevitably be something pleasant, such as stopping a game or no longer giving treats.

Thus anything that an animal either desires or wishes to avoid can be used to provide either reinforcement to encourage a response or punishment to weaken its motivation, depending on context.

## Evaluation of commodities

Potential sources of positive reinforcement and negative punishment to be used in training, and which can be scored and ranked by owners, include:

- Desirable foodstuffs
- Enjoyable activities
- Favourite toys
- Preferred companions
- Favourite places to be or things to have.

From a functional point of view, what is important is how these things are used. However, from an ethical perspective it may be that certain forms are more or less acceptable; see Barry (2008) for a useful review of the ethics of dog training, which can also be used as a basis for work with other species.

For the treatment element of a behaviour consultation, it is often useful to check how highly the patient values different commodities. This not only allows the scaling of rewards according to the task and response, but also the checklist can serve at least two other important functions:

- It allows different reinforcers to be used strategically within a behaviour modification plan, i.e. different rewards can be used to reward different behaviours being trained at the same time. This results in a better rate of learning (**differential outcome effect**). The instruction to the owners should ask them to rank the reinforcement used and generally to use the most potent reinforcement for their pet for the most difficult learning tasks
- It provides a safeguard against accidental punishment during training. When rewards are used in training, an expectancy develops in the subject about the consequences of its action. If this expectancy is not met the consequence may actually be detrimental, since, from the animal's perspective, it has been punished (a form of relative negative punishment). For example, for a dog that loves pieces of hot dog and quite likes cheese, if its owner starts by using only hot dog in the early stages (perhaps because they want to motivate the dog) but later in the training tries to switch to something like cheese, there is a real danger that the dog's performance will slip back at least temporarily and this may seriously undermine the confidence of the trainer. This phenomenon is also important when considering the training history of an animal believed by the owner to be an under-achiever or 'stupid'.

It is also important to recognize that the value of a reinforcer is not fixed but can be manipulated and can vary with the state of the animal. For example, if an owner comments that their pet is not really motivated by anything, placing the animal on a fixed meal-time feeding schedule (and possibly reducing its allowance

if it is safe to do so) and eliminating certain luxuries that may currently be freely available will often increase their value and utility within a few days. Training should then be scheduled for shortly before feeding time, when appetite is likely to be at its greatest. Trying to use food after a meal is likely to be less effective, but if the animal is too hungry this can also result in problems. If the stimulus being used is too arousing, the animal may have difficulty focusing on the task for which the owner is trying to train it.

## Absence of reward

Another important implication of the concept of rewards and punishment being relative terms and linked partly to expectancy is that *there is no such thing as reward-only training*. Although some trainers claim to use only positive reinforcement, what they usually mean is that they do not use physical punishment. This claim also indicates that perhaps they do not fully understand the processes of reinforcement and punishment and so, rather than being a sign of a good trainer, may in fact be a sign of a more limited trainer. It is important to be aware that *the absence of an expected reward is a form of punishment*, otherwise it is quite easy to be unaware of when inappropriate punishment may be being applied (by the trainer or inadvertently by the owner) and how this might be affecting the animal's performance.

### Extinction

The consistent omission of a reward ultimately leads to the loss of the reinforced association, a process referred to as extinction.

Extinction of a learned response does not result in a simple decline in the response. The response often intensifies before it starts to disappear and this is believed to be a sign of frustration. This 'worsening before it gets better' (or **extinction burst**, as it is known) limits the value of this method clinically because:

- Most owners will not tolerate a worsening of the problem, even if this is explained in advance
- The frustration may result in undesirable emotional changes leading to behaviours such as aggression.

The magnitude of the extinction burst is dependent on the temperament of the individual and the previous level of reinforcement, being more intense when rewards have been given on an occasional basis for the behaviour (as happens with most learned problems, such as attention seeking) rather than every time. Such an intermittent schedule also makes extinction a much more drawn out process as the animal is used to not being rewarded some of the time, making it initially difficult for the animal to ascertain that reinforcement has stopped (further details relating to schedules of reinforcement are given later in the chapter). Nonetheless this technique can be used clinically – for example, with certain forms of attention-seeking behaviour and excitability to inappropriate stimuli – but it is not without risk and each case needs to be assessed on its merits, with appropriate precautions in place. In some cases it is worth getting the owner to reward the problem behaviour more frequently before the extinction programme begins, in order to make the elimination run more smoothly (see previous comment relating to the effect of the preceding level of reinforcement). In practice it also helps if the procedure is combined with rewarding a behaviour that is incompatible with the problem behaviour (see later section on Counter-conditioning). It is also worth noting a few other precautions concerning the use of extinction.

- If reinforcement is inadvertently given during the extinction burst, the more intense form of the response may become learned – the exact opposite of what is usually desired.
- Some behaviours, such as play, are self-reinforcing and so it is not possible to remove the reward and still allow the behaviour.
- It is essential to identify all sources of reinforcement for the pet since some may not be apparent to the owner, such as eye contact even without speaking to the pet.

Apparent failure of an extinction programme usually means that the behaviour is self-reinforcing or that reinforcement has been provided from another source, or the programme has been given insufficient time to take effect.

### Inadvertent reinforcement

Recognition that reinforcement and punishment go together like two sides of a coin does not mean that an emphasis on the use of reinforcement is not a useful thing, nor that the two processes of punishment and reinforcement are equal. Indeed they are not. Given that when we train an animal we want it to do something specific, only the use of rewards specifically guide the animal to the desired goal; punishment simply says what was done was wrong and gives no information about how to get it right next time. (However, information that the right response has not been provided can be useful and will be explained later in the chapter.)

While both negative reinforcement and punishment use aversive stimuli, there are important differences between them (Figure 5.1).

It is important to recognize these differences, as it is possible otherwise to apply inappropriate reinforcement inadvertently.

*Example 7:* **Many owners try (quite understandably) to comfort their pet when it is distressed. By doing this they may be relieving the distress but may actually negatively reinforce certain behaviours that they find undesirable. In the case of fears this can give rise to a condition known as a *pseudo-phobia*, where the animal is not actually scared but has learned to appear as such in order to gain attention. It is for this reason that the best advice is often to ignore the behaviour if it is safe to do so. In other situations, the message that the animal receives is that the behaviour it is engaging in at the time is appropriate, thus increasing the behaviour rather than decreasing it.**

| Stimulus property | Punishment | Negative reinforcement |
|---|---|---|
| Application and removal of the stimulus | Aversive stimulus is applied to stop ongoing behaviour and inhibit its recurrence in similar circumstances; it is removed when the undesired behaviour has stopped rather than when a specific behavioural goal expressed | Aversive stimulus is removed when the desired behaviour is achieved in order to increase the likelihood of the desired behaviour in similar circumstances; any inhibition of ongoing behaviour that occurs when the stimulus is applied is coincidental |
| Intensity of the stimulus | Aversive tends to be quite intense, in order to have long-term effects on behaviour (i.e. prevent recurrence) | Aversive is usually quite mild, since its aim is to make things unpleasant but still allow the animal to operate as it makes other behaviour choices that will lead to its termination |
| Length of stimulus application | Aversive tends to be applied briefly, though may be applied serially; prolonged application is likely to evoke a serious compromise of welfare and significant emotional disturbance given the intensity of the stimulus | Aversive may be applied for prolonged period initially, but the animal quickly learns to avoid this by performing the desired behaviour as it anticipates what will result in its removal |
| Successful outcome | Successful use depends on application being contingent upon problem behaviour | Successful use depends upon termination being contingent upon desired behaviour |

**5.1** Differences between punishment and negative reinforcement.

Alternatively, an owner may think that they are applying punishment when they are not.

*Example 8:* **It is not uncommon for owners to respond inappropriately towards their dog when it is on the lead and shows awareness of someone close by. The increased arousal may be misunderstood as an intention to be aggressive (when it may be just as likely to be an invitation for play). As a result the owner may jerk on the lead, scold the dog and perhaps pull it closer and so the dog decides that it does not wish the unknown individual to approach (in the dog's mind the unknown individual is associated with the application of an unpleasant stimulus by the owner). The dog may then begin to growl in an attempt to eliminate the predictor of this aversive stimulus. Unfortunately, this appears to confirm the erroneous prediction of the owner that the dog was going to be aggressive because of the approaching individual, rather than because of their own action, and they conclude that they were right to jerk the lead and may continue to do so until the approaching individual has passed. Contrary to the owners' belief, they have not** been punishing the dog for its behaviour, but rather building a classically conditioned response (approaching individual predicts uncomfortable jerk on the lead, which leads to irritability). The individual passes in their own time and the behaviour of both the owner and the dog ceases. This sets up a spiral of attempted but ineffective 'punishment' that only makes the problem worse. This problem can often be identified by the mixed messages sent by the dog (mixing play bows with aggressive threats, together with the complete cessation of response once the stimulus has passed) when presented with new individuals in a new area. Treatment involves addressing the misguided behaviour of the owner as well as reconditioning the dog to enjoy the approach of others.

## The problem with 'gentle punishment'

It is not uncommon for mild aversives to be applied in the mistaken belief that they are a form of gentle punishment, but the reality is that punishment has to be of an appropriate intensity to be effective and what is appropriate will depend on the individual being punished. Such assessments need to be made with skill and attention to detail, and are not without their own risks. The use of so-called gentle punishment is perfectly understandable for an individual who does not want to harm their pet, but unfortunately the use of aversive stimuli in this manner can have several detrimental effects and can result in greater harm in the long term.

- It is not effective (if it were, the owner would not be seeking help for the problem). It may disrupt the behaviour in the short term (in much the same way as any novel stimulus can interrupt ongoing behaviour), but it does not result in a long-term change in behaviour or stop the initiation of the behavioural sequence.
- The lack of efficacy means that the owner is more likely to have to repeat the 'gentle punishment' on a frequent basis, giving the animal conflicting information about their relationship and what they should be doing at the time and potentially producing emotional disturbance.
- The initial disruption of the problem behaviour misleads the owner into thinking that their actions have been successful and actually negatively reinforces their own behaviour, making them more likely to use this long-term ineffective strategy in future, including in other contexts.
- Frequent exposure to initially 'gentle punishment' can result in habituation to this experience, resulting potentially in a response by the owner of gradually increasing severity without significant effect (especially in light of the negative reinforcement of the owner's behaviour). Ultimately very severe punishments may be applied without them being effective or the owner necessarily being aware of how aversive their behaviour has become.

- Attempts at punishment may induce a fear or anxiety response when previously there was none. As mentioned earlier, this is particularly common when owners are concerned at what their pet might do when out on the lead. The result is a confused dog that is being trained to display aggression in social contexts.
- In the case of behaviours that feature anxiety and fear, the attempted application of punishment will intensify the fear and so most likely exacerbate the problem. This is not uncommon in dogs displaying what owners believe are irrational fears, or dogs that are 'supersubmissive' (i.e. roll over and possibly urinate when an individual approaches even in a non-threatening manner; see Chapter 10).
- The frequent use of mild aversives can result in irritability and increase the probability of a defensive aggressive response, with potentially catastrophic consequences.
- Interaction with the owner (even if they are trying to scold the animal) may inadvertently provide reinforcement for the problem if the behaviour is socially motivated, for example in the case of attention-seeking behaviours. Thus this form of attempted punishment actually makes the problem worse.
- When ineffective attempts at punishment are made, the animal is focusing on how to avoid the aversive stimulus. In some cases it may be that freezing, ignoring the owner, running away or some sort of display of aggression will achieve an end to the encounter. As a result these responses are conditioned by negative reinforcement leading to, at best, an animal that appears stubborn and, at worst, an individual that is a danger to itself and others.

The attempted application of punishment is not without potential risk to both the handler and the animal, and its appropriate use is technically quite difficult. Its misuse is a serious welfare concern, much more likely to create further behavioural or emotional problems, and disrupts the animal–owner bond. It is for these reasons that in most situations punishment is inadvisable, and it should only be considered after careful assessment of a given case. By definition, a measure of the effect of punishment is that the behaviour decreases in the long term or stops. If punishment is applied inappropriately and the behaviour continues, the punishment should be stopped.

## Common problems with positive reinforcement

Some owners are concerned about the use of food in training. They often believe that their pet will get fat and greedy or that they are just 'bribing' the pet to behave. It is important to reassure them that this is not the case if food is used correctly. Owners should be encouraged to see the food used for training as the pet's 'salary' provided on a daily basis. *Any food used in training, including treats, should be considered part of the daily ration and not an addition to it!*

### Lures

Problems can arise if no clear distinction is made between the use of food as a 'reinforcer' and as a 'lure'. Lures are often used to encourage a behaviour in the early stages of training and may be used to reward the behaviour as it is guided towards its goal (**shaping**). They may be a useful aid to gain attention, but in dogs that are highly food motivated the use of food as a lure may actually interfere with its attention to the task. If a behaviour occurs spontaneously and with enough frequency, it is often better to reward these occurrences rather than use lures initially. An efficient training programme should, however, involve the fading of food both as a lure and in many cases as a reward too. A hand gesture can usually replace the gesture that involves food (initially the food is shown, then it is held within the hand and finally it is no longer in the hand). Clickers (see Example 4 above) can be used to provide conditioned reinforcement, with food following as the primary reinforcer on a more intermittent basis.

### Non-contingent reinforcement

If positive reinforcement is given inappropriately in training, undesirable behaviours may be reinforced (begging or pestering at the table are obvious examples of this). There are other more insidious effects of random or excessive positive reinforcement. The effect of such non-contingent reinforcement is to deprive the animal of control in its environment, i.e. it does not know which behaviours will reliably elicit a reward. This can result in generalized anxiety and perhaps unfocused behaviours that attempt to obtain rewards. So, far from being harmless, the titbit given now and again just for being 'cute' can actually lead to serious problems. Like most humans, animals are happier when they have reliable control over certain aspects of their environment and so asking them to undertake something first is actually good for them. The use of clearly identifiable cues that predict when reinforcement is available is known as **stimulus discrimination** and is a very important part of training. It allows a reliable contingency to be set up, which means training becomes more efficient, and it gives the animal more control over its environment, which improves its welfare.

### Frequency of reinforcement

Other common problems with positive reinforcement relate to the frequency of its use. The rules governing when reinforcement is given are called the **schedule of reinforcement**. If rewards are given every time, this is called **continuous reinforcement**, the alternative being an **intermittent schedule**. Continuous reinforcement is useful initially in helping the animal to understand what is required during the early stages of training, but a switch to an intermittent schedule as soon as practical should be encouraged. This transition should be gradually managed, by dropping out rewards for the worst of the acceptable responses. There are various forms of intermittent reinforcement but the most commonly used one in practice is the **variable ratio**, in which a behaviour is reinforced on average only a fraction of the occasions that it has been requested. The fraction can be expressed as a ratio; for example, if on average half of the responses are reinforced the ratio is 2:1. Other schedules include **variable duration**, which requires the behaviour to be performed for differing lengths of time before a reward is given. This can be useful in behaviours such as a 'stay' where the duration is an important component of the goal.

While it may seem intuitively better to reward every occurrence of the correct behaviour (continuous reinforcement) once the animal has learned what is expected, this is not necessarily the case.

- Such a schedule very quickly becomes predictable; and predictability, like control, is another very important factor governing animal behaviour. Something that is highly predictable does not require much attention and so is not attended to as well as something that is also rewarding but less predictable (complete unpredictability is not a good thing). Thus, in order to maintain the interest of the animal in the task, it is best to move on to a variable schedule as soon as possible.
- If an animal is on a continuous reinforcement schedule and then not rewarded, it is in effect being punished by the lack of an expected reinforcement (negative punishment). The efficiency of training is compromised.
- Animals that are maintained on a high reinforcement schedule may also fail to develop fully their potential mechanisms of coping with non-reward (or unmet expectations, which includes novelty). Due to this lack of capacity these animals are at greater risk of developing stress-related problems as a result (see Chapter 13).
- An intermittent schedule will use less food and this often means that training sessions can be more frequent, or if necessary last longer, before the animal is satiated. Thus there is greater potential for progress in a given time with an intermittent schedule.
- By using a variable schedule of intermittent reinforcement, it also is easier to improve and maintain high levels of reinforcement. By focusing the delivery of rewards on the occasions when performance is best, a process known as **differential reinforcement**, the response is shaped towards these higher-end displays (see 'The Ten Tasks of a Trainer', below, for details of which parameters can be used to define the quality of a response). Such guidance is not available with continuous reinforcement unless larger quantities are used.

While intermittent reinforcement is preferable to continuous reinforcement, it is not the case that less is necessarily more. It is important that reinforcement is provided frequently enough and with sufficient intensity (i.e. the rewards are worth working for, from the animal's perspective) to maintain the motivation for the behaviour. In the case of cats, special treats such as dried fish generally work much more effectively than part of the cat's ration; but in the case of the dog, all of its daily allowance can be used readily as a powerful tool for behaviour modification, assuming that it has not lost its appetite as a result of stress.

Intermittent reinforcement requires particular consideration in certain circumstances:

- A problem behaviour learned through intermittent reinforcement is generally harder to eliminate, especially if the animal has been slowly conditioned to accept very low rates of reinforcement
- If the intermittent schedule has an identifiable pattern (differential reinforcement), this may be detected by the animal, even if it is not recognized by the trainer, leading to particular patterns of response (see section below on Stimulus control and discriminative stimuli). Examples of problems arising from inadvertent differential reinforcement include:
  - The cat that only attacks one member of the family (the one who gave it treats to end the game when it got too rough)
  - The dog that pesters one person more than another (the former individual using food more often in an attempt to quieten it down)
  - The cat that is more vocal at night when one individual is there but causes no problem when they are not (e.g. the partner who has to travel a lot).

Generally a high schedule of reinforcement is used initially for any new behaviour that is being established, but the rate should be gradually reduced as the behaviour becomes more reliable, and where possible food should be replaced with alternatives (such as social contact or the opportunity for a preferred form of play) as the behaviour becomes established. For many behaviours there are different dimensions to the end goal (e.g. the time taken for the animal to respond initially; the time taken to complete the behaviour) and each of these elements may need to be trained separately, with a higher schedule used each time the focus shifts to a new aspect of the behaviour. However, high-level and important responses, such as an effective emergency recall, should always be rewarded.

As with many practical aspects of instruction, it is easy for the competent trainer or counsellor to over-look how these features of behaviour modification can be and frequently are misapplied in practice by the less experienced owner. The theory is relatively simple and generally well understood, but the practical application often proves more problematic. For example, many owners end up using clickers as signals for a given behaviour rather than as a reinforcer, due to a lack of clarity about their role.

## Stimulus control and discriminative stimuli

The signals or cues that indicate what is wanted behaviourally from the animal at any given time and its consequences are called **discriminative stimuli**. The behaviour is said to be under **stimulus control** if a given discriminative stimulus indicates that only when it is present is there any chance of reinforcement. Rewarding at other times will actually reduce learning by reducing the contingency between the stimulus and reinforcement. It is not surprising, then, that if several tasks need to be taught at the same time it is best if different rewards are used for the different actions (**differential outcome effect**) as well as different cues.

The most commonly recognized discriminative stimuli are verbal commands, but these are not always appropriate or used appropriately and it is important to appreciate that the cue chosen by a trainer may not necessarily be the same as the one attended to by the animal if there are other more significant or reliable predictors of the outcome. For example, in the case of a dog asked to come when called, the body language of the owner in combination with the tone of the request may be a better predictor of a reward than simply the word 'come'. An angry tone of voice while giving the command is often a good predictor of some form of punishment, perhaps reducing the likelihood that the animal will obey the command. It is therefore important to pay attention to:

- The method of communication used during training
- What different discriminative stimuli may be operating in any given context (i.e. why the animal will not perform reliably in some contexts, such as with one individual and not another)
- What may be the best discriminative stimuli for a given task.

The choice of cue will vary with context and patient but, while there is a tendency to focus on verbal signals, it is important to appreciate that dogs (and probably cats as well) are more likely to attend to and respond to visual cues, given the choice between the two (Mills, 2005). In some training programmes aimed at reducing anxiety, it may be relevant first to train the animal to relax on a specific mat (which is not used in any other context) so that the mat becomes a conditioned stimulus for emotional relaxation (**conditioned safety signal**), before desensitization begins. By not using it in other contexts for anything else, the contingency is improved.

The concept of the discriminative stimulus and stimulus control is an essential one for owners to appreciate, as it forms the basis of an animal's under-standing of what is being requested. Many owners have the mistaken belief that non-human animals understand language in a similar way to humans, but this is simply not the case. As a result of their pet not being able to pick out the clear signals that indicate the right thing to do (because the owner is talking *at* the pet and not communicating with it), the animal will often fail and this leads to mistaken beliefs that the animal is stubborn, stupid, or trying to dominate them. As a result owners may get very frustrated and angry or attempt to teach them 'who is boss', to the detri-ment of the animal's wellbeing and its relationship with its owner. The failure in communication is then perpetuated, together with the cycle of unintentional abuse that follows.

The clarity of communication of the discriminative stimulus also provides the animal with security by letting it know what it can expect at certain times and so is important in reducing the anxiety that is an undercurrent to many behavioural problems.

As with the other features of learning, discrimination can have a downside if not fully recognized. If different members of a family respond differently to a pet's behaviour, there is a good chance that the animal will learn to behave differently towards them as a result. For example, a pet may learn that an aggressive display results in retention of its food and the chance to eat in peace in the case of the children, but isolation and loss of its supper in the case of the parents. The display therefore becomes more frequent when children are around without an adult. Similar situations may arise in relation to attention-seeking behaviour, with the identity of the individual becoming the discriminative stimulus for the behaviour.

## Losing a response

There are many reasons why a previously established response may be lost, leading to a problem situation, and these are rarely if ever due to 'stubbornness', as many owners would believe. Examples include forgetting, extinction, counter-conditioning and stress-induced dishabituation.

### Forgetting
If a learned response is not occasionally rehearsed and reinforced accordingly, the animal may simply forget what it has learned. One study on the long-term follow-up of treatment of noise fears in dogs with a counter-conditioning and desensitization programme (Levine and Mills, 2008) found that after 12 months there were the beginnings of signs of relapse. At least some retraining is to be advised on an occasional basis. (Counter-conditioning and desensitization are explained in more detail in the section on specific behaviour modification techniques later in this chapter.)

### Extinction
As already noted, if a learned response is not occasionally reinforced (i.e. it is taken for granted) it will eventually disappear. This is not uncommon with obedience commands after they have initially been learned, as the owner believes that the dog 'knows what he should be doing', but forgets to give the dog an incentive.

### Counter-conditioning
In this case an alternative behaviour may be inadvertently being reinforced. For example, the owner asks their dog to sit but then lets it stand to take its reward, because they have offered it too far in front of the animal. The animal learns that 'sit' is a request to wriggle about a bit and then stand.

### Stress-induced dishabituation
Until recently this phenomenon has been largely ignored in the veterinary literature, but its importance is being increasingly recognized. When an individual is subjected to chronic stress, the acceptance of what was established through habituation (for example, during the socialization period) may no longer occur, i.e. the animal forgets that these things are not important. This phenomenon can explain the onset of a wide variety of fears later in life when there is no history of a clearly aversive event to undo the previous training. In these cases, it is essential that the background stress in the animal's environment (e.g. a change in household dynamics, such as a divorce, an individual leaving home or bereavement) is addressed and the pet is provided with consistency again, before reconditioning is attempted. These changes may not seem relevant to the owner, as they may have adapted to them, but their pet may adapt at a different rate and so a careful history, probing for such risk factors, is often essential to uncover these events.

## Building a behaviour modification protocol: the Ten Tasks of a Trainer

In order to train an animal it is necessary not only to understand how the processes described above operate in real life, but also how to set things up so that they operate as expected. In order to do this it is necessary to have a clear idea of what the *functional end goal* of the programme is, i.e. what we want to achieve in an overall general sense as opposed to what we want to 'stop'. For example, in the case of a dog that jumps up on people, it is about establishing manners rather than merely stopping it from jumping up; in the case of a dog with separation anxiety, the owner wants it to be relaxed when they go out rather than distressed; and so on for other issues. It is the functional goal of the programme that determines the number and range of specific exercises that may be necessary within a given programme.

The majority of behaviour therapy programmes consist of multiple exercises (e.g. counter-conditioning *and* desensitization; see later) and may require foundation training too, i.e. exercises that generally reduce anxiety by increasing predictable structure in the animal's life or that form the basis of the specific modification exercises (e.g. a reliable 'lie down and stay'). Each of these component exercises has its own specific physical end goal, i.e. a goal that can be assessed behaviourally, even if it is primarily focused on bringing about an emotional change.

Nonetheless, whether it is obedience training or behaviour therapy, there are ten key questions that should be answered for each exercise in order to ensure that a clear protocol is built that can be implemented and assessed efficiently. The answer to each of these questions needs to be clearly communicated to the owner so that the animal will learn (i.e. be trained) efficiently.

### Ten Questions
The ten key questions to answer in order to design an efficient training programme are summarized in Figure 5.2. Each question is considered in more detail below.

1.  **Is the animal 'fit for training'?**
    a.  Is the animal physically fit enough?
    b.  Is the animal psychologically fit?

2.  **What is the physical end goal of training and how is it defined?**
    a.  Focus the owners on what they want the pet 'to do', not on what they want to stop.
    b.  The end goal should be physically recognizable.

3.  **What is the best way to get the animal's attention?**
    a.  What gets its attention without inappropriately arousing it?

4.  **What is going to be the cue for the new behaviour?**
    a.  Define the discriminative stimulus, which has stimulus control.
    b.  Initially build the new response in a calm and quiet environment.

5.  **What is going to be used to help the animal to make the decision that is wanted?**
    a.  What is the benefit *versus* cost of doing what is being requested?
    b.  What is the cost *versus* benefit of doing something else?
    c.  The reinforcer should be:
        i.  Of an appropriate magnitude
        ii.  Relevant
        iii.  Delivered according to an agreed schedule dependent on the stage of training.

6.  **What is being done to convince the animal it is making the right choice?**
    a.  Consider possible conditioned reinforcers to help provide feedback.

7.  **Which dimension of the behaviour is most important?**
    a.  Topography.
    b.  Error/success rate.
    c.  Frequency.
    d.  Duration.
    e.  Latency.

8.  **What is the best way to build up the behaviour?**

9.  **What level of generalization is required?**
    a.  Remember to make allowances as the response shifts into a new environment.

10.  **How can I monitor the programme?**
    a.  Homemade diary or some other means.

**5.2** Ten key questions to answer in order to design an efficient training programme.

## 1. Is the animal 'fit for training'?

There are two elements to answer here, and the answers may affect the prognosis for the end goal, or even the choice of specific end goal:

a) Is the animal physically fit enough?
b) Is the animal psychologically fit?

*(a) Physical fitness:* If an animal is in any pain or has some physical limitation such as poor hearing or eyesight, its performance will be compromised until these issues are either addressed (e.g. through the use of analgesics) or accommodated (e.g. designing a programme based on visual and tactile communication for a dog that is deaf; see Eaton, 1997 for a good resource on training the deaf dog). In the author's opinion the effect of chronic and subacute musculoskeletal pain, especially in relation to hip dysplasia, is grossly underrated.

*(b) Psychological fitness:* Animals that are highly stressed (e.g. temperamentally anxious or highly aroused – excitable or restless) much of the time are not good learners: it is very difficult to learn new tasks when highly emotionally aroused, and every individual has their own optimal level for performance. In this case a careful assessment needs to be made of the underlying reason for the lack of relaxation and this may need to be addressed before training begins. Common sources of psychological unfitness include:

- Inconsistent behaviour by an individual or between individuals in the home (e.g. sometimes the animal is allowed on the furniture and sometimes it is not, with no clear indication to the animal when this can be differentiated, similarly with greeting behaviour, enforcement of commands and so on)
- General disruption in the home (e.g. troublesome teenagers, marital strife, moving home, a family member leaving home)
- An imbalance between the diet and exercise regime. Many dogs and cats do not receive either an adequate volume of exercise (i.e. duration of imposed exercise) or exercise of an appropriate nature (e.g. off-lead exercise in the dog, or intensive play in the cat), given their caloric intake. This can result in not only obesity but also frustration, due to the lack of opportunity to exercise (exercise has a calming effect in many species). In the case of cats it is worth noting that exercise typically should consist of multiple small bouts, usually focused on play (2 minutes or less perhaps), while in dogs fewer longer bouts are preferable. Many mature animals do not exercise themselves for the sake of exercise, though they may seek out activities that are enjoyable
- Frustration as a result of a lack of stimulation. Many animals left on their own or subjected to quite strict management regimes require some additional stimulation. It is preferable to identify specific frustrations (e.g. lack of an opportunity to chew in a dog on a high-concentrate diet and no chew toys) and address these, rather than simply assume the animal is 'bored' and think that any attempted enrichment will be adequate.

Stress can arise for many other reasons when the needs of the animal are not met, and a deeper review of its husbandry (see Chapters 3 and 4) may be required. In some cases psychoactive medication or pheromone therapy may be required, to reduce the problem if chronic or get the animal into a suitable frame of mind for training, but this should not be done without consideration of the necessary management changes possible and necessary first. Reducing anxiety medically should enhance learning, but it must be remembered that some anxiolytics (e.g. benzodiazepines) may inhibit memory. It has been suggested that selegiline may increase sensitivity to reward and so be useful in certain clinical contexts as an aid to training (Mills and Ledger, 2001).

Older animals in particular need careful assessment and may take longer to train even if otherwise healthy.

### 2. What is the physical end goal of training and how is it defined?

Owners will usually focus on what they do not want the animal to do, but they need to understand that the focus should not be on stopping the problem but rather on establishing acceptable behaviour, since training and behaviour modification are about establishing new responses, i.e. looking forward, not trying to undo the past. This also gets the owner into a more positive mindset.

The physical end goal is exactly what the animal must do to do the right thing. It is important to have a clear and precise idea of what you want to achieve, so you have a goal to work towards. This goal should be a *behaviour* and not a vague state, e.g. 'We would like the dog to sit when greeting people' is clearer than 'We want him to be OK when people approach'. It may be necessary to qualify the physical goal further, to ensure a distinction is made between a relaxed response and one associated with a high level of emotional arousal.

### 3. What is the best way to get the animal's attention?

Any animal can be distracted and so it is important to know what will get its attention. Many animals do not 'know' their name as such, especially if it has been used in a variety of ways by the owner (e.g. it is not uncommon for owners to use the animal's name in a disapproving tone of voice as a reprimand for problem behaviour).

When managing an established problem it is often useful to employ some form of novelty (e.g. a new sound) to get the animal's attention, but getting the intensity right for the given patient is key. What may be necessary for one may be overwhelming for another. It also needs to be appropriate to the training task and not be used in a way that results ultimately in habituation and being ignored.

### 4. What is going to be the cue for the new behaviour?

This is not the same as the answer to the last question. The cue should be delivered once the animal is in a receptive state, so it is not wise to use a request (such as 'sit') as the attention-getting device. If nothing else, the animal may have missed the first part (or all) of the request by the time it has focused its attention.

In most cases the animal is going to need a *discriminative stimulus*, i.e. a clear signal to indicate when it should do the desired behaviour. It is important that this is presented in a way that does not adversely affect the desired stimulus control; for example, if a command is issued several times, the animal learns not to respond to the first occasion.

- Dogs, and probably cats as well, are much more sensitive to visual rather than verbal cues.
- The signal need not necessarily come from the owner. For example, the cue could be a sit command, but it would be better if it were the approach of people that triggered the response.
- It is best to avoid commands used previously, as these have a lot of history (i.e. are not often

reliable predictors of the current goal; if they were, the problem would not exist) and it is easiest to build an association between novel events as this sets up a new relationship between events (contingency).

- It is best to avoid building a new response initially in an environment where an animal may be distracted (such as that in which the problem behaviour occurs), though this will often need to be addressed eventually (see Question 9) and so it is important to have a method of keeping the animal focused on the task that will not undermine the exercise later.

### 5. What is going to be used to help the animal to make the decision that is wanted?

At any given time an animal may choose to do any one of a whole range of possible actions. The skill of training is to convince the animal to do what is desired initially and for this experience to convince it to do the same in future. The animal always has a choice.

There are two components to the decision-making process for an animal, assuming the decision time has been clearly cued (see questions above):

a) What is the benefit–cost of doing what is being requested?
b) What is the cost–benefit of doing something else?

Thus if a cued behaviour has little benefit (e.g. no additional reward) or a high cost (e.g. the pain involved in sitting when suffering from hip dysplasia), it may easily lose out to the alternative. The aim is to make the requested behaviour as desirable as possible; and only then, and if necessary, should the alternative be made less desirable to help the animal make the desired choice.

From this it should also be apparent why it is more efficient (quite apart from being more conducive to the animal's welfare) to focus on *reinforcing* the right behaviour, since it is only reinforcement that guides the animal precisely to the goal. Punishment, at best, simply blocks one of many undesirable alternatives, leaving it open for the animal to fail in a different way the next time.

Not only may the reinforcer need to be of an appropriate magnitude, but also attention needs to be paid to its relevance and the schedule of reinforcement being used, both of which can affect the motivation (see earlier section).

- A continuous schedule is often used initially but rapidly moved to an intermittent one based on differential performance, to allow shaping.
- It is preferable where possible to use ethologically relevant rewards for the behaviour, e.g. social reinforcers (such as playing with the owner) for social behaviours (such as coming when called), since it engages compatible behaviour systems and so makes learning easier.

Latent inhibition may be used to help the animal to perform reliably in an aversive environment, by initially training it do what is wanted with rewards away from the problem situation (see also Question 9 on generalization of the response).

**6. What is being done to convince the animal it is making the right choice?**
Once the animal has made a decision, it should not be assumed that the goal will be achieved – especially if the goal involves some considerable effort. It may start off on the right track but give up. It is useful to provide the animal with feedback on its decision until the time the goal has been achieved. This part of the process is often overlooked.

- Conditioned reinforcers, such as 'good boy' if properly trained (see section on Contingency and contiguity above), can be very useful at this point, but so can visual reinforcers such as the mat that is brought out at feeding time (i.e. that predicts a large reward).
- The conditioned reinforcer can also be used to give feedback when things go wrong, since if it is reliably present when a reward is going to be delivered, its absence or withdrawal can be used to indicate no reward, i.e. that a wrong decision has been made. One method that exploits this element is known as 'syn-alia training' (developed by Kayce Cover), in which a repetitive sound such as an 'X' sound is used to communicate with the animal during its performance of an operant response (i.e. a behaviour that will be rewarded or punished). The 'X' is initially paired with a reward (in much the same way as a clicker), but during training the intensity of the sound can be varied to provide more quantitative feedback (a more excited and louder sound indicating that the animal is getting closer to the end goal). If the animal makes a wrong decision the sound is stopped and only started again when the animal's response starts to move towards the goal again.

However, it is important when using feedback during the response to make sure this does not distract the animal from its task.

**7. Which dimension of the behaviour is most important?**
Learned behaviour has a number of quantifiable dimensions. It is important to focus on them individually and in order, with the most important one addressed first. Trying to do too much often results in a lack of focus and attention to detail, with failure as a consequence. There are five dimensions to a response, and not all may be relevant to a given situation but they are all described below.

**Topography:** This is the general form of the response. A change in topography means that a new behaviour is being established. For example, in the case of a dog who jumps up to greet people, a change in topography is the primary goal, i.e. to replace jumping up with a more acceptable behaviour, such as sitting.

**Error/success rate:** This reflects the reliability of the response in a given situation. For example, for a dog with a poor recall, increasing its reliability (increasing success) is usually the first priority. In the case of an animal with a separation problem, the number of occurrences of the problem, relative to the number of opportunities (times left alone, which would normally provoke the problem), is a good measure to focus on. Similarly, in the case of two cat housemates who do not get on, it may be most useful to focus on reducing the number of lapses (ideally zero) that occur as they are slowly reintroduced to each other during a controlled and proscribed programme of specific duration. Only when there has been success a certain number of times should the exposure be intensified.

**Frequency:** This is the rate at which the behaviour occurs. It is not necessarily related to the error rate, since the frequency reflects the actually intensity of the behaviour during a specific bout rather than its context. For example, a measure of frequency is the number of times the desired behaviour can be comfortably cued in a 10-minute training session without causing early signs of distress, such as a decline in one of the other dimensions or a behaviour like yawning or nose-licking (see Ladder of Aggression in Chapter 2).

**Duration:** This describes the time engaged in the behaviour and is perhaps most important when training some sort of relaxed stay. The aim may be to gradually increase the animal's capacity to tolerate a particular circumstance, as occurs in systematic desensitization.

**Latency:** This refers to the delay before response is made. For example, every dog should be trained to stop on command and focus on its owner. This single command can be a lifesaver. Having established a clear stop signal, the most important thing is then to ensure that it happens instantly and so the latency to respond is the focus of behaviour modification.

**8. What is the best way to build up the behaviour?**
The answer to this question depends on the answer to the following: does the end goal exist in some form or other at present? That is to say, is the pet being asked to perform a task that it already shows at least some of the time?

- Yes:
  - Look to reward its occurrence in the right context if possible. By definition, rewarding behaviour increases the chance of its recurrence in the same situation and so the desired behaviour will become more frequent with time
  - Put the behaviour on cue and use the cue to introduce it into the desired situation (e.g. operant counter-conditioning)
  - Shape the behaviour if it is only a rough approximation of the end goal, i.e. reward approximations of the end goal to increase their expression and then stop rewarding those approximations that are less close in order to guide the behaviour towards the end goal (e.g. systematic desensitization).
- No:
  - Encourage the behaviour to occur in some form (e.g. respondent counter-conditioning or behavioural luring).

## 9. What level of generalization is required?

It is often desired that the new behaviour be reliably elicited in a range of contexts (stimulus generalization). This does not necessarily happen automatically and indeed for dogs most responses are initially learned in quite a specific context. This means that when the environment is changed even slightly, performance may dip, at least temporarily (something as subtle as the owner changing posture from standing to sitting or wearing sunglasses, or a change in voice, can affect the reliability of response to novel obedience commands (Fukuzawa *et al.*, 2005)). This is normal and it is important that owners are aware of it and adjust their expectations accordingly. It is particularly important to be aware of the need to generalize the response to different individuals, e.g. for a dog to learn to sit instantly in response to a request from anyone, including a child.

The amount of 'proofing' required (exposure in different environments necessary for the behaviour to become reliable even in a novel environment) varies with both the individual animal and the behaviour being established, and so each case needs to be assessed on its own basis. In general it seems that, if training proceeds in a variety of contexts initially, generalization occurs more readily; whereas if the animal is trained in only a limited number of places that become familiar, generalization may be more limited.

This does not mean that training should always begin in a range of settings, as it may be necessary to have tight controls over the context in the early stages in order to help the animal to focus on the task in hand. In this circumstance, the need for specific generalization exercises needs to be identified to the client early on and proscribed, once the animal's response is suitably reliable.

When the goal is for the animal to perform a particular behaviour in a situation that it might find otherwise aversive (e.g. to lie down in its safe haven when there are fireworks) these stimuli should be introduced gradually, not only because it helps the animal to maintain focus on the task in hand, but also because it helps the animal to generalize its response without making an error that could set it back.

## 10. How can I monitor the programme?

The five different dimensions (see Question 7) of the behaviour to be established can all be measured objectively and relatively easily. Those dimensions of the goal that are relevant need to be precisely defined, together with how they can be assessed, and it is usually preferable to focus on the establishment of a specific dimension of the new behaviour (progress) rather than the decline of the undesirable behaviour (regression), which may be much more varied and less coherently defined. For example, in relation to each of the dimensions described the following might be a way of assessing progress:

- **Topography**
  - Record what behaviour was shown when cued. The owner may need to be provided with clear descriptions or images of different forms of response as a point of reference. See elsewhere in this book for descriptions of different postures and behaviours; see also Aloff (2005) and Handelman (2008) for good pictorial representations of dog behaviour, and UK Cat Behaviour Working Group (1995) and Leyhausen (1979) for useful descriptions relating to the cat.
- **Error/success rate**
  - Record each possible eliciting context and calculate (on a daily or weekly basis) in what proportion of eliciting contexts the animal showed appropriate behaviour.
- **Frequency**
  - Record the number of times the behaviour occurred in a particular time period (e.g. number of times a dog sat successfully when meeting people in a staged training session of 10 minutes duration).
- **Duration**
  - Record how long the animal managed to perform the behaviour (an approximation of duration in which the owner counts may be used if necessary, so that they can still watch their pet while recording).
- **Latency**
  - Record the time between the cue and the animal either interrupting what it was doing, starting to respond or completing the response (depending on the stage of training reached).

A homemade diary will suffice in many situations, depending on the programme being recommended. In the diary, the owner assesses the response according to a given criterion or criteria each time. The change in the response over time can then be plotted relatively easily to demonstrate how progress is being made. This is often important, as many owners left to their own devices will only recognize progress once the problem has completely disappeared and so give up if this goal is not reached quickly. However, showing owners at each follow-up the progress that they are making will give them more motivation to continue through what may be a very challenging time. The plot also allows the identification of dips (acute or chronic), which can be discussed and remedied in good time before the programme is undermined.

Worked examples of this process in relation to different types of exercise are given in Figures 5.3 to 5.5 (see later), but it is important to appreciate that the success of any specific programme will often depend on laying appropriate foundations, by establishing simple reliable responses and an appropriate emotional state, before this is applied to the more challenging circumstances that form the basis of the owner's complaint. This means creating relaxation where there was anxiety, creating calmness where there was excitability, and creating acceptance where there was fear. Only with these in place can the correct behavioural and emotional responses begin to be applied in the problem context. Later transition needs to be gradual and is dependent on the rate of progress made by the patient at each level.

Progress is not always smooth and owners should be made aware that they may encounter sticking points during the programme, but it is important that they persist and seek additional help if progress is not as might be predicted.

## Specific behaviour modification techniques

A couple of techniques are frequently used in the management of a wide range of behaviour problems: counter-conditioning and systematic desensitization. While they can be used separately, they are often used in combination, but it is important to distinguish between them in order to ensure that the training tasks necessary for each to work efficiently are identified.

**Counter-conditioning** is the process whereby an animal is trained to perform a behaviour or response that is incompatible with the problem response when the animal is presented with the problem-evoking stimulus.

- **Classical** (or **respondent**) counter-conditioning uses an unconditioned response, such as eating treats or playing.
- **Instrumental** (**operant**) counter-conditioning (also called **response substitution**) uses a conditioned response such as a 'sit–stay' as the training goal.

In order for this technique to work, it is essential that the motivation to perform the incompatible behaviour is greater than that for the problem behaviour when the two are elicited at the same time. To achieve this, the problem scenario is often phased in gradually along a gradient of distractibility, in much the same way that it is during systematic desensitization. In other words, good control of the stimulus gradient so that the animal can respond properly is necessary to ensure progress with the treatment programme.

**Systematic desensitization** is a training exercise involving graduated exposure and habituation to an arousing stimulus that can lead to problem behaviour, the result of which is to raise the threshold at which the animal responds inappropriately. It therefore involves increasing the animal's ability to control its response, so that it elicits a desired rather than problematic behaviour.

The theory behind both of these techniques is relatively easy to understand, but there can be serious problems with client compliance. These usually arise from the client trying to do too much too soon, and a lack of clear instruction. It is important to set realistic goals and ensure that each of the Ten Questions above is addressed. The examples in Figures 5.3, 5.4 and 5.5 show how this might be done to build a programme, firstly in relation to two situations associated with 'obedience' requests and secondly in relation to these three most commonly used behaviour therapy techniques (classical and operant counter-conditioning and systematic desensitization).

| *Presenting complaint:* | Will not sit on command | Takes initiative in inappropriate circumstances |
|---|---|---|
| *Programme goal:* | *To establish obedience* | *To teach animal to wait for instruction from its owner before action (e.g. 'Learn to Earn' / 'Nothing in Life for Free')* |
| *Training exercise:* | *Obedience training* | *Sit and wait before the door is opened* |
| 1. Fitness for training | (i) Rule out medical complications such as hip dysplasia, deafness, etc. <br> (ii) If animal seems unable to focus, check management (including diet) and address relevant factors, if necessary with assistance of pheromonatherapy or psychopharmacology | |
| 2. Physical goal | Sit on command | Sit at doorways to receive desired reward (i.e. access through the door) |
| 3. Attention | Dog's name | Possible use of a 'shaker can' to interrupt forging ahead, followed by dog's name to orientate dog towards owner |
| 4. Cue | 'Sit' spoken in a clear, calm and consistent way | 'Sit' spoken in a clear, calm and consistent way, followed by a release command such as 'Go on' |
| 5. Decision aid | Food reward *versus* no food, initially on a continuous schedule <br> Once dog is reliable, reinforcement provided on differential basis to improve performance | Verbal praise (previously conditioned reinforcer) and opportunity to go through the door *versus* no access and prolonged wait (response cost) <br> Schedule will be intermittent from the outset, as the dog will probably make errors in the waiting phase initially |
| 6. Encouragement | Maintaining eye contact and attention on dog | Verbal 'Wait' command, which may need prior training focusing on duration |
| 7. Primary dimension | Latency to respond | Success rate, i.e. tendency to sit in front of doors rather than try to forge ahead |
| 8. How to build up behaviour | Either wait till dog is about to sit and then pair command with action and reinforcement; or lure behaviour | Wait for dog to sit before opening door; owner goes ahead, release command issued variable time afterwards (to reduce predictability of release). Ultimately the sit command should be faded out so dog spontaneously sits at the door and waits to be 'given permission' to go through |
| 9. Generalization | Start by involving all members of the family and recording their individual progress <br> Work initially in a quiet area and then move to more distracting environments, but expect slight relapse in performance at these times and so lower criteria for reinforcement | |
| 10. Monitoring | Record time to respond | Record number of opportunities encountered and number of times exercise needs to be rehearsed at each door before dog performs required response |
| Comments | | This is only one of several exercises within the programme |

**5.3** Examples of obedience training programmes.

| Presenting complaint: | Separation anxiety | Giving injections difficult |
|---|---|---|
| Programme goal: | Classical counter-conditioning | Operant counter-conditioning |
| Training exercise: | Remain calm as owner leaves | Sit and take treats on instruction as injection is given |
| 1. Fitness for training | (i) Rule out medical complications (see Chapter 1 and specific problem chapters) <br> (ii) If animal seems unable to settle and temperamentally anxious, check management and address relevant factors (if necessary with assistance of pheromonatherapy or psychopharmacology) | |
| 2. Physical goal | Lie on mat when requested to 'settle down' | 'Sit' on command |
| 3. Attention | Animal's name | Interaction with animal |
| 4. Cue | 'Settle down' and presentation of training mat | Visual gesture such as hand moving over head with treat |
| 5. Decision aid | Food treats *versus* no food treats when relaxed <br> Pre-trained on mat away from problem situation | Food treats fed several times to reinforce good sit in clinic |
| 6. Encouragement | Provision of treats within toy that animal has to work to remove; plus use of a cue to help dog discriminate the training departures from longer real-life ones | Food used as lure to shape behaviour |
| 7. Primary dimension | Duration of relaxed posture | Focusing on reduced latency for behaviour will encourage animal to pay attention to trainer |
| 8. How to build up behaviour | Ensure treat is highly desirable so elicits strong motivation to engage with task <br> Set clear criteria for acceptable behaviours (e.g. okay for dog to prick ears and interrupt chewing for up to 5 seconds but must remain on mat) and for reliability required before progressing to longer durations (e.g. 10 repetitions without failure) | Luring with differential reinforcement of continued sitting associated with quicker responses <br> Slower responses not rewarded; animal released and request repeated |
| 9. Generalization | Response trained in a consistent location on mat to facilitate more rapid increase in duration | Owner to be encouraged to train animal in wide range of contexts with different people if desired |
| 10. Monitoring | Success rate in relation to increasing duration | Duration of focus on owner giving treats |
| Comments | Increasing duration slowly represents element of systematic desensitization | |

**5.4** Examples of counter-conditioning training programmes.

| Presenting complaint: | Firework noise sensitivity |
|---|---|
| Programme goal: | Systematic desensitization |
| Training exercise: | Reduce sensitivity to firework noises |
| 1. Fitness for training | (i) Rule out medical complications (see Chapter 1 and specific problem chapters) <br> (ii) If animal seems unable to settle and temperamentally anxious, check management and address relevant factors (if necessary with assistance of pheromonatherapy or psychopharmacology) |
| 2. Physical goal | Maintain relaxed posture when firework recordings played |
| 3. Attention | Animal's name |
| 4. Cue | 'Settle down' and presentation of training mat |
| 5. Decision aid | Habituate to reduce initial reactivity if possible with sound being played as background noise at low level that does not cause overt anxiety or prompt any change in owner's behaviour <br> Animal rewarded with gentle calm interaction from owner when lying on designated training mat *versus* no interaction from owner if moves off mat |
| 6. Encouragement | Owner interaction or access to favoured toys without drawing any attention to sound stimulus |
| 7. Primary dimension | Topography – aim is to maintain relaxed posture; owner must be aware of signs of low-level anxiety, e.g. nose licking, yawning, increased blink rate |
| 8. How to build up behaviour | Gradually increase volume at rate the animal can accept <br> Set clear criteria for acceptable behaviours and for behaviours indicating caution and need for further repetition of sound without intensification of stimulus and reliability required before progressing to longer durations (e.g. 10 repetitions without failure) <br> Best if training is little and often rather than prolonged |
| 9. Generalization | Response trained in consistent location (preconditioned safe haven) to facilitate more rapid progress by utilizing classically conditioned relaxation response |
| 10. Monitoring | Success rate used to monitor progress and determine point at which stimulus intensity may be increased |
| Comments | Pre-training is a form of classical counter-conditioning |

**5.5** Example of systematic desensitization training programme.

## Conclusion

Behavioural management is an integral part of veterinary practice and an understanding of the principles is essential to good animal management and client care. Recognition of this is important: a veterinary surgeon would not refer a complicated orthopaedic case without understanding principles involved in the treatment, and the same standard should be applied to the behavioural case. Although the application of the science of training can be a specialized skill beyond the scope of the 'average' veterinary surgeon, the basic principles should not be seen as a specialty. Animal training is not a difficult skill to develop, especially when there are so many opportunities to interact with and learn from animals on a daily basis.

## References and further reading

Aloff B (2005) *Canine Body Language: A Photographic Guide Interpreting the Native Language of the Domestic Dog*. Dogwise Publishing, Wenatchee, Washington

Barry J (2008) *The Ethical Dog Trainer: A Practical Guide to Canine Professionals*. Dogwise Publishing, Wenatchee, Washington

Brammeier S, Brennan J, Brown S, *et al*. (2006) Good trainers: how to identify one and why this is important to your practice of veterinary medicine. *Journal of Veterinary Behavior: Clinical Applications and Research* **1**, 47–52

Eaton B (1997) *Hear, Hear! A Guide to Training a Deaf Puppy*. Holmes & Sons, Andover

Fukuzawa M, Mills DS and Cooper JJ (2005) More than just a word: non-semantic command variables affecting obedience in the domestic dog (*Canis familiaris*). *Applied Animal Behaviour Science* **91**, 129–141

Handelman B (2008) *Canine Behavior: A Photo Illustrated Handbook*. Woof and Word Press, Norwich, Vermont

Leyhausen PM (1979) *Cat Behavior: the Predatory and Social Behavior of Domestic and Wild Cats*. Garland Series in Ethology, New York

Levine ED and Mills DS (2008) Long term follow-up of the efficacy of a behavioural treatment programme for dogs with firework fears. *Veterinary Record* **162**, 657–659

Lindsay SR (2000/2001/2005) *Handbook of Applied Dog Behavior and Training. Vols 1–3*. Iowa State University Press, Ames, Iowa

Mills DS (2005) What's in a word? Recent findings on the attributes of a command on the performance of pet dogs. *Anthrozoos* **18**, 208–221

Mills DS and Ledger R (2001) The effect of oral selegiline hydrochloride on learning and training in the dog: a psychobiological interpretation. *Progress in Neuropsychopharmacology and Biological Psychiatry* **25**, 1597–1613

UK Cat Behaviour Working Group (1995) *An Ethogram for Behavioural Studies of the Domestic Cat (Felis silvestis catus L.)*. Universities Federation for Animal Welfare, Potters Bar

---

### Client handouts (bsavalibrary.com/behaviour_leaflets)

- Down–stay mat exercises
- Headcollar training
- How to find a good trainer
- Ladder of Aggression
- 'Leave it' exercises
- Litterbox training
- Muzzle training
- 'Nothing in Life is Free'
- Playing with your dog – toys
- Playing with your kitten
- Puppy socialization: getting used to new people
- Recall exercises
- Sit–stay exercises
- Teaching your dog to go to a place on command
- Treating a fear of car journeys using desensitization and counter-conditioning
- Treating a fear of the veterinary clinic using desensitization and counter-conditioning
- Treating a noise fear using desensitization and counter-conditioning
- Treating separation anxiety in dogs

# Preventive behavioural medicine for dogs

## Wayne Hunthausen

## Introduction

Behaviour problems are still one of the most common causes of death and abandonment of companion dogs in industrialized countries and it seems that pets under one year of age are at the highest risk. Preventing behaviour problems is much easier, safer and more successful than treating them. To accomplish this, the family must be educated about normal canine behaviour, humane training methods and strategies for shaping behaviour. It is important for them to understand that, in addition to providing food, shelter and medical care for their pet, they must also provide for its social and behavioural needs. If this is not done, problems can arise that are frustrating for the family and weaken the bond with the pet. Failure to resolve the problems is likely to lead to abandonment or euthanasia because of undesirable behaviours that could have been prevented.

What constitutes a problem for one family may not necessarily be a problem for another. An individual's tolerance or acceptance of an animal's particular behaviour will depend on that person's previous experience, culture and ideas about what constitutes acceptable behaviour. Some people do not mind when an animal rules their lives, while others feel they must have complete control of the pet.

Problem behaviours tend to be those that are disruptive to the household or potentially dangerous. While the behaviours may be socially unacceptable or undesirable, in many cases they are often normal behaviours. In some cases, completely eliminating such behaviours may not be possible or even mentally healthy for the pet, but they can usually be modified to be more socially acceptable by altering the time, place, duration or target of the behaviours. The family needs to understand why its dog behaves in certain ways and how to respond appropriately. A little basic understanding of the nature of dogs and their needs can be very helpful in dealing with behaviour problems (see also Chapter 3).

Key concepts for raising young dogs include:

- Providing for the pet's needs (nutrition, health care, social interaction, mental stimulation, exercise)
- Setting the pet up to succeed (close supervision, safe confinement when necessary, begin training in quiet non-distracting situations)
- Not taking good behaviours for granted (actively look for and reward desirable behaviour)
- Being consistent (establish rules and boundaries that the whole family will support)
- Avoiding harsh or inappropriate punishment (avoid anything that will weaken the bond between family members and the pet).

## Pre-selection advice

Choosing a pet that is most likely to be a good fit for the family is the first step in preventing problems. It is beneficial if the selection of a dog involves some forethought, rather than being an impulsive decision based solely on emotional factors or the latest trend in fashionable breeds. Pet selection counselling is a service that should be offered by all veterinary surgeons and should include advice on choosing a pet based on breed characteristics, lifestyle, expectations and personal preferences.

A questionnaire may help to clarify the family's needs and expectations (see client handout). The consultation should include a discussion of breed characteristics, such as the tendency to vocalize, get along with children, guard territory and house soil. Social, mental, exercise and grooming needs should also be covered. The family should be cautioned about adopting a dog from a working breed, for example, that requires substantial mental and physical exercise if they have a relatively sedentary lifestyle. It is also important to appreciate that the choice of a given breed is not a guarantee of certain characteristics: there is enormous variation within breeds.

Other important issues include advice about the best age to purchase a pet, its socialization needs, what to look for in the temperament of the sire and dam, choice of sex, where to obtain the pet and how to assess the kennel, breeder and individual animals. In addition, the family will need advice on preparing for the new arrival, including topics such as confinement training, housetraining, feeding, toys and health care requirements.

## Introducing the puppy into the household

### Socialization

The first few months of an animal's life are the most important for social development. Puppies that do not have adequate social interaction with humans during the early months of their lives are likely to grow up to be unsociable adults that exhibit undesirable avoidance or aggressive behaviour. This can usually be avoided by providing plenty of opportunities for social contact with a wide variety of people very early in life.

Social interaction must be provided as soon as the puppy is obtained and continued into its adulthood. It is best for the pet to meet as many people and other animals as possible in a wide range of circumstances and settings in an unthreatening way. This should be done without overwhelming the puppy. The family should ensure that the pet meets people of both sexes, all ages and a wide variety of appearances. A pet that grows up within a restricted social group may not be comfortable when later exposed to people who appear or act differently from those people to whom it was exposed early in life. Socialization should start with simple, quiet introductions and gradually widen to include more people in more robust situations as the pet becomes more comfortable.

Early socialization can be achieved in the family's home, or in the homes of friends who do not have dogs that spend a significant amount of time in parks or other areas where they are likely to pick up infectious agents and bring them into the home. There are no hard and fast rules regarding when a puppy is safe to take out of the home: as it progresses through its vaccination schedule, the family can be advised initially to carry it into new environments and later allow it to walk on sidewalks and, eventually, visit parks. The factors that determine at what age a puppy should be allowed more exposure to situations with potential pathogens include age, vaccination status, health and, especially, the incidence of infectious disease in the area. This will vary from situation to situation and will require a subjective judgement by the veterinary surgeon.

To promote socialization, the family can be sent home with a small bag of 'socialization biscuits' (see **client handout**). The bag should also contain some information on the concept of socialization and a reading list, along with instructions telling the family that they themselves may not give the treats: they must only be given by new people the puppy meets. To make new introductions a positive experience for the puppy, each new person should be asked to hand it a biscuit or a few pieces of its food. This teaches the pet to look forward to having hands reach out toward it and thus helps to prevent hand-shyness. As soon as the young puppy has learned to sit on command, family members should request it to sit every time it meets a new person and then ask that person to give a piece of food. This helps to prevent the problem of jumping up on people during greetings.

## Meeting other pets and children

Puppies should be introduced to other pets and children in a calm, non-stressful environment. If the pet is exceptionally exuberant, a bit of exercise to wear it out prior to the introduction may help. Initial introductions should only be attempted with pets and children that are calm and unaggressive. A relaxed, calm tone of voice is more conducive to successful introductions than anxious, excited tones. Adult supervision is very important and the puppy should never be left alone with young children. Resources that might be guarded should not be available during introductions with children or other pets. Keeping a lead or light line on the puppy (and on any pet it is meeting) may also be helpful. Another excellent way to provide opportunities for socialization is to enrol the pet in well run puppy socialization classes at an early age.

## Experiencing new environments

The puppy also needs to learn all about the environment in which it will live as an adult. Without adequate exposure during early life, novel situations may elicit fear and aggression when the pet is exposed to them later in life. The puppy should experience a wide variety of sights, sounds, odours and situations, such as car rides, traffic, bicycles, noisy vacuum cleaners, hair dryers (Figure 6.1) and lawnmowers. It is vital that the habituation process begins at an early age. Ideally, the breeder should begin the process, but breeders who are raising puppies in quiet rural environments may find it impractical to expose young pets to sufficient stimuli early in life. For them, tape recordings of various urban and environmental sounds can be recommended.

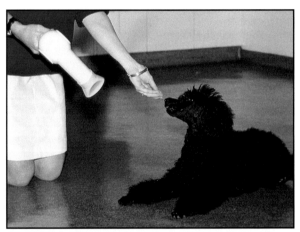

**6.1** A young poodle puppy receives a treat while being exposed to a hairdryer.

## Pheromone therapy

Pheromones may be a helpful aid for socializing puppies. Studies on the use of pheromones in puppies by Denenberg and Landsberg (2008) showed that the pheromone product DAP® (see Chapter 21) may be helpful in reducing fear and anxiety and can have positive effects on socialization and adapting to new situations and environments.

## Handling

A puppy needs to learn to accept and look forward to all types of handling that it will encounter throughout its life. Family members should introduce it to brushing, bathing, nail trimming and other procedures in a calm way without causing any anxiety or resistance.

They should 'play vet' at home from time to time: someone should check the ears, inspect the eyes, open the mouth and handle the pet in all ways that the veterinary surgeon will need to do during a formal examination. This should be carried out when the pet is relaxed and without using any type of force. The puppy should always be rewarded with praise or a small piece of puppy kibble for allowing examination and being relaxed. The best time to start habituating the pet to physical handling is at a time when the puppy is already quiet and calm, not after play or before meals when it is aroused.

If a pet seems to be exceptionally guarded when first introduced to something new, it is best to back off and resume with milder, less intimidating situations. If the pet resists a certain type of handling, the person should stop, handle more gently and then proceed very slowly until it becomes well accustomed to the milder handling and accepts it. Food, toys and praise can be given as rewards to the pet when it is calm during exposure to these situations, so that it begins to look forward to them. The rewards should not be given if the pet exhibits aggressive behaviours as part of a fear response. Once it is comfortable with mild stimuli, it can be introduced to stronger or more complex stimuli and situations. On no account should a situation (such as nail trimming) proceed to the point where the pet bites, growls or flails about and the procedure has to stop. In that case the pet learns that aggression or other undesirable behaviours can control the person's behaviour.

## Preventing aggression

Aggression is one of the most serious behaviour problems that may have to be faced (see Chapters 17 and 18). Once established, aggressive behaviour can be difficult and dangerous to correct. On the other hand, reducing the tendency to show aggressive behaviour is relatively easy, safe and successful in most cases. Since many people are quite naive about dog social behaviour, it is imperative that important issues concerning social behaviour and training are discussed early on.

Training plays a very important role in allowing the family to gain control of the puppy. Those who have good verbal control of their pets are less likely to encounter aggression during confrontational or competitive situations. All dogs should go through puppy training classes at 2–4 months of age, and again during adolescence. Young puppies can easily be taught command responses, using food-lure-reward training.

Until the puppy has learnt to perform command responses dependably, care should be taken to avoid repeatedly giving a command in distracting situations during which it is not likely to respond. Repeated non-compliance may weaken the pet's response to commands. For some puppies, headcollars may be beneficial in helping to establish and maintain control. The family should be guided away from the use of pinch collars and choke collars, since these can cause aggressive behaviour.

## Learning and rule setting

### How dogs learn

There are some important basic principles to understand when attempting to train an animal or modify its behaviour (see Chapter 5). One that is often underestimated is that behaviour is controlled by consequences. Operant conditioning is the primary method by which dog training is achieved. If the consequence is pleasant, the behaviour is more likely to be repeated; and conversely, if the consequence is unpleasant, the behaviour is less likely to be repeated. Timing is critical. The consequence should occur during or immediately following the behaviour. The longer the interval between the behaviour and the consequence, the slower the learning.

### The pet's name

The pet's name is important for training and should not be used as rebuke. It is helpful always to say the pet's name before giving an obedience command. This attracts the pet's attention and provides the opportunity to use a visual signal in addition to the auditory cue to elicit a response.

### Tone of voice

Dogs are non-verbal communicators and so they rely to a great extent on human body language and tone of voice to help them understand what is intended.

- Speaking in a gruff or harsh tone may convey displeasure, regardless of the words that are used, and has been shown to produce less reliable responding (Mills *et al.*, 2005).
- Conversely, speaking in a pleasant tone may convey approval, no matter what is said, and produces more reliable responding (Mills *et al.*, 2005).
- Higher-pitched tones encourage movement and are helpful for teaching commands such as 'come'.
- Low tones tend to decrease movement and are helpful for teaching a dog to 'stay', or to stop a behaviour such as jumping up on someone (McConnell, 1991).

### Punishment

Punishment is a poor training tool and should be avoided. Punitive practices such as swatting the pet, thumping it on the nose, squeezing the muzzle, rubbing the face in a mess or anything that causes pain or fear should never be used. It is extremely important during the early months of the pet's life to avoid any interactions with people that make it anxious or fearful. Pets that are raised using harsh punishment run the risk of growing up to fear hand movements and are likely to bite. Punishment may also produce enough anxiety to slow learning. Finally, when punishment is the sole training tool, it does not provide the pet with any information about what acceptable behaviours are (see Chapter 5). It should be emphasized to the family that reinforcement for appropriate behaviour is the only way a puppy learns what is required of it.

## Teaching the pet that the family is in control

Soon after the pet is adopted, family members should begin to teach it that they are in control. This can be done by using obedience commands to control resources. The pet should learn to defer to family members by responding to a command before receiving anything. Once the puppy learns to sit, family members should request that the pet sit before receiving food (Figure 6.2), play, toys and social attention. Once it learns to stay, it should learn to wait and get permission from family members to move about with them. This can be done by periodically asking the pet to do a one-second stay and wait for a release before following the person around its environment (e.g. entering/leaving rooms, stairways, long hallways, the home). Teaching the pet to hesitate, focus on a family member and wait for further instructions before any activity helps to diminish impulsive, unruly social behaviour.

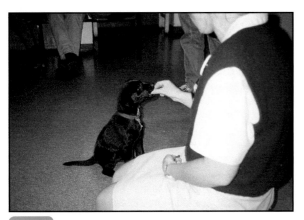

**6.2** Using a food treat to teach a puppy to sit.

If family members set boundaries, are consistent and in control, they will reduce the risk of anxiety in the puppy. They should avoid allowing the pet to demand social interaction. Pushy behaviour such as whining, pawing and nudging for attention should be ignored. This will not only reduce attention-seeking behaviour but also teach the puppy that calm quiet behaviours get attention while pushing, pawing and whining behaviours do not. The strategy is not to curtail the amount of attention the pet receives, but to control how and when it receives it. In time, the family will have dependable control. Controlling resources and using command responses are safe, humane ways of show-ing the puppy what to do and who takes precedence.

This approach is preferable to the potentially inhumane methods of exerting physical control by using scruff shakes, throwing the puppy on its back or pinning it against the ground as it struggles – techniques that are derived from a misunderstanding of the evolution of the dog–human relationship and can lead to fear, avoidance and aggression.

### Food and object guarding

Dogs should learn to be comfortable eating their dinner when humans are nearby. This can be accomplished easily and safely when the pet is young.

Dinnertime should be a social time for the family and the pet. A family member should occasionally sit on the floor with the food bowl in their lap, hand feeding and gently stroking the pet. Small pieces of canned food, meat or cheese can be slipped into the bowl as the pet eats. Visitors who are present during the puppy's dinnertime can drop small pieces of moist dog food into the bowl as they walk by. The puppy will learn not only to tolerate but actually to look forward to having people nearby during its dinnertime.

A popular misconception is that it is necessary to remove the bowl repeatedly from the pet during dinnertime to prove that the family member controls the food. This will not only irritate the pet but may lead to aggression. Teaching a puppy to relinquish a bowl of food is a reasonable strategy only if it learns that there is a benefit to having the bowl taken away, and this can be done if the bowl is traded for a tasty treat, piece of meat or cheese.

To prevent object guarding, family members should occasionally trade toys for treats. When the pet has a toy in its mouth, they can hold a piece of puppy kibble or small treat in front of its nose and say 'drop it' as the pet opens its mouth to take the food. When the pet finishes eating the food, they should request it to sit and then give the toy back. Eventually, the family members will be able to give the command and move a hand toward the puppy without food and have it drop an object from its mouth.

The above approach is only safe for puppies without problems. Older dogs with established food- or object-guarding aggression issues can be difficult and dangerous to treat. Feeding the pet in a room by itself and a visit to a behaviour consultant are warranted for these pets (see Chapter 17).

## Confinement training

A fundamental strategy for preventing undesirable behaviour is to keep the pet out of trouble by providing adequate supervision so that it does not have the opportunity to misbehave. Confinement training is necessary to prevent problems when a family member is not available to supervise. This is required until the pet is trained to eliminate in an appropriate area, to occupy itself with toys instead of being undesirably destructive, and is beyond the adolescent exploratory phase. While it is preferable for the pet to wander around freely with family members for socialization, it is not realistic to expect the family to be constantly on the alert so that the pet does not stray and get into trouble. Using a lead attached to a belt to keep the pet nearby or putting a bell on its collar will help with supervision.

The confinement area should not be used as a punishment area where a dog is scolded and contained if it misbehaves. Possible choices for a confinement area include a dog-proof room, crate, run or exercise pen.

There is a common misconception that puppies and dogs innately desire to be in a 'den'. A puppy should actively be trained to accept and look forward to staying in its confinement area. The pet's dinnertime provides an excellent opportunity for training, as the pet can be fed in the confinement area. A puppy can be taught to go into its quarters on command by repeatedly tossing pieces of dry food into the area for it to chase, while giving a command cue such as 'go to your room' before the food is thrown. It will eventually learn to go to this place when it hears the command. To make further positive associations with the area, toys and biscuits should frequently be left there for the pet to wander in and find.

The pet should be allowed to become used to short confinement periods first and then these can be lengthened gradually. Vocalizations should be ignored: the pet should not be released when it is barking or whining. If it is time to release the pet but it continues to vocalize, a family member should distract it by making a noise (not loud enough to frighten the pet) while out of sight, such as whistling, stomping the floor, or slapping the wall, to draw the pet's attention towards the sound and encourage it to be quiet for at least 10 seconds before it is released.

If a crate is used, it should be big enough for the dog to stand up and turn around in comfortably. The pet should not be left inside for longer than it can control elimination, or longer than about 4 hours during the day on a daily basis. When done correctly, a crate can be a safe, secure and humane place to confine a pet and an aid for travel. Use of a crate is inappropriate if the pet is confined for longer than 4–5 hours every day when the family is away from home, if it voids in the crate or if crating causes severe anxiety. Those who are out for long periods each day should make certain that their pet receives sufficient exercise and adequate social attention when they are at home or should consider employing a dog-walker.

## Housetraining

Housetraining is one of the more important tasks since most dogs spend a considerable amount of their lives inside the home. Dogs that are not successfully trained may be banished to live outdoors or may be removed from the home. The overall goal of housetraining is to teach the puppy when to eliminate, where to eliminate and on what surface to eliminate. The process involves reinforcing elimination behaviour in a desirable location, while preventing the behaviour in undesirable locations, for a sufficient amount of time that the appropriate behaviour becomes well entrenched. The whole process may take anywhere from several weeks to many months, depending on the consistency of the family members and the pet's capacity for learning. The family should be able to complete housetraining within a relatively short period, usually within 3 months, if they are consistent and patient.

### Reinforcement of elimination in a desirable area

The first step is to teach the pet where it is acceptable to eliminate. To do this, the pet must be guided to the chosen elimination area and the family member should mildly praise pre-elimination behaviours, such as sniffing, and heartily praise it as soon as it eliminates. The family member can also provide a small food reward immediately following elimination to strongly reinforce the behaviour in the desired location. The opportunity to eliminate outdoors should be given frequently, especially after eating, drinking, napping, playing and before confinement periods.

One way of determining how often to take the pup to its elimination area is to take the pet's age in months and add one hour; for example, a 3-month-old puppy should be taken out to eliminate about every 4 hours. It is often desirable to use a phrase (e.g. go potty, be quick, hurry, take care of business, go pee) as the puppy begins to eliminate. This can place the elimination behaviour under verbal control, which is useful in cold weather and when the puppy is away from home.

If the pet is taken indoors immediately after eliminating, a puppy that wants to stay outdoors might see this as a punishment. In such cases, it may be beneficial to provide some play or a short walk before returning indoors. Other puppies would rather be indoors, especially if the weather is inclement, and so going back indoors may be reinforcing.

### Provision of a consistent feeding schedule

The family needs to set up a relatively fixed feeding schedule. Food should be offered for about 30 minutes, two to three times daily, at the same time every day. By controlling the time at which the pet eats, the family will have some control over when it eliminates, which hopefully will be a time when they will be available to take it outdoors. The last meal should be finished about 4 hours prior to bedtime. Water should be available all day but removed just prior to bedtime, unless the pet requires access to water throughout the night due to a health problem.

### Prevention of elimination in undesirable areas

One the most important facets of housetraining involves preventing the development of the habit of eliminating in the home. The pet must be very closely supervised for an adequate number of weeks until elimination in an appropriate area has been satisfactorily reinforced. To accomplish this, the pet must be kept within eyesight 100% of the time when it is in the home. When it cannot be supervised, it should be confined to a small area, such as an exercise pen, or placed outdoors. Baby gates or a lead can be used to prevent the pet from wandering away when family members are busy. Confining a puppy to a sleeping kennel when it cannot be watched is a common way to prevent the pet from house soiling during training, but family members should be counselled not to overuse this method. The pet should not be confined to a small sleeping area for longer than it can physically control elimination, or for more than 4–5 hours during the day on a constant schedule. Until the puppy has not eliminated in the home for at least 4–8 *consecutive* weeks, it should not be considered housetrained or allowed to wander off unattended. Once a sufficient amount of time has passed and the puppy is exhibiting control, it can gradually be given unsupervised freedom in the home.

## Dealing with mistakes

No matter how closely a pet is watched, mistakes are bound to happen. If the house soiling repeatedly occurs in one area, an objectionable habit may readily become established. To prevent this, urine and faecal odour should be removed from soiled areas with an effective commercial deodorizing product. Fabric and carpets should be soaked with the product, since merely spraying the surface is not likely to be as effective. Closing doors or moving furniture over frequently soiled areas will prevent access to those areas.

The pet can be taught to avoid some areas by making them unpleasant. Upside-down mousetraps, balloons set to pop when disturbed and motion-activated alarms can be successful in teaching a pet to avoid an area. However, these items should only be used when the positive approach alone has failed, and the aversive stimulus should be acceptable given the pet's temperament. For a very sensitive young puppy, any aversive stimulus could potentially cause unwanted anxiety and should be avoided.

Another way to prevent resoiling is to change the behavioural function of the areas. Since a dog usually will not eliminate in an area where it eats, sleeps or plays, food bowls, water bowls, the pet's bed or toys can be placed in areas where it has soiled in order to stop elimination in those places.

Punishment is often overused and relatively ineffective, and is not required for successful housetraining. It must be discussed with all families, because it is a common practice that is usually used in an inappropriate manner. The family member should understand that physical punishment, harsh reproach and rubbing the pet's nose in urine or faeces are unacceptable and may break the bond between them and the pet. A sharp noise such as a quick stomp of the foot, a loud handclap or a sharp thump on a tabletop can be used (without saying anything) to interrupt the pet when it is caught in the act of eliminating in an inappropriate area. The sound should be just loud enough to stop the behaviour without frightening the pet and, if possible, should not be directly associated with the person. The interruption should only be given during the unwanted behaviour. The pet should then be taken to the area the family has chosen as an appropriate elimination area and praised for completing its eliminations there.

## Destructive behaviour

All puppies and most adolescent dogs have a high propensity for chewing on just about anything they find around the home. The best way to handle this behaviour is to provide consistent supervision or confinement, and teach the pet to chew on acceptable objects. This can be done by providing a safe environment for the puppy with a variety of appealing toys to chew. Providing lots of exercise and mental stimulation is also very important, since an active, under-stimulated puppy is more likely to engage in exploratory behaviour and destructive chewing.

## Encouraging proper chewing habits

A variety of safe, interesting toys should be provided (see **client handout**). The family should observe the pet's interest in the toys to decide which are the most appealing to it. Toys that are made of durable rubber are most practical (Figure 6.3). Particularly good choices are ones that have cavities or depressions that can be packed with small amounts of food to capture the pet's attention. Spreading a light coat of meat juice, canned dog food, peanut butter or cheese on the toys will help to make them attractive. Freezing a toy containing moist food will provide an additional challenge for the dog and lengthen the time it spends with the toy.

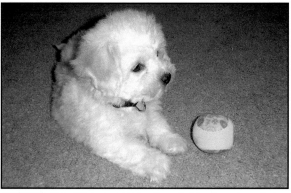

**6.3** Providing puppies with suitable chew toys helps prevent unacceptable chewing behaviour.

The pet should have a moderate number of toys, but no more than about 80% of them should be available at any one time. A few toys should be removed from time to time and replaced with ones the pet has not seen recently. Periodically rotating the toys will maintain an interest in them. The pet can have 'Monday toys', 'Tuesday toys' and so on. The family should be encouraged to look for and reward acceptable chewing behaviour with praise or food as often as possible. A piece of kibble or a small treat can be tossed next to the pet as it chews on a toy. This further reinforces the behaviour, in a way that does not happen when it chews on non-toy objects around the home.

## Discouraging unacceptable chewing and stealing

Even with an exceptional selection of tempting chew toys, there will be objects around the home that are tempting for the pet to chew. Until the pet can be trusted not to chew the family's possessions, it must be under supervision or confined to a safe area. Supervision or confinement may be necessary for up to 24 months of age for some pets. Giving the pet old shoes, towels and other items that are similar to objects that should not be chewed should be discouraged. As the pet grows older and is allowed more freedom around the home, the family may need to take extra care to prevent mistakes.

The pet can be taught to avoid certain objects by making them taste bad. Commercial anti-chew sprays, oil of citronella or a small amount of cayenne pepper may act as a successful deterrent when applied to objects. The pet can also be kept away from areas or objects that need to be protected by using a motion-activated alarm when it cannot be supervised. The pet should not be punished if caught in the act of chewing a family member's possessions. A sharp noise can be used to interrupt the behaviour, and a chew toy can then be given to it.

'Stealing' can be stopped by teaching the pet that the family's possessions taste bad. Several objects should be chosen and sprayed with a bitter or hot spray. They should then be placed in areas where the puppy will find them and pick them up. The objects should periodically be moved to different areas around the home so that the pet learns that they taste bad no matter where they are found. They should be resprayed as needed. After about 2 weeks (and every 2 weeks thereafter), those objects should be replaced with several different, sprayed objects.

## Play-biting

Play-biting is a natural behaviour commonly exhibited by puppies, but some are quite intense and have poor bite inhibition, making the behaviour a considerable annoyance (or worse). Family members should not engage in rough play with the pet, wear gloves to permit hard bites, or encourage the pet to attack and bite hands or feet. Likewise, harsh or physical corrections should be avoided. The pet should not be struck, thumped on the nose, have its lips squeezed against its teeth in a painful manner, shaken by the scruff, forcefully rolled it on its back or have a fist pushed into its mouth to stop it from play-biting.

Puppies should receive frequent opportunities for exercise, including romps in the garden, walks and 'fetch' games. Pets that receive lots of aerobic exercise will have less energy with which to play-attack people. Soft, inhibited bites and mouth–hand contact during play may be permitted, but family members should respond to any bite that has enough force to be even mildly uncomfortable by yelling 'ouch', immediately stopping play and walking away from the pet.

It may also be helpful to teach the pet to stop play-biting on command. This can be done by giving a command, such as 'enough', as the pet is biting. If the pet stops, it should be rewarded with a small, very tasty piece of food. If it continues the biting, the person should respond with an instructive reprimand. This is done by immediately saying 'enough' with sufficient volume that the pet backs away, but not loud enough that it is frightened. Eventually, the pet will stop biting every time the command is given. For this to work, the family members must be very consistent in their responses and have precise timing. 'Monkey in the Middle' games (described below) in the garden will teach puppies to run up and sit by family members instead of biting at their feet. Head halters may be helpful for some puppies.

## Jumping up

Jumping up on people is a common problem that can be controlled with training and management. Training against this problem should begin right away. The young puppy should be taught to sit on command when it is 6–8 weeks old and then asked to sit before it gets anything it wants or needs. Recall games such as 'Monkey in the Middle' (two or more people repeatedly call the puppy back and forth between them and ask it to sit) can be very helpful. If the pet is behind a baby gate, a person can make multiple approaches to the gate. Each time the pet jumps on the gate the person ignores it, turns and walks away. Once the pet does not jump up during the approach, it can be asked to sit for a treat. This is repeated until the pet readily sits during each approach. The gate can then be removed and the repeated greetings can continue.

Holding a treat at nose level for the puppy as a door is opened and a person enters may help to get the pet's attention for a sit before it jumps up. Puppies should be frequently trained to sit during greetings and approaches throughout the home and garden, especially at doorways and gates. This should initially be done in quiet situations with family members, then with visitors. Training should also be done during greetings on walks. Once the pet is doing well, the food is gradually phased out.

The pet should never get any attention when it jumps up on someone. Petting, light scolding or pushing the pet away may reinforce the behaviour. When the pet jumps up, the person should quickly turn and walk away.

Leads can be helpful for control during greetings. Stepping on the lead will prevent the puppy from jumping up and provide an opportunity to have the pet sit for a reward. Finally, confinement or a lead tie-down may sometimes be the best option for the young untrained pet during exciting social situations.

## Puppy socialization and training classes

### Puppy classes

Puppy training classes can be very helpful for teaching families how to understand their pet's behaviour and can help them to teach their puppies basic good manners. They provide a great opportunity for providing information that will help to prevent behaviour problems and educate them on all aspects of raising a puppy. Besides obedience training for younger dogs, they provide important socialization opportunities during a critical period in the puppy's life (Figures 6.4 and 6.5).

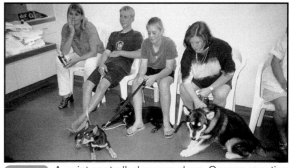

**6.4** A quiet controlled puppy class. Owners practise asking their puppies to stay whilst on the lead as the puppies wait for their turn to play.

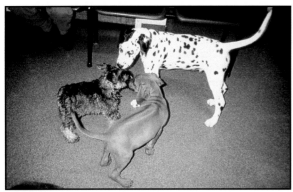

**6.5**  Classes enable socialization with other puppies of different breeds, colour, shapes and sizes.

Puppy classes in the veterinary practice provide benefits beyond those that pets and owners receive. They help to solidify the relationship between owners and the veterinary staff. Owners feel more comfortable coming into the practice if their pet enjoys the visit and the staff know them personally.

Practices that do not offer their own classes should give advice for evaluating a puppy class before signing up (see Chapter 5).

- A good puppy class trainer should stress positive reinforcement methods for shaping behaviour.
- The environment should be clean and there should be requirements to ensure that puppies are up to date on vaccinations and free from parasites.
- There should be ample time for socialization during the class and an age limit or size limit so that small puppies are not frightened by larger ones during play periods. (To prevent small puppies from being overwhelmed during play sessions, the author's hospital offers a separate 'Petite Puppy Class' for small breeds.)
- Topics should include obedience training, socialization, humane methods for shaping behaviour, handling tolerance, prevention of behaviour problems and how to deal with potential problems (see below).
- As a bonus, the presence of a qualified person to discuss health and nutrition increases the value of the course.

Topics for puppy classes include:

- Responsible pet ownership
- Health care
- Normal canine behaviour
- Appropriate methods for training and shaping the pet's behaviour
- Socialization to other puppies and people
- Teaching puppies to accept gentle handling from humans
- Basic obedience commands (see Chapter 5)
- Prevention and problem solving for issues that are common to young puppies, such as housetraining, biting, jumping up on people, unruliness, chewing and scratching.

Puppy classes are usually run as a 4–8-week course designed to help 8–16-week-old puppies become sociable and manageable pets. For the most part, the training is done off-lead and should be reward based, training the puppy to perform a task to obtain a reinforcement. With this approach, force or physical pressure is not necessary.

There is usually a maximum of eight puppies per class, with one to two instructors. All puppies must have had their first vaccinations against distemper, hepatitis and parvovirus at least 10 days before starting at puppy classes. Applicants should be screened and shelter puppies should not be allowed into class until they have been out of the shelter and disease-free for 2 weeks. Some practices begin classes with a 'puppy-free' session to allow the family to concentrate on basic information and have questions answered without distractions.

Family members are taught about how dogs learn and how they perceive the world, and are introduced to aspects of responsible pet care including nutrition, dental care, bathing, grooming, housetraining and worming. Basic obedience commands, such as sit, come, stay and down, are taught. The pet also should learn how to walk on a lead without pulling. Family members should be taught how to handle their puppies, give pills, trim nails and do basic physical manipulations.

A very important part of the class sessions involves social interaction. Each class may be started with a 5-minute period during which the puppies are allowed to play with each other, and the session ends with a 5-minute period during which handlers interact with all the puppies.

### Confidence building

In each class there will usually be many different types of puppy, ranging from the very pushy and confident to the very timid. The shy or timid puppy needs encouragement but should never be forced to interact. If it feels more comfortable under a chair or behind a barrier during play sessions, it should be allowed to stay there until it feels more confident. In some classes, it may be helpful to divide large exuberant puppies from smaller ones during play and social sessions. It is essential that the puppy does not become more frightened by larger or more confident puppies being allowed to harass it or even accidentally trample on it during play.

It is usually best to avoid giving the puppy attention while it is hiding as this may reinforce the hiding behaviour. Anxious pups that are ignored are usually more likely to venture out and interact. Most of these puppies develop confidence by the second or third week and it is very rewarding to watch them discover the joys of socializing. Some small shy puppies may benefit from repeating the course and the author has not found the age disparity to be problematic. The odd puppy, however, may remain shy and fail to interact much with the other puppies throughout the course. It should be monitored closely over the course and extra counselling with the family will probably be needed if its behaviour does not improve.

### Assertiveness

Varying degrees of assertiveness can be observed in a group of puppies. Most puppies exhibit some form of testing behaviour (not to be confused with social or dominance aggression) and usually the puppies sort it out themselves. Ideally, they teach each other when it has gone too far, but this is not always the case. It is the persistently pushy puppy or the one that uses aggression to control others that should raise most concern. Unfortunately, these puppies usually continue to 'win' their interactions with the other puppies and so they do not get the appropriate negative feedback to curb the behaviour. These puppies need careful supervision in their interactions to make sure that their behaviour is appropriate, with people as well as with other dogs. If the problem seems to be accelerating, further advice from a qualified veterinary behaviourist or applied animal behaviour consultant should be sought.

## Puppy parties

An alternative to formal puppy classes is to have 'puppy parties.' These are informal, less structured socialization sessions at the practice. They can be held in the reception area during evening or weekend hours when the practice is not open for regular business. Puppies and families attend for social interaction with each other and the veterinary staff. Handouts and puppy-raising information can be provided at these times, but without careful management they can create problems if animals are left to be free.

A study using canine pheromones in puppy classes showed that puppies exposed to DAP® (see Chapter 21) and those in placebo groups were significantly different with respect to degrees of fear and anxiety (Denenberg and Landsberg, 2008). Longer and more positive interactions between puppies, including play, were evident in dogs in the DAP® groups. Data from follow-up telephone surveys indicated that puppies in the DAP® groups were better socialized and adapted faster to new situations and environments, compared with puppies in the placebo groups.

## Veterinary visits

The puppy's vaccination visits provide a timely opportunity to provide important behaviour information to the family that they will need to raise a pet in a way that maximizes its behavioural potential. The veterinary surgeon and the practice's support staff should set aside time to discuss housetraining, destructive behaviours, socialization, training, handling techniques and prevention of problem behaviours (see Chapter 2). Since there are so many health and behaviour topics to cover, placing a checklist in the puppy's medical file will help the practice to keep track of which topics have been covered in previous appointments and which remain to be addressed.

Exceptional care should be taken to ensure that the initial visits to the veterinary practice are as pleasant as possible. Minimal restraint during a veterinary examination works best. Rough handling or excessive force is never recommended, as this can cause fear and lead to aggressive responses. During a veterinary examination, the owner should be taught how to restrain and handle their young pet properly (see Chapter 2). If they practise gentle handling at home whenever the pet is calm and quiet, it will help future veterinary visits.

If the pet becomes over-anxious at any stage, the examination should be stopped and not continued until the pet relaxes. If the puppy is exceptionally fearful, frantic and does not relax, the visit should stop altogether (unless a medical or other urgent issue makes this impractical) and the owner should be instructed to bring the pet back once or twice daily during the following week to receive special treats from the staff. It is amazing how much the pet's behaviour can change in a relatively short time with this approach.

## Conclusion

The importance of providing families with the tools and information they need to raise their pets properly cannot be overemphasized. Puppies that are raised by educated owners are more likely to exhibit appropriate and acceptable social behaviour, and less likely to develop behaviour problems. By helping to accomplish this, veterinary staff will ensure a long-lasting rich relationship between the family, the pet and the practice. This results in a well behaved pet with a strong bond with the family and helps to ensure that the pet will stay in the home.

## References and further reading

Ackerman L, Landsberg G and Hunthausen W (eds) (1996) *Dog Behavior and Training: Veterinary Advice for Owners*. TFH Publications, Neptune, New Jersey

Bailey G (1998) *Good Dog Behaviour*. Harper Collins, London

Denenberg S and Landsberg G (2008) Effects of dog-appeasing pheromones on anxiety and fear in puppies during training and on long-term socialization. *Journal of the American Veterinary Medical Association* **233**, 1874–1882

Dunbar I (1991) *How to Teach a New Dog Old Tricks*. James and Kenneth Publishers, Berkeley, California

Dunbar I (2004) *Before and After Getting Your Puppy*. New World Library, Novato, California

Dunbar I (2006) *Sirius Puppy Training* [DVD]. James and Kenneth Publishers, Berkeley, California

Dunbar I (2007) *Sirius Puppy Training*. [DVD] James and Kenneth Publishers, Berkeley, California

Fisher J (ed.) (1993) *The Behaviour of Dogs and Cats*. Random House, London

Fogle B (1990) *The Dog's Mind*. Viking Penguin, New York

Fox MW (1978) *The Dog: Its Domestication and Behaviour*. Garland STPM Press, New York

Freedman DG, King JA and Elliot E (1961) Critical period in the social development of dogs. *Science* **133**, 1016–1017

Houpt KA (1985) Companion animal behavior: a review of dog and cat behavior in the field, the laboratory and the clinic. *Cornell Veterinarian* **75**, 248–261

Hunthausen WL and Landsberg G (1998) *American Animal Hospital Association puppy behavior pamphlets*. American Animal Hospital Association, Lakewood, Colorado

Landsberg G, Hunthausen W and Ackerman L (2003) *Handbook of Behavior Problems of the Dog and Cat, 2nd edn*. Saunders, Edinburgh

Markwell PJ and Thorne CJ (1987) Early behavioural development of dogs. *Journal of Small Animal Practice* **28**, 984–991

McConnell, PB (1991) Lessons from animal trainers: the effect of acoustic structure on an animal's response. In: *Perspectives in Ethology*, ed. P Bateson and P Klopfer, pp. 165–187. Plenum Press, New York

McConnell P and London K (2003) *Way To Go! How To Housetrain a Dog of Any Age*. Dog's Best Friend Ltd, Black Earth, Wisconsin

McCune S, McPherson JA and Bradshaw JWS (1995) Avoiding problems: the importance of socialisation. In: *Waltham Book of Human–Animal Interaction: Benefits and Responsibilities of Pet Ownership*, ed. I Robinson, pp. 71–86. Pergamon Press, Oxford

Miller DD, Staats SR, Partlo C *et al.* (1996) Factors associated with the decision to surrender a pet to an animal shelter. *Journal of the*

*American Veterinary Medical Association* **209**, 738–742

Mills DS, Fukuzawa M and Cooper JJ (2005) The effect of emotional content of verbal commands on the response of dogs. In: *Current Issues and Research in Veterinary Behavioural Medicine – Papers Presented at the 5th International Veterinary Behavior Meeting, Purdue University Press, West Lafayette, Indiana*, pp. 217–220

Mills DS (1997) Using learning theory in animal behavior therapy. *Veterinary Clinics of North America: Small Animal Practice* **27**, 617–636

Salman MD, Hutchison J and Ruch-Gallie R (2000) Behavioral reasons for relinquishment of dogs and cats to 12 shelters. *Journal of Applied Animal Welfare Science* **3**, 93–106

Scidmore K and McConnell PB (1996) *Puppy Primer.* Dog's Best Friend Ltd, Black Earth, Wisconsin

Scott JP (1962) Critical periods in behavioral development. *Science* **138**,

949–958

Scott JP and Marston MV (1950) Critical periods affecting the development of normal and maladjustive social behavior in puppies. *Journal of Genetics and Psychology* **77**, 25–60

Seksel K (1997) Puppy socialization classes. In *Veterinary Clinics of North America: Small Animal Practice* **27**, 465–477

Seksel K, Mazurski E and Taylor A (1999) A. Puppy socialisation programs: short and long term behavioural effects. *Applied Animal Behaviour Science* **62,** 335–349

Silvani P and Eckhardt L (2005) *Raising Puppies And Kids Together – A Guide For Parents.* TFH Publishers, Neptune, New Jersey

Weston D and Weston R (1997) *Your Ideal Dog.* Hyland House, South Melbourne, Victoria, Australia

Yin S (2004) *How to Behave So Your Dog Behaves.* TFH Publications, Neptune, New Jersey

---

## Client handouts (bsavalibrary.com/behaviour_leaflets)

- Adopting a rescue dog: the pros and cons
- Avoiding house soiling by dogs
- Canine behaviour questionnaire
- Down–stay mat exercises
- Environmental enrichment for dogs in animal shelters
- Handling exercises for puppies and kittens
- Headcollar training
- How to find a good trainer
- Ladder of Aggression
- 'Leave it' exercises
- Muzzle training
- 'Nothing in Life is Free'
- Pet selection questionnaire
- Playing with your dog – toys
- Puppy socialization: getting used to new people
- Recall exercises
- Redirected aggression in dogs
- Request for information on problem behaviours
- Sit–stay exercises
- Teaching your dog to go to a place on command
- The newly adopted rescue dog: preventing problems
- Treating a fear of car journeys using desensitization and counter-conditioning
- Treating a fear of the veterinary clinic using desensitization and counter-conditioning
- Treating separation anxiety in dogs
- What your dog needs
- Your puppy's first year

# 7

# Preventive behavioural medicine for cats

## Kersti Seksel

## Introduction

Cats are a popular pet in many countries. For example, it is estimated that in the UK in 2008 18% of households owned cats. Although in Australia in 2005 around 25% of households owned cats, while the owned cat population is increasing in many parts of the world it has been in steady decline in Australia since 1999. As the demographics of society change, with more and more people living in busy single-person households, cats appear to be the ideal pet: small, clean, independent, low care and cute as well. However, although cats may appear to be 'lower maintenance' than dogs, they are not a 'no-care' pet (see Chapter 4).

Unfortunately the number of cats surrendered each year to shelters has not diminished appreciably. The many reasons that lead to surrender are incompletely understood but most studies indicate that misunderstanding and failing to accommodate normal feline behaviour are major contributing factors. Studies indicate that house soiling is the most common reason for surrender of cats, followed by problems with other pets and aggressive behaviours (Salman *et al.*, 2000). Dogs and cats were more likely to be relinquished if there was another pet in the household, especially if that other pet had been acquired in the previous year. One survey of cat owners indicated that the most common problem behaviours identified are fear of strangers and intercat aggression. Spraying or other elimination problems featured much less prominently than is apparent from the number of referrals to veterinary behaviourists.

## Prevention of problems

Behaviour is influenced by three main factors:

- Genetic or inherited characteristics
- Learning from previous experiences
- The current situation.

The key to preventing problems is to help owners to understand why the cat behaves in the way it does and to help them to manage, modify or accept the behaviours.

Many feline behaviours that are problematic for owners are in fact normal behaviours. Most people view feline behaviour anthropocentrically and have unrealistic expectations of their cat. This leads to misunderstanding of the motivation for the behaviour and to the breakdown of the human–cat bond. Veterinary surgeons need to educate clients and teach them to see the world from the cat's perspective. Owners who understand their cat's behavioural development, its needs and feline ways of communication are better able to prevent some behaviour problems (or problem behaviours) from occurring.

Education should focus on three key areas:

- Selection
- Socialization
- Stimulation.

It is important for all involved with a cat to appreciate what is desired from the outset. Kittens that make the best pets are generally approachable and friendly and do not mind being picked up or handled. They do not get distressed when separated from littermates and are not frightened of people. They allow handling of the paws, head and body without excessive struggling. Being picked up is not natural for cats and so kittens do need to be taught that being picked up is something that their owners expect of them. With this in mind, measures can be taken to maximize a developmental path towards this goal.

## Selection

Selection of the most appropriate pet for the household is the first step in the prevention of problems. This involves helping owners to decide whether a cat is the most appropriate choice of pet and also providing advice on selection of the breed, gender, age and so on.

To increase the likelihood that the kitten will develop normally into a well behaved cat that is suitable for the average cat owner, the selection of a kitten for the family should be based on temperament and good health, not appearance – even if it is proposed to show or breed the cat.

Studies have indicated that the temperament of the father has a large influence in determining the temperament of the kitten as far as boldness and timidity in its response to humans are concerned. This is not to say that the queen may not have a similar influence, but it is easier to isolate and identify the influence of the father experimentally (he has no input after mating) and there have not been any studies to determine the influence of the queen. Nonetheless, an outgoing and friendly queen will teach the kittens how to behave by her example as well. Ideally a prospective kitten owner should meet and interact with the tom and the queen, as well as their siblings and previous issue. However, this opportunity is rarely available.

The ideal time to home a kitten is after its first vaccinations at around 7–9 weeks of age (Bradshaw, 1992). If kittens are not homed until after this age, or if they go to homes where they may not experience a wide variety of situations, special measures may be necessary to ensure adequate socialization.

## Socialization

Pets that fit into human society need to be socialized. Socialization is the term used for the process by which individuals learn and perform behaviours expected of them by society. In the case of dogs and cats, socialization is a special learning process whereby the puppy or kitten learns to accept the close proximity of members of its own species as well as members of other species.

In the first 4 weeks of life it is essential that kittens have social contact with the queen. If this is prevented a variety of behavioural, emotional and physical abnormalities may develop. From studies it is now known that cats that have been isolated during the sensitive socialization period are more likely to be hyperactive, antisocial and fearful of people and other cats (Bradshaw, 1992). They can also be slow to learn even simple associations, such as the location of food. Handling kittens for as little as 20 minutes a day can help to substitute for some of the stimulation provided by the queen (Bradshaw, 1992), but anecdotal evidence in hand-raised kittens suggests that they may have difficulty controlling bite strength and sheathing of claws, though the relative importance of specific factors remains unknown. Lack of socialization, as may be shown by inappropriate responses to people or other animals, is one of the many issues that lead to abandonment of pets.

To develop into normal, friendly and confident adults, kittens need regular handling and to be exposed to many novel situations in an unthreatening manner during the sensitive socialization period. Kittens that do not have the opportunity to interact with other cats and humans during the socialization period may later exhibit undesirable behavioural responses, such as aggression or avoidance, to other cats or people, or abnormal 'bonding' to people.

## Stimulation

During the socialization period it is important to expose the young kitten to as many new things as possible in an unthreatening way. The kitten needs to play and have contact with people other than just the immediate family and it should be exposed to children as well as adults.

Through play, kittens develop confidence and learn how to interact and communicate. They learn body language and communication skills. Play behaviour is affected by the time of weaning. When development proceeds normally, weaned kittens show a reduction in social play and an increase in object

play at around 8 weeks of age. Studies have shown that kittens that are weaned early show an earlier increase in the frequency of object play (Martin and Bateson, 1988).

Exercising the mind as well as the body is an important aspect of keeping cats healthy and looking after their welfare. Indoor cats require more active enrichment, which means providing them with mental as well as physical stimulation. Ways to provide complexity and variety should include the provision of suitable toys (Figure 7.1) and activities that allow the kitten to use its senses of sight, hearing, smell, taste and touch. Toys need to be changed at regular intervals, even daily, for the kitten or cat to maintain interest. Additionally, the kitten may first need to be taught how to play, and then encouraged to play with toys.

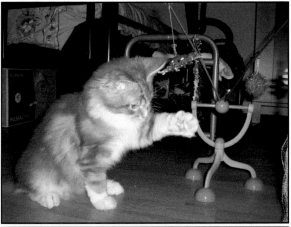

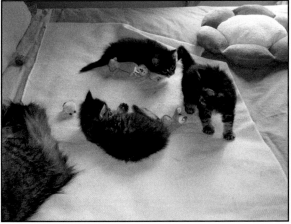

**7.1** Toys for kittens allow both mental and physical stimulation.

Foraging devices that allow exploratory activity, simulate normal predatory behaviours and stimulate the senses are important. Hiding dry food in different places around the house and letting the kitten 'hunt' for dinner provides excellent mental as well as physical exercise.

An indoor garden filled with grass, catnip or catmint can provide sensory stimulation as well as tactile stimulation, though some cats become over-aroused by catnip and can appear aggressive to owners who interact inappropriately with them at this time. Plants also provide fibre and may prevent the cat eating potentially toxic indoor plants.

Cat flaps can provide a degree of freedom by allowing access to a safe outside enclosure for visual and olfactory stimulation. (See Chapter 4 for additional information on enrichment.)

## Kitten socialization and training

Setting boundaries for acceptable and unacceptable behaviour as soon as a kitten has entered its new home is important. Rewarding appropriate behaviour is the key to a well mannered cat. Behaviours that are unacceptable to the owner should be ignored and more acceptable behaviours substituted by using rewards rather than punishment. Behaviours that might be cute when a kitten is little will not necessarily be acceptable when a fully grown adult cat expresses the same behaviour. It is important to make owners aware that potentially problematic behaviour does not disappear on its own, but it may become more noticeable as the cat grows up.

Although the advantages of puppy training are now well established and accepted, many people still do not appreciate that kittens also benefit from classes that focus on early handling and socialization. It can be of advantage to the veterinary clinic to run its own kitten classes, an example of which is Kitten Kindy®, an early socialization, training and education programme developed in Australia by the author and designed to help owners and kittens start off properly together. The goal is to prevent problem behaviours and to educate owners on all aspects of raising a kitten and living with a cat in the family. An additional benefit is the establishment of a close bond between the cat, the owner and the veterinary practice.

Kitten Kindy® classes are designed for kittens aged 8–10 weeks. A maximum of six kittens should partake in the classes at any one time, with two instructors.

The classes allow kittens to explore novel environments, learn to accept other kittens, play with toys and develop confidence in new surroundings. Hand-raised kittens or kittens from small litters appear to benefit especially from these social interactions.

The classes also aim to teach owners about normal feline behaviour so that behaviours that may be problematic are prevented, or at least understood. The classes focus on how to interact appropriately and play with a kitten.

### Class structure

The structure of kitten classes should be tailored to suit each individual veterinary practice and the aim should be to recruit the kittens at the time of their first visit. Kitten Kindy® classes are generally run for 1 hour a week and the course is conducted over 2–3 weeks. They can also be conducted over one night but this does not allow any follow-up except over the phone. Owners of cats over 14 weeks of age should be encouraged to attend, but without their cat; this way they too can learn about feline behaviour.

Kittens need to learn in a safe unthreatening environment. They are not small puppies and, although the basic principles are the same, there are some important differences. Cats communicate differently and their socialization period ends earlier than that of dogs. Many are also less food motivated and it may be necessary to find other rewards. Although some kittens respond well to food (especially treats rather than their normal food) and praise, others are more motivated by a game such as hide-and-seek.

The rewards must be varied, as some kittens are very timid and may not be used to eating from the hand. Kittens can also appear to be very fussy about their food and owners need to understand that cats are careful about what they ingest. Small tasty treats such as dehydrated liver, barbecued chicken, cheese, raw minced meat or yeast extract spread (e.g. Vegemite) can all work well as rewards. It helps to start teaching any exercises when the kitten is most responsive, for example just before a meal. As kittens have short concentration spans each session must be fun and should be kept short.

### Introductory class

Each class should be about one hour in length and ideally the first class is 'kitten free'. This allows people to concentrate without distraction. It allows everyone in the group to meet each other and the person running the class can give a formal or informal presentation to set the scene. Owners' questions can be answered and cover common behaviours that may be problematic to them.

Explaining the principles of encouraging appropriate behaviours (reward appropriate behaviour and ignore inappropriate behaviour) is an important part of the education process. Handouts covering the problems that have been discussed, such as litter training, biting and scratching, should be distributed. Many practices have developed their own handouts or use or adapt the many that appear in textbooks.

### Kitten class one

Kittens should arrive in cat carriers or cages and owners should not let them out until asked by the class instructor. In class one, owners can be shown how to handle kittens appropriately and how to massage them to relax them. Kittens need to learn to accept the attention that people want to give them, such as being picked up, stroked or patted for long periods of time, and how to play appropriately. They can be taught to come and sit on cue, using food rewards and praise.

Owners need to be taught that cats will behave like cats. In many multi-cat households, although the cats may accept living together they may not be part of a bonded group. This means providing separate places for the cats to eat, rest, play and eliminate. Cats do not share and they do not queue. When they want to eliminate, they want to do it immediately. This means providing enough litter trays for the number of cats (and one to spare), as they will not wait until a tray is free.

### Kitten class two

In this class owners can be shown how to groom their kitten, give medications, trim the nails and check the ears (Figure 7.2). Kittens can also be taught to walk on a lead or accept a harness.

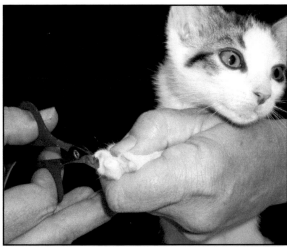

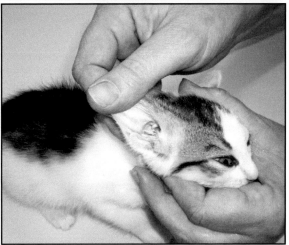

7.2 Kitten classes should teach the owner how to check a kitten's ears and trim its nails.

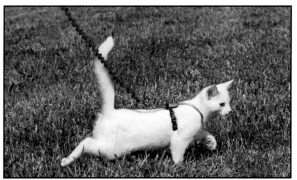

7.3 A kitten can be trained to walk in a harness. (Premier's "Come With Me Kitty™" harness and bungee leash, courtesy of Premier Pet Products.)

Many owners need to be taught how to play appropriately with their kitten and not to use human body parts (hands, fingers, feet and toes) as toys. Suitable toys should be available to demonstrate their use during the class.

A 'graduation' ceremony with a certificate can complete the class.

## Topics to cover

Many behavioural and medical issues can be discussed during kitten classes. The emphasis should be on preventive medicine (see Chapter 9).

Behavioural topics such as litter training should be covered, as well as how to prevent problem behaviours from developing. Topics that could be discussed include urine spraying, scratching furniture, appropriate play behaviour and dealing with aggressive behaviours. Owners can be helped to recognize normal body language and when the cat is feeling happy or approachable or when it should be left alone. Kitten owners find explanations of cat body language, cat communication and feline senses fascinating.

As the demographics of society are changing, meeting the needs of indoor cats is also an important topic. This may include training a kitten to walk in a harness (Figure 7.3) or creating appropriate and safe outdoor enclosures for cats.

## Kitten problem behaviours

The most common complaints that owners have with their kittens usually reflect the fact that they do not understand normal feline behaviour or have misconceptions about how a cat should behave.

### Exuberant play

There are several types of play recognized in kittens, such as social play, object play and locomotory play (see **client handout**). It is possible and probable that these may each have separate motivations, different developmental courses and different evolutionary origins. Play may have more than one function.

Feline play begins at around 3 weeks of age, generally at the beginning of the weaning process. It starts as gentle pawing, then progresses to biting, chasing and rolling as coordination improves. Social play increases from 4 to 11 weeks of age and then starts to decline.

A classic sign of play is the arched back and tail (out and down). Play often begins with a pounce and ends with the chase. Kittens may face off, bat each other, stand on their hind legs and leap. Kittens generally have four play periods per day and spend up to an hour a day playing by the time they are 9 weeks of age (Robinson, 1992). Male kittens appear to play more with objects than do female kittens with no male littermates. Solitary play declines by 4 months of age (Bradshaw, 1992).

Cats, especially as young kittens, appear to have boundless energy. However, these energetic periods are limited to about 9% of the day; they tend to be short and aerobic and are interspersed with long periods of rest. Unfortunately these energetic periods do not always coincide with when owners have the time or inclination to interact with their kittens. Owners need to encourage appropriate play and provide appropriate outlets for this energy.

### Toys

Toys that move can help to redirect exuberant play but games should never involve the use of human body parts (hands, fingers, toes). Toys that encourage the kitten to chase, run, stalk and pounce should always be on the end of poles and dangle freely to avoid inflicting damage on owners (Figure 7.4).

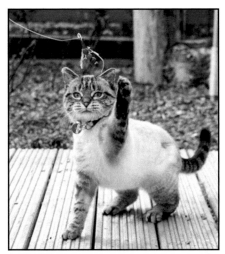

**7.4** Moveable toys should dangle freely to avoid damage to the holder. (Courtesy of D. Mills.)

There are many commercial toys available and some will be more interesting or appealing to the owner than the cat. Commercially available toys can provide stimulation, but simple toys such as hair scrunchies, paper bags and cardboard boxes can keep many kittens occupied and happy for hours.

Toys should be changed regularly, even daily, to maintain interest. Although it may appear that a cat loses interest, re-presentation of the same toy 5 minutes later may result in the resumption of play. For safety, toys need to be checked regularly for loose parts and damage.

### Climbing
Cats often appear to prefer vertical space over horizontal space (see Chapter 4). For many cats this may mean providing more places to climb up to rather than lots of room to run around. This vertical space requirement seems to increase with the number of cats in the household.

Kittens should be provided with suitable things to climb, such as posts or shelving (Figure 7.5). They also need places to hide and resting places up high. However, these places should have easily accessible escape routes in multi-cat households.

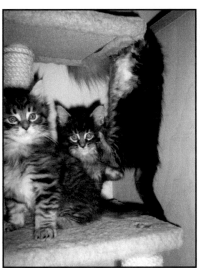

**7.5** Kittens on a climbing tower.

Indoor cats generally require more active enrichment, which means more thought needs to go into how to provide them with sufficient mental as well as physical stimulation (see Chapter 4).

### Play-related aggression
Play-related aggression behaviour is likely to be associated with owner-facilitated learning, orphaning, early weaning or hand raising and absence of appropriate stimuli during the sensitive period for modulating responses. In cats, social play is seen between 4 and 12 weeks of age and is replaced by social fighting by 14 weeks of age. The kitten may stalk, chase, pounce and lie in wait for people passing by and then bite as well as scratch. The targets may be moving objects, people or another cat, especially an older one, in the household.

It is sometimes difficult to recognize play-related aggression, as some cats play more roughly than others and do not retract their claws when they swat. It is important to differentiate between play-related aggression and aggression that has another basis, such as fear (see Chapter 19 for more information).

Because play is a normal part of the kitten repertoire, the aim is to redirect unacceptable aggressive play behaviour to more suitable objects rather than trying to stop the behaviour completely. Providing the cat with appropriate toys is helpful, but the toys need to be changed at regular intervals for the cat to maintain interest. Additionally, the cat may first need to be taught how to play, and then encouraged to play with toys. Often the behaviour occurs at predictable times and locations and if these are noted other activities can be substituted at those times and places to encourage a different activity.

Rough play, especially using hands or other body parts, should be discouraged. Whenever the cat plays in this manner, play should be interrupted or suspended and the cat's attention should be directed to appropriate toys instead.

Any punishment, such as smacking, or squirting the cat with a water pistol, may actually encourage the behaviour and increase the cat's arousal. Punishment should be avoided as it may lead to other problems, such as fear aggression.

Providing the cat with a regular routine that involves interactive playtime involving toys 2–3 times daily for 5–10 minutes is important to provide a natural outlet for the behaviour. A second kitten, preferably one that is not very young, may also help to teach more appropriate play behaviour.

### Scratching
Scratching is a normal behaviour in cats. They scratch to communicate with each other and use the marks as both visual and scent markers. To prevent problems with inappropriate scratching, a kitten should be taught to use and have access to a suitable scratching post.

The post should be covered with a suitable material (loose weave like hessian or carpet). Some cats like to scratch on vertical surfaces, others on horizontal surfaces (see Chapter 4), but the kitten or cat has to be able to rip and shred the material. It should not be replaced when it is worn and torn as this may discourage the cat from using the post. At least some of the old material should be left attached to the scratching post or to the new scratching post to attract the cat to the area.

The scratching post should be stable, so that it will not fall over or rock while it is being used, and tall enough for the cat to stretch out fully. Attaching toys on strings can make it more interesting. Some cats are attracted to the post if catnip is used but this will depend on the individual cat. A post may need to be changed to accommodate the increasing size as a kitten grows. If several cats share a home, then several posts in several locations should be provided.

The scratching post should be placed where the cat will use it, usually a prominent area or directly in front of where the cat has already started to scratch. Unacceptable areas that have previously been scratched need to be covered so that the cat no longer has access to the area. Over time the scratching post can gradually be moved to another spot.

Empty cardboard boxes can be used as scratching areas and also make good toys for kittens.

## Litterbox problems

Cats are usually considered clean creatures and most cats take to using a litterbox easily. The following suggestions will help to prevent problems (see also **client handout**).

- Place the litterbox somewhere that is easily accessible for the kitten. That means not in a downstairs bathroom if the kitten spends most of the day upstairs.
- Place the box away from the kitten's food (no one likes to eat near the toilet).
- Place the box in a quiet area away from busy passageways or other traffic areas.
- Clean the box daily. Cats do not like dirty toilets any more than humans. This is especially important for covered boxes.
- Offer the kitten a selection of different litters, then provide the one that is most frequently used.
- Place the kitten in the litterbox after it has eaten. Most kittens want to empty their bowels and bladder within 30 minutes of eating.
- Schedule feeding at set times.
- Reward the kitten after it has eliminated in the litterbox. A tasty treat with praise can be an effective reward.
- If there is more than one cat in the household, the rule of thumb is one litterbox per cat and one extra. Each box should be in a different location. If the boxes are side by side in the same room, this can lead to one cat 'guarding' them so that the other cats do not have easy access.
- Any 'accident' should be cleaned with warm water and enzymatic washing powder and not ammonia-based disinfectants.

## Aggression when patted or handled

Owners find it very distressing when their kitten suddenly bites or scratches after tactile stimulation of variable duration. The kitten may swipe or bite if the petting stops, or if the stroking is carried out for a prolonged period. The cat may stiffen, or lash with the tail, and may or may not give a warning bite while being patted. Some cats appear to be content just sitting on a lap as long as no stroking or other tactile stimulation occurs. Owners are most commonly bitten or scratched on the hands and arms in these situations.

Kittens need to be taught to accept being stroked or patted, as prolonged periods of social grooming are not part of a cat's normal social interactions. Kittens may be taught gradually to tolerate longer periods of stroking but it takes time and patience. Some never learn to tolerate patting and this needs to be explained to owners. It is also important to teach owners how to stroke or pat cats in an appropriate way without over-stimulating them. Owners find it difficult to comprehend that some cats actually solicit attention and then attack when it is given. In many cases the cat may want to be nearby, but does not want to be stroked.

If the kitten can accept a short period of stimulation of, say, 3 minutes but not 4 minutes, it should be stroked slowly for only 2 minutes. Using a brush rather than a hand can be useful initially. The period of stroking should always be below the kitten's current threshold for non-tolerance of stimulation and it should be rewarded with food treats or play. The time can be increased gradually over a period of days or weeks until the kitten tolerates longer and longer periods. The stroking should always be stopped before the kitten shows signs of excessive arousal. These sessions should be conducted at a predictable time each day.

Owners should never punish a cat that is aggressive when patted or handled as this may lead to more aggression, since the animal is already aroused and over-stimulated. In the author's experience the synthetic analogue of a feline facial pheromone (see Chapter 21) has been useful in some cases when sprayed on the owner's hands prior to handling the cat.

## Fear/anxiety-related aggression

Cats learn to be fearful of certain situations, especially if they have had a bad experience (e.g. rough handling, noises, smells at veterinary hospitals) with no opportunity to escape. Inadequate or lack of socialization and handling prior to 12 weeks of age may contribute to the cat's responses to people. Inadequate or lack of socialization with other cats early in life may contribute to the cat's responses to other cats.

Some kittens are fearful of people, places, other cats, or various stimuli such as noises or odours. The aggressive behaviour may be a combination of offence and defence (see Chapter 19). The kitten will initially attempt to avoid the stimulus (if that is an option) and give many warning signals such as hissing, spitting, growling, piloerection, or flattening its ears against the head and showing a low or crouched body position (see Chapter 4). Pupillary dilatation is common. It may try to flee or attack, depending on the circumstances. Aggression is usually the last resort but is often very violent and the behaviour may become learnt.

The first step is to teach the kitten to be calm and relaxed. This can be done by offering it a tasty treat such as vegemite, chicken, or dehydrated liver. If the kitten eats, it is usually a good indication that it is not too anxious. While the kitten is eating, the fear stimulus (e.g. a person) is gradually introduced at a distance. The initial distance should be great enough not to cause any fearful response from the kitten. If the kitten continues to take food, the person may approach the kitten very slowly. The time frame for the gradual approach may vary from days to months, depending on the severity of the problem. The kitten should not be forced to interact in any way, as that would exacerbate the fear. Punishment or forced restraint would aggravate the situation and should be avoided: it may lead to an increase in anxiety and impede learning.

The synthetic analogue of feline pheromone, Feliway®, either as a spray or in a diffuser, may also be beneficial and can be used at home as well as in the veterinary hospital. Both Feliway® and Felifriend® (see Chapter 21) can be sprayed on to wrists and hands prior to handling to help to decrease arousal levels.

## Introducing a new kitten

Owners often find the best way to introduce a new kitten is time consuming and want to rush the process.

### Households with resident cats
When introducing a new kitten into a household with resident cats, the owners should always keep in mind that this introduction is not the choice of any of the cats – it is the owner's choice. The cats do not have a say about whether another cat will come into the household or which cat. Introductions should be slow and supervised (for details, see Chapter 4 and the **client handout**). Several Feliway® diffusers (see Chapter 21) should be dispersed around the house for about a week before the introduction of the new kitten.

Owners should be informed that, although most cats can learn to tolerate another cat in their environment, they may never actually develop a close relationship where allogrooming (mutual grooming) occurs. Owners should watch the interactions of an older cat and kitten: if one of them is actively avoiding the other or if hissing or spitting occurs, they should be separated and the integration process started again more slowly. In some cases it may be necessary to have some time of separation that allows the older cat to rest undisturbed. In other situations, having the kitten wear a quick-release cat collar with a large bell on it will keep the older cat aware of the kitten's location and allow avoidance if wanted. Cats should never be punished for exhibiting aggressive or fearful behaviour around the other cat as that may lead to an increase in the undesirable behaviours.

Even when cats have successfully integrated, it is important that each cat has a separate station for eating, drinking, sleeping and eliminating so that problems do not arise.

### Households with children
The cardinal rule is never to leave young children alone with any pet. Adult supervision of all children under 6 years of age with pets means one adult per child and one adult per pet. This applies regardless of whether the pet is a puppy or a kitten, as accidents with either can occur in a split second. Young kittens can be easily frightened as well as accidentally injured.

When introducing a kitten into a household with children, the advice given above about introducing a kitten to a home with other cats can provide a useful basis.

It is ideal to choose a kitten that has already had friendly experiences with children, such as in the breeder's home. (If adopting an older cat, it is important to gain as much information about the cat's life as possible and assess the response of an older cat to children before accepting it into the home.)

Prior to the arrival of the kitten, children should understand that it is a living and feeling animal and not a toy. It can be beneficial for children to have positive supervised socialization experiences with other cats before the new kitten is brought home. The kitten should always be treated gently and quietly. The child should be praised for being involved and demonstrating the correct actions; and the kitten should be praised for being calm and compliant.

Periods of interaction should be relatively short and can be interactive (play) or passive (stroking). All interactions should occur when the kitten is awake and children should be taught not disturb kittens that are resting.

Children should be taught how to stroke a kitten and, depending on the age of the child, this may initially involve modelling of the behaviour. This can be accomplished by an adult first demonstrating the behaviour and then holding the child's hand while gently stroking. The kitten should be rewarded for staying calm and relaxed when being stroked. A tasty treat can be used as well as quiet praise.

It should not be assumed that, once the behaviour has been demonstrated, the child will remember the correct order, appropriate place to pat the kitten or action required. The skill may need a longer period of assistance before the child is fully able to demonstrate it. Only once the child begins consistently to stroke the kitten correctly, and the kitten is calm and relaxed with the contact, may the parent modelling be gradually withdrawn, but the child's and kitten's interactions should always be closely supervised.

Young children need constant and close supervision when in contact with pets. They do not have the skills or understanding of how to interact appropriately with a pet. The child may have no concept of the pain they may be inflicting on a pet when they handle it roughly and they may not be able to recognize the early signs of concern or aggression from the cat, such as tail flicking or stiffening.

## References and further reading

American Association of Feline Practitioners (2004) *Feline Behavior Guidelines*. AAFP, Hilsborough, New Jersey [obtainable online from www.aafponline.org]

Australian Companion Animal Council (2006) *BIS Shrapnel report: Contribution of the Pet Care Industry to the Australian Economy, 6th edn.* ACAC, Sydney

Beaver BV (2003) *Feline Behavior: a Guide for Veterinarians.* WB Saunders, Philadelphia

Bowen J and Heath S (2005) *Behaviour Problems in Small Animals: Practical Advice for the Veterinary Team.* Elsevier Saunders, Edinburgh

Bradshaw JWS (1992) *The Behaviour of the Domestic Cat.* CAB International, Wallingford

Houpt KA (1998) *Domestic Animal Behavior, 3rd edn.* Iowa State University Press, Ames, Iowa

Landsberg G, Hunthausen W and Ackerman L (2003) *Handbook of Behaviour Problems of the Dog and Cat.* Butterworth-Heinemann, Oxford

Martin P and Bateson P (1988) Behavioural development in the cat. In: *The Domestic Cat: the Biology of its Behaviour*, ed. DC Turner and P Bateson, pp. 9–22. Cambridge University Press, Cambridge

Overall KL (1997) *Clinical Behavioral Medicine for Small Animals.* Mosby, St Louis, Missouri

Robinson I (1992) Behavioural development of the cat. In: *The Waltham Book of Dog and Cat Behaviour*, ed. C Thorne, pp. 53–64. Pergamon Press, Oxford

Salman M, Hutchison J, Ruch-Gaille R *et al.* (2000) Behavioral reasons for relinquishment of dogs and cats to 12 shelters. *Journal of Applied Animal Welfare Science* **3**, 93–106

Seksel K (2001) *Training Your Cat.* Hyland House, Flemington, Melbourne, Australia

Seksel K (2004) Prevention of future behaviour problems: kitten classes. *European Journal of Companion Animal Practice* **14**, 101–104

Seksel K (2008) Preventing behavior problems in puppies and kittens. *Veterinary Clinics of North America: Small Animal Practice* **38**, 971–982

## Client handouts (bsavalibrary.com/behaviour_leaflets)

- Avoiding aggression in cats
- Avoiding house soiling by cats
- Avoiding urine marking by cats
- Environmental enrichment for cats in animal shelters
- Feline behaviour questionnaire
- Handling exercises for puppies and kittens
- Introducing a new cat into the household
- Litterbox training
- Pet selection questionnaire
- Playing with your kitten
- Request for information on problem behaviours
- Taking your cat in the car
- Treating a fear of car journeys using desensitization and counter-conditioning
- Treating a fear of the veterinary clinic using desensitization and counter-conditioning
- What your cat needs
- What your cat needs: multi-cat households

# 8

# Management problems in dogs

## Ellen Lindell

## Introduction

Dogs are usually adopted to improve the wellbeing of the people in the household. Responsible dog owners begin to train their puppies soon after they are adopted. Yet despite training, as dogs mature they often exhibit behaviours that, albeit normal, are deemed to be socially unacceptable. Although it is appropriate to reassure the client that a particular behaviour is normal, the behaviour should be addressed if the client is concerned.

Training guidelines are widely available in the form of books, DVDs, television programmes and on the internet. This information is of necessity general in nature. The relationship that veterinary practices have with their clients and patients allows them to offer personalized information and prescribe safe, effective treatment plans. In some cases, an unacceptable behaviour may be eliminated entirely. Other innate behaviours will be difficult to modify, but can still be managed.

## Evaluation of the patient

### History
Dogs mature socially, and behaviour problems develop, during the year that follows the final puppy visit. A juvenile behavioural wellness examination should be scheduled specifically for 12–18-month-old dogs that are physically healthy.

Using a screening checklist (see e.g. **client handout**), clients may tick any of the behaviours that they would like to discuss. If indicated, an in-depth behavioural consultation can be scheduled. Even though a problem might appear to be related to management or training, it is important to collect a behavioural history and to screen for underlying anxiety and aggression.

Some clients tolerate mild aggression. It is the responsibility of the veterinary surgeon to counsel clients regarding the implications of aggressive behaviour, and to emphasize the need to diagnose, evaluate and treat this potentially serious condition.

### Diagnosis
The client complaint combined with information gained through passive observation will be used to confirm a diagnosis of normal but undesirable behaviour. Anxious dogs may be very active or very subdued and it is important to identify any postures that suggest fear or aggression (see Chapter 2).

The owner's response to any unacceptable behaviour should be noted. Owners are often not aware that their gestures, including pushing or scolding, can actually reinforce undesirable behaviour.

Before assigning a behavioural diagnosis, a physical examination should be done to confirm that there is no medical basis for the problem behaviour.

## Treatment

The behaviours described in the following sections are considered to be normal canine behaviours. Therefore the use of psychotropic medication is generally not indicated. The diagnosis must be reconsidered if an appropriately applied behavioural and environmental modification protocol does not result in adequate control.

An effective treatment plan should emphasize preventing access to the unacceptable behaviour while teaching and rewarding appropriate behaviour (see Chapter 5). For most situations, positive punishment techniques will not be emphasized. In particular, punishment-based techniques may be contraindicated in a patient that has been diagnosed with an anxiety-based condition, as even mild corrections can exacerbate anxiety.

Treatment recommendations presented in this chapter may need to be adjusted or eliminated in the face of aggression. For example, it might not be possible for a client to apply a head halter safely if a dog behaves aggressively during handling (see Chapter 17 for advice on this matter).

## Prognosis

The problematic behaviours discussed in this chapter could be virtually eliminated through stringent attention to management. In theory, it is possible to deny a dog the opportunity to engage in these behaviours. In practice, however, owners may find it difficult or tiresome to follow through with the necessary preventive measures. The outcome of a case, therefore, depends largely on owner tolerance and compliance.

## Follow-up for management problems

Owners should be encouraged to maintain a behavioural diary to document progress. A table format is ideal (Figure 8.1).

Clients should generally be contacted by the practice (not necessarily the consulting clinician) in 1 week to address any technical questions and to be reminded that any increase in the problem behaviour is likely to be temporary.

A recheck visit should be scheduled for week 2 or 3 to review the behavioural diary. There should be some steady improvement at this point. If not, the behaviour modification protocol should be reviewed to confirm that the owner has been able to follow treatment recommendations as outlined. It is equally important to determine that the techniques are being applied at an appropriate pace. Finally, the diagnosis should be reconsidered.

At a 6–8-week recheck, progress should be noticeable if compliance has been good. The need for long-term management should be discussed. Monthly rechecks should be planned until the client is satisfied with the resolution.

## Problems of obedience

See also Chapter 5 for obedience training.

## Poor response to commands

People expect their dogs to obey basic commands. A lack of response can be frustrating and even dangerous, particularly when a dog does not come when called.

### Evaluation

When a client complains that their dog is not obedient, a physical examination should be done. A dog cannot obey unless it is physically able to perceive and process a command. The dog should be assessed for evidence of hearing impairment or visual deficits. It should be noticed whether the dog is neurologically appropriate as it moves about the examination room. It is worth asking about the dog's ease of housetraining. Difficulty in learning this basic task may reflect a central nervous system abnormality such as hydrocephalus. Dogs that have difficulty with a specific demand should be assessed for their physical ability to complete the required action: for example, a dog that does not sit readily may have hip pain.

If physical findings are within normal limits, the owner should be asked to demonstrate the dog's response to two or three basic commands (Figure 8.2). The delivery of the commands as well as the dog's reaction should be observed. If a dog appears fearful, the history should be reviewed for signs of underlying anxiety.

|  | No. of items stolen | Owner response | Task 1: Settle exercises – length of session | Task 2: Leash time – enforced supervision | Comment (change routine/ overall mood) | Any new behavioural concerns? (aggression, barking) |
|---|---|---|---|---|---|---|
| Monday |  |  |  |  |  |  |
| Tuesday |  |  |  |  |  |  |
| Wednesday |  |  |  |  |  |  |
| Thursday |  |  |  |  |  |  |
| Friday |  |  |  |  |  |  |

**8.1** Sample behavioural diary for a dog that steals items.

| Appropriate | | Inappropriate | | |
|---|---|---|---|---|
| *Delivery* | *Response* | *Delivery* | *Response* | *Interpretation of response* |
| Calm Friendly tone Moderate volume | Relaxed Ears forward Watches owner | Physically forces dog Harsh tone Loud volume | Cowers Tail tuck Ears back Backs away Averts gaze | Fearful – assess delivery of commands |
| Clear discreet cue | Correct response to first cue Single response per cue | Vague cue | Incorrect response Multiple responses to single cue | Dog does not understand command Communication or reinforcement error |

**8.2** Evaluation of the delivery and response to basic commands.

### Treatment

***Attention:*** Owners should be instructed to attract their dog's attention before giving a command. Examples include squeaking a toy, rattling a treat bag, or tapping on the floor. Shouting a command at the dog is not an appropriate way to gain attention.

Owners may have been advised to give a command once and then physically force the dog to obey. Training techniques that rely on coercion can be problematic for both owners and their pets. Many dogs wait for physical prompts and do not respond on their own. Fearful dogs may shy away or even snap when physically confronted.

It should be noted that dogs suffering from anxiety might have difficulty attending to commands. Anxiety should be managed as a priority, so that obedience/command training can be successful.

***Comprehension and cues:*** A dog cannot obey unless it understands the meaning of the command as issued. Dogs follow body language and some may not recognize a verbal command that is given without visual cues. The subtle body language used when luring a dog with food can be a salient cue for many dogs.

***Use of reinforcers:*** Both the value and the timing of the reinforcer affect learning. A dog may not perform a difficult task for a low-value reward. Responsiveness is likely to be poor if rewards are not presented at the time that the task is completed.

Clients often express a desire to 'wean' their dogs from treats. To maintain excellent performance, the dog does not need to be weaned from food rewards. Rather, the frequency of the reward needs to be adjusted. (See Chapter 5 for more information on learning and training protocols.)

***Context:*** Dogs are usually taught basic commands in specific contexts. For training to progress, owners should teach their dogs to respond while the context varies. The dog that obeys commands in a quiet training arena will not necessarily be compliant when running in the park.

As the context changes, the frequency and value of the reward may also need to be adjusted until a consistent high level of performance has been attained in that new context. Then the frequency of the reward or the value may be lowered.

***An essential command – the recall:*** Clients commonly complain that their dog does not come when called. They are appropriately concerned knowing that a failure to respond to this important command could jeopardize their dog's life. There are several explanations for a dog's poor recall response (see Chapter 5 for terms used below).

- Inadvertent positive reinforcement.
  - The dog that ignores the 'come' command may gain an opportunity to do something more pleasurable, such as pursue a squirrel. It then has a chance to play 'tag' as its owner attempts to capture the dog.

- Inadvertent punishment.
  - When a dog obeys only to be removed from the play arena, it will be less eager to respond in the future. Similarly, the dog that is routinely called so that its owner may leave for work soon learns that responsiveness leads to the unpleasant consequence of being left alone. To avoid this effect, whenever a dog responds to the 'come' command it should receive a short period of play or training before being brought indoors.
- Incomplete training.
  - Lead restraint is essential until the dog reliably comes when called.

See **client handout** for tips on teaching the recall.

## Pulling on the lead

When a client complains that their dog is pulling, it is important to enquire about the dog's posture. A dog that is pulling forward aggressively requires a different treatment than a dog that is enthusiastic but friendly.

It is tempting to respond to a dog's forward pull by tugging back on the lead. Dogs nearly always pull harder in response to this resistance, especially if they continue to move forward. Extendible leads may further exacerbate pulling problems. The dog that expects to explore at will may resist being reined in. The goal should be a controlled loose lead walk without pulling.

Chapter 5 (Example 8) explains the risk of inadvertent reinforcement when a dog is scolded and its lead jerked because the owner misinterprets the dog's interest in an approaching person or another dog, anticipating aggression when the dog's intention might in fact be playful.

### Treatment

Acute management includes the use of halters and harnesses. Management in the long term includes positive reinforcement or negative or positive punishment.

***Halters and harnesses:*** In many situations immediate resolution of pulling can usually be accomplished through the use of devices that mechanically prevent pulling. A head halter offers excellent control (Figure 8.3a).

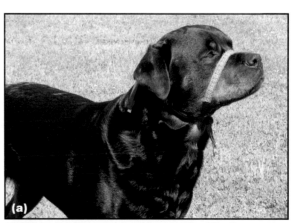

**8.3** **(a)** Dog wearing a head halter (Gentle Leader®). (continues) ▶

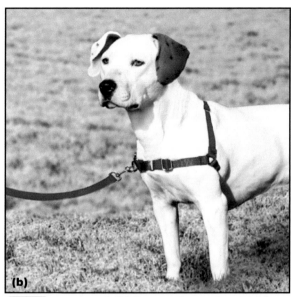

**8.3** (continued) **(b)** Dog wearing an Easy Walk® harness. (Courtesy of Premier Pet Products.)

Another useful tool is a body harness designed specifically to reduce pulling (Figure 8.3b). Harnesses are safe, well tolerated and particularly suitable for dogs with medical conditions that preclude the use of neck collars. With the proper use of a head halter or control harness, improvement in the dog's behaviour while walking on a lead should be very rapid.

*Behaviour modification:* For owners who prefer not to use a halter or harness indefinitely, a behaviour modification strategy can be used. During training, the owner should refrain from tugging or snapping the lead. It is helpful to think of the lead as a safety net that serves to prevent the dog from slipping away.

- Positive reinforcement: come on back.
  - This exercise may be practised even on an extendible lead. Several times on each walk, without pulling on the lead, the owner should call the dog, reward it with some delicious treats or a gentle tug on a toy, and then release the dog to again sniff and explore.
- Negative punishment: going nowhere.
  - This is a time-consuming but effective technique. The owner should stop walking every time the dog begins to pull. The dog therefore learns that the consequence of pulling is the loss of the walk or of forward movement. It is helpful to offer a cue immediately before halting. The cue should be a novel sound or word (cluck or 'oops') that is not aversive on its own. The neutral cue will signal to the dog that the walk is about to end.
  - As a practical measure, the negative punishment protocol may be combined with positive reinforcement of basic commands. When the owner needs to move on due to time constraints, a 'heel' command may be used. Properly taught, this command signals the dog to walk beside its handler while

maintaining an attentive posture. During the 'working' phase of the walk, there should be no sniffing or exploring.
- Positive punishment: a word of caution.
  - Many owners purchase chain or prong-style choke collars hoping that collar corrections will reduce pulling. A punishment-based technique can exacerbate underlying aggression and cause physical injury, such as Horner's syndrome. If a dog is snapped by a collar each time it pulls toward a person, it may behave more aggressively as it associates the approach of the person with the discomfort of a collar snap. The continued use of corrective techniques without a behavioural change is an indication that the pet has not learned the task desired.

> **BSAVA is opposed to the use of training aids that administer pain and to those that use an electric current to help control behaviour, in the absence of good evidence that these devices do not also cause pain.**

### Prognosis and follow-up
The prognosis for resolving problems related to obedience is very good.

A 1-week follow-up call can serve to answer any specific questions about the treatment recommendations. The owner should be invited back 2–3 weeks later to re-evaluate their delivery of commands and the dog's responsiveness.

Considerable skill is required to apply reinforcers appropriately. Many clients will benefit from the services of a professional obedience trainer. It is important to meet and observe local trainers so that clients can be referred to them with comfort and confidence.

### Prevention
Owners should be encouraged to pursue obedience training beyond basic puppy class. Continued education fosters communication between owners and their dogs, thereby improving responsiveness.

## Problems of reactivity

Enthusiastic responses may be welcomed as newly adopted dogs adjust to the household. Puppies are routinely petted even when they greet people by jumping up. Owners often respond to a puppy's bark by politely asking 'what would you like?' Rewarded behaviours are not only repeated but may be exhibited with increased intensity as the rewards are delivered on an inconsistent, i.e. intermittent, basis.

### Jumping on people
As a dog grows larger, or when it is muddy, jumping up is no longer acceptable. Commonly recommended strategies such as kneeing, pushing or shouting often result in increased enthusiasm on the part of the dog. Many dogs behave as though physical intervention is a form of play.

When an owner complains that a dog is jumping up on visitors, it is important to be sure that the behaviour represents excitement rather than a negative emotional response such as fear or aggression. Separation-related anxiety should be ruled out if the history suggests that jumping on family members is part of an exaggerated greeting.

### Treatment

Acute management includes physical restraint (collar-and-lead, halter or harness). Long-term management includes counter-commanding and withdrawal strategies.

*Lead restraint:* Immediate resolution of jumping up can often be accomplished through lead restraint. If the dog is wearing a buckle collar or standard harness, just enough tension should be applied to stop the dog's upward motion.

A head halter can improve control still further and should be recommended in households with young children, infirm or elderly adults, or very large dogs. With the head halter in place, gentle pressure on the lead will prevent the dog from jumping up and return its focus to the handler.

*Behaviour modification:* Although lead restraint may be continued indefinitely, a behaviour modification protocol can be designed to reduce the dog's tendency to jump up in the first place.

- Counter-commanding.
  - This technique involves asking the dog to perform a behaviour that is incompatible with jumping up. For example, the dog could be asked to 'sit' before it is petted. During greetings, a clearly visible treat or toy can be held in front of the dog to attract its attention and improve its response to the 'sit' command. The reward is given as soon as the dog sits.
- Withdrawal.
  - An alternative strategy for treatment of jumping up is to remove reinforcement by ignoring the dog until it is calm. This technique should only be used by physically fit adults, or when treating young puppies and small dogs. The target of the jumping behaviour should be silent and still, fold their arms, and look away until jumping ceases.
  - Once the dog has stopped jumping it can receive positive reinforcement by being petted. If the dog again jumps up as the person reaches to pet it, the person should withdraw quietly and refrain from petting until the dog settles.
  - Owners should be advised that this technique can result in a temporary increase in the intensity of the jumping as the behaviour is extinguished.

*Refractory cases:* Some dogs are so excited about greeting a person that they cannot pay attention to any treat or command. These patients can benefit from a desensitization and counter-conditioning (DSCC) strategy (see Chapter 5) that gradually reduces their arousal level.

Before beginning the desensitization process, owners should practise the counter-conditioning strategy in the absence of the stimulus. Sit–stay or down–stay exercises are well suited to this process (see **client handouts**). Once the dog can stay reliably, a 'place' (see **client handout**) should be set up several feet away from the entrance. At this increased distance, it will be easier for the dog to stay while people enter.

An excellent tool for working through this protocol is a device that automatically rewards the dog for sitting (or lying down) quietly at a designated location and also allows the owner to dispense treats remotely (Figure 8.4). Initially, a gate or tether should be used so that the dog does not leave the area and rush to the door.

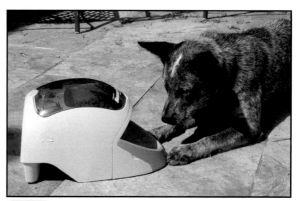

**8.4** Dog lying quietly in front of a Manners Minder™ remote treat dispenser.

Once guests have settled and the dog is sitting quietly, it may be led to meet the visitors. With its arousal level down, the dog should be able to sit for its greeting.

### Prognosis and follow-up

The prognosis for controlling jumping up is very good. Owners should be consistent. If the dog is intermittently invited to jump up, then the behaviour will continue indefinitely.

Owners should be called after 1 week to address any questions or concerns about the treatment plan. A recheck visit might be scheduled after 2–3 weeks. During this visit, staff members can knock and enter the consulting room to simulate a greeting.

### Prevention

Jumping up can easily be prevented by teaching dogs to sit for their privileges.

## Barking

Normal dogs bark for many different reasons and in most cases barking serves as a form of communication. The behaviour increases through social facilitation and owner reinforcement.

### Evaluation

When an owner expresses concern that their dog is barking excessively, it is important to establish a diagnosis. Barking is a clinical sign associated with several serious behaviour problems (Figure 8.5).

| Cause | Relevant history | Character of bark |
|---|---|---|
| Separation-related anxiety | Owner absent | Monotonic and perhaps high pitched |
| Compulsive behaviour | No clear trigger | Repetitive; monotonic |
| Territorial/fear-based aggression | External trigger – usually person or animal | High arousal; difficult to interrupt, lower pitched perhaps with growling |
| Noise phobia | External trigger Prior history of fear | High arousal; fast pitched barking |
| Cognitive decline | Senior dog Concurrent behaviour changes | Monotonic |

**8.5** Some causes of barking, with underlying pathology.

If there is no behavioural pathology, barking may be treated as a normal but sometimes unacceptable behaviour. It is important to learn the contexts or triggers for the patient in question. Dogs frequently bark in response to doorbells, passing people or dogs, and assorted noises. They may bark during work, play or while greeting.

When family members attempt to relax, dogs may bark in order to gain their attention. Attention-seeking behaviours and their treatment are discussed later in this chapter.

### Treatment
There are certain situations in which barking becomes an emergency. For example, a client may be threatened with eviction due to their barking dog. Unfortunately, behaviour modification to reduce barking usually takes time.

**Collars:** Automatic anti-bark collars can be useful in certain circumstances for dogs that have been assessed and that do not have an anxiety disorder or a tendency to exhibit aggressive behaviour. These devices may be effective when used for rapid relief at selective times, such as when a baby is napping, but should not be used in the long term without concomitant behaviour therapy.

The theory behind anti-bark collars is that they work by delivering an appropriately timed punishment in response to the bark. Whatever the stimulus used for punishment (whether it be a mild electric current, an ultrasonic tone or a burst of unpleasant spray such as citronella), it must be sufficiently unpleasant to the dog for it to suppress the behaviour in the long term, and so the use of any such device is not without potentially serious welfare implications. Interestingly, Juarbe-Diaz and Houpt (1996) found that citronella collars were at least as effective as electric current collars (and so probably at least as aversive) but were perceived by the owners to be more acceptable.

All anti-bark collars should initially be used with supervision, to be certain that the dog's reaction to

this mild level of punishment is appropriate and that there is no extreme fear response. Since dogs can habituate to mild punishment, anti-bark collars should be paired with a behaviour modification technique such as counter-conditioning (Wells, 2001) so that the dog learns to be silent. The owner should also understand that in many cases the dog only learns to inhibit barking while wearing the collar, but will bark when the collar is not on or may bark if the stimulus is extremely intense even while wearing the collar.

### *Behaviour modification:*

- Counter-conditioning.
  - Dogs that bark in predictable situations or in response to known triggers such as passers-by may be treated effectively by using counter-conditioning (see Chapter 5). The dog learns to respond to the stimulus in a new manner. For instance, a dog that barks to alert the family to a passer-by can learn to pick up a toy and play.
  - Dogs that are motivated by food can be taught to go to a 'place' for a treat instead of barking (see **client handout**). When a person passes the house, the dog can be sent to 'place' for a food reward. The remote-operated treat dispenser discussed in the previous section can be used to encourage the dog to lie quietly in place.
- Owner-based punishment.
  - People often yell in response to a dog's barking. Shouting is likely to arouse the already excited dog further and may increase rather than decrease the intensity of barking behaviour.
  - Many owners have tried shaking noisy coin-filled cans to interrupt barking. With proper timing and intensity of application, these cans may interrupt a bark, but they may also increase arousal and fear. In any case, they increase the noise level in an already noisy environment and are not generally recommended.
- Using a head halter to teach 'quiet'.
  - It may be helpful to fit the dog with a head halter and drag line that is worn indoors for control. When the dog attempts to bark inappropriately, it can be interrupted with a gentle tug to the lead that closes the mouth and given a verbal command such as 'quiet'. When silence is achieved, the headcollar is released and the dog is praised. Over time the dog should learn that the verbal phrase ('quiet') indicates that the mouth will be closed and the dog should become quiet on its own. In some patients the use of food rewards will enhance compliance.

### Prognosis and follow-up
The prognosis for controlling learned barking is fair to good. When owners are not available to offer the necessary reinforcement, dogs are self-rewarded

for barking. For example, dogs that bark at passing people are rewarded when the 'trespasser' leaves. To improve prognosis and perhaps improve outcome, it may be necessary in some cases to restrict access to areas that stimulate barking when the dog is at home alone.

Owners should be contacted at the end of the first week to confirm that mechanical devices are being used appropriately and to be sure that there has been no evidence of fear or aggression.

After 2–3 weeks, some reduction in barking can be expected. A recheck should be scheduled in 1 month. If improvement is not considerable by that time, the diagnosis should be reviewed to confirm that there is no behavioural pathology.

### Prevention

During wellness examinations, it is worth discreetly inquiring about barking. Barking that has not been highly reinforced may be more amenable to therapy. Since barking can reflect a number of serious behaviour problems, early identification is important.

## Excitability

It is not uncommon for owners to complain that their dogs are easily stimulated or that they just never relax. It may be challenging to distinguish those animals that are highly responsive and over-reactive, or between very active and hyperactive.

### Evaluation

Fear or anxiety can contribute to excitability and dogs with anxiety disorders may be hypervigilant. They cannot focus on the owner or the task at hand when they are scanning for danger.

Clinical hyperactivity is an uncommon condition in dogs. A diagnosis of hyperactivity should be restricted to those dogs that exhibit excessive activity despite adequate exercise. A hyperactive dog rarely rests, even in the relative absence of external stimulation. A physical examination often reveals an elevated heart rate, respiratory rate and baseline temperature.

In some cases of hyperactivity, the administration of a stimulant such as methylphenidate produces a normalization of physiological parameters as well as behavioural calming (Overall, 1997). However, this result is not always obtained and may not effectively diagnose the problem. Dietary sensitivity should be assessed in dogs that appear clinically hyperactive (see Chapter 22).

One of the features of reward-based training is that some dogs learn to offer a variety of behaviours spontaneously. Behaviours that are rewarded haphazardly can be offered at such high frequencies that the dog might be considered excitable.

It is very important to determine whether the dog's need for activity, social interaction, mental stimulation and environmental enrichment are being met on a daily basis. In some cases the environment is not providing for the pet's needs and the hyperactivity is based on attempts to fulfil those needs. In other situations, inconsistent interactions between owner and pet lead to hypervigilance and reactivity.

### Treatment

It is important to determine that the owner is providing the dog with adequate exercise.

*Physical containment:* Until behaviour modification is well underway, some form of physical containment may be needed to prevent the dog from accessing stimulating situations. For instance, many dogs will lie relatively quietly if restricted with a lead or crate. If the owner reports that the dog becomes agitated when restrained in this manner, then the presence of an underlying anxiety disorder should be considered and investigated. Confinement should not be presented as punishment. In some cases teaching the dog how to be confined comfortably or restrained may be appropriate. For some dogs the use of a headcollar or body harness indoors will facilitate calmness and increase owner control.

*Behaviour modification:* It can be helpful to ask clients to draw up a list of contexts in which they perceive that their dog becomes overly excited. A structured training session or play period can be initiated before the anticipated activity burst.

The excitable dog can benefit from learning to down–stay/settle on command (see **client handout**). A relaxation mat (Figure 8.6), crate or exercise pen provides a cue that it is time to settle. When possible, the 'settle' cue should be presented in anticipation of a stimulating situation. If the dog is already excited, the owner should gain its attention and then ask it to lie down. Although a lure may be needed initially, dogs that have routinely practised down–stay/settle exercises readily assume that position.

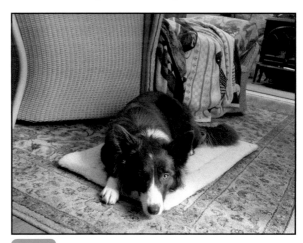

**8.6** Relaxing on a 'settle' mat.

It is essential that the pet's daily needs for exercise, play, social interaction and mental stimulation have been met prior to asking the pet to settle and stay. Consistent interactions and clear expectations for how these things are obtained should also be put in place.

### Prognosis and follow-up

The prognosis for controlling excitable behaviour may only be fair to good. Certain breeds and certain individuals are more energetic, responsive or reactive than others. Owner expectations may not be compatible with their dog's disposition. In some cases, avoidance of extremely stimulating environments might be the only practical way to manage the situation.

Owners should be called in 1 week to address any concerns about working through a relaxation technique. A follow-up visit should be scheduled in 2–3 weeks. Owners may be advised to bring their 'settle' mat along so that their dog's ability to lie quietly can be assessed. After 1 month, if progress is insufficient the dog should be re-evaluated for evidence of clinical hyperactivity or anxiety.

### Prevention
Pre-adoption counselling is an invaluable service. Clients often lack information about breed-typical behaviours. Temperament assessments can be incorporated into initial wellness examinations so that owners develop realistic expectations for their new dog, but the predictive value of these is variable.

Owners of very active young dogs should attend advanced training classes to teach the dogs to channel their energy. Both exercise and structured quiet time should be incorporated into the daily routine.

## Problems of self-regulation

Dogs are considered to be family members and in many ways they are treated as children. Parents monitor their children, for reasons of safety and to educate them regarding appropriate behaviour. Dogs also need guidance and supervision. They do not mature socially until they are well over 1 year of age.

Owners routinely correct their dogs when they exhibit unacceptable behaviours. The behaviours nevertheless increase in intensity, generally in response to inconsistent or inadequately timed corrections. Furthermore, inappropriate punishment can also cause fear, which prevents learning and carries the risk of fear-based aggression.

A strategy that emphasizes supervision, prevention and instruction rather than correction may initially seem labour intensive but there will be long-term benefits.

### Inappropriate play
By definition, play should be fun for all participants. Owners will often accept rough play in small dogs and puppies. Once the dog grows larger, the game is not usually fun for the human participants any longer. When physical or verbal corrections are used to subdue a dog, the intensity of the behaviour often increases rather than decreases.

### Evaluation
Owners of dogs that play inappropriately may present with a complaint of aggression. An aggression screen should be used to confirm that there is no evidence of owner-directed aggression in other contexts (see Chapter 17).

The owner should be questioned regarding the dog's posture when playing. If the behavioural history supports a diagnosis of inappropriate play and not owner-directed aggression, the owner should be asked to prepare a video recording of a typical play session (it is important to provide guidelines and clearly specify that no one should be put in harm's way for the purpose of the recording). The diagnosis will be confirmed if the dog's postures are consistent with play.

### Treatment
Owners should discontinue games that involve physical contact – no wrestling or chasing the dog. Risky play should be replaced with lead-walking, training games and fetch. Young children must be supervised when playing with dogs.

***Behaviour modification:***

1. **Establish guidelines for safe play.**
- Initiation and termination of play:
  - A clear signal should be used to invite the dog to play. For example, the owner might say 'playtime' and then present the dog with a special toy or move to a specific play area. To terminate the session, another clear cue such as 'all done' should be given, and the toy removed.
- Monitor arousal:
  - Dogs that are quickly over-stimulated by play are best controlled if play bouts are kept brief. In some cases, owners may be able to recognize subtle signs of arousal. For example, the dog may begin to direct its attention away from a toy to the owner. The dog may jump up, mouth, bark at, or begin to circle the person. Play should be interrupted immediately, at the first sign that the nature of the game has changed. The owner should quietly withdraw
  - Another way to lead a dog from excited play is to use a training game. A container of food treats is kept nearby. The container is shaken to attract the dog's attention, then the dog is asked to follow some familiar, fun commands in order to earn the treats.
- Rules of contact:
  - Many people enjoy wrestling with their dogs but it must be understood that if a dog is permitted to wrestle with some people, it may attempt to wrestle with all people – including small children. Therefore, rough play should be discouraged. Dogs should not be permitted to chase people. The act of chasing may elicit predatory behaviour, which poses a risk to small children.
2. **Interactive play.**
- Most dogs will catch, chase, or push a ball with little encouragement. For dogs that are reluctant to relinquish following the retrieve, a bucket of balls can be used. As one ball is returned, the next one is tossed. Gentle tug games may be played with dogs that do not exhibit aggressive behaviour (Rooney *et al.*, 2000).

- Owners should be encouraged to create games that involve object play or structured sports. Fly ball and agility (Figure 8.7) offer great opportunities for athletic dogs.
- Other options include teaching the dog to 'find' toys that have been hidden by the owner.
3. **Object play.**
- Many toys that encourage solitary play are available for dogs. Most of these are toys that dispense food and encourage chewing behaviour. For many dogs these will occupy their time and may decrease requests for interactive play with owners.

| Diagnosis | Owner at home? | Target of damage |
|---|---|---|
| Separation-related anxiety | No | Multiple small items or points of egress |
| Compulsive disorder | Yes/No | Usually single target item |
| Noise/storm phobia | Yes/No | Points of egress; could target small items |
| Territorial aggression | Yes/No | Points of egress |

**8.8** Some causes of destructive behaviour, with underlying pathology.

cavity should be performed. Underlying pain can also contribute to anxiety. If the dog is actually ingesting the items in question, medical conditions contributing to polyphagia should be ruled out and the client should be asked about any recent diet changes.

Destructive behaviour in normal dogs develops as a consequence of inadequate supervision. Dogs left unattended to explore their environment will discover interesting items to chew. When owners find damaged property, they often shout or chase after the dog, either of which can exacerbate the problem.

### Treatment
A management programme that combines supervision with ample access to appropriate chew toys can be implemented immediately. During the initial phase of supervision, it may be helpful to fit the dog with a head halter. When the dog attempts to chew inappropriately, it can be interrupted with a gentle pull on the lead and then given an appropriate toy.

For those times when adequate supervision is not possible, the dog should be contained in a relatively dog-proof environment. This environment could be a large dog crate or a gated area with access to appropriate chew toys. Confinement should not substitute for adequate supervision and a dog should not be put in confinement unless its needs for exercise, attention and stimulation have been met or will be met later in the day.

***Appropriate chew items:*** Novel toys should be provided. Favoured toys that are rotated every 5–7 days are likely to remain interesting. Chewable toys (Figure 8.9) can be enhanced with the addition of food such as peanut butter or soft cheese. Toys should be large enough that they cannot be swallowed.

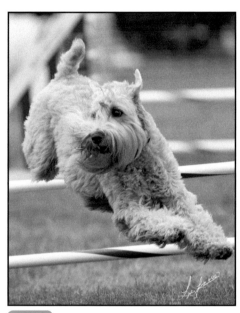

**8.7** Performing at an agility event.

### Prognosis and follow-up
The prognosis for teaching a dog to play appropriately is excellent once guidelines have been established.

A follow-up visit should be scheduled in 2–3 weeks. This visit can be used to discuss appropriate alternative games. In 1 month, to ensure that all participants are indeed having fun, owners can be invited to bring a new video recording of them playing with their dog.

### Prevention
The veterinary surgeon is in an excellent position to prevent the development of inappropriate play behaviour. Behavioural wellness consultations should include information about appropriate games, toys and dog sports.

## Destructive behaviour

### Evaluation
Destructive behaviour is a common presenting complaint but it is a clinical sign, not a diagnosis. Several behavioural rule-outs are listed in Figure 8.8.

When the behaviour represents a new or sudden change for an individual dog, an underlying medical condition should always be considered. A thorough physical examination with special attention to the oral

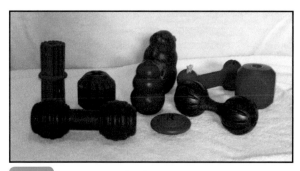

**8.9** Assortment of safe chew toys.

*Repellents:* There are several ways to render favoured but unacceptable items less attractive to the dog. The simplest method is to paint the objects in question with an offensive flavour. Bitter products are commercially available. Homemade recipes often include spicy ingredients such as cayenne pepper. These deterrents are generally safe, but many dogs appear unaffected by offensive flavours.

*Punishment devices:* Automatic or remotely controlled positive punishment devices to discourage chewing are available. Timing is essential. It is appropriate to interrupt the dog as it reaches for the item, but it is not appropriate to punish a dog after it has finished chewing an item (see Chapter 5). Delayed punishment can create anxiety or aggression. A correction should startle the dog without causing undue fear. An appropriate toy should be immediately available so that the dog can be praised immediately following the interruption.

Remote-activated citronella collars deliver a mild punishment or distraction in the form of a citronella spray. The owner can administer a correction from an inconspicuous location. A bonus to this method is that other items that the dog has favoured may be sprayed with a citronella-based product. The dog is likely to associate the scent with the unpleasant sensation of the spray and avoid these scented items.

Automatic devices have the advantage of accurate timing. Automatic citronella collars are activated when the dog approaches a disc that has been placed near a favourite target item. Other effective devices include motion sensors that emit either a piercing sound or a burst of air. Automatic mats that emit sounds upon contact prevent the dog from approaching a target area, but in some cases the dog only learns to leave the items alone when the device is present.

### Prognosis and follow-up

Normal destructive behaviour with no underlying anxiety can usually be treated quite successfully. If the dog is highly motivated to chew, long-term maintenance will require that the dog always has access to novel toys.

Owners should be contacted after 1 week to confirm that they are not relying on punishment alone and that corrections are not causing undue fear. They may have further questions about the selection of appropriate chewable items.

After 2 weeks, a follow-up visit can be scheduled to confirm that the behaviour is improving and that there is no apparent behavioural pathology. After 4–6 weeks, if the dog has responded nicely, a very gradual removal of correction devices may be initiated, followed by a gradual reduction of supervision. Clients should be reminded that their dog will always need access to interesting and appropriate chew toys.

### Prevention

The development of destructive behaviour is largely preventable. Young dogs need supervision, selective confinement and plenty of appropriate chew toys. A dog that does not tolerate confinement should be evaluated for a potentially serious anxiety-based condition.

## Stealing

A popular pastime for many dogs is to steal items. Targets include favourite possessions of family members, children's toys that resemble dog toys, or food items. Although food items are generally eaten promptly, toys and other items are frequently presented to the family.

When a person spots the dog with a stolen item, a chase often ensues. The dog is rewarded by the attention and is afforded an opportunity to 'play'. Therefore, much to the owner's chagrin, the behaviour is soon repeated on a routine basis. In many situations the owner will punish their dog after repossessing the item. This punishment can elicit fear without diminishing the stealing behaviours and the dog may respond aggressively in the future if it is approached while in possession of a valuable item.

### Evaluation

If food items are targeted, particularly if the behaviour is of sudden onset, it is important to explore the possibility of a physical cause for this new behaviour. Owners should be asked whether there have been any recent changes in the type or quantity of food provided to the dog. Medical conditions that affect digestion, absorption or appetite should be ruled out.

Behavioural rule-outs for stealing include attention-seeking behaviour, lack of appropriate play and interactive outlets and compulsive behaviour.

### Treatment

Initial treatment requires supervision to prevent successful access to frequently targeted items. A lead and headcollar can be used to interrupt the dog immediately and effectively.

*Behaviour modification:* Owners must avoid inadvertently reinforcing the behaviour. The dog should not be chased. It can simply be ignored if an item is not valuable and presents no danger to the dog.

Alternatively, the owner can teach the dog to relinquish stolen items. The reward for relinquishing should be a food treat, which is presented in a calm, quiet manner. Although this strategy could teach the dog to steal with increased frequency, the risk is low. The dog is rewarded not for taking but for returning. Furthermore, the motivation to steal items is usually to play or gain attention. The offer of a titbit of food is probably less valuable than the game of chase.

If stealing persists, owners may use one of the automatic or remote punishment devices described in the previous section. The dog should be provided with assorted appropriate toys as well as ample opportunity for owner-initiated interactive play. In other situations keeping a journal may show that stealing is common at certain times of day or when the owner is engaged in other activities. Arranging alternative activities at those times may diminish stealing behaviours.

### Prognosis and follow-up

The prognosis for controlling stealing is very good if owners are consistent. There should be noticeable improvement in 2–4 weeks.

### Prevention

All newcomers to the home should be supervised so that any attempt to steal food or property can be interrupted immediately.

## Digging

Dogs dig in the garden for many reasons. On warm days, they may dig to create cool sleeping surfaces. Management may simply involve offering a wading pool and shaded bed. Digging can be predatory behaviour when creatures such as grubs or moles lie beneath the surface. Treating the area to eliminate the pests may be the solution.

The main diagnostic rule-outs for this behaviour are anxiety secondary to separation and compulsive behaviour. In most cases, digging is a self-rewarding normal behaviour.

### Treatment

Digging can be managed in the same manner as destructive behaviour, i.e. with a combination of supervision and environmental enrichment.

*Environmental enrichment:* Enriching the environment can be accomplished by simply hiding a variety of toys throughout the garden. The toys should be rotated regularly. If digging can be tolerated in a part of the garden, treats and toys can be buried in that location. The dog must be able to distinguish clearly between the acceptable area and the area where digging is not permitted. In some cases the provision of a digging box, similar to a child's sandpit, may be appropriate.

*Punishment devices:* A remote-activated citronella collar can be used to interrupt the dog as it begins to dig. A commercially available motion sensor that attaches to a garden hose can be used to prevent dogs from accessing attractive digging spots. These punishment-based techniques will be most effective when the dog receives the correction every time it engages in the behaviour and when an appropriate alternative activity is immediately accessible.

### Prognosis

As with all self-rewarding behaviours, the prognosis for control is only fair unless adequate supervision can be maintained.

## Attention-seeking behaviour

It is quite normal for a dog to solicit attention from humans. When the behaviour is excessive it often becomes an imposition and a problem. The dog's response to its owner's exasperation is often to exhibit an assortment of behaviours that might serve to appease the owner, yet the behaviour will continue at another time and these appeasement behaviours are considered to be problematic as well.

### Evaluation

The presenting signs for this condition vary widely. Typical complaints include barking, pawing at the owner, stealing personal items, chewing inappropriate items, chasing lights and shadows, house soiling, over-grooming, licking the floor or a person, limping, or vomiting.

It is important to exclude relevant medical conditions. For instance, although a dog may limp in order to attract attention, it may not be possible to assign a behavioural diagnosis until after an orthopaedic and neurological examination. However, many dogs with attention-seeking lameness will cease the behaviour in the absence of the owner, for example if walked by the clinician alone. The nature and scope of the medical workup will be based on signalment and clinical signs.

Behavioural rule-outs include anxiety-based conditions:

- Compulsive disorder – the behaviour is exhibited whether or not the owner is nearby (see Chapter 20)
- Separation anxiety – the owner finds evidence of the behaviour, which is exhibited only in the real or virtual absence of the owner (see Chapter 14).

The diagnosis is based largely on context: attention-seeking behaviour is exhibited in the presence of the owner, particularly when the owner is engaging in an activity that does not include the dog. There should be historical evidence that the owner has interacted with the dog when the dog demonstrated the behaviour. Owners unwittingly offer reinforcement by touching, speaking to, or even closely watching the dog. The value of the owner's company may be sufficiently rewarding that verbal or even physical reprimands are tolerated.

### Treatment

The owner should be educated about appropriate reinforcement. Successful treatment requires that owners discontinue reinforcement of the undesirable behaviour. Where possible, the dog should be ignored whenever it engages in the attention-seeking behaviour. It is essential to prepare owners for an extinction burst: the behaviour may escalate for a few days before it finally ceases (Chapter 5).

There are circumstances in which intensification cannot be tolerated. Some behaviours cause injury or damage to the dog (e.g. pad chewing), to a person, or to property. Instead of completely ignoring the dog, the owners should ask it to engage in an acceptable behaviour prior to interacting with it. For example, the dog can be asked to sit or lie down for a quiet minute before its ball is tossed.

A lead and head halter will improve compliance. A gentle pull on the collar can interrupt barking, chewing or jumping. Tension should be released as soon as the dog appears calm. Once the dog is calm, it can be asked to sit–stay for a minute before earning future attention.

*Behaviour modification:* Clients should be advised to create a daily routine that includes both structured exercise and a reward-based training session to encourage the dog to engage in owner-directed activity.

After interaction based on the owner's schedule, the dog can be asked to 'rest' as discussed in the section on excitability, above. This may be accomplished through the down–stay exercise (see **client handout**) or by using a crate or exercise pen to signal that there will be no interaction for the moment.

It is often possible to anticipate situations in which the dog is known to be needy. For instance, many dogs seek attention when their owners attempt to relax after dinner, or when they talk on the phone. Before engaging in the activity that the dog finds problematic, owners can prepare a food-filled toy, or put the dog into its settle spot.

### Prognosis and follow-up
The prognosis for control of this normal learned behaviour is very good.

A follow-up phone call after about 5–7 days can be used to remind the owner that the behaviour may increase before it fades. Substantial improvement can be expected over a 2–4-week period. If problems continue, the diagnosis should be re-evaluated.

### Prevention
Prevention is best accomplished by incorporating a discussion of learning theory into new patient visits so that owners avoid inadvertently rewarding undesirable behaviours. Programmes such as 'Learn to earn' and 'Nothing in Life is Free' (see Chapter 18 and **client handout**) teach dogs to perform an appropriate behaviour before receiving attention. Owners should be helped to establish routines that assure ample opportunities for appropriate exercise, play and training.

## Roaming
Owners are often surprised when their dogs stray from their gardens. Certain breeds, such as hounds, are more inclined to wander than others. Intact dogs are apt to roam while searching for a mate. Behavioural rule-outs for dogs that leave the property include territorial aggression and anxiety-based behaviour. Separation-related anxiety, fears and phobias can cause a dog to panic and run away. There is, of course, a risk that the dog could be injured or that the dog could injure another animal or person, or damage personal property.

### Treatment
A lead should be used until the dog's responsiveness to commands has improved. A dog with a history of roaming from the property needs secure confinement. Toys and bones can be hidden in the confinement area to encourage the dog to explore its own property. Interactive play should be incorporated into the daily routine. Neutering males and spaying females may further reduce the desire to roam, if it is sexually related.

Obedience training should be emphasized for dogs that roam while hiking with their owners. While walking on a long line or extendible lead, the dog should be called frequently and rewarded with a ball toss, a treat, or a tug on a toy. Varying the nature of the prize will serve to maintain a prompt, eager response. The owner needs to remain more interesting than the surrounding environment.

### Prognosis and follow-up
The prognosis for control is only fair unless the owners adhere to rigid management. The motivation to explore is very high for many individuals.

A follow-up visit should be scheduled in 2–4 weeks for the purpose of observing the dog's responsiveness to a recall command in a controlled environment.

### Prevention
It may be difficult to prevent roaming in a predisposed individual, though excellent foundation obedience may prevent reinforcement of running off.

Electric containment systems for both cats and dogs are available. These typically involve a buried wire which is in communication with an electronic collar worn by the animal. An electric pulse is administered to the animal's neck if it does not retreat. The collar should emit an audible tone or a vibration before an electric pulse is applied. This signal then acts as a reliable predictor that allows the animal to avoid the actual pain stimulus in future. The use of training systems that employ electric current is controversial, with both proponents and opponents arguing their case on animal welfare grounds. In fact, electronic training systems are banned in some countries. Proponents argue that the fence systems are very reliable and not subject to the same risk of human error that is encountered with owner-operated electric collars, and that if properly trained, the animals can learn rather quickly to retreat at the sound of the beep. They suggest that the discomfort involved in this training is more than outweighed by the improved quality of life the animal can enjoy from greater access to free exercise. One problem is that they do not prevent other animals or humans from entering the space. Therefore, animals that are contained with these devices should always be supervised. Although using appropriate traditional boundary fences for containing a dog are recommended, in some environments they are not allowed or are impractical. If electronic systems are to be used they should be combined with some visible marker to help the animal and humans passing by recognize the limits of the boundary. Visual markers also help to prevent the urge to rush through and get 'locked outside' the system, by the collar aimed at containing it. Electric fences may not be suitable for dogs with certain anxiety disorders, including noise phobias, and with certain types of aggressive behaviour such as territorial aggression. The ethical arguments are complex but it is better to assist owners determined to use such a system than just to leave them to it.

> **BSAVA is opposed to the use of training aids that administer pain and to those that use an electric current to help control behaviour, in the absence of good evidence that these devices do not also cause pain.**

## Inappropriate chase behaviour
Dogs with no behavioural pathology chase moving objects to some degree and chasing may have its roots in play, fear, or even predatory behaviour.

Puppy aptitude tests can attempt to grade puppies on their chasing motivation. Obedience enthusiasts may seek a puppy that shows an interest in chasing moving objects.

Left unchecked, or in the hands of an inexperienced owner, this self-rewarding behaviour can have serious consequences. With physical maturity, coordination improves and the dogs are more successful at reaching their targets.

### Evaluation
When a client expresses concern about a dog chasing people, animals or vehicles, the dog should be evaluated for signs of fear-based or territorial aggression as well as predatory behaviour.

### Treatment
A lead should be used both for safety and to prevent the dog from gaining an opportunity to chase. Rather than snapping the leash, the owner should apply just enough tension to stop the dog from moving forward, then release the tension. A head halter will improve control.

*Behaviour modification:* Long-term treatment involves improving the dog's responsiveness to its owner. As with all training, initial practice is done in a quiet environment. It is helpful to teach a dog to 'leave it' on command (see client handout). While on lead-walks, the dog should be frequently asked to 'sit' and 'leave it'. When the dog responds consistently, practice is continued in the presence of stimulating distractions.

If arousal is high, a systematic desensitization and counter-conditioning protocol should be designed. Sit–stay exercises (see client handout) can be used to teach dogs to relax while focusing on the owner. Triggers that elicit a chase must be introduced gradually over a series of sessions. At the onset of a session, the dog must be far enough from any trigger to be able to maintain a sit–stay with attention to the owner.

If the owner suggests that a long-term goal is to have the dog run off-lead, the dog must respond to both a 'come' and a 'lie down' while it is in motion. Both commands should initially be practised while the dog is playing close to the handler. A long line can then be used to assure safety as the dog is taught to respond from increasing distances.

Clickers can be very helpful for this type of training (see Chapter 5). Initial conditioning involves pairing the sound of the clicker with a delicious treat. Next, the owner should 'click' the dog the moment it offers a correct response. Immediately following the click, the owner should bring the reward to the dog.

### Prognosis and follow-up
The prognosis for control of chasing while off-lead is only fair. Unsupervised access to triggers must be prevented, as the potential for accidental injury is high. Owners must understand that no conditioning is absolute. If small pets or children are targeted, the dog should remain on-lead in public areas.

A follow-up visit should be scheduled in 2–4 weeks to determine whether the dog's responsiveness has improved and to confirm that the owners are following safety guidelines.

### Prevention
Prevention should be emphasized. Young dogs should be supervised and restrained so that they cannot successfully chase people or vehicles. With a combination of consistent training and lack of opportunity, chasing is less likely to develop.

## Predatory behaviour

### Evaluation
Dogs that chase moving objects are often said to have a high 'prey drive'. Their behaviour may be not actually predatory but rather a reflection of other forms of arousal. Targets of such pursuit include not only wildlife but cats, other dogs, active children, joggers and inanimate objects such as cars or vacuums. While in pursuit, dogs may vocalize, exhibit piloerection, and may even redirect a bite to a family member who attempts to restrain the dog from chasing. But this does not mean that the animal is behaving in a predatory way. A high level of arousal suggests that the behaviour may be based on excitement (play, which is self-reinforcing) or underlying fear.

By contrast, true predatory behaviour is exhibited without affectation: there is no posturing or growling prior to the attack. It involves a chase and a hard bite and the dog is generally calm immediately afterward. A small dog, cat or other pet may be targeted, particularly if it moves suddenly. Pets that appear to get along nicely can be killed by a predatory housemate. Infants are at risk, as are young children that are running and screaming.

### Treatment
Predatory behaviour is treated similarly to chase behaviour. Excellent obedience skills are needed. Safety restrictions must be absolutely enforced, including the use of a lead in public areas. If children are targeted, a muzzle may be needed as well.

In the home, children and small pets should never be left alone with a dog that has exhibited predatory behaviour. Excessive staring, whining or arousal in the presence of infants, small children and small pets should be taken seriously.

Remote-correction devices are sometimes used in an attempt to reduce predatory behaviour. Both the timing and intensity of the correction are critical. Otherwise, the owner risks introducing a component of fear, thereby exacerbating the problem. Remote-correction collars may lead to a false sense of security. If the collar malfunctions or the dog is overwhelmed by the stimulus, the dog could ignore a correction, with dire consequences. If such devices are being considered, their use must be under expert supervision.

### Prognosis and follow-up
The prognosis for completely eliminating predatory behaviour is poor. The behaviour may improve while a dog is on-lead or under direct supervision of the owner. Left unsupervised, this self-rewarding, innate behaviour is likely to resurface.

Follow-up calls should be used to ensure that there has been progress with training and to remind the client about the need for lifelong management. Dogs that have killed small animals of any type should not be permitted to run off-lead with small dogs. Predatory behaviour is socially facilitated and, as such, may be more readily exhibited at locations such as dog parks where several dogs congregate.

### Prevention

Certain individual dogs will be predisposed to exhibit this instinctual behaviour more readily. Using a lead until obedience training is well established may prevent inadvertent reinforcement of predatory behaviour.

## Coprophagia

This behaviour may reflect normal exploratory behaviour, particularly in young puppies, and is less likely to reflect a serious medical or behavioural condition, but it is generally considered repulsive to owners. It is normal for a dam to ingest the faeces of her puppies.

### Evaluation

When a patient presents with a complaint of coprophagia, it is important to determine whose faeces are being ingested. A medical workup is indicated for the dog that presents for eating its own faeces. Some dogs seek out the stool of other dogs or other animals. If the faeces of a particular household dog are targeted, that dog should be worked up medically as well.

Medical conditions or medications that can affect appetite, digestion or absorption could contribute to coprophagia. Owners should be asked whether they have noticed any changes in the consistency, volume or frequency of bowel movements that might suggest a medical basis for the behaviour. A physical examination should include the evaluation of body score and coat quality. Baseline laboratory data should include a faecal evaluation for intestinal parasites and a TLI to screen for maldigestion.

If the behaviour is recent in onset, careful questioning may uncover an underlying trigger. Changes in the type of food or the quantity of food can be particularly relevant. If food is less available or less satisfying to the dog, hunger may trigger it to eat faeces.

It is also helpful to learn whether there has been any recent change in the environment or routine. A recently fenced garden may mean fewer supervised walks and more opportunity for exposure to faeces. A change in time spent alone may result in behaviour changes secondary to separation-related anxiety.

The owner's response to watching a dog ingest its faeces may serve to reinforce the behaviour. Many owners rush over in a futile attempt to interrupt the dog. The dog that seeks attention will be more likely to eat faeces if it can expect the owner to appear.

Coprophagia can become a compulsive behaviour. Support for this diagnosis would include evidence of underlying anxiety. Owners will report that the dog spends its time scavenging for faeces at the expense of routine sniffing or playing.

### Treatment

Treatment for coprophagia initially involves preventing access. Owners should clean up after their dogs immediately. Dogs should not be free to play until after they have defecated. Lead-walking, using a head halter for improved control, and increased supervision when outdoors should prevent ingestion. Basket muzzles must be used with caution: many dogs will still attempt to pick up faeces and owners will be unhappy if they must clean a faeces-soiled muzzle.

***Behaviour modification:*** One very helpful behaviour modification strategy is to teach the dog to 'leave it' (see **client handout**). The dog is rewarded for turning to its owner immediately after defecating.

***Aversive flavours:*** Several commercial products are available to render the faeces unpalatable. Aversive substances such as hot sauce or cayenne pepper may also be used. The efficacy of these products is generally not good. Some dogs are not deterred in the first place, while others quickly habituate to the taste. Furthermore, unless every batch of faeces contains the product, the dog will continue to be rewarded (more forcefully through negative reinforcement, as paradoxical as it may seem) by the occasional prize of untainted stool.

For some dogs, a punishment-based strategy that uses a remote-activated citronella-based collar may be effective. The owner must be prepared to use the collar every time the dog reaches to pick up the faeces and it should only be used in conjunction with a reward-based recall training programme.

### Prognosis and follow-up

The prognosis for resolution of coprophagia in the absence of the owner is only fair. The prognosis for control with supervision and good hygiene is good.

An initial follow-up appointment may be scheduled in 1–2 weeks. The owner should be asked to demonstrate the dog's response to 'leave it'. If a correction-based method is used, the need for long-term management should be reviewed to include supervision.

### Prevention

Owners can teach newly adopted dogs to defecate on cue so that faeces can be cleared up immediately.

## References and further reading

Braem MD and Mills DS (2007) How does additional verbal information influence a dog's obedience to a command? *Proceedings, 6th International Veterinary Behaviour Meeting and European College of Veterinary Behavioural Medicine* pp. 144–145

Juarbe-Diaz SV and Houpt KA (1996) Comparison of two antibarking collars for the treatment of nuisance barking. *Journal of the American Animal Hospital Association* **32**, 231–235

Lindell EM (1997) Diagnosis and treatment of destructive behavior in dogs. *Veterinary Clinics of North America: Small Animal Practice* **27**, 533–547

Miller P (2001) *The Power of Positive Dog Training.* Howell Book House, New York

Overall KL (1997) *Clinical Behavioral Medicine for Small Animals.* Mosby, St Louis, Missouri

Rooney N, Bradshaw JW and Robinson I (2000) A comparison of

dog–dog and dog–human play behavior. *Applied Animal Behaviour Science* **66**, 235–248

Simpson B (1997) Canine communication. *Veterinary Clinics of North America: Small Animal Practice* **27**, 445–464

Wells DL (2001) The effectiveness of a citronella spray collar in reducing certain forms of barking in dogs. *Applied Animal Behaviour Science* **73**, 299–309

Yin S and McCowan B (2004) Barking in domestic dogs: context specificity and individual identification. *Animal Behaviour* **68**, 343–355

## Client handouts (bsavalibrary.com/behaviour_leaflets)

- Adopting a rescue dog: the pros and cons
- Avoiding house soiling by dogs
- Canine behaviour profile
- Canine behaviour questionnaire
- Down–stay mat exercises
- Environmental enrichment for dogs in animal shelters
- Handling exercises for puppies and kittens
- Headcollar training
- How to find a good trainer
- Ladder of aggression
- 'Leave it' exercises
- Muzzle training
- 'Nothing in Life is Free'
- Playing with your dog – toys
- Puppy socialization: getting used to new people
- Recall exercises
- Redirected aggression in dogs
- Request for information on problem behaviours
- Sit–stay exercises
- Teaching your dog to go to a place on command
- The newly adopted rescue dog: preventing problems
- Treating a fear of car journeys using desensitization and counter-conditioning
- Treating a fear of the veterinary clinic using desensitization and counter-conditioning
- Treating separation anxiety in dogs
- What your dog needs
- Your puppy's first year

# 9

# Management problems in cats

## Rachel Casey

## Introduction

In this chapter, a range of miscellaneous behavioural presentations shown by cats, with widely diverse aetiological origins, diagnostic criteria and treatments, are discussed. Scratching, cats moving away from home, activity during the night and predatory activity are all behaviours that generally have a largely ethological origin. 'Inappropriate' play and attention seeking are behaviours that generally develop because of specific operant learning, in either development or adulthood. Pica and retained nursing behaviours are not within the normal behavioural repertoire of the adult domestic cat and appear to arise during the developmental period. Because of their diverse aetiologies, each of these presentations is considered separately below.

It is important to remember that behavioural presentations are not diagnoses. When presented with an animal displaying a particular behaviour, there are usually several possible reasons why the behaviour could have developed and often combinations of more than one factor that have contributed to its current form and context. Evaluating individual patients involves investigating these factors through observation of the patient and comprehensive history taking. Similarly, treatment options are not prescriptive for an individual behavioural presentation but dependent on the individual factors of each case. Clinicians should be wary of following advice suggesting that a prescriptive approach can be followed for the treatment of a descriptive category of behaviour.

## Scratching

Scratching, or clawing, is a normal part of the behavioural repertoire of the domestic cat, but where this occurs inside the house on items of furniture, owners can perceive the behaviour as a problem. Inappropriate scratching is rarely a behaviour that primarily leads owners to seek referral (<1% of cases in the clinical population referred to the University of Bristol) but owners more often mention this behaviour as an additional problem during consultations. General population surveys suggest that scratching in an undesirable location occurs much more commonly than referral rates might suggest. For example, it was reported by 60% of 120 cat owners surveyed in the USA (Morgan and Houpt, 1990); and in a regional survey of 109 cat

owners in the UK 72% reported the behaviour, though only 10% of these considered it to actually be a 'problem' for them (R Casey, unpublished data). In the USA 15% of indoor cat owners considered scratching a problem (Heidenberger, 1997). Owners are often only concerned about the behaviour where scratching occurs excessively or happens to be directed towards valued household items. Scratching can also lead to relinquishment in extreme cases. In a recent study, 7% of owners reported that they relinquished their cats to UK rescue centres for 'behavioural reasons' and of these only 1% did so primarily because of scratching (Casey et al., in press).

### Behavioural biology

Scratching behaviour, whether it occurs in an 'appropriate' (usually outside or on a scratching post) or 'inappropriate' location from a human perspective, is considered to have two different functions for cats. The behaviour may originate as a mechanism to maintain the claws for predation, or as a mechanism for providing an olfactory and visual communicative signal (Bradshaw, 1992). In both cases, scratching has an important function for cats and they are highly motivated to display the behaviour.

The action of scratching removes the blunted outer claw sheaths, and exercises the ligaments involved in the protraction of claws during hunting. Cats appear to be motivated to maintain nail health even when predatory behaviour is not shown. Those with limited access outside will therefore require suitable surfaces to be provided inside (see Chapter 4). To perform this function, the ideal substrate is one that has a vertical grain or thread, is high enough for the cat to reach and drag its nails down, and stable enough for it to lean into. This does not necessarily need to be a vertical site: some cats prefer to scratch on horizontal surfaces such as the top of fences or carpets, or lie upside down and scratch at the underside of beds. Where scratching is used to work the nails, there is generally a small number of preferred locations. Once sites are established, cats tend to prefer these to other locations.

Although the full meaning of scratching as an olfactory and visual signal to a cat is currently unknown, it does tend to occur in multiple significant locations. For example, cats scratch on fence posts where other cats patrol past, or at the bottom of the stairs where individuals within a multi-cat household pass each other. As with other olfactory signals used by cats, such as urine spraying, one function of scratch marking for the cat may be in providing a signal to other cats, with the aim of reducing the chance of face-to-face meetings. However, it is also likely that the signal provides information for the marking cat itself whether or not it lives with other cats, indicating locations of emotional significance within its environment. This is a highly adaptive mechanism, as it may provide the cat with an indication as to where it needs to remain vigilant, and where it can remain relaxed, giving it greater predictability and control over its environment.

Once scratching has become an established behaviour, for either of the reasons above, its occurrence is often influenced by the reaction of owners. Since most owners dislike their cat scratching on carpets or furniture, they will often react to the behaviour by, for example, shouting at the cat. Many cats may find this response aversive and this may lead to changes in the presentation of the scratching. Cats may change their location to one that is less obvious to owners, or scratch when owners are not present. They may also associate the response of the owner not with their own action of scratching but with other aspects of the context. This may lead to them continuing scratching, but also being anxious about their owner whilst they are close to the sofa, for example. Some individuals appear to find scolding not as punishing, but as reinforcing. In these cases, the occurrence of scratching can develop into a behaviour used by cats to achieve a response from their owners. In evaluating the patient, it is important to distinguish these different factors in the development of the behaviour, as treatment protocols will vary for different motivations.

## Evaluation and diagnosis

### Presenting signs and history

As with any other behaviour 'problem', investigation of a scratching case primarily involves identifying the circumstances that led to the development of the behaviour, and any that have influenced its development, or altered its function, for the cat.

Identifying the current function of the behaviour involves either observing the cat or asking for detailed information from the owner. The circumstances in which scratching is initiated should be noted, as well as the learnt consequences of performing the behaviour for the cat. As discussed earlier, it is important to determine the location of scratching, as locations that are 'significant' are more likely to indicate a marking function. Significant areas are likely to be locations where the cat is anxious or vigilant because of a perceived threat or unpredictable element to the environment. Commonly this might be a location where cats from different social groups need to pass each other in order to reach valued resources, but may also be a location where, for example, the cat may be anxious about an unpredictable response from owners. Where cats scratch in one or two distinct locations they may be scratching to work their nails, in which case the reason for this choice of site

should be investigated. As discussed earlier, scratching mainly in the presence, or absence, of owners may indicate that the behaviour has been modulated by owner response.

Finding out whether the cat has an acceptable scratching surface that fulfils its criteria for working its nails is also a useful starting point. In many cases the owner either has no scratching post, or has one that is not covered with suitable material, is too short or in a location not preferred by the cat. Another line of enquiry, especially if a suitable scratching surface is provided, includes evaluating the cat's ability to access the site. For example, access may be restricted by the presence of other cats in a multi-cat household, particularly where there is more than one social group. If a post is sited in the core area for one group, its use by another is likely to be inhibited. Equally, historical and observational evidence that the cat is anxious about the presence of people might be significant if the post is located in a busy part of the household.

Bearing in mind that the current presentation of behaviours may not reflect their original reason for development, asking owners about the history of the development is important for a full diagnosis. The development of scratching into an attention-seeking behaviour will only occur in cats that value owner attention and have had the opportunity to learn that this behaviour is successful at achieving it. Where this is the main current motivation for inappropriate scratching, the behaviour will tend to occur when the owner is present and, in most cases, when they are engaged in some activity that takes their attention away from the cat.

### Client attitudes, beliefs and behaviour

Owners often have highly anthropocentric views of a pet's behaviours and many will believe that their cat scratches to 'get back at them' or to be 'deliberately naughty'. Although such ideas are nonsensical, it is important to ascertain how the owner perceives the cat's behaviours in a completely non-judgemental manner during history taking. Understanding their perceptions of the problem is also valuable when explaining the cat's behaviour to the owner, as it enables the veterinary surgeon to emphasize aspects of the behaviour that were misinterpreted or misunderstood, thereby improving compliance with treatment advice (Casey and Bradshaw, 2008a).

Evaluation of how owners regard the behaviour of their cat will also provide useful indicators as to their likely compliance in following particular treatment protocols, particularly those that require a degree of effort on their part. Often it is those owners that value their possessions and home, or have recently acquired new soft furnishing, who seek help for this behaviour, since these factors increase their motivation to deal with the problem. Some people may react to the behaviour intermittently. For example, they may tolerate scratching if they are relaxed or it occurs on a surface they do not value, but shout at the cat if it makes a noise whilst they are trying to concentrate. As with dogs, this type of inconsistent response can lead to anxiety about owners.

**Differential diagnoses**

To summarize, to make a diagnosis in a cat that presents with scratching behaviour, the veterinary surgeon must distinguish between the following motivations:

- Scratching to work nails and predatory apparatus
- Scratching as a marking behaviour
- Scratching that developed for one of the reasons above, but has become an attention-seeking behaviour
- Scratching behaviour that developed for other reasons and has changed in presentation due to anxiety about owner response.

Signs typical of each causal factor are summarized in Figure 9.1.

## Treatment

Treatment protocols depend upon identification of the factors contributing to the development and maintenance of the behaviour: there is no 'prescriptive' approach to all cases with this presentation.

### Scratching to work nails

Where a suitable scratching surface is not available, treatment clearly involves provision of such a surface. Owners need to be advised of the criteria used by cats for preferred scratching surfaces, and also advised on suitable locations. Initially, the existing surface preferred by the cat may need to be covered over (e.g. with thick plastic) whilst scratching on the new surface is established. The new scratching post should be located near the unacceptable site of scratching, at least initially, but can later be gradually moved to a preferred site once use is established.

Where access to a suitable scratching site is the problem, the reason for inhibited access needs to be identified. For example, in a multi-cat household a suitable scratching site can be provided within the core area of each identified social group.

### Scratching as a marking behaviour

As with urine spraying, the resolution of scratching behaviour depends on identifying the reason why the location of marking is of significance to the cat. For example, in a multi-cat household a cat may scratch at the bottom of the stairs where it needs to pass cats from different social groups to reach important resources or entrance/exit points. Resolution will involve changing the specific characteristics of the environment such that the cat no longer needs to do so, for example by providing important resources within core areas, providing alternative entrance/exit points or providing three-dimensional space, such as high shelves, in passing places so that cats can avoid direct contact.

### Scratching behaviour influenced by owner response

Whether owner response is perceived by the cat as aversive, positive or both, it is important for owners to be instructed not to respond when their cat claws at furniture. As this is likely to be difficult for owners if valuable items are being damaged, specific advice should be given as to how the environment can be adapted to enable cessation of punishment (for example, temporarily replacing particularly valuable curtains with old ones). The specific treatment of cats that have learnt to scratch as an attention-seeking behaviour is covered in more detail in the later section on general attention-seeking behaviours.

### Declawing

Although restricted in the UK, as it is considered an 'unnecessary mutilation', declawing is still conducted in many other countries. This option has welfare implications and owners should be strongly

| Motivation | Location | Timing | Presentation | Historical development |
|---|---|---|---|---|
| Working nails | Usually few locations with suitable substrate | Often unrelated to owner activity, unless modified by owner response | Usually relaxed when scratching; may also play and facial rub in scratching area | Sudden onset may be associated with loss of other suitable sites, or restricted access to them |
| Marking | Significant locations, associated with unpredictable elements in environment | May initially occur after anxiogenic situation, but usually becomes more routine over time | Rarely also facial marking in scratching area. In early stages may be rapid short bouts of scratching which becomes less anxious-appearing over time | Onset associated with anxiogenic situation (e.g. changes in multi-cat household) |
| Development into attention-seeking response | Increasingly in close proximity to owner | Occurs when owner present, particularly if their attention is not on cat | Cat *may* be relaxed if behaviour reliably predicts positive owner response, but often signs of anxiety where owner response is variable, resulting in emotional conflict | As for working nails or marking, plus history of owner reaction/punishment |
| Additional anxiety about owner punishment | May move to locations away from or inaccessible to owner, or rapidly shift between locations in avoidance | May be more when owner is absent, or in short, rapid bouts when owner present | Cat is often anxious and will move away rapidly with any owner movement, or rapidly shift between sites. May be anxious about owner in other contexts | As for working nails or marking, plus history of owner reaction/punishment |

**9.1** Scratching behaviour: signs useful for differential diagnosis.

discouraged from this course of action by an explanation of the function of scratching behaviour and ways to manage the behaviour successfully. With accurate diagnosis of cause, treatment of this behaviour is relatively easy for owners to follow and generally very successful, making this type of surgery unnecessary.

## Prognosis

Casey and Bradshaw (2008a) reported that owner compliance in following treatment protocols for inappropriate scratching behaviour was not significantly different from other behaviour problems. Provided that owners comply with advice, treatment protocols for scratching are generally very successful.

## Prevention

Routine scratching in inappropriate locations for working nails is easily prevented by enabling the behaviour in an appropriate site. This is through providing a suitable surface, either inside or outside, and ensuring that the cat has adequate access to it (see Chapter 4). Owners should be advised that allowing the cat to use 'old' furniture for scratching may lead it to use other furniture, which may be unacceptable at a later time.

Prevention of scratching as a signalling behaviour can be achieved through reducing the risk of anxiety about cats in other social groups, for example by enabling the creation of safe core areas and access to important resources. Owners should also be advised not to respond when cats scratch on inappropriate surfaces, to avoid the possibility of reinforcing the behaviour or causing anxiety in the cat. If inappropriate scratching does occur, immediate redirection by preventing access to the inappropriate surface and providing easy access to a suitable surface will generally prevent further recurrence.

## Roaming

Cats sometimes disappear from their homes for long periods, causing their owners a great deal of distress. These absences may be due to hunting trips, an entire male or female cat searching for mates, being trapped because of human activity (e.g. in a garage), or perhaps having difficulty getting back home through the territory of another cat. In some cases, cats permanently move away to another area or house, becoming effectively lost to their owners. Where cats are identified, owners may repeatedly attempt to pick up their cat and return them home.

Cats will generally choose to move away from their core area if they no longer perceive this to be safe. This may result from a single traumatic event, or chronic anxiety about aspects of the environment. Finding another location that proves to be safer and more suitable as a core area is often also a factor. Moving from one site to another may be sudden or gradual: in the latter case owners may report that their cat has spent progressively less and less time at home, and ultimately has not returned home at all.

A common factor in cats moving core areas is the presence of other cats in their original home, in either the same household or neighbouring households. Dispersal of cats is a normal response to increased population density, and migrating to a new territory is likely to be perceived by the cat as a better option than being constantly anxious about the threat of other cats or some other source of specific fear or anxiety in its original home.

## Evaluation and diagnosis

### Presenting signs, history and differential diagnoses

Evaluating cases of repeated roaming involves identifying those particular aspects of the environment that the cat finds anxiogenic or aversive, or identifying an entire cat that is looking for a mate. Observation and history taking will give information as to how the cat responds to conspecifics in the household and neighbourhood. In addition, the possibility that the cat is anxious about interaction with people should be investigated by evaluating their socialization experience, their response to family members and unfamiliar people, and changes in interactions prior to bouts of roaming. Interaction with other pets in the household should also be investigated. In some cases, moving away is associated with a sudden aversive event, such as a party, loud noise or start of building work: these types of events are generally identified with careful history taking.

### Client attitudes, beliefs and behaviour

Owners often take their cat leaving home very personally and ascribe anthropocentric causes. Part of the clinical process should involve educating them as to the factors that have contributed to their pet's altered patterns of behaviour, to maintain the owner–pet bond and enhance compliance to treatment programmes (Casey and Bradshaw, 2008a). Where poor tolerance by the cat of enforced close handling by owners is considered to be a contributory factor to the roaming, client expectations of interactions with their pet need to be explored.

### Risk evaluation

Roaming is likely to increase the risk of road-related injuries in cats (Rochlitz, 2003a,b). Roaming and mating by entire cats increases the cat population.

## Treatment and prognosis

Treatment is determined by the underlying cause of the behaviour. Affected animals that are not to be used for breeding should be neutered or spayed. Merely shutting the cat inside is unlikely to be a long-term solution, and may well compromise the welfare of the cat as it is unable to escape a perceived threat. Where a cat is unable to maintain a safe core area from other cats, establishing a core area in a specific part of the house and preventing access by other cats may help to make the cat feel more secure. If the cat is avoiding social contact with people, changing how owners interact with their cat (not approaching the cat but positively reinforcing approaches by the cat itself) is generally a very successful treatment. Where other aversive events have led to the cat moving away from home, then either avoiding repetitions of these events or desensitization and counter-conditioning the cat to their occurrence are required. From clinical experience, the use of feline facial pheromone fraction 3 (Feliway®) (see Chapter 21) may be useful *in conjunction with behaviour therapy* to alter the cat's perception of a core area; using it alone without addressing the cause of anxiety, however, may lead to increased distress in the cat. Anxiolytic medication may also be indicated in some cases. Medication is used in conjunction with behaviour therapy in cases where the threshold at which the animal responds to a perceived threat or the particular circumstances of the case make desensitization and counter-conditioning difficult to start alone. It is inappropriate to use medication alone to maintain an animal in an environment without addressing the source of perceived threat.

Prognosis for changing the behaviour will depend on the reason for cats moving away from their core area, the threshold and severity of response, and the owner's ability to implement the suggested treatment programmes.

## Prevention

In most cases, cats show some signs of anxiety about their environment before leaving home. Ensuring that such signs are recognized by owners and that the source of perceived threat is addressed will reduce the desire of the cat to find an alternative core area.

## Hiding

Owners may also become concerned when their cat spends excessive amounts of time hiding or avoiding interaction, particularly if this is a change from their normal behaviour. Withdrawal and hiding (Figure 9.2) is a normal and common behavioural response to a perceived threat (Casey and Bradshaw, 2005). By finding a hidden away or high place to avoid an aversive situation, cats are able to 'cope' better in their environment. Hiding behaviour in a rescue shelter environment results in reduced behavioural (Kry and Casey, 2007) and physiological (Hawkins, 2005) measures of stress.

As with roaming, cats will hide for extensive periods if there is an aspect of their home environment that causes them anxiety, or where they have a specific fear response to something present in their environment for prolonged periods. Cats that are fearful of unfamiliar people, for example, may spend prolonged periods hiding whilst visitors stay in the owner's house. Anxiety caused by unpredictable activity of other cats, not perceived as part of the same social group, may also lead to prolonged hiding.

It is important to remember that, although hiding and roaming are perceived as problems by owners, these behaviours are actually resolutions for perceived problems by cats themselves. Hence, merely preventing cats from showing these avoidance responses is likely to compromise welfare further.

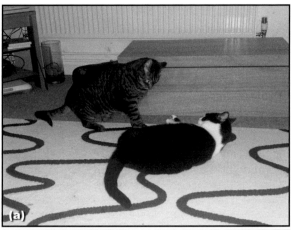

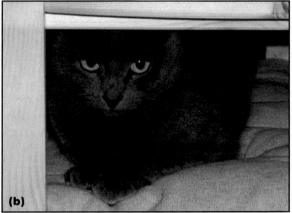

**9.2** **(a)** Conflict between cats within a household can be one factor in causing individuals to spend prolonged periods hiding, or move away from their home. (Courtesy of A. Seawright.) **(b)** Hiding is a normal coping response and provision of hiding opportunities is important in helping animals cope with, and adapt to, novel environments. Where prolonged hiding occurs, the continued source of anxiety should be investigated.

## Evaluation and diagnosis

### Presenting signs, history and differential diagnoses

Resolution involves identifying the source of perceived threat with thorough history taking. This may involve, for example, investigating whether times of hiding are associated with particular periods of human activity, specific noises, or periods when other cats are active in the house.

### Client attitudes, beliefs and behaviour

Owners need to understand hiding behaviour from their cat's perspective, as they may take avoidance as a personal slight. They should be clear that hiding is their cat's way of trying to cope with an adverse environment and that resolving this situation should involve reducing the perceived threat, not preventing the hiding. Some owners seek out their cat when it is hiding, try to retrieve it and give reassurance. Understanding that this will only make the cat more anxious (especially where it is hiding to avoid the owner) is an important aspect of owner education in such cases.

### Risk evaluation

Where cats spend prolonged periods hiding, they may not be accessing important resources adequately. For example, they may either not eat enough, or, because they can only access food intermittently, eat excessively when they do get access and sometimes also vomit. This type of situation can lead to long-term changes in satiety control.

Restricted access to water can also lead to problems in cats spending prolonged periods hiding. Inadequate fluid intake is an important risk factor for feline idiopathic cystitis (FIC), particularly in combination with chronic stress (Seawright *et al.*, 2008), and may also contribute to the development of renal disease.

Restricted access to the outside or to indoor litterboxes also increases the risk of FIC, because of urinary retention. Cats may also select an alternative toileting site that does not involve moving too far away from a safe hiding place, resulting in inappropriate toileting problems for the owner. Frustration and increased signs of stress can also arise where cats value owner attention but cannot access their owners due to anxiety about other aspects of the environment.

### Treatment and prognosis

As preventing access to hiding sites is likely to increase anxiety and compromise welfare, the first step is to identify the cause(s) of fear or anxiety for the cat so that either this threat can be removed or reduced, or a programme of desensitization and counter-conditioning can be initiated. The location where the cat is hiding may be the only place in the house where it feels safe; thus the first stage is to increase this area, so that there is one part of the house that the cat can establish a core area.

Where anxiety is due to the presence of other cats, for example, this may mean excluding other cats from one room. The hiding place within this area should be retained, so that the cat can retreat if sounds or scents predictive of the original threat occur. Use of Feliway® in this area may be of benefit, provided that the source of threat is removed. The extent of the area in which the cat feels safe can then gradually be increased.

Where hiding is from people, desensitization and counter-conditioning programmes can be very successful if conducted in a slow and careful manner, initially rewarding the cat with a tasty treat for emerging from its hiding place when there is a person sitting quietly ignoring the cat. The person needs to start this process far enough away that the cat feels safe enough to emerge. Over time, the cat can be rewarded for moving gradually further from its hiding place. People should not approach or interact with the cat other than as part of these desensitization sessions, or any progress will be undone.

Prognosis for changing the behaviour will depend on the source of perceived threat, how easy it is to enable the cat to avoid contact with the threat in the short term, and the owner's compliance in following the suggested treatment programmes.

### Prevention

As with any behavioural sign of anxiety or fear, prevention begins with appropriate socialization. Research has shown that fear behaviours are significantly less likely to occur in cats from rescue shelters given a programme of additional handling as kittens, even a year after homing (Casey and Bradshaw, 2008b). Ensuring that early signs of anxiety are identified by owners, for example by asking questions at routine check-ups, will make treatment easier.

## Predatory behaviour

The cat is a specialized solitary hunter, with sensory as well as behavioural attributes attuned to this function (see Chapter 4). Indeed, the reason why the cat became a domesticated species is likely to have been due to its hunting prowess, making it somewhat ironic that many people now find the consequences of its hunting activities distasteful. The effect of cat predation on populations of birds and rodents is widely debated (e.g. Woods *et al.*, 2003). Whilst this should be a concern, it is also important to note that hunting is a natural behaviour for the cat, for which some outlet must be provided. Hence, cats that are restricted from hunting, such as indoor cats, will still be motivated to show predatory types of activity, which need to be directed into play (see Chapter 19). Since cats still maintain the drive to hunt despite satiety, purely ensuring that a cat has plenty to eat will not necessarily stop predatory behaviour (though a hungry cat will tend to increase the amount of time spent hunting). Cats that are not hungry will still hunt, but not eat their prey. Although it is often assumed that young cats hunt more, this is not necessarily the case: Peachey and Harper (2002) found no effect of age on hunting behaviour.

### Evaluation and diagnosis

Generally where owners seek help for a cat showing predatory behaviour, they have seen the cat return with prey items (Figure 9.3) or find the remains within the house. Owners may perceive bringing prey back to the house as 'bringing them a present', but cats will naturally return with prey to eat it in their safe core area.

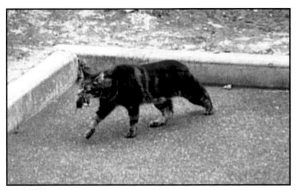

**9.3** Many are concerned by the tendency for cats to predate local wildlife, but the management of this problem without compromising the welfare of cats is challenging. (Courtesy of D. Mills.)

Suitable substrates and effective motor patterns for predatory behaviour are learnt in development. Hence, individual cats often have a preference for a particular type of prey. Some cats seek unusual 'prey', such as cuddly toys, raiding other houses in the neighbourhood and bringing them back to their core area. This behaviour is likely also to be reinforced by the initial response of owners.

## Treatment and prevention

Because cats are highly motivated to show some form of predatory behaviour, preventing any opportunity to do so will compromise their welfare and can contribute to a range of behavioural and physical problems, such as aggression to owners and obesity (Heath, 2005). Preventing cats from damaging wildlife populations, therefore, should focus on either decreasing the success of hunting forays or redirecting their desire to hunt into other activities.

There is some evidence that wearing a bell or sonic device on the collar makes hunting trips less successful (Nelson et al., 2005). The wearing of a plastic 'bib' on the neck has also been shown to reduce hunting success (Calvera et al., 2007), but it seems likely that this device will affect other patterns of behaviour and will also reduce the visual field when jumping downwards, hence adversely affecting welfare.

Reducing the access of cats to the outside at times when preferred prey species are most active may also reduce hunting success. Most rodent species are active overnight and birds active during the day, so cats with a preferred prey species can be allowed out when their particular prey are not active. However, cats may adapt to this and hunt at other times, or hunt other species, if they are highly motivated to do so.

Redirecting predatory responses into play can also help to reduce the extent of hunting. This is particularly important if cats are restricted inside when they have previously been out hunting, to avoid the development of frustration related behaviours. Play activity is particularly important. This should be in short, regular bouts, with toys that are distant from the owner's body but attract the cat's attention with movement (e.g. 'fishing rod' type toys, or table tennis balls; see Chapter 4). Laser pens are popular and can gain a cat's interest, but can lead to further frustration because there is nothing for the cat to 'get hold of'. This can be ameliorated by 'leading' a cat with a point of light to a 'prey item', such as a prawn wrapped up in a piece of paper. Playing with hands, or moving feet under the duvet, is not appropriate, as it can lead to aggressive behaviour being directed at these parts of the body.

Food-based enrichment can also be used to increase the proportion of their time budget that cats are engaged in independent activity (see Chapter 4). Commercial 'food balls' are available, which drop pieces of dried food as the cat manipulates them (empty plastic drink bottles with small holes cut in are a cheap alternative). Hiding food parcels in different parts of the house can also engage the cat's interest. Making the hiding places progressively more difficult to find and access will use up more of the cat's mental and physical energy.

## Nocturnal activity

Research on the activity patterns of domestic cats is not conclusive (Fitzgerald and Turner, 2000). Although cats are often described as crepuscular (active mainly at dawn and dusk) it is likely that patterns of activity are adapted to environmental circumstances. Hence, feral cats are likely to show crepuscular patterns of activity because these are the times of greatest prey activity. Cats in a domestic environment appear to be generally able to adapt their pattern of activity around that of their owners. However, cases do present where owners are disturbed by activity of their cats in the middle of the night.

### Evaluation and diagnosis

In evaluating such cases, history taking is directed towards differentiating the potential causes of the presentation. These include a number of medical conditions, which may be the sole reason for the behavioural change, or precipitate a change that is subsequently reinforced through owner response. Examples of possible differentials for changes in behaviour overnight are shown in Figure 9.4.

| **Physiological and pathological causes** |
|---|
| Onset of oestrus in entire female or response to oestrous female in entire male<br>Changes associated with ageing (e.g. cognitive dysfunction)<br>Osteoarthritic pain<br>Hyperthyroidism<br>Cushing's disease<br>Skin irritation (e.g. flea infestation)<br>Gastrointestinal pain or changes in motility<br>Lower urinary tract disease and associated urgency and pain<br>Seizure activity (general or partial)<br>Causes of polydipsia/polyuria<br>Pyrexia<br>Hyperaesthesia |
| **'Behavioural' causes** |
| Established pattern of activity (e.g. going out to hunt) inhibited, causing frustration<br>Pattern of activity interrupted by presence of other cats (e.g. entering through cat door and preventing household cat going outside)<br>Owner presence associated with inhibition of agonistic behaviour by other cats, leading to seeking owner proximity when other cats are active<br>Change in feeding pattern causing changes in toileting activity<br>Lack of sufficient stimulation during day<br>Activity initiated for other reasons (medical or behavioural) reinforced by owner response (e.g. getting up to feed cat)<br>Change in activity in other pets (e.g. rodents) precipitates behaviour |

**9.4** Examples of medical and behavioural factors that may contribute to a change in nocturnal activity patterns in domestic cats.

Medical causes should clearly be investigated. Although most have distinctive additional signs on further investigation, the first signs noticed by owners may be changes in nocturnal activity. For example, vocalization and increased activity are often associated with the pain of toileting with FIC. Because they are asleep at the time, owners may not realize that the first occurrence of activity at night is associated with toileting, and hence asking about changes in toileting routines during the daytime, and other signs such as haematuria, is important in history taking. The initiating bout of cystitis could have occurred some time ago, if the behaviour has subsequently been reinforced by owner response, so other changes in behaviour around the time of changes in nocturnal activity should be investigated. So-called cognitive dysfunction (see Chapter 12) may initially only present as changes in sleep–wake patterns.

Where interactions between cats are suspected to be a factor, observation of interactions during the day is helpful. For example, if the owner inhibits any chasing behaviour by scolding other cats and the 'victim' remains in close proximity with the owner (as this is predictive of not being chased), they may seek to do the same when aggressors are active during the night.

Although many factors appear to initiate this behaviour, it is often maintained and reinforced by owners waking up and interacting with their cat. Equally, any changes in routine that may have frustrated expected patterns of activity in the cat should be investigated in the history.

## Treatment and prognosis

By the time owners seek referral the behaviour is often well established, with the cat having an established routine of getting the owner up in the early hours so that it can have a bowl of food or a game, or be let outside. Treatment largely depends on the factors that have initiated the behaviour and any that have maintained or reinforced it over time. Identification of these factors enables a specific programme of treatment to be devised for the individual case.

For example, a cat that has its activity outside restricted by the arrival of another cat in the neighbourhood may require additional stimulation inside the house. Additional cover around entrance and exit points may also facilitate its passage outside. Alternatively, an agreement can be made between owners to allow cats out at different times of the day or night. In many cases, stimulating additional activity during the day is useful, for example through play sessions and the use of food enrichment devices.

Although the use of a timed feeder may give owners a temporary respite, the author would not recommend this due to the probability of further reinforcing a learnt response.

## Attention-seeking behaviour

Attention-seeking behaviours are those that a cat has learnt are successful at achieving an owner response, which it perceives as reinforcing. Only 3% of a population of 61 cats referred to a university behaviour clinic had attention seeking as the owners' primary complaint (R Casey, unpublished data). In a general population survey, 45% of 113 owners reported that their cats showed one or more attention-seeking behaviours, though only 6% of these perceived the behaviour as a 'problem' (R Casey, unpublished data), suggesting that these behaviours are widely tolerated by owners. Since cats need to be motivated to achieve owner attention, only those cats that value social contact with their owner will learn attention-seeking behaviours.

Attention-seeking behaviours can be very variable in form, depending on what each cat finds will achieve a response. Like dogs, many cats will have a range of different behaviours, which they use in different circumstances and in response to different discriminative stimuli. For example, a cat may gain attention by jumping on the owner's lap when they are sitting down, but need to climb up their leg to get a response if they are standing talking on the phone. Cats are often very good at identifying behaviours that owners cannot ignore, and which always 'work' by achieving a response even when the owner is occupied with something else. For example, an owner might find a particular pitch of their cat's vocalization very annoying or endearing, or always needs to react when the cat walks along the mantelpiece wobbling their best china vases.

Although less common than in dogs, cats might solicit attention when they are anxious about other events in the environment. This occurs where owners have previously responded to signs of anxiety by giving their cat 'reassurance'. Cats can also gain owner attention to achieve specific resources, such as food, or being let out of the house.

## Evaluation and diagnosis

A wide range of behaviours can develop into attention-seeking behaviours if a cat learns that their performance is successful at achieving owner response. In evaluating a cat, therefore, the context of the behaviour and how its performance has been modified over time are often more important than the specific presentation shown. Cats need to learn which behaviours are successful at achieving attention in each circumstance: often behaviours are originally shown for other reasons, but become attention seeking as the cat learns the consequence of its performance. For example, inappropriate sexual behaviour can be directed towards soft furnishings, owners, or other items. As in the dog, these behaviours develop initially when male cats reach sexual maturity. If reinforced by owner response at this time, the behaviour can continue to be directed at inappropriate substrates.

In the history-taking process, it is important to identify the schedule of reinforcement (see Chapter 5) that owners have inadvertently used to train their cat to show a particular attention-seeking behaviour. Behaviours that have been intermittently reinforced (i.e. owners sometimes react to the cat and sometimes do not) will be more resistant to extinction programmes in treatment than those where the owner has responded on every occasion. Often there is a mixture of different reinforcement schedules. For example, an owner may initially respond every time the behaviour is shown, and later only do so intermittently. Equally, different members of the household may respond to the behaviour differently, which will often result in differential frequency and intensity of the behaviour toward different family members.

Attention-seeking behaviours will obviously only occur when owners are present and tend to increase in intensity or change in nature when owners are busy with other things. Cats, like dogs, may identify specific cues that predict the withdrawal of owner attention, such as the phone ringing, or the theme tune of the owner's favourite TV programme, and start to show an attention-seeking behaviour on these cues.

In some cases, owners perceive that they are 'punishing' their cat for showing a particular behaviour, but the cat finds their response reinforcing. For example, urine spraying can become an attention-seeking behaviour where owners consistently scold the cat for spraying, and the cat perceives this response as reinforcing.

By the time cases of attention seeking are seen clinically, owners have often tried a range of ways of stopping the behaviour. They have frequently been advised to use punishers, such as water-pistol sprays, when the cat shows the undesired behaviour. In occasional cases, cats find even these responses still reinforcing, and continue to increase the frequency of the behaviour. In some cases, the cat associates showing the behaviour with the aversive outcome and inhibits the undesired behaviour, in which case this approach may appear to be successful, but often the motivation to achieve owner attention is merely directed into different behaviours, as the underlying cause has not been addressed. In most cases where cats have a mixture of positive and negative outcomes in response to showing the same behaviour, they develop signs of emotional conflict. The increased arousal associated with an uncertain outcome often leads to the behaviour being shown at an increased intensity, or may result in the development of displacement activities. Cats with emotional conflict generally appear more anxious and 'desperate' when showing attention-seeking behaviours, or may show approach–avoidance patterns before showing the behaviour. Non-judgemental history taking is important to ascertain from the owner exactly how they have responded to the cat at different stages of the development of the behaviour.

It is also important in the history taking to attempt to ascertain what types of interaction are provided and what types of interaction the cat prefers. If the cat is not receiving appropriate and adequate social interaction with family members and play and exploratory stimulation, this must be identified and changed.

## Treatment

Treatments aimed at directly inhibiting the performance of an attention-seeking behaviour are not recommended. Although these are sometimes described as 'interrupters' of behaviour, they do not address the underlying reason for the initiation of the behaviour and therefore have little more than a transient effect on the behaviour if the cat perceives them as punishing. The dangers of using this approach are that the behaviour is directly reinforced if the cat finds the response reinforcing, or that the cat finds them aversive and develops a state of emotional conflict about interacting with its owner.

Since the behaviours originate because they are successful for the cat at achieving attention, treatment involves a combination of stopping this reinforcement and actively reinforcing desired behaviours with attention. Applied consistently, this treatment protocol is very effective. In order for owners to be consistent in their responding, however, it is important to give them specific advice about how they can realistically not respond to behaviours that may have become extreme in nature. Preventing the cat from having the opportunity to show the undesired behaviours is not a long-term solution, as it will not have the opportunity to learn that there is no longer a consequence to the behaviour. Instead, the environment needs to be controlled, such that the cat is able to show the undesired response but the owner is able to not respond. For example, if a cat seeks attention by wobbling the china on the mantelpiece, the owner could remove the valuable items and replace them with cheap plastic items temporarily, so that they can carry on watching TV whilst the cat knocks them off. Where urine spraying has been maintained as an attention-seeking behaviour, asking owners to not replace their curtains for a while, so they do not need to respond to the spraying, would be effective. The specific advice given to each owner will vary with the type and range of behaviours shown by their cat and their particular circumstances; in every case, however, some opportunity to extinguish this response will present itself after discussion with the owner.

Before treatment is started, owners need to be made aware that the intensity and possibly frequency of the behaviour is likely to increase initially before declining. Where cats have learnt that a particular behaviour reliably 'works' to achieve a particular outcome, they will experience frustration when it no longer works. Owners who are not prepared for this will be more likely to give up in the early stages of treatment, but starting to ignore attention-seeking behaviours and then giving in will effectively train cats to try even harder, because eventually a response is achieved, and makes the behaviour more difficult to extinguish in the future (i.e. they start to use an intermittent reinforcement schedule). All family members need to be clear about the protocol before it is started: ideally they should start at a time when they are not too busy or stressed, and when more than one family member is present to remind each other not to respond.

It is also very important to explain to owners the importance of reinforcing desired behaviours with attention and how to interact properly with their cat. Since these behaviours develop because the patient is highly motivated to achieve owner attention, not providing a mechanism for them to achieve this will lead to high levels of frustration and make extinguishing the undesired behaviour much more difficult. Owners need to be counselled as to when they should start and finish interactions with their cat, and how to respond should the cat start showing the undesired behaviour during an interaction. They may also need advice on how to solicit appropriate behaviours from their cat and how to have meaningful interactions. Often owners assume all cats would prefer petting and stroking as interaction and this may not be the case. Owner education on appropriate play and physical interactions with their pet will help to keep attention-seeking behaviours from recurring.

## Prognosis

The prognosis for attention-seeking behaviours is generally extremely good, as long as owners understand the principles of treatment, and family members apply them consistently. Getting the owner to start to follow this protocol during the consultation is often useful, as it enables the veterinary surgeon to remind them if they are not responding appropriately.

## Prevention

Education of kitten owners as to appropriate interactions with their cat and the power of inadvertent reinforcement is likely to reduce the incidence of attention-seeking behaviours. Owners should be advised to be consistent in how they interact with their kitten, and to use attention to reinforce desired, and not undesired, behaviours.

## Inappropriate play

Playing by cats may be inappropriate because it occurs at an unwanted time, or in an unwanted context, or because the play is rough in nature and causes injury. Interactions between cat and owner are strongly influenced by learning outcomes; hence, where cats value social interaction, including play, the types of behaviour that achieve interaction will be reinforced and thereafter more likely to occur. For example, if owners ignore their cat when it brings a toy, but respond when it jumps off the kitchen work-surface on to their shoulder, the cat will differentially learn to show the latter behaviour.

The nature of play behaviour is strongly influenced by experiences in the developmental period. In kittens, play is considered to be partly a mechanism for developing and refining the appropriate motor skills for predation (Bradshaw, 1992). During this period, they are also likely to be learning about suitable substrates for these behaviours. Initially, kittens will play with any objects around, such as leaves and twigs, but the queen will direct these motor sequences to the appropriate substrate by returning with prey items. It is likely, therefore, that inappropriate play with kittens, such as waggling fingers on the back of the sofa, may lead to the establishment of play routines in adults directed at humans.

## Evaluation and diagnosis

In evaluating a case, it is important to establish the motivation for showing the behaviour and how this may have changed over time. In many cases that present at referral level, the behaviour has become well established and has modified as a result of changing owner response. Many owners initially reinforce behaviours in kittens that appear 'cute' but alter how they respond as the kitten becomes an adult cat. Hence, many owners will laugh when a kitten pounces on their feet under the duvet and encourage the kitten by moving their feet around more. As the kitten gets older, the owner may no longer respond to their cat, which may try to establish the interaction harder, perhaps by jumping on feet as they emerge from the duvet. Since owners usually respond to this, the cat will learn to show just this behaviour rather than the original game. However, when the 1-year-old cat jumps on their bare feet as they get out of bed, owners generally respond by punishing the cat. Often they do not relate this behaviour to the games they played with their kitten, and perceive that their cat has suddenly become 'vicious' or aggressive toward them.

The changed consequence of the behavioural sequence for the cat at this stage will commonly induce a state of emotional conflict. In other words, the cat has an established pattern of behaviour that has been reinforced, which it remains motivated to show, but having arrived at the owner's feet it becomes anxious about their response and this may lead to an increased intensity of the behaviour.

In taking a history, therefore, it is important to ascertain how the owner responded when the behaviour first started, as well as how they respond currently, in order to help to differentiate those cats that find the interaction reinforcing or fulfilling a need for activity, and those where there is also conflicting anxiety. Observing the cat, either directly (if safe to do so) or via video footage, is useful. Cats that are anxious tend to be more aroused and may dash out, leap on their owner and then immediately run away again. It is also useful to determine how the owner plays and interacts with the cat to meet its social and interactive needs on a daily basis.

Often a sudden increase in frequency or intensity of this type of behaviour is associated with other changes in the cat's environment. For example, if the owner has changed jobs and has less time to play, the cat will be more likely to seek out interaction opportunities. Equally, curtailment of other activities of the cat (e.g. reduced ability to go outside to hunt because of the activity of another cat) can lead to an increase in owner-directed behaviours. These factors should be investigated in the history, as successful treatment programmes include strategies to ameliorate the effect of such changes.

## Treatment

Treatments aimed at purely stopping inappropriate play are ineffective and often counter-productive. Making a loud noise, throwing things at the cat, or squirting it with water tends to increase anxiety and hence arousal, often resulting in an increased intensity of response. These attempts at treatment focus on teaching the cat what not to do, but without giving information on the preferred behavioural patterns.

Changing the cat's behaviour relies on it learning that the current pattern of interaction has no consequence, but that more appropriate ones have a positive outcome. Often cats that develop this type of behaviour are very owner-focused because they have limited other opportunities for activity. Particularly where the history indicates that changes in opportunity to show other aspects of the behavioural repertoire are a factor in the development of the behaviour, providing the cat with adequate enrichment is an important aspect of treatment (see Chapter 4). Encouraging activities that are independent of the owner is particularly useful, such as providing feeding enrichment devices (Figure 9.5) or hiding food around the household rather than in one bowl.

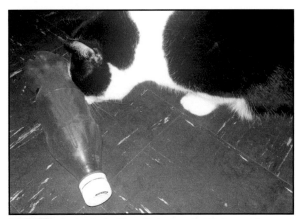

**9.5** A plastic bottle with holes slightly larger than kibble makes an effective puzzle feeder. (Courtesy of A. Seawright.)

The owner should be encouraged to play with the cat appropriately, using toys that are distant from the body (Figure 9.6). Some owners make the mistake of trying to 'distract' a cat that is starting to play inappropriately by waving a toy at them, which tends to reinforce the original behaviour. Instead, these play sessions should be initiated when the cat is relaxed and not seeking interaction. In this way, the cat learns that play sessions do occur regularly, but not when it tries to initiate them.

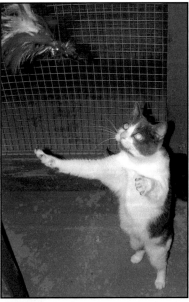

**9.6** Controlled periods of playing initiated by the owner will help reduce the occurrence of attention seeking. (Courtesy of E. Blackwell.)

Owners need to be able not to respond when the cat does initiate inappropriate play. Any movement or shouting will tend to reinforce the response, as these behaviours are 'predatory play' in origin. Particularly

in severe cases, this can be very hard for owners. Rather than expect them to stand still as their cat sinks its teeth into their ankle, it is important to ensure that owners are prepared; for example, wearing several layers of clothing, such as socks and jeans, or wellington boots under trousers, will enable them to not respond. Ideally the additional layers should not be too apparent to the cat, as some may learn that jumping on owners' legs only works when they are not wearing their protective layers.

### Prognosis
The prognosis for this behaviour is generally very good, even in extreme cases, but very dependent on owner compliance. It is helpful to keep in contact with the owner after the consultation to ensure that they are responding consistently and to support them through the period when frustration may temporarily increase the intensity of bouts.

### Prevention
Every kitten education session for owners and the first vaccination consultations for kittens should include some advice about how to interact and play with cats appropriately (see Chapter 2). The development of this type of behaviour can be completely prevented with suitable early advice to owners.

## Retained juvenile nursing behaviours

Sucking behaviour is normal in kittens when feeding. Kneading with the paws is another element of the feeding response, as this encourages milk letdown by the queen. In some individuals, these juvenile behaviours are retained into adulthood. Often such behaviours are tolerated, and even liked, by owners, which probably accounts for why so few affected cats appear in clinical populations. However, cases sometimes appear where the owner dislikes the behaviour, or the sucking results in the ingestion of hairs that cause gastrointestinal disturbance.

In feral cats, suckling can continue until the cat is 6 months old (Houpt, 1982) and tends to decline gradually over that time as the kitten is gradually weaned. In the domestic environment, kittens are often weaned suddenly, or at least have a truncated weaning period, as they are usually homed to owners between 6 and 12 weeks of age. This sudden weaning may be implicated in the retention of sucking and kneading behaviours into adulthood. Anecdotally, such behaviours appear to occur more in cats that were hand-reared as kittens, but no long-term studies have verified this supposition.

### Evaluation and diagnosis
In evaluating cases, it is useful to try to establish the early history of the pet, and ascertain which factors have contributed to the reinforcement of the behaviour and its retention into adulthood. The current context in which the behaviour occurs may help to identify the factors that are important in the maintenance of these behaviours. For example, if the behaviour only occurs during interactions with owners, it is likely that owner interaction is an important reinforcer.

## Treatment and prognosis

Where these behaviours are retained due to owner response, they can usually be extinguished relatively rapidly by instructing owners to interact with their pet only when the behaviour is absent.

## Prevention

To enable juvenile nursing behaviours to be extinguished naturally with weaning, owners need to be careful not to reinforce them through social attention to the kitten.

## Pica

Pica is the ingestion of non-food materials. Materials ingested may include fabrics (such as wool and cotton), plastics and paper. Although eating grass and plants comes strictly under the definition of pica, ingesting these materials probably has a different motivation in the majority of cases. Ingestion of plant material is thought to enable gastrointestinal motility and transit.

Owners seek help at referral centres for these behaviours relatively rarely. Out of 6089 cats relinquished to rescue shelters in the UK in 2001, no owners reported pica as the main reason for relinquishment (Casey *et al.*, in press). However, 6% of 113 cats in a general population survey in the UK were reported by owners as eating or chewing non-food items (R Casey, unpublished data). In the USA, Morgan and Houpt (1990) reported that 7% of 120 cats chewed fabric and 42% ate houseplants in a non-clinical population.

Cats that are weaned early (2–4 weeks of age) appear to be particularly prone to develop this behaviour (Bradshaw *et al.*, 1997), suggesting that weaning experience is important in the development of pica. In the 'natural' situation, the process of weaning is a gradual one, with offspring becoming progressively more independent, both emotionally and nutritionally, from maternal care. However, in the domestic environment offspring are removed from their mothers, and generally also from their familiar social and physical environment, relatively suddenly. These differences in early experience are likely to be significant in the development of pica, particularly as the occurrence of 'abnormal' or repetitive oral behaviours appears to be a characteristic of early or sudden weaning across species (Latham and Mason, 2007).

In addition, there appears to be a genetic predisposition to show pica, with an increased incidence in Oriental breeds (Bradshaw *et al.*, 1997) and some indication of familial inheritance (Bradshaw *et al.*, 2002). The development of pica therefore appears to be precipitated by the occurrence of a high level of stress early in life in susceptible individuals.

### Evaluation and diagnosis

In cases of pica, investigating the origin and development of each case is useful, as well as the context in which the behaviour currently occurs. In some cases, especially where identified in kittens, pica may occur only in the presence of owners, specifically during periods of inadequate stimulation, or during periods of anxiety or emotional conflict. However, in most cases that reach referral level the behaviour is well established, such that the cat actively seeks out its preferred material and will ingest this whenever the opportunity presents itself, a state that some authors describe as 'compulsive' (see Chapter 20). In these cases, it is important to identify the extent to which such behaviour is interfering with nutritional intake or gastrointestinal function.

### Treatment and prognosis

In cases where pica is precipitated in a specific context, the particular factors that lead to the onset of behaviour need to be identified. Treatment is often more difficult where the behaviours occur in multiple contexts or whenever a suitable substrate is available (i.e. it occurs apparently 'compulsively'). Explaining the origin of the behaviour to owners often helps them to empathize with their cat better, and will often help them to stop becoming irritated or using punishment. The use of punishment of any sort is not advised, as this will only act to increase the cat's anxiety.

In most cases, where cats eat normally as well as ingesting non-food materials, it is important to remove availability of the preferred substrate, so that the opportunity for pica is reduced. It is also helpful to make eating normal food as positive as possible, for example by using palatable food and using interaction and play during feeding. Generally increasing enrichment and stimulation for the cat is also likely to be useful, as a recent epidemiological study suggested that cats kept indoors only are at a greater risk of showing pica (Casey and Murray, unpublished data). In some extreme cases, complete inability to access the preferred substrate leads to high levels of distress and poor or no ingestion of normal food materials. With these cats, controlled access to small pieces of the material (which are likely to pass through the gastrointestinal tract) mixed with food means that the cat will gain essential nutrients. Over time, the amount of the substrate mixed with food can be very slowly reduced.

### Prevention

There is some evidence that the timing and style of weaning in kittens may have an impact on the development of abnormal oral behaviours. The emphasis on early homing to maximize socialization with people should be balanced against the possible adverse effects of removing a kitten from maternal care too early or suddenly. Given the likely familial inheritance, it is also important not to breed from affected individuals.

## Conclusion

The title of this chapter ('Management problems') reflects the fact that many behaviours shown by cats are perceived by owners as problems because they impact on their lifestyle, household or routine management of their cats. From the cats' perspective, these behaviours are often either normal species behaviours that are finding an outlet in a domestic environment, or behaviours that the cat has learnt to display either to avoid a perceived threat or to achieve a valued resource. In investigating such problems, it is essential to approach each case as an individual 'story' and work out why a particular cat started to show a specific behaviour, and how it may have become altered or reinforced over time because of changing events in its environment, such as the behaviour of the owner.

## References and further reading

Bradshaw JWS (1992) *The Behaviour of the Domestic Cat.* CAB International, Wallingford

Bradshaw JWS, Bale V and Casey RA (2002) Pica in Siamese cats: association with other behavioural abnormalities. *BSAVA Congress Scientific Proceedings*, p. 609.

Bradshaw JWS, Neville PF and Sawyer D (1997) Factors affecting pica in the domestic cat. *Applied Animal Behaviour Science* **52**, 373–379

Calvera M, Thomas S, Bradley S and McCutcheon H (2007) Reducing the rate of predation on wildlife by pet cats: the efficacy and practicability of collar-mounted pounce protectors. *Biological Conservation* **137**, 341–348

Casey RA and Bradshaw JWS (2005) The assessment of welfare. In: *The Welfare of Cats*, ed. I Rochlitz, pp. 23–46. Springer, Dordrecht

Casey RA and Bradshaw JWS (2008a) Owner compliance and clinical outcome measures for domestic cats undergoing clinical behaviour therapy. *Journal of Veterinary Behavior: Clinical Applications and Research* **3**, 114–124

Casey RA and Bradshaw JWS (2008b) The effects of additional socialisation for kittens in a rescue centre on their behaviour and suitability as a pet. *Applied Animal Behaviour Science* **114**, 196–205

Casey RA, Vandenbussche S, Bradshaw JWS and Roberts MA (in press) Reasons for relinquishment and return of domestic cats (*Felis silvestris catus*) to rescue shelters in the UK. *Anthrozöos*

Fitzgerald BM and Turner DC (2000) Hunting behaviour of domestic cats and their impact on prey populations. In: *The Domestic Cat: the Biology of its Behaviour, 2nd edn*, ed. DC Turner and P Bateson, pp. 152–175. Cambridge University Press, Cambridge

Hawkins K (2005) *Stress, Enrichment and the Welfare of Domestic Cats in Rescue Shelters.* PhD Thesis, University of Bristol

Heath S (2005) Behaviour problems and welfare. In: *The Welfare of Cats*, ed. I Rochlitz, pp. 91–118. Springer, Dordrecht

Heidenberger E (1997) Housing conditions and behavioral problems of indoor cats as assessed by their owners. *Applied Animal Behaviour Science* **52**, 345–364

Houpt KA (1982) Ingestive behaviour problems of dogs and cats. *Veterinary Clinics of North America: Small Animal Practice* **12**, 683–692

Kry K and Casey RA (2007) The effect of hiding enrichment on stress levels and behaviour of domestic cats (*Felis sylvestris catus*) in a shelter setting and the implications for adoption potential. *Animal Welfare* **16**, 375–383

Latham NR and Mason GJ (2007) Maternal deprivation and the development of stereotypic behaviour. *Applied Animal Behaviour Science* **110**, 84–108

Morgan M and Houpt KA (1990) Feline behaviour problems: the influence of declawing. *Anthrozöos* **3**, 50–53

Nelson SH, Evans AD and Bradbury RB (2005) The efficacy of collar-mounted devices in reducing the rate of predation of wildlife by domestic cats. *Applied Animal Behaviour Science*, **94** 273–285

Peachey SE and Harper EJ (2002) Aging does not influence feeding behaviour in cats. *Journal of Nutrition* **132**, S1735–S1739

Rochlitz I (2003a) Study of factors that may predispose domestic cats to road traffic accidents: Part 1. *Veterinary Record* **153**, 549–553

Rochlitz I (2003b) Study of factors that may predispose domestic cats to road traffic accidents: Part 2. *Veterinary Record* **153**, 585–588

Rochlitz I (2005) Housing and welfare. In: *The Welfare of Cats*, ed. I Rochlitz, pp. 177–203. Springer, Dordrecht

Seawright A, Casey RA, Kiddie J *et al.* (2008) A case of recurrent feline idiopathic cystitis: the control of clinical signs with behaviour therapy. *Journal of Veterinary Behavior: Clinical Applications and Research* **3**, 32–38

Woods M, McDonald RA and Harris S (2003) Predation of wildlife by domestic cats *Felis catus* in Great Britain. *Mammal Review* **33**, 174–188

## Client handouts (bsavalibrary.com/behaviour_leaflets)

- Avoiding aggression in cats
- Avoiding house soiling by cats
- Avoiding urine marking by cats
- Complementary therapies in behaviour problems
- Environmental enrichment for cats in animal shelters
- Feline behaviour questionnaire
- Handling exercises for an aggressive cat
- Handling exercises for puppies and kittens
- Introducing a new cat into the household
- Litterbox training
- Playing with your kitten
- Request for information on problem behaviours
- Taking your cat in the car
- Treating a fear of the veterinary clinic using desensitization and counter-conditioning
- What your cat needs
- What your cat needs: multi-cat households

# 10

# House soiling by dogs

Katherine A. Houpt

## Introduction

House soiling is the preferred term for elimination in the house. It has also been called inappropriate elimination, but this implies that it is an inappropriate behaviour of the dog when it is almost always a normal canine behaviour, though in a place the owner finds objectionable. Canine house soiling can be subdivided into:

- Defecation
- Urination
- Marking with urine.

Middening, or marking with faeces, is much less frequent in the dog than in the cat. Other behavioural problems contributing to house soiling include separation anxiety, submissive and excitement urination, cognitive dysfunction and walk prolongation; these are considered at the end of this chapter.

Although only 9% of cases referred to a veterinary behaviour clinic are primarily house soiling, the problem is much larger. Approximately 20% of dogs house soil and this can be a reason for relinquishment to a shelter (Wells and Hepper, 2000). 'Submissive' urination affects about 9–12% of dogs adopted from a shelter (Spain et al., 2004).

## Evaluation of the patient

### Presenting signs and history

The presenting signs are the presence of urine or faeces in the house and that is usually the presenting complaint, but the owner may present the dog as spiteful or stupid.

Important facts from the history are:

- Is the dog urinating, defecating, or both?
- Is this a new problem or just a continuation of a problem?
- When does the behaviour occur (time of day, and in owner's presence or absence)?
- Are any medical problems evident or need to be tested for? For example, if the dog has renal disease it may be producing more urine and unable to wait until access to the appropriate location is provided. Polyuria could be iatrogenic; if the dog is being treated with corticosteroids it will also be producing more urine.

Pertinent questions include:

- Where is the animal soiling?
- Is the urine found in the dog's bed? This indicates incontinence or excessive restriction. A map with the soiled spots is sometimes helpful
- How does the owner react when they find the urine or faeces?
- When outside, what substrate does the dog prefer for defecation and for urination?
- Does the owner accompany the dog outdoors or watch closely to verify elimination?
- When does the dog soil in the house (when the owner is home, when they are gone, overnight)? The answer to timing may help to point the diagnosis and treatment in the correct direction. For example: elimination when home alone may be due to an anxiety problem or lack of access; elimination overnight may indicate that the dog is required to wait too long before outdoor access is provided again in the morning
- What is the dog's daily schedule, including meals, walks, play time and number of opportunities to eliminate outside? If the dog is fed and not given the opportunity to defecate outside within the next hour, it may defecate indoors. Dogs that are fed free choice may not have predictable elimination patterns, making house soiling more likely if the owners work away from home. Dogs should have at least five opportunities to eliminate a day.

### Evaluation of all areas of behaviour

A complete history should also cover other areas and, if appropriate, questions should be asked to reveal whether the dog has aggressive or other behaviour problems. The most relevant to house soiling are separation anxiety (see Chapter 14) and cognitive dysfunction (see Chapter 12). For urine marking, the most relevant are aggression and anxiety.

- Aggressive dogs may be more likely to urine mark. The act of urinating may occur between the time the dog sees another dog (or even a prey animal) and the time it becomes aggressive. The act or the odour of the urine may increase his confidence.
- Dogs that appear to be socially dominant, rather than fearful, also tend to mark socially significant objects in the house such as beds, couches and curtains.
- Anxiety may cause other dogs to urine mark.

## Client attitudes, beliefs and behaviour

### Owner misconceptions

Owners are more likely to have misconceptions about elimination problems than any other. They believe the dog knows it did the wrong thing and often believe the dog is trying to 'get even' with them. This belief often creates anger and disappointment towards the pet, which may undermine the treatment programme.

### Problem owner behaviours

Few owners would think to punish aggression hours after it occurred, but they will punish elimination in the house say 2 hours after the elimination occurred. This is probably because the 'evidence' remains. They will not only punish the dog verbally, but may also rub its nose in the excrement as well as strike the animal. This often results in the dog assuming 'appeasing' body postures when the owner discovers the elimination in the house, leading the owner to assume that the dog is acting 'guilty'. It is imperative that owners should understand the temporal relationship between the action and the punishment and be counselled not to punish the dog when they do not witness the indoor elimination.

## Risk evaluation

The greatest risk to the dog is that it will be punished severely or inappropriately, or relinquished to a shelter. House soiling may recur when there is illness or a social or temporal change in the dog's environment resulting in changed access to the proper elimination location.

## Defecation and urination

### Behavioural biology

Elimination indoors may be adaptive, yet unwanted, in cases where access to the outdoors is restricted or unavailable at the times the dog needs to eliminate. Even after the access difficulties are resolved, a learnt component to the behaviour may contribute to ongoing house soiling.

### Substrate preference

Substrate preference appears to be as common a cause for canine defecation problems as for feline urination problems. In the case of dogs, hygiene of the area can also be a problem if the dog is restricted to a small area in which to eliminate and the owner fails to clean up after it.

Dogs are vulnerable when they squat to defecate and this may be partly responsible for defecation in the house, where they feel safer. Dogs that have been raised in a kennel on concrete may have a preference for (or only feel safe when) defecating on that surface. Another common substrate preference is for wood shavings, if that is what was available to the dog. The owner may take the dog for long walks over grass, bare earth, asphalt and concrete only to have the dog defecate in the house.

Many problems of defecation result when the owner and dog move from an urban to a rural environment or *vice versa*. Dogs accustomed to sidewalks or streets may refuse to defecate on grass or soil and eventually defecate wherever they happen to be when rectal pressure becomes too great. More common is refusal of country dogs to defecate on concrete in the city, where not only is the substrate different but also the volume of noise, the vibrations, and even the odours are very different from those in the country or the suburbs.

### Breed differences

Toy dogs such as Bichon and Maltese appear in the author's clinic quite frequently for house soiling problems. The reasons are unclear, but two hypothetical ones are: early experience, and small core area. Maltese, like other toy breeds, are susceptible to hypoglycaemia if they fail to eat after as little as 12 hours. For this reason the Maltese breed association advocates transferring them to their new homes at 12 weeks of age rather than earlier. The difficulty in housetraining results because the owner of the dam may have made no effort to housetrain the puppies, simply keeping them on wood shavings or papers, and allowing them to eliminate at will. The puppy not only fails to learn to go outside; it also learns a substrate preference of which the new owner may be unaware. The second hypothetical reason for the difficulty in housetraining small-breed dogs is that they probably have a small core area, proportional to their body size, so that they are willing to eliminate within 2 metres of their resting place, whereas a Labrador Retriever would not eliminate within 4 metres.

Beagles and Basset Hounds are difficult to housetrain. This is not only a clinical impression, but is substantiated by a survey of veterinary surgeons and obedience judges who ranked over 70 breeds on various characteristics, including ease of housetraining and trainability, aggression, barking and destructiveness. Ease of training and ease of housetraining seemed to cluster together, so that obedience-trained breeds such as Poodles and Border Collies were also easy to housetrain (Hart and Hart, 1988).

### Evaluation of differential diagnosis

There are myriad medical conditions that can cause house soiling. These include:

- Problems that cause an increased volume of faeces, such as a diet change
- Problems that cause an increased frequency of defecation, such as diarrhoea or colitis
- Problems that influence control, such as neurological problems.

Even arthritis may cause house soiling, because the dog is reluctant to walk and reluctant to flex its spine to defecate.

For defecation problems, a faecal examination for parasites, as well as a complete blood count and chemistry screen, should be performed. Bile acids should be measured pre- and post-prandially to assess for liver disease.

Medical causes of urination in the house are even more numerous. Problems that cause polyuria include renal failure, diabetes mellitus, pyometra, hyperadenocorticism and diabetes insipidus, and iatrogenic causes such as the use of corticosteroids that increase thirst. Problems that cause an increased frequency of urination include lower urinary tract disease, bladder calculi, prostatitis and abdominal masses. Problems of control include urethral incompetence or neurological problems of the spinal cord or brain.

A urinalysis, a complete blood count and a chemistry screen, as well as measurement of water consumption, should be done. If an adrenal problem is suspected, the urine creatinine:cortisol ratio should be calculated. Incontinence in older dogs, usually spayed bitches, should not be confused with voluntary urination and will present as soiled areas associated with the dog resting or sleeping.

## Treatment

### Housetraining an adult or adolescent dog

Many of the problems of house soiling turn out to be a lack of housetraining. In this situation, the owner must begin again as if the dog were a puppy (see client handout). It should never have a chance to make a mistake, so it should be taken out frequently (at least every 2 hours) but for a short time (5 minutes is usually adequate). If the animal eliminates, the owner should immediately praise it and give it a small, delicious treat or play with it for a while. Although the act of elimination itself should be rewarding, because bladder or rectal tension is relieved, there is no harm in giving an exogenous reward. The reward might be perceived as being for elimination at that time and in that place, which is also the goal. In addition, by pairing praise with a treat, the praise itself should become rewarding. The owner should accompany the dog outside, preferably on a lead, so that they will be close to the animal when it eliminates. Most owners will give the dog a treat when it returns to the house, which teaches the dog to return to the house, but not that eliminating outside is rewarded.

A few dogs will not eliminate on-lead. In this case, an exercise pen could be used to accustom the dog to using the place the owner has chosen and to keep the animal close to the owner.

A technique that works well to ensure that the dog does not eliminate in the house is 'umbilical cording'. The dog is tethered to the owner, or close to the owner, so that it cannot move more than a metre or two away. This serves two purposes: the dog is less likely to eliminate in an area it cannot leave; and the owner will learn the signals the dog gives indicating that its bladder or rectum is full. Circling while sniffing is a common signal of impending defecation and the dog with a full bladder may pant or stare at the owner. It is known that dogs innately attempt to communicate with humans when they cannot solve a problem: they will look at a human, especially their owner, when they cannot reach a goal, such as food that is out of reach or behind a barrier (Hare *et al.*, 2002). The aim of housetraining is to have the dog communicate with the owner in order to reach an outdoor elimination area rather than choosing an indoor elimination site.

Punishing the dog after it has eliminated will not help to housetrain it. In fact, it may teach the dog, at worst, to fear the owner or, at best, to be out of sight of the owner when it eliminates. If the dog is eliminating

or just about to do so, startling the dog should cause it to tighten its external anal or urethral sphincters, thus allowing the owner to take the dog outside, where it can eliminate. See Chapter 6 for information on housetraining puppies.

### Substrate preference

If possible, the preferred substrate should be provided or, if necessary, the surface the dog is accustomed to should be gradually replaced by the new substrate. For example, wood shavings can be scattered in the area where the owner prefers the dog to defecate and not be replenished if the dog begins to use the proper area. If necessary, a piece of sod with grass could be used in the city and, as it disintegrates, the dog will be gradually habituated to concrete as a substrate. Although dogs will urinate, and especially mark, in the same place, they usually chose a fresh place to defecate each time.

### Multi-dog households

There are several problems that arise when house soiling occurs in multi-dog households. One problem is identification of the dog responsible; the second problem is that more than one dog may be eliminating.

If defecation is the problem, a non-toxic indigestible coloured substance, such as crayon, can be fed to the dogs. Each dog will be fed one colour, so that the colour that appears in the faeces found in the house will identify the culprit.

When urination is involved, determining which dog is responsible is much more difficult. Dyes excreted in the urine can stain furnishing fabrics. If this is a serious concern, a video camera can be used to monitor or, better yet, record the dogs' behaviour. Sometimes removal of the dog suspected of soiling will confirm the suspicions, or will exonerate the dog if eliminations are still found in its absence. In other situations, if the problem is urine marking due to social conflicts, separation of the dog may result in a decrease in marking behaviour due to a change in the social situation, but without identifying the culprit.

## Marking

### Behavioural biology

Marking behaviour is primarily a male problem. Presumably marking is a means of olfactory communication between dogs. When a dog is marking indoors it usually voids only a small amount of urine, generally placed on vertical surfaces and running downward. The locations may or may not have social significance.

### Evaluation of differential diagnosis

It is necessary to differentiate between indoor urination for emptying the bladder and marking. This is usually done by focusing on the amount of urine voided: marking tends to result in a smaller amount of urine voided, while house soiling entails the dog emptying its bladder. Because marking occurs primarily in male dogs, castration is recommended; castration reduces marking in 50–80% of male dogs and virtually cures marking in 40% (Neilson *et al.*, 1997).

## Treatment

If the dog has already been castrated, behavioural measures will be necessary. The owner should strive to prevent outdoor marking as much as possible, by letting the dog urinate only once when it first goes outside and once before it comes in. The scent of other dogs should be avoided, because that may increase the motivation to mark. This will necessitate lead-walks, which will also increase the owner's control.

Favourite indoor marking spots can be booby trapped with a pile of empty drink cans that will fall on the dog, a motion detector that will sound an alarm, or, for a smaller dog, a motion-activated compressed air canister that will frighten it away. Additional supervision or keeping the dog out of areas that are frequently targeted may also help to improve the problem. In multi-dog households, the relationship between the dogs should be considered as it possibly contributes to ongoing urine marking. An outdoor scent post could be provided so that the dogs can engage in the behaviour with impunity.

Soiled areas should be cleaned with an enzymatic cleaner in an attempt to remove odour. Owners should be discouraged from using repellents, because they often either do not repel or merely encourage the dog to eliminate elsewhere.

## Prognosis

The prognosis for improvement for house soiling problems is very good. At the author's clinic, 84% of cases were improved (according to the owners). Of the treatments suggested, owners were least likely to paper train or crate train their dogs (see below), to clean soiled areas, or to increase the dog's exercise, but they were willing to take the dogs outside more frequently. Puppies had a much better prognosis than older dogs, but adolescent dogs were least likely to have improved.

## Follow-up

Initial follow-up should occur 7–10 days after the consultation, either in person or by telephone. At this time owner journals can be examined and discussed and any changes in elimination location noted. Hopefully a decrease in indoor elimination and an increase in outdoor elimination will be noted. If progress is being made, the interval between trips outdoors can be increased but indoor supervision should continue. If the dog has learnt to signal the need to eliminate, tethering can be decreased.

If there has been no change in the elimination patterns, the treatment plan should be reviewed and followed up a week later. If no change has been noted by then, the diagnosis and treatment plan and possible contributory medical issues should be re-evaluated.

## Prevention of the problem

Prevention of house soiling is by housetraining (see also Chapter 6). Two common methods are crate training and paper training.

## Crate training

Crate training is probably the ideal way to housetrain puppies. The puppy is introduced to a plastic crate or cage by being fed in it, tossing toys into it and eventually being closed in for short periods. After a few days it should be possible to restrain the puppy in the crate for a few hours. *The rule of thumb for length of time between elimination opportunities is an hour for each month of the puppy's life plus one for small-breed puppies, or plus two for large-breed puppies.* Thus a 2-month-old Labrador should be able to wait 4 hours to eliminate, but a Toy Poodle only 3 hours. The puppy should be taken outside to eliminate and should be praised and given a treat if it does so. It should also be taken outside after each meal and play period, but should be in the crate at all other times.

Not only is crate training an easy method of housetraining, but it also habituates the dog to being in a crate, which can be used later when travelling. The crate should enable the dog to turn around but should not be much larger: if it is too large, the dog may eliminate at one end and stay at the other.

## Paper training

Another method should be used by those owners who must leave their puppy for longer than a few hours, because if the puppy is confined too long it will eliminate in the crate and then may learn that the crate is an acceptable place to eliminate. If the puppy must be left for more than 4 hours, it should be placed in a pen with its crate open at one end and its food and water nearby. The entire pen can be covered with newspapers; when the puppy begins to use a given area, the paper in other areas can gradually be removed. With this method, the puppy is being paper trained.

There are pros and cons to paper training. The pros are that the puppy can be trained even in very cold or rainy weather and in later life will be able to use paper when it will be unable to go outside for long periods. Paper training is especially useful for small apartment-dwelling dogs whose owners are reluctant to go outside at night. One of the cons is that it may be difficult to transition the dog from paper to ground. One approach is to move the papers gradually towards the door and then put a slightly soiled paper outside where the dog is to eliminate. A litterbox for dogs and pellets of newspaper have been marketed and puppies can be trained to use it. The texture of the pellets may make it difficult to entice adult dogs. Commercial paper pads similar to disposable nappies are marketed, but unless they are held down in a frame, dogs are more likely to play with than to eliminate upon them.

## Other behaviour problems contributing to house soiling

### Separation anxiety

Visceral signs of separation anxiety (see Chapter 14) occur in 31% of cases (Yeon *et al.*, 1999). These can be salivation, urination, defecation or, rarely, vomiting. The owner complains that the dog will have recently urinated outside, but will urinate indoors within an hour of the owner's leaving. This is so frequent an occurrence that it could indicate a suppression of antidiuretic hormone owing to the stress of isolation.

Dogs may defecate when left alone and may then walk through the faeces, which is more likely to happen if the dog is caged. The owner has to bathe the dog each day, as well as clean up the faeces, increasing the owner's stress associated with a dog exhibiting behaviour problems.

Treatment for separation anxiety is addressed in Chapter 15. Briefly, teaching the dog to tolerate separation from the owner is the goal. The owner should ignore attention-seeking behaviour, not allow the dog to lie in contact with the owner, give departure cues and not leave, leave the dog with a long-lasting chew toy, teach the dog to stay when the owner is out of sight, and practise desensitization to departures that initially are very brief but increase very gradually in duration. Psychopharmacological treatment with fluoxetine helps to reduce many of the signs of separation anxiety, such as vocalization and destructive activities, but unfortunately does not substantially reduce urination or defecation (Simpson *et al.*, 2007). Clomipramine does reduce urination and defecation, probably because of its anticholinergic effects (King *et al.*, 2000), and is often the drug of choice for dogs that urinate or defecate as part of the separation anxiety syndrome.

## Submissive urination

Young dogs frequently urinate when approached. The stimulus may be proximity or a gesture, such as reaching over the puppy to pet it, or can be to a specific person. This behaviour is believed to be derived from the reflex response of neonatal puppies to maternal licking in the urogenital area. When they are 2 weeks old they can eliminate spontaneously, but may become conditioned to urinate when approached by a larger or more threatening being.

Submissive urination is usually presented as a problem in a young dog that is otherwise house-trained. The puppy crouches down or even lies on its side, exposing the abdomen, and urinates. Although derived from neonatal behaviour, it may have become a gesture designed to appease and thus avoid conflict both with familiar and unfamiliar individuals.

The clue to solving submissive urination is to determine the stimulus. The usual stimulus is a person approaching, especially a large, loud-voiced person. For that reason, men are more likely to be the stimulus. A hand over the dog's head is the next most common stimulus, or raised voice. Of course, any genetic problem causing malformation of the urinary tract or gastrointestinal tract may also cause house soiling. Springer Spaniels may have more of these problems than other breeds.

The worst response by the owner is punishment. The dog is already attempting appeasement, and punishment will only increase its anxiety and intensify fear.

The best treatment is to eliminate or desensitize to the stimulus (see Chapter 5). The large person should not approach the dog, a hand should not be raised over its head, and so on. Usually the problem will dis-

appear with time, unless the dog is inappropriately punished for submissive urination. The dog can be taught to respond to commands and then those commands are used in the situations where submissive urination is likely to occur. This consistency will help to build the dog's confidence: it learns that if it sits when told to do so, it receives praise or a treat and frightening things do not happen. If the problem persists, sympathomimetic drugs, such as phenylpropanolamine, can be used to increase sphincter strength.

## Excitement urination

A related problem is the dog reacting to visitors with wagging tail and jumping up while urinating. In this case the young dog may not be frightened, but rather too focused on a possible playmate to tighten its sphincters.

Teaching the dog an alternative response, such as lying down in a designated place when visitors come, and gaining control of the dog's behaviour in general should be sufficient to eliminate the problem.

## Cognitive dysfunction

Dogs over 12 years old may present for cognitive dysfunction: 20% of dogs of that age have one or more signs and two-thirds of 16-year-old dogs have signs (Neilson *et al.*, 2001). The common signs of cognitive dysfunction fall into five categories: disorientation; inactivity; sleep/wake problems; house soiling; and disinterest in social interactions (see Chapter 12). If an older dog that has been perfectly housetrained for years begins to soil in the house, cognitive dysfunction should be among the differential diagnoses if other medical problems have been eliminated. The aetiology is believed to be accumulation of beta amyloid in the brain.

Treatment for cognitive dysfunction should focus on retraining lost responses after appropriate medical intervention, which should include selegiline (L-deprenyl) (Campbell *et al.*, 2001) and an anti-oxidant diet, as well as environment enrichment (Milgram *et al.*, 2005).

## Walk prolongation

Some dogs learn that their walks will end as soon as they eliminate. Consequently they do not eliminate, in order to have a longer walk, and may then eliminate when back in the house. To solve the problem the owner should either walk the dog for a few minutes after it eliminates or require elimination prior to initiating a walk.

## References and further reading

Campbell S, Trettien A and Kozan B (2001) A noncomparative open-label study evaluating the effect of selegiline hydrochloride in a clinical setting. *Veterinary Therapeutics* **2**, 24–39

Hare B, Brown MS, Williamson C and Tomasello M (2002) The domestication of social cognition in dogs. *Science* **298**, 1634–1636

Hart B and Hart LA (eds) (1988) *The Perfect Puppy: How to Choose Your Dog by its Behaviour*. WH Freeman, New York

King JN, Simpson BS, Overall KL *et al.* (2000) Treatment of separation anxiety in dogs with clomipramine: results from a prospective randomized, double-blind, placebo-controlled, parallel-group, multicenter clinical trial. *Applied Animal Behaviour Science* **67**, 255–275

Milgram NW, Head E, Zicker SC *et al.* (2005) Learning ability in aged beagle dogs is preserved by behavioural enrichment and dietary fortification: a two-year longitudinal study. *Neurobiology of Aging* **26**, 77–90

Neilson JC, Eckstein RA and Hart JL (1997) Effects of castration on problem behaviours in male dogs with reference to age and duration of behaviour. *Journal of the American Veterinary Medical Association* **211**, 180–182

Neilson JC, Hart BL, Cliff KD and Ruehl WW (2001) Prevalence of behavioural changes associated with age-related cognitive impairment in dogs. *Journal of the American Veterinary Medical Association* **218**, 1787–1791

Simpson BS, Landsberg GM, Reisner IR *et al.* (2007) Effects of Reconcile (fluoxetine) chewable tablets plus behaviour management for canine separation anxiety. *Veterinary Therapeutics* **8**, 18–31

Spain CV, Scarlett JM and Houpt KA (2004) Long-term risks and benefits of early-age gonadectomy in dogs. *Journal of the American Veterinary Medical Association* **224**, 380–384

Wells DL and Hepper PG (2000) Prevalence of behaviour problems reported by owners of dogs purchased from an animal rescue shelter. *Applied Animal Behaviour Science* **69**, 55–65

Yeon SC, Erb HN and Houpt KA (1999) A retrospective study of canine house soiling: diagnosis and treatment. *Journal of the American Veterinary Medical Association* **35**, 101–106

## Client handouts (bsavalibrary.com/behaviour_leaflets)

- Avoiding house soiling by dogs
- Canine behaviour questionnaire
- Cognitive dysfunction syndrome
- Headcollar training
- Questionnaire to assess separation anxiety
- Request for information on problem behaviours
- Treating separation anxiety in dogs
- What your dog needs
- Your puppy's first year

# 11

# House soiling by cats

## Jacqueline C. Neilson

## Introduction

The deposition of urine or faeces in inappropriate locations is the most common behavioural problem for which cat owners seek professional advice. Data collected in 2003 from behaviour referral practices in three different countries found that feline elimination problems constituted 48% (Australia), 60% (Canada) and 66% (United States) of their feline caseload, respectively (Denenberg *et al.*, 2005). The actual incidence of house soiling in the general feline population is unknown but, in a survey of 800 cat owners, 11% cited inappropriate elimination as a behavioural problem with their cat (Borchelt and Voith, 1986). Another study examining behavioural problems after adoption from a shelter found that house soiling was the most common problem identified after adoption, with 9% of the cats exhibiting the behaviour within 3 months of adoption (Marder *et al.*, 2007).

The terms **periuria** and **perichezia** derived from Latin roots (*peri* = around, *uria* = urination, *chezia* = defecation) can be used to describe the condition of urinating or defecating around the home. Unfortunately, universally accepted diagnostic terminology does not exist to describe problems with feline house soiling. When a cat exhibits periuria or perichezia, the veterinary surgeon's goal is to establish whether the cat is doing this with the intent of evacuating its bladder or bowels (a toileting/latrine activity) or if it is using the excrement as a communication tool (a marking activity). This chapter will use the following definitions:

- **Inappropriate toileting**: urine or faeces deposited inappropriately with the intent of evacuating the bladder or bowels

- **Marking**: urine or faeces deposited with the intent of communication
- **Spraying**: form of urine marking where the cat stands with tail erect and twitching and forcefully ejects urine in a caudal stream against a vertical surface.

The term **house soiling** will encompass both inappropriate toileting and marking behaviours. In other literature, however, the term inappropriate elimination may be used as a synonym for house soiling or inappropriate toileting.

## Evaluation of the patient

### Presenting signs and history
In cases of house soiling the history will include the deposition of urine or faeces in what the owner considers to be an inappropriate location. It is critical for the veterinary surgeon to discern whether the problem involves urine, faeces or both. Due to the relative ease of cleaning inappropriately deposited cat faeces, owners may not include the perichezia in the historical profile. However, this information may be helpful in the diagnostic process, as the presence of perichezia is often indicative of a toileting problem.

A complete history is essential for the proper diagnosis and treatment of feline house soiling problems and should include the information listed in Figure 11.1. Factual, objective information is more helpful than owners' interpretations of their cat's intentions or behaviour. In cases where an in-home evaluation is not possible, a map of the house showing soiled locations and the core living areas of the cat(s) may be very useful.

| Historical data | Clinical relevance |
|---|---|
| Medical history | To identify if an appropriate medical evaluation has been completed. A history of FLUTD may elucidate a primary medical cause for the house soiling |
| Dietary history | A change in diet may contribute to elimination problems |
| Type of excrement involved (urine and/or faeces) | Faeces rarely associated with marking in domestic cat, so presence of perichezia is often indicative of inappropriate toileting problem |
| Frequency of house soiling | Allows for assessment of severity of problem. May elucidate patterns that indicate triggers. Helps to assess treatment progress |

**11.1** Important historical data of clinical relevance for cats with house soiling. (continues) ▶

| Historical data | Clinical relevance |
|---|---|
| Any identifiable triggers for house soiling | May elucidate primary underlying problem (e.g. intercat aggression) and provide treatment guidance |
| Locations where house soiling is discovered | Urine discovered on vertical surfaces (sprayed) is most likely marking. Urine discovered on horizontal surfaces could be either marking or inappropriate toileting. Faeces deposited on very prominent raised surfaces (e.g. middle of dining room table) may indicate faecal marking |
| Substrates where house soiling occurs | If there is a substrate pattern for the house soiling (e.g. urine always found on soft absorbent substrates) then inappropriate toileting diagnosis is suspected. If a substrate pattern is absent (urine discovered on a variety of surfaces) then a marking diagnosis is suspected |
| Owner's response to finding periuria/ perichezia | Allows veterinary surgeon to identify inappropriate owner responses (e.g. delayed punishment) and advise owners against those techniques |
| Typical elimination behaviour patterns of the cat when it uses the box (pre-digging; sniffing; covering; time spent in box) | May elucidate a problem with litterbox or litter if the cat is abandoning or abbreviating species-typical elimination behaviour patterns |
| Litterbox history (box style, box size, box location, litter type, box cleaning regime, any changes in litterbox management) | May elucidate litterbox issues that could contribute to litterbox rejection such as an inadequate cleaning regime, an unfavourable litter, etc. |
| Social and environmental history (intercat relations; significant social or environmental changes; addition of another pet, e.g. dog) | A causative relationship may be suspected if onset of house soiling coincided with a significant social change such as move to new home or addition of new family member |
| Culprits witnessed | Identification of cats involved in the house soiling very important if medication is going to be part of the treatment programme |
| General temperament of household cats | Can help to identify social or environmental issues that may be playing a role in the house soiling |

**11.1** (continued) Important historical data of clinical relevance for cats with house soiling.

All the history information is valuable, but it is extremely important to ask questions about the litterbox(es) and household social interactions. Studies in cats show a strong preference for finely granular material (clumping litter) over other types of litter (Borchelt, 1991). In relation to litterbox hygiene, in addition to the client being asked how often they scoop the litterbox, they should specifically be asked how often they dump, wash the litterbox and refill it with new litter. Inadequate litterbox hygiene is suspected to be a leading cause of litterbox rejection and subsequent inappropriate toileting.

It is important to recognize that it is not the number of litterboxes *per se* in the home that is important, but rather the number of litterbox sites. An owner may have three boxes, but if they are all next to each other they really comprise only one (somewhat larger) site.

Social interactions between cats can often be one of the precipitating factors for marking *or* inappropriate toileting. A cat may avoid the litterbox because it gets attacked when it attempts to use the litterbox or trapped after using the box. A cat in these circumstances may simply develop a safer elimination area elsewhere in the home (inappropriate toileting).

Alternatively, a cat that lives in a hostile environment may start urine marking secondary to territorial issues or anxiety. The client should be questioned carefully regarding relationships between animals and for signs of covert tension (such as staring) and overt tension (such as hissing, growling and fighting). Since social tension between cats may be very subtle and therefore missed by owners, clinical observation of the cats (which can be via video recording) or detailed questioning may be necessary to assess properly the social atmosphere in multi-cat households (see Chapter 19 for additional diagnostic and treatment

information for intercat aggression). Questions should also encompass other animals in the household, since the presence of dogs may influence litterbox usage for some cats. It is useful to document the frequency of the house soiling, as this can be useful in ascertaining treatment success.

It is important to remember that cases of house soiling may have different initiating factors and maintenance factors. For example, a medical disease such as an episode of painful and urgent urination secondary to a bout of feline idiopathic cystitis (FIC) may initially cause a cat to toilet inappropriately on the rug. However, that same cat may prefer the texture, location or rapid clean-up of the soiled rug and will maintain its new toileting spot for a behavioural reason when the FIC bout resolves.

## Client attitudes, beliefs and behaviour

When a cat house soils, some owners mistakenly believe that their cat is vindictive or spiteful. In fact, marking behaviour is considered to be a normal feline communication tool. Inappropriate toileting occurs due to preferences or aversions and is not motivated by personal grievances.

Some people still believe that only male cats will urine mark. Although the incidence of urine marking is higher in male cats than in female cats, all domestic cats regardless of their gender or neutering status can urine mark.

A common human response upon discovery of periuria or perichezia is to punish the cat. Since owners rarely catch the cat 'in the act', this punishment is often significantly delayed from the actual moment of house soiling, rendering it ineffective. Owners should be advised against punishment, which is more likely to exacerbate than resolve house soiling.

## Identifying the culprit

In multi-cat households, owners often blame one cat for the house soiling without solid evidence. It is important not to assume that, just because a problem started when a new cat was introduced, the new cat is necessarily the culprit. Confirmation of participation in house soiling may be particularly important in cases where treatment is targeted at a particular cat (e.g. drug therapy). Segregation of the cats may help to identify the guilty party, but segregation may have such a significant impact on the environment that the house soiling is modified or resolved. Video surveillance provides the best evidence with minimal environmental or social impact, but it does require equipment and expertise to set up the surveillance system.

## Urination

A fluorescein dye test can be used to identify those participating in periuria. If their urine is alkaline, the urine of cats given oral fluorescein (10 mg/cat) will fluoresce with a bright yellow-green colour when viewed with a fluorescent black light for about 24 hours after administration. The owners can give the oral fluorescein to one cat in the household and then scan any new deposits in the 24 hours post administration for strong fluorescence, thereby confirming their participation. Since untreated urine will also fluoresce, the owner must become familiar with normal fluorescence so that they can appreciate the enhanced fluorescence. If using this test, is important to remember that the fluorescent qualities of sodium fluorescein vary with solution pH (low fluorescence in acidic solutions) and if the cat's urine is acidic this test will produce false negative results. Also, owners should be advised that fluorescein-treated urine may be visible to the naked eye on certain fabrics, creating unsightly staining that is resistant to cleaning.

## Defecation

To identify the culprit of inappropriate defecation, shavings of different coloured **non-toxic** crayons can be added to some moist food for each cat. For example, in a two-cat household, Cat A can be given purple crayon shavings and Cat B green crayon shavings. If the faeces deposited on the carpet contain green crayon shavings, Cat B is a confirmed participant.

## Risk evaluation

Risk factors have been identified for the three major diagnostic categories, but there are some contradictory data and some risk factors have almost certainly not yet been identified.

- Risk factors for *medical diseases* (e.g. obesity as a risk factor for diabetes) are established and can be found elsewhere.
- Several risk factors for *marking* have been postulated, though few have been substantiated with data. Three risk factors for marking that have been substantiated are gender (male > female) and neuter status (intact > neutered) and living in a multi-cat household (Pryor *et al.*, 2001a).

- Risk factors for *inappropriate toileting* have been postulated to include litter granule size, litter scent, box style, box size, box location, box cleaning regime, significant social or environmental change and the presence of more than one cat in the home. While some or all of these factors may be important to an individual cat, none has been found consistently across studies to be a significant risk factor for inappropriate toileting (Horwitz, 1997; Sung and Crowell-Davis, 2006).

Faeces and urine can carry zoonotic disease and so their presence around the house may pose risk to those humans who come in contact with the deposited excrement.

The consequences of house soiling can be serious and include significant property damage and dissolution of the human–animal bond. In one study (Patronek *et al.*, 1996), over 23% of the cats relinquished to shelters had daily or weekly incidents of house soiling, suggesting that house soiling is a significant contributing factor to feline relinquishment. Some house soiling cats get banished to the outdoors, where their expected lifespan is shortened due to inherent risks associated with an outdoor life. Finally, some owners request euthanasia for their house soiling cat, believing that rehoming and banishment outdoors are not viable options.

Even with successful control of the house soiling, relapse is possible. The likelihood of relapse is a function of the presence of initiating triggers. For example, if a heavily soiled box was the initiating trigger for inappropriate toileting and the owner's box cleaning lapses, there may be a relapse of litterbox aversion. Or if a cat suffering from FIC had an episode of inflammation with concurrent painful urination in the litterbox, this may trigger another bout of inappropriate toileting, specifically periuria. A cat that urine marks in response to the sight of cats outside the home may relapse if new neighbours move in with outdoor cats. Management of house soiling is an ongoing process that requires constant assessment of circumstances and appropriate interventions.

## Evaluation of differential diagnosis

Primary and secondary tiers of diagnosis exist for cats with house soiling. In the first tier, it should be established whether the cat is experiencing one of three main diagnostic categories:

- A *medical* problem
- *Marking* behaviour (communication)
- *Inappropriate toileting* behaviour (selection of another toileting spot).

The latter two are behavioural diagnoses and are diagnoses of exclusion. In other words, medical problems need to be ruled out prior to establishing a diagnosis of inappropriate toileting or marking. It should be borne in mind that these are not mutually exclusive diagnoses: a medical problem can contribute to a behavioural problem.

The secondary tier of diagnosis is to identify the motivational causes behind the behavioural expression:

- If the cat is *marking*, the aim should be to try to establish whether the marking is a result of conflict between household cats, or a disruption in routine, or visualization of animals outside the home, or other causes
- When considering *inappropriate toileting*, the second tier of diagnosis is trying to establish what preferences or aversions are contributing to the problem. For example, is the cat avoiding the litterbox due to, say, poor box hygiene, box location, box style or intercat aggression, or has the cat established a preference for another location or substrate?

Confirming the first and second tiers of diagnosis helps to target treatment effectively.

### Medical differential diagnosis

As well as physical problems in accessing the litterbox, the medical differential list for house soiling includes any medical condition that causes increased urgency or frequency or painful urination or defecation. While primary urinary or gastrointestinal system diseases are most commonly suspected, it is important to include other systems that may impact litterbox usage, such as the musculoskeletal system (e.g. arthritis) and neurological system (e.g. senility).

The signalment of the cat and initial physical examination will help to direct diagnostic testing, but every cat with periuria should have a minimal database of urinalysis via cystocentesis and imaging studies of the lower urinary tract (Figure 11.2).

- In cats less than 10 years of age, these two tests will capture the majority of primary medical conditions, namely FIC, urolithiasis and crystalluria.
- A geriatric cat with periuria will be more likely to have organ failure, neoplasia or metabolic disease and so bloodwork (CBC, chemistry panel and thyroid) should be included in the primary diagnostic workup in a cat more than 10 years of age.

Tynes *et al.* (2003) compared the urinalysis results of urine-spraying cats with results for cats with no reported periura. There were no differences between the two groups, suggesting that cats that spray urine are unlikely to have primary medical contributing factors. Another study (Frank *et al.*, 1999) found that 24% of cats presented with vertical urine marking (spraying) had crystalluria. They found a similar incidence (20%) of crystalluria in a control group of cats without urine marking. The similar prevalence of crystalluria in marking (affected) and non-marking (control) cats may suggest that crystalluria is not a risk factor for marking. However, these studies did not examine whether there was a causative association between the crystalluria and the marking.

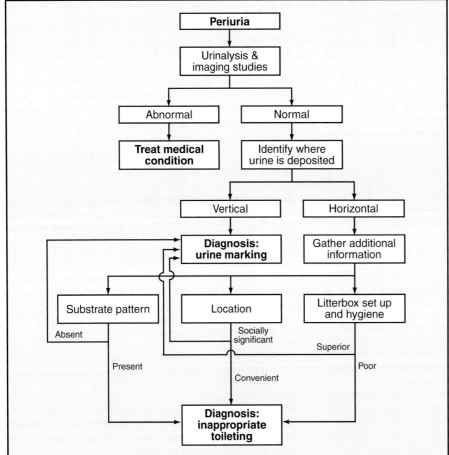

**11.2** Diagnostic algorithm for periuria.

Medical treatment for any concurrent disease is considered good general veterinary practice and therefore should be pursued regardless of its impact on the marking. Some personal communications and anecdotal reports suggest that an occasionally spraying cat with a concurrent primary medical aetiology discontinues the marking when the medical condition is addressed, and so diagnostics and appropriate interventions are always advised.

Any identified primary medical conditions should be treated, but it should be remembered that cats with medical problems may have concurrent behavioural problems, and so a comprehensive programme that considers both the medical and behavioural components for the periuria or perichezia is advised. A cat with perichezia should have a physical examination that includes a digital rectal examination and a faecal analysis.

Periuria is a common clinical sign of cats with FIC, with over 90% of cats with FIC exhibiting periuria. Stress has been implicated in the pathogenesis of FIC. Environmental stress results in activation of the sympathetic nervous system that may initiate or aggravate a bout of FIC. Therefore stress reduction is critical in the management of this condition (Buffington *et al.*, 1999).

## Marking

### Behavioural biology

Urine marking is considered a normal communication behaviour in both male and female cats. Sexual sterilization drastically reduces the incidence of urine marking, with 90% of intact males showing a significant decreasing in marking behaviour after castration (Hart and Barrett, 1973), but 10% of castrated male cats and 5% of ovariohysterectomized female cats are estimated to engage in urine marking (Hart and Cooper, 1984). Cats that mark are perhaps best described as being in a state of heightened emotional arousal. In some cases, that arousal may be due to territorial behaviour or anxiety/stress. In other cases, the urine marking may be secondary to a positive state of emotional arousal. When a cat examines another cat's urine mark, it generally will not show defensive behaviour, active retreat or distress, suggesting that the information encoded in the urine mark is not intended to repel or deter but instead to share information.

The classic urine-marking cat will back up to a vertical surface and stand with an erect quivering tail, treading its hind feet and forcefully expelling urine on to that vertical surface. This 'spraying' posture is diagnostic for urine marking, since cats do not toilet in this standing posture unless they are suffering from musculoskeletal or neurological abnormalities that limit their ability to squat. Urine-marking cats can also deposit urine on a horizontal surface, in a squat posture. These horizontally marking cats are more difficult to discern from inappropriately toileting cats.

Although it has been reported that marking cats deposit small volumes of urine, objective data to support this claim are lacking. To address this question the author measured the volume of urine deposited by cats engaged in vertical marking and compared it with the volume of urine deposited by cats toileting in the litterbox and found that there was no difference in the average volume of urine deposited. Therefore urine volume should not be used as the sole diagnostic criterion and, in reality, may not be particularly helpful in establishing a diagnosis for periuria.

## Diagnosis

The criteria that the author finds most helpful in distinguishing horizontal urine marking from inappropriate toileting are the location and substrate. The periuria location for cats that are marking is driven by social significance, not by qualities that would make that location a good toileting site. In general:

- Cats that are *marking* do not show a substrate pattern for their periuria
- Cats with *inappropriate toileting* do exhibit a substrate pattern (e.g. always on soft absorbent substrates)
- Cats that are *marking* are content with their litterbox and use it for evacuation of the bladder and bowels, so owners often report normal litterbox usage
- Cats with *inappropriate toileting* engage in typical toileting behaviours in location(s) other than their designated litterbox.

### Perichezia

Although the use of faeces to mark has been described in the literature, the author finds this to be a rare occurrence in the clinical population. If perichezia is part of the clinical presentation, in the vast majority of cases it will indicate that the cat has a diagnosis of inappropriate toileting. However, it is important to note that a lack of perichezia does not aid in the diagnosis, as many cats with inappropriate toileting characterized by periuria continue to use the litterbox for defecation.

## Treatment for marking

A **client handout** featuring treatment suggestions for urine marking is provided.

### Acute management strategies

Segregation in one room or zone can help to contain the marking behaviour until treatment can be successfully instituted. If specific triggers for the behaviour can be identified, such as visualization of outdoor cats or guests in the home, then those triggers should be avoided.

### Surgery

Cats that mark should be neutered. Castration significantly decreases marking behaviour of intact males. Oestrous female cats show an increase in urine marking and this can be addressed by ovariohysterectomy.

### Environmental management

Creation of a peaceful, enriched environment is indicated in the treatment of urine marking (see also Chapter 4). Stray cats and neighbourhood cats should be discouraged from entering the territory of the resident cat. For example, if the owner feeds stray animals in the garden, this should be discontinued. The owner may need to block the view from windows if their cat is aroused by the presence of other cats outside the home. If there is tension between cats in a household, this should be addressed (see Chapter 19). An 'environment of plenty' should be created in multi-cat households: this involves creating multiple feeding areas, multiple elimination areas, multiple scratching stations and multiple single-cat sleeping perches throughout the home. Positive interaction time (e.g. playing with a toy, grooming) should be provided to each cat on a daily basis.

Environmental management of soiled areas and litterboxes may help to reduce marking and should be implemented in all cases. Providing one litterbox per cat plus one additional box, scooping waste from boxes daily, changing boxes weekly and cleaning soiled areas with an enzymatic cleanser significantly reduced the incidence of vertical urine marking in a population of affected cats (Pryor *et al.*, 2001a).

If there are only a few target spots, the owner can attempt to make those areas aversive by covering them with aluminium foil, or placing upside-down contact paper (sticky side up), vinyl carpet runner (nub side up) or citrus scent at the sites. Alternatively, the cat's food and water can be placed at the soiled sites after proper cleaning. The owner should be warned that making the soiled areas aversive may simply result in the cat choosing another location to mark. An alternative option is to create 'kitty urinals' at the chosen spots by placing a plastic tub on end (Figure 11.3). This urinal option does not stop the urine-marking behaviour but may offer a reasonable compromise for some owners, as it prevents urine damage to the home and simplifies clean-up.

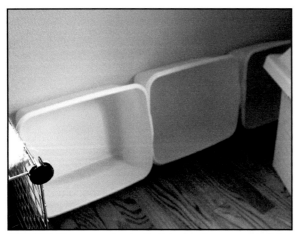

**11.3** These empty plastic tubs leaning up against the wall where the household cat routinely sprays allow the cat to continue to spray without damaging the home.

Other forms of marking such as 'bunting' (facial marking) and scratch marking should be encouraged. To encourage scratch marking, scratching posts or pads should be placed around the home, with the highest concentration in areas where the marking is occurring.

### Pheromone therapy

Feliway® is the synthetic analogue of a feline facial pheromone that is purported to have three principal functions: assisting in spatial organization, enhancing intercat relations and providing emotional stabilization (see Chapter 21). The product is available for delivery in a plug-in device and as a spray (and recently as a plug-in mat in some countries).

Several studies have supported the efficacy of Feliway® in reducing urine marking, whether of recent onset (less than 3 months) or chronic. Cats with recent-onset marking have the best response to Feliway®, with full cessation of marking in 96% of affected cats reported in one 28-day study (Pageat, 1996). Treatment success in cats with chronic urine marking was lower, but still impressive (see Chapter 21).

While full cessation of marking is the best outcome, reduction in marking is also considered a positive outcome and studies have repeatedly shown high success rates with Feliway® treatment, with greater than 75% of households experiencing a significant decrease in urine marking (Hunthausen, 2000; Mills and Mills, 2001). Most cats respond within a month of treatment implementation, with some responding within just a few days. Incidence of relapse after cessation of Feliway® treatment has not been reported, with the exception of a study that tracked urine marking for 4 weeks following completion of a month of treatment with Feliway® (Frank *et al.*, 1999). In that study, there was no evidence of a relapse within the 4 weeks post treatment. Long-term therapy may be necessary, especially if other treatment recommendations are not successfully implemented.

### Drug therapy

Drug therapy has been used to help to control urine marking (Figure 11.4). Historically hormones and benzodiazepines were prescribed but these are no longer considered the first choice of treatment, due to lower efficacy and greater side-effect profiles. Current drug research and therapy is focused on serotonergic drugs to manage/control urine marking. Drug availability and applications may vary between countries, so it is prudent to stay abreast of the authorization status of the drugs in their respective countries and inform owners before using drugs 'off-label'.

| Drug name | Dose | Frequency | Route |
|---|---|---|---|
| Fluoxetine | 0.5–1.0 mg/kg | q24h | Oral |
| Clomipramine | 0.25–0.5 mg/kg | q24h | Oral |
| Paroxetine | 0.25–0.5 mg/kg | q24h | Oral |
| Amitriptyline | 0.5–1.0 mg/kg | q12–24h | Oral |
| Buspirone | 0.5–1.0 mg/kg | q12h | Oral |
| Cyproheptadine | 0.5 mg/kg | q24h | Oral |
| Diazepam | 0.2–0.5 mg/kg | q12h | Oral |

**11.4** Drug options for treating feline urine marking (ranked in order of author's preference, with fluoxetine being the most preferred based on experience and available studies: Hart *et al.*, 1993; Dehasse, 1997; Kroll and Houpt, 2001; Pryor *et al.*, 2001a; Landsberg and Wilson, 2005).

Prior to instituting drug therapy a physical examination, CBC, chemistry panel and urinalysis should be conducted to evaluate the cat's ability to metabolize and excrete the medication and establish baseline values for future reference.

The two drugs that have the most information published regarding their efficacy in the treatment of urine marking are clomipramine and fluoxetine (Dehasse, 1997; Pryor *et al.*, 2001a; King *et al.*, 2004; Landsberg and Wilson, 2005). The relative treatment success for both of these drugs is comparable and it is high, with approximately 80% of treated cats having a significant (> 75%) reduction in urine marking when receiving the medication. Response to treatment can be rapid, within days of initiating, but continued treatment shows a steady incremental increase in efficacy. Studies have evaluated cases on drug therapy up to 32 weeks and found that urine marking is controlled over these prolonged treatment durations (Hart *et al.*, 2005). Side effects are usually mild and self-limiting but may include lethargy, gastrointestinal upset and paradoxical anxiety. Severe or persistent side effects may warrant dose reduction or termination of treatment.

***Route of administration:*** The recommended route of administration for the medications discussed above is oral (see Chapter 21). To date, studies on fluoxetine, amitriptyline and buspirone all suggest that delivery via the transdermal route does not achieve plasma levels of active drug anywhere near that achieved with oral administration (Ciribassi *et al.*, 2003; Mealey *et al.*, 2004; see also Chapter 21). Since most of these medications are quite bitter and owners will be expected to administer daily doses for several months, it is important to provide them with instructions and tools to aid in medicating. Proper pilling technique can be demonstrated and use of a pill gun may be helpful in some cats. Other tips may include use of commercially available treats with pockets for pill placement, dispensing empty gelatine caps into which the pill can be inserted prior to pilling, having the medication compounded into a fish-flavoured liquid or suggesting that the owners mix pills with canned cat food. In some cases it may be useful to precondition the cat to handling and pill administration, using food rewards, so that the cat will tolerate medication administration.

***Duration of treatment with medication:*** If a medication is effective at controlling the urine marking, appropriate duration of treatment is debatable. If significant environmental and behavioural modifications are achieved, attempts to discontinue drug therapy may be made after 2–3 months of successful control. However, extended therapy is probably necessary if the trigger stimuli persist in the environment. Hart *et al.* (2005) found that where the only prescribed intervention was drug therapy, most cats relapsed when drug therapy was withdrawn after 32 weeks of treatment. However, it is worth noting that a second course of treatment was as successful as the first course at controlling the marking. Cats that require long-term treatment should receive regular (every 6–12 months) physical examinations and laboratory evaluations. The author has seen a few cases that experienced an unexplained leucopenia during drug therapy with selective serotonin reuptake inhibitors; in all cases it was reversible with discontinuation of medication.

***Discontinuing drug therapy:*** In people treated with serotonin-enhancing medications, some experience a 'discontinuation syndrome' associated with abrupt drug withdrawal (Haddad, 2001). This syndrome includes signs such as light-headedness, headaches, irritability, anxiety and nausea. Most reactions start within a few days of stopping medication and are mild and short-lived (1 week), so no treatment is necessary. However, in cats, if discontinuation syndrome exists, this short period of anxiety or irritability/anxiety may initiate a problem with other cats or cause a relapse in marking. Therefore, while it is not physiologically necessary to wean cats off serotonin-enhancing medications, it may be prudent to consider weaning the cat off the medication over 2–4 weeks via dose reduction, or reduction in frequency of dosing. If there is a relapse in marking during the weaning process, there should be a return to the lowest effective dose and treatment should be maintained for another 2–4 months before attempting to wean the cat again. It should be noted that, even after prolonged successful treatment periods, Hart *et al.* (2005) found that urine marking returned in most cats upon discontinuation of medication.

## Prognosis

Since marking is considered a normal feline communication behaviour, unless specific inciting triggers can be identified and altered, at best marking may be considered controlled rather than 'cured' through the use of pheromones and perhaps medication.

## Inappropriate toileting

### Behavioural biology

The standard feline elimination sequence includes selection of a location, digging a shallow depression, squatting to deposit excrement in that depression, sniffing excrement and finally covering the excrement. Not all cats engage in all steps of the elimination sequence, and one or more of the steps may be missing if they are inappropriately toileting, but the ultimate purpose, to evacuate the bladder or bowels, is accomplished.

Inappropriate toileting can be triggered by medical causes, stress, aversions or preferences. Any medical condition that results in elimination with increased frequency, volume or pain may trigger inappropriate toileting. Veterinary surgeons should keep in mind that inappropriate toileting initiated by a medical cause may persist secondary to behavioural causes even after resolution of the medical problem. For example, a cat with diabetes may start to urinate on carpets and develop a preference for that substrate as a toileting spot due to its characteristics (absorbs well, convenient location, readily cleaned) that is maintained even when the diabetes is stabilized.

Aversions and preferences often coexist, as the aversion drives the cat out of the box and a preference for something or somewhere else is established.

- Aversions can develop to any aspect of the litterbox experience. If the cat is repelled by any aspect of the elimination experience, it may be driven to another elimination spot, resulting in inappropriate toileting.
- Preferences can include anything that encourages a cat to use another toileting site due to its attractiveness, for example a substrate preference or easier accessibility.

## Diagnosis

The two most compelling pieces of information that lead to a diagnosis of inappropriate toileting in a cat are:

- Identification of some factor that makes it unpleasant or difficult for the cat to use the designated litterbox
- The presence of a substrate pattern at the inappropriate sites.

When a cat ceases to use the litterbox completely, the diagnosis of inappropriate toileting is straightforward. However, most cats that toilet inappropriately still use the litterbox periodically for elimination, making this an unhelpful historical finding since cats with marking also continue to use the litterbox. Differences in the litterbox behaviour patterns of cats with inappropriate toileting versus cats without inappropriate toileting do exist, with inappropriately toileting cats spending less time in the box digging in litter than cats without elimination problems (Sung and Crowell–Davis, 2006). These differences are helpful when trying to establish overall patterns and suspected aetiologies, but their use in individual cases is limited.

## Treatment for inappropriate toileting

A **client handout** is also provided.

### Acute management protocols

In situations where clients are intolerant of inappropriate toileting, it may be beneficial to restrict the cat to a confined area devoid of any of the substrates that may be attractive for inappropriate toileting. For example, the cat may be contained in a laundry room that has no carpets if it has been inappropriately toileting on carpet in the home. The cat should be provided with all necessary items in this zone, including food, water, resting perches, scratching stations, litterboxes and social engagement periods (if desirable to the cat). For some cats and owners, this segregation can be very stressful, resulting in exit attempts and vocalization on behalf of the cat and guilt and distress for the owner. In these cases, confinement may not be an acceptable acute management protocol.

### Long-term treatment strategies

The treatment for inappropriate toileting should focus on identifying and providing very attractive litterboxes while reducing the attractiveness or accessibility of inappropriate target spots.

There are several components of the litterbox experience that may affect its usage, including hygiene, litter type and depth, box style and location. While there are data to suggest general feline preferences for some of these factors, unique individual preferences may exist and testing various options in the home of the inappropriately toileting cat will elucidate the most attractive box for the cat in question. Personal preferences are assessed by offering the cat new options in addition to its current litterbox set up. The various options are offered in a row and essentially the cat can inspect the choices and indicate its preferred set up by choosing that box for most of its eliminations (Figure 11.5). These options can also be offered in a sequential manner by introducing one new variable in the test box every 3–5 days, with owners retaining any preferred choice after each variable is introduced (Figure 11.6). Once all factors have been tested and preferences established, that box option should be maintained.

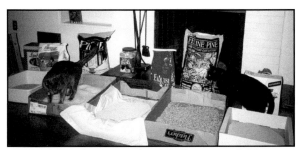

**11.5** This litterbox 'cafeteria' offers several different litter options for cats to select their preferred substrate for elimination.

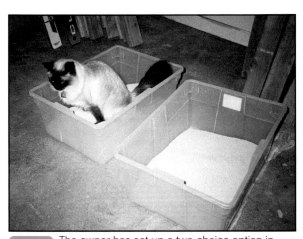

**11.6** The owner has set up a two-choice option in which every parameter is the same except the litter. The cat has chosen the litter in the box on the left and the owner will retain this litter option and then test it against other litters and other box parameters in future weeks.

Based on the case history and identified common feline preferences, the veterinary surgeon may be able to guide owners as to the most important factors to alter in each case. The amount of time needed to complete this process will depend upon whether the owner offers all options at once or elects to offer options sequentially. Time to treatment success also depends upon the ability of the veterinary surgeon to identify and prioritize changes.

*Hygiene and odour control:* If there has been a lack of appropriate hygiene, educating clients about proper litterbox cleanliness is imperative. Cats are considered to be fastidious creatures. Certainly they spend a good portion of their time on grooming and appear to be repelled by heavily soiled litterboxes.

Reducing offensive odours may be important in litterbox management. Scooping waste out of the box regularly (daily or twice daily) can help to achieve odour control but, considering that the average cat eliminates approximately five times (2–4 urinations and 1 defecation) in a 24-hour period (Sung and Crowell–Davis, 2006), keeping the box totally free of excrement is not practical for most owners. The frequency of complete litterbox changing (dump litter, wash box with soap and water, fill box with new litter) depends on the type of litter, the number of cats and the individual cat, but a minimum cleaning schedule involves changing non-absorbable/non-clumping litter weekly and scoopable/absorbable litter at least monthly.

Different brands of litter incorporate different substances to facilitate odour control, but there is a lack of independently conducted peer-reviewed clinical trials to evaluate claims of efficacy. Recent research has established that litter with activated carbon is used more often by cats than litter with baking soda, suggesting that it was preferred, most likely secondary to superior odour control (Neilson, 2008a).

*Litter type:* When given a variety of litter options, cats preferentially use finely particulate sand-like clay-based ('clumping' or 'scoopable') litter for elimination (Borchelt, 1991; Neilson, 2001). Therefore initial treatment could include testing a clay clumping litter in the row of litterbox set-up options.

The impact of fragrance additives in litter is not clear. Horwitz (1997) found scented litter to be a risk factor for elimination problems; but Sung and Crowell-Davis (2006) found that scented litter was not associated with elimination problems. The aroma and intensity of the fragrance may both be a factor in a cat's response to it. There is a lack of published information on feline scent preferences but recent data suggest that cats avoid citrus scents (Neilson, 2008b). Therefore current recommendations include avoiding citrus-scented litters; and if a cat with a toileting problem has historically been offered scented litters, providing an unscented litter option is advised.

*Litter depth:* Enough litter should be provided in the box so that the cat has the ability to perform the digging and covering associated with a normal elimination sequence.

*Litterboxes:* Litterboxes should be located throughout the home in areas that are easily accessible but not excessively noisy or highly trafficked. If a cat has chosen one or two areas in the house for inappropriate toileting, its new 'attractive' litterboxes should be placed at those locations. If the box is then used by the cat, it can be moved gradually (2.5 cm per day) to a more appropriate permanent location if necessary.

If intercat aggression is having an impact on the ability to use the litterbox, rooms with more than one entrance/exit might be good choices for litterbox placement. A standard recommendation is to offer at least as many litterboxes as there are cats in the home, plus one additional box, and the boxes should be in separate locations.

It is currently recommended that the box should be at least 1.5 times the length of the cat (Figure 11.7) and a trend for preferential use of the largest box offered has been shown (Neilson, 2008c).

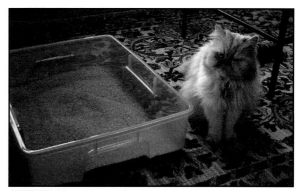

**11.7** The ultimate litterbox for most cats: large, clean, and with clay-based clumping litter.

To individualize treatment recommendations, attention should be paid to the inappropriate sites chosen by the cat. Anecdotal evidence suggests that most cats prefer uncovered boxes, but if a cat selects covered nooks for inappropriate elimination, then that particular cat may prefer a covered litterbox.

Owners should be cautioned against disturbing the cat when it is using the litterbox and should not attempt to give medications or perform other aversive actions. Children and other pets should not be allowed to harass the cat when it is using the litterbox.

*Reducing attractiveness/accessibility of inappropriate target spots:* The soiled areas should be cleansed with an enzymatic cleanser. Sometimes the cat will have to be confined away from areas in the house where it has chosen to eliminate. Alternatively, those soiled areas can be made aversive with plastic, aluminum foil, etc.

### Drug therapy
If anxiety is associated with the inappropriate toileting, anxiolytic drug therapy may be instituted. However, in most cases drugs are neither necessary nor indicated for successful treatment.

### Punishment
The owner should avoid punishing the cat when soiled areas are discovered. If the animal is caught during the event, the owner can use a startle technique to stop the behaviour, but should appreciate that this will not solve the problem and in the case of nervous cats it may exacerbate the issue.

### Prognosis
With good owner compliance, most cases of inappropriate toileting can be resolved successfully. The shorter duration of problematic behaviour may be linked with treatment success. Recurrent inciting medical issues may cause relapses.

## Follow-up

Owners should be encouraged to record the number of inappropriate toileting or marking incidents in a log to objectively evaluate treatment response. If they are having trouble finding urine deposits, a fluorescent black light will illuminate them as fluorescent yellow-green spots. Owners should be advised that they may need to differentiate other organic material from the urine stains.

Follow-up can be by phone or email but a visit to the home may be preferable if compliance with treatment recommendations is questionable. The initial follow-up should be at 1 week after initiation of treatment; thereafter, barring any problems, every 2–4 weeks should be adequate. If the cat is on drug therapy, regular rechecks (every 6 months) are advised, with routine blood testing (CBC, chemistry panel) every 6–12 months.

## Prevention

Neutering is the single most effective way to prevent urine marking. Since marking behaviours tend to increase with an increase in feline population density, limiting the number of cats in the environment or providing abundant resources in the home may reduce the likelihood of marking. Early identification and resolution of intercat aggression issues may also help to reduce urine marking.

Provision of attractive litterboxes is the best way to prevent inappropriate toileting. While cats may have individual preferences, the majority of cats would consider a large, uncovered, clean box with clay clumping litter in an easily accessible yet private site to be desirable.

## References and further reading

Borchelt PL (1991) Cat elimination behaviour problems. *Veterinary Clinics of North America: Small Animal Practice* **21**, 257–264

Borchelt PL and Voith VL (1986) Elimination behaviour problems in cats. *Compendium on Continuing Education for the Practicing Veterinarian* **8**, 197–207

Buffington CAT, Chew DJ and Woodworth BE (1999) Feline interstitial cystitis. *Journal of the American Veterinary Medical Association* **215**, 682–687

Ciribassi J, Luescher A, Pasloske KS *et al.* (2003) Comparative bioavailability of fluoxetine after transdermal and oral administration to healthy cats. *American Journal of Veterinary Research* **64**, 994–998

Dehasse J (1997) Feline urine spraying. *Applied Animal Behaviour Science* **52**, 365–371

Denenberg S, Landsberg G, Horwitz D and Seksel K (2005) A comparison of cases referred to behaviourists in three different countries. In: *Current Issues and Research in Veterinary Behavioural Medicine*, ed. D Mills *et al.*, pp. 56–62. Purdue University Press, West Lafayette, Indiana

Frank DF, Erb HN and Houpt KA (1999) Urine spraying in cats: presence of concurrent disease and effects of a pheromone treatment. *Applied Animal Behaviour Science* **61**, 263–272

Haddad PM (2001) Antidepressant discontinuation syndromes: clinical relevance, prevention and management. *Drug Safety* **24**, 183–195

Hart BL and Barrett RE (1973) Effects of castration on fighting, roaming and urine spraying in adult male cats. *Journal of the American Veterinary Medical Association* **163**, 290–292

Hart BL, Cliff KD, Tynes VV and Bergman L (2005) Control of urine marking by use of long-term treatment with fluoxetine or clomipramine in cats. *Journal of the American Veterinary Medical Association* **226**, 378–382

Hart BL and Cooper L (1984) Factors relating to urine spraying and fighting in prepubertally gonadectomized cats. *Journal of the American Veterinary Medical Association* **184**, 1255–1258

Hart BL, Eckstein RA, Powell KL and Dodman NH (1993) Effectiveness of buspirone on urine spraying and inappropriate urination in cats. *Journal of the American Veterinary Medical Association* **203**, 254–258

Horwitz DF (1997) Behavioural and environmental factors associated with elimination behaviour problems in cats: a retrospective study. *Applied Animal Behaviour Science* **52**, 129–137

Hunthausen W (2000) Evaluating a feline facial pheromone analogue to control urine spraying. *Veterinary Medicine* **95**, 151–156

King JN, Steffan J, Heath SE *et al.* (2004) Determination of clomipramine for the treatment of urine spraying in cats. *Journal of the American Veterinary Medical Association* **225**, 881–887

Kroll T and Houpt KA (2001) A comparison of cyproheptadine and clomipramine for the treatment of spraying cats. *Proceedings, 3rd International Congress on Veterinary Behavioural Medicine*, pp. 184–185

Landsberg GM and Wilson AL (2005) Effects of clomipramine on cats presented for urine marking. *Journal of the American Animal Hospital Association* **41**, 3–11

Marder AR, Engel JM and Hekman JP (2007) Feline behaviour problems reported by owners after adoption from an animal shelter. *Proceedings, 6th International Veterinary Behaviour Meeting and European College of Veterinary Behavioural Medicine – Companion Animals*, pp. 183–189

Mealey KL, Peck KE, Bennet BS *et al.* (2004) Systemic absorption of amitriptyline and buspirone after oral and transdermal administration to healthy cats. *Journal of Veterinary Internal Medicine* **18**, 43–46

Mills DS and Mills CB (2001) Evaluation of a novel method of delivering a synthetic analogue of feline facial pheromone to control urine spraying by cats. *Veterinary Record* **149**, 197–199

Mills DS and Munster C (2003) Litter depth preference in the domestic cat. *Proceedings, 4th International Veterinary Behaviour Meeting*, pp. 201–202

Neilson JC (2001) Pearl vs. clumping: litter preference in a population of shelter cats. In: *Abstracts from the American Veterinary Society of Animal Behaviour*, Boston, p. 14

Neilson JC (2008a) Litter odor control: carbon vs. bicarbonate of soda. In: *Proceedings, ACVB/AVSAB 2008: Scientific Paper and Poster Session*, pp. 31–34

Neilson JC (2008b) Scent preferences in the domestic cat. *Proceedings, ACVB/AVSAB 2008: Scientific Paper and Poster Session*, pp. 42–45

Neilson JC (2008c) Is bigger better? Litterbox size preference test. *Proceedings, ACVB/AVSAB 2008: Scientific Paper and Poster Session*, pp. 46–49

Pageat P (1996) Functions and use of the facial pheromones in the treatment of urine marking in the cat, interest of a structural analogue. *Proceedings and Abstracts, 21st WSAVA Congress*, pp. 197–198

Patronek GJ, Glickman TJ, Beck AM, McCabe GP and Ecker C (1996) Risk factors for relinquishment of cats to an animal shelter. *Journal of the American Veterinary Medical Association* **209**, 582–588

Pryor PA, Hart BL, Bain MJ and Cliff KD (2001a) Causes of urine marking in cats and the effects of environmental management on frequency of marking. *Journal of the American Veterinary Medical Association* **219**, 1709–1713

Pryor PA, Hart, BL, Cliff KD *et al.* (2001b) Effects of a selective serotonin reuptake inhibitor on urine spraying behaviour in cats. *Journal of the American Veterinary Medical Association* **219**, 1557–1561

Sung W and Crowell-Davis SL (2006) Elimination behaviour patterns of domestic cats with and without elimination behaviour problems. *American Journal of Veterinary Research* **67**, 1500–1504

Tynes VV, Hart BL, Pryor PA *et al.* (2003) Evaluation of the role of lower urinary tract disease in cats with urine-marking behaviour. *Journal of the American Veterinary Medical Association* **223**, 457–461

White JC and Mills DS (1997) Efficacy of synthetic feline facial pheromone analogue (Feliway) for the treatment of chronic non-sexual urine spraying by the domestic cat. *Proceedings, 1st International Conference on Veterinary Behavioural Medicine*, p. 262

---

**Client handouts (bsavalibrary.com/behaviour_leaflets)**

- Avoiding house soiling by cats
- Avoiding urine marking by cats
- Cognitive dysfunction syndrome
- Feline behaviour questionnaire
- Introducing a new cat into the household
- Litterbox training
- What your cat needs
- What your cat needs: multi-cat households

# 12

# Behaviour problems in the senior pet

## Gary M. Landsberg and Sagi Denenberg

## Introduction

Advances in veterinary medicine in recent years have greatly helped to increase the longevity of pets and so veterinary surgeons and owners are now encountering an increasing number of age-related medical and behavioural problems. Over a 40-year period, the number of senior pets increased from about a quarter to a third of the population (Watson, 1996). Many publications have defined senior pets as 7–11 years of age. However, with more pets living into their senior years, the American Animal Hospital Association (AAHA) Senior Care Taskforce has suggested that it might be more accurate to consider dogs and cats as middle aged at 50% of their lifespan and senior at 75% of their expected life span (Epstein *et al.*, 2005).

Ageing itself is not a disease, but it is associated with a reduced ability to cope with physiological and environmental stressors. The pet's immune system becomes increasingly compromised, the risk of neoplasia increases and degenerative (ageing) processes begin to affect the organ systems.

While the incidence of medical problems increases with age, the percentage of reported behaviour problems may actually decrease (Cantanzaro, 1999). This may be due to the fact that the serious problems associated with genetics and early experience are likely to be reported within the first 1–3 years, and that these are either successfully managed or the pet is euthanized or rehomed. In addition, medical problems of older pets may mask underlying behaviour problems, when in fact these problems can arise concurrently. Most important is that many behaviour changes go unreported. In a study by Hills Pet Nutrition (2000) about 75% of owners of dogs over the age of 7 reported at least one behavioural sign consistent with cognitive dysfunction syndrome (CDS), yet only 12% reported the signs to their veterinary surgeon. Diagnosis and treatment of CDS are discussed below.

## Patient evaluation

### Presenting signs and history

Since behavioural signs may be the first or only sign of many medical conditions, identifying all behavioural signs should be a major focus of every old-age evaluation (Figure 12.1), either by questioning the owners directly or with the aid of a questionnaire. In fact, the identification and monitoring of CDS, sensory loss and pain often relies entirely on behavioural signs. Along with the physical examination, collection of *all* behavioural and *all* medical signs can help to determine what diagnostic workup is most appropriate. In addition, the veterinary surgeon should determine whether any medications (prescription, over-the-counter or natural) are being taken that might be contributing factors to the behavioural changes.

| Condition or category | Clinical signs |
|---|---|
| Disorientation | Less responsive to stimuli<br>Decreased recognition of familiar people, pets or places<br>Gets lost in familiar locations<br>Goes to wrong side of door (e.g. hinge side) |
| Interactions and social behaviour | Decreased or increased interest in social contact with familiar people or pets<br>Decreased greeting behaviour<br>Newly exhibited fear, avoidance or aggression toward familiar people or pets |
| Sleep/wake cycle | Restless sleep or waking at night<br>Increased daytime sleep |
| House soiling | Indoor elimination at random sites (including sleeping areas) or in view of owners<br>Decreased or no signalling<br>Goes outdoors, eliminates indoors upon return |
| Activity: increased, decreased, stereotypic (displacement), repetitive | Increased wandering, pacing, restlessness<br>Decreased exploration<br>Depression or apathy<br>Staring, fixation or snapping at objects<br>Licking owners or household objects |

**12.1** Signs of cognitive dysfunction or brain ageing. (continues) ▶

| Condition or category | Clinical signs |
|---|---|
| Anxiety/agitation | Inappropriate vocalization<br>Increased irritability, aggression<br>Aimless pacing and wandering<br>Increased or new fears or phobias<br>Separation anxiety |
| Self-hygiene | Increased self-directed grooming<br>Decrease grooming behaviour |
| Reduced learning and memory loss | Decreased responsiveness to known commands or tricks<br>Decreased ability to perform tasks<br>Inability or slow to learn new tasks (must retrain) |
| Appetite | Increased volume or speed of eating<br>Decreased interest |
| Decrease responsiveness to stimuli | Not coming for verbal commands/treats<br>Less responsive or altered responses to visual, auditory and olfactory stimuli |

**12.1** (continued) Signs of cognitive dysfunction or brain ageing.

When owners report behavioural signs in a senior pet, especially those that have recently emerged, medical conditions must first be ruled out. Medical conditions of virtually any organ system can affect behaviour (Figure 12.2). Central nervous system (CNS) disease can lead to aggression or changes in interaction with owners, other people and other pets. Pets with impaired vision or hearing may become anxious and fearful. Urinary tract disorders can lead to house soiling and an altered sleep/wake cycle. Pain and irritation (such as pruritic skin disease and anal sacculitis) can lead to aggression and changes in interactions.

In some cases the medical problem may not be the sole cause but may be a contributing factor. This might occur in a dog that avoids certain people due to fear, but is aggressive when it is in pain or less mobile. Also there may be more than one health problem or a combination of medical and behavioural factors. For example, a dog with loss of vision and hearing can become anxious due to a reduced ability to cope with environmental changes.

Even when medical problems are diagnosed and controlled, there can be a learned component that may also need to be addressed. A cat that soils outside the litterbox due to lower urinary tract disease may develop an aversion to its box; a dog that begins to eliminate indoors due to cystitis or diabetes may learn to use a new indoor area; and a dog or cat that becomes aggressive because of a painful condition, such as arthritis or otitis, may continue to use aggression as a means of removing a perceived threat. These cases would need both medical treatment and behavioural guidance.

## Client attitudes, beliefs and underreporting

There are several reasons why owners might not report changes in behaviour in older pets. Firstly, they must be made aware that a change in behaviour, even if it seems subtle or insignificant, is not necessarily a normal part of ageing and that it could be an early sign of a medical problem, including CDS (Figure 12.1). Secondly, owners may not be aware

| System | Possible causes | Possible behavioural signs |
|---|---|---|
| Nervous system | CNS diseases; infectious diseases; neoplasia; toxins; degenerative diseases; diseases that affect CNS oxygenation (e.g. respiratory, cardiac, intracranial causes); seizures; endocrinopathies; pain | All signs of DISHA (see page 131); aggression; irritability; fear/anxiety; avoidance; reduced activity or interest in exercise; coprophagia; altered response to stimuli; appetite; vocalization; stereotypic/displacement (e.g. snapping) |
| Musculoskeletal | Disc and spinal diseases; degenerative diseases; arthritis; pain | All signs of DISHA; reduced activity or interest in exercise; aggression; avoidance; self-hygiene; vocalization; altered response to stimuli |
| Sensory | Loss of vision (cataracts, glaucoma, etc.); loss of hearing | All signs of DISHA; fear/anxiety/phobia; aggression; avoidance; vocalization; altered response to stimuli |
| Digestive system | Dental diseases; hepatic diseases; infectious/inflammatory; constipation; nutritional imbalances; pain | Reduced appetite; aggression; avoidance; house soiling; night walking; stereotypic: pacing, licking; coprophagia |
| Urogenital | Renal diseases; urinary tract infection; hormonal abnormalities; tumours; urolithiasis; urinary incontinence | Polyuria/polydipsia; aggression; house soiling, marking; mounting; pacing; sleep/wake changes |
| Endocrine | Diabetes mellitus; insulinoma; diabetes insipidus; hypothyroidism; hyperthyroidism; hyperadrenocorticism; hypoadrenocortism | All signs of DISHA; polyuria/polydipsia; appetite – increased/decreased; activity – increased/decreased/apathy; irritability; aggression; house soiling, urine marking; sleep/wake cycle; stereotypic – licking; restlessness – pacing; vocalization; coprophagia |

**12.2** Examples of medical conditions leading to behavioural signs.

that there may be effective treatments for these problems and that early intervention is the best way to improve, stabilize or at least slow the progress of the problem. In addition, some owners may be concerned that the problem may be terminal and choose to cope with the signs rather than possibly allow the pet to face euthanasia (Stewart, 1999). Therefore it is essential for the veterinary surgeon to inform pet owners of the importance of early reporting of these changes. The **client handout** explains CDS and behavioural problems in senior pets and gives advice on prevention and treatment.

## Risk evaluation

As pets age, there is an increased risk of degenerative diseases, tumour development and immune system compromise. For example, the risk of arthritis in senior cats approaches 90% by age 11 and is a common finding in aged dogs (Clark and Bennett, 2006); and periodontal disease in dogs between 7 and 8 years of age is reported to have a prevalence of 95% and is a common finding in aged cats (Harvey, 1988). In addition, diseases such as diabetes, sensory loss, Cushing's disease in dogs, hyperthyroidism in cats and cognitive dysfunction become increasingly more common. Veterinary surgeons should be cognisant of the increased risks related to breed and sex, such as neoplasia in Boxers and prostate disease in male dogs.

It is essential that all middle-aged and senior pets are carefully screened to ensure earliest possible detection of these conditions, since early diagnosis and intervention provide the best opportunity to resolve the condition, decrease the risk of complications, slow the progress of some diseases and improve quality of life and perhaps longevity. For healthy pets, this screening should include annual physical examination of middle-aged pets and twice-yearly examination of senior pets, a comprehensive questionnaire to identify all medical and behavioural signs (no matter how subtle) and laboratory screening. Particular attention should be paid to pain assessment, sensory loss and neurological evaluation. More frequent assessments and monitoring should be instituted for pets with pre-existing conditions and those on medication.

The risk for developing CDS increases with age. While breed and size do not seem to be factors, in a study of 325 geriatric dogs there was a trend towards increased prevalence in smaller dogs; in addition females and neutered dogs were significantly more affected than males and entire dogs.

## Diagnosis

In general, behaviour problems of senior pets are diagnosed and treated in the same manner as those of any other age and these are discussed in other chapters. However, due to age and the likelihood of concurrent medical problems, initially the focus will need to be on ruling out possible medical problems before considering a diagnosis of CDS.

Retraining of senior pets may need to progress more slowly and may require more repetitions and rewards (see Chapter 5). In addition, the choice and doses of behavioural medications may need to be adjusted (see Chapter 21). Finally, in senior pets the success of managing behaviour problems may be lower due to limitations such as medical conditions, loss of memory and decreased ability to cope with new experiences. When medical problems cannot be resolved, long-term environmental management changes may be required. Below are some specific considerations when presented with some of the common complaints in senior pets.

## Senior pet behavioural problems

Studies from veterinary behavioural practices have found that the following problems in older dogs were most commonly referred: aggression toward people 27%; aggression toward other dogs 5–17%; separation anxiety 29%; inappropriate elimination 3–23%; excessive vocalization 1–21%; phobias and anxiety 9–19%; night-time walking 8%; compulsive behaviour 5–8%; and CDS 7% (Landsberg, 1995; Horwitz, 2001). In a study of three veterinary behaviour referral practices in Canada, the United States and Australia, approximately 25% of dogs over 7 years of age had a diagnosis of CDS (Denenberg *et al.*, 2005). The higher prevalence in the 2005 study may be due to increased awareness of CDS since the diagnosis was first introduced into the veterinary literature in the mid 1990s (Milgram *et al.*, 1993). In addition, when CDS is diagnosed by the general practitioner, referral is often unnecessary. Similar studies in older cats found that 73% of cases were for house soiling, 6% were for aggression, vocalization or restlessness, and 4% for excessive grooming (Landsberg and Araujo, 2005).

## Aggression

Aggression may have multiple causes. In the senior pet, the clinician must first rule out medical causes (e.g. pain, sensory deficits, or diseases affecting the CNS) and perform a behavioural assessment, determining when the problem first began (i.e. whether there were any signs of aggression at an earlier age) and whether there were any changes in the environment at the onset of the aggression. When the aggression is between family pets, it is possible that they can no longer effectively communicate with each other due to alterations in their health, sensory function or mobility. Some combination of health problems, CDS and altered behavioural responses often contributes to the problem.

### Treatment

If the problem persists after diagnosing and treating medical problems, the behavioural programme will need firstly to focus on identifying the underlying cause and preventing exposure to the aggression-evoking stimuli. If medical factors (e.g. pain) can be controlled or improved, and the pet is neurologically and physically capable of learning, desensitization, counter-conditioning and drug therapy can often be utilized (see Chapters 17 to 19 for treatment protocols).

## Anxiety, fears and phobias

Anxiety, fears and phobias can result from the pet's lack of ability to cope with situations, noises, environment and interactions. Although the problem may have an entirely medical cause, the anxiety may have been pre-existing at a level that the owner and pet could tolerate but along with concurrent medical problems the summation of effects might induce clinical signs. Senior pets are less able to cope with change and can therefore become more anxious when the environment or household is altered. Medical problems such as CDS or sensory loss may cause the pet to become more anxious and fearful, develop hyperattachment and separation anxiety, or even become aggressive. Once the pet begins to display fear and anxiety, owner responses may unwittingly aggravate the problem. For example, owners who try to calm their pet with attention may actually reinforce fearful and anxious behaviours, which in turn may make it more difficult for the pet to cope with owner departures. Owners who are frustrated or anxious or who punish their pet will also increase its fear and anxiety.

### Treatment

Treatment should focus on using reinforcement-based techniques to train the pet to settle and drugs, pheromones or products that might help to calm the pet or treat underlying CDS. As with aggression, the ability to improve or control underlying medical problems will have an impact on outcome. Treatment for anxiety is covered in more detail in other chapters.

## House soiling

House soiling is the most common problem in senior cats (see Chapter 11) and is also a frequent complaint of owners of senior dogs (see Chapter 10). Medical causes should be the first consideration in a senior pet that was previously housetrained. CDS may be a contributing factor in, or the cause of, house soiling in both dogs and cats. The history is a critical component in diagnosis, since any indication of increased drinking, urine volume, urine frequency or discomfort when eliminating would indicate a medical cause. The pet that eliminates indiscriminately around the house may have incontinence, pain, control issues or CDS, as opposed to a pet that consciously eliminates in one or two selected indoor locations.

### Treatment

Many senior pets may require environmental modifications to help them to cope better with their ailments (e.g. dogs might require a dog door, dog walker, indoor toilet area, ramps, confinement or diapers; cats might need a change in litterbox location, an increase in number of boxes, more frequent cleaning, or easier access to boxes). When underlying medical problems can be improved or resolved, behaviour management and retraining to use appropriate sites for elimination might be possible (see Chapters 10 and 11).

## Pacing and repetitive behaviours

Pacing and other repetitive behaviours, such as licking, may develop in older pets. Often the restlessness and aimless pacing is more noticeable at night. Pacing can be accompanied by vocalization,

panting, attention seeking and salivation.

Before considering CDS as a cause, the first step is to rule out sensory loss, pain, neurological impairment and metabolic disorders, and especially in the case of oral behaviours (e.g. licking or pica) any form of gastrointestinal disease.

## Problems with sleep/wake cycles

Sleep/wake cycle alterations are commonly reported in senior dogs and cats. However, since cats may be more active at dusk and dawn, the history will need to identify when the problem first appeared. Medical problems (especially pain, sensory decline and conditions that might lead to more frequent elimination) as well as CDS must be ruled out. Pets that sleep more during the day and receive reduced enrichment or stimulation are more likely to wake at night. In addition, the behavioural history should focus on any change in daily routine or a decrease in daytime activity.

### Treatment

Treatment should focus on making sure the pet has a stimulating daily routine that includes sufficient exercise and mental stimulation (e.g. feeding toys) during the day. In addition, the owner must avoid reinforcing the behaviour. Determining why the pet is waking may be essential to treatment success, since medical therapy may be required to resolve the underlying cause (e.g. cystitis, Cushing's disease, diabetes, CDS), while some problems such as chronic renal failure may lead to continued night waking. Drugs that help to reduce anxiety or induce sleep may also be useful on a short-term basis (see drugs and natural products below).

## Disorientation

Disorientation may have many presentations. To determine whether the problem is CDS, the physical examination and diagnostic tests should focus on ruling out any other CNS diseases, sensory loss, or metabolic diseases that might be contributing to the signs.

## Vocalization

Vocalization may be a problem when it occurs at inappropriate times (e.g. at night), when there are no obvious inciting stimuli or when it is prolonged or stereotypic. Pain, discomfort, CNS disease and sensory loss are some of the more common medical differentials. The history should focus on whether there are external stimuli to which the pet is responding (e.g. neighbouring pet, people across the street, fireworks, thunderstorms), the age of onset of the first signs and the owner's response to the vocalization. Regardless of the cause, many owners further aggravate vocalization by their responses, whether reinforcement (which would increase the behaviour) or punishment (which would not address the underlying cause and could add to the pet's anxiety).

### Treatment

After ruling out and treating any medical causes, owners must be taught to focus on reinforcing non-vocal behaviours, to keep the pet sufficiently occupied and enriched (response substitution) and neither to reinforce nor to punish the undesirable vocalization.

## Cognitive dysfunction syndrome

CDS is a neurodegenerative disorder of senior dogs and cats that is characterized by gradual cognitive decline and increasing brain pathology. Because there are sufficient similarities between dogs with CDS and humans with early Alzheimer's disease (AD), dogs are used as models for human brain ageing. (Cummings *et al.*, 1996a; Adams *et al.*, 2000).

To determine whether a dog or cat might be showing signs of CDS, veterinary surgeons must rely almost entirely on history supplied by the owner. Only with careful questioning is it likely that signs would be detectable in the earliest stages of development. The diagnosis is initially based on clinical signs represented by the acronym DISH: **D**isorientation; alterations in social **I**nteractions with people or other pets; changes in **S**leep/wake cycles; or **H**ouse soiling.

The acronym has been extended to DISHA, since an alteration in **A**ctivity level is a common finding in dogs with CDS. Initially the alteration in activity may be an increase in rest or sleep and a decreased interest in social interactions, but this may progress to restlessness, night waking, pacing and other stereotypic or repetitive behaviours. Studies in humans with AD and other forms of age-related frontal lobe dysfunction show that patients may have anxiety, agitation and sleep/wake cycle disturbances associated with their dementia (Senanarong *et al.*, 2004). Similarly many of the problems in senior pets that are most commonly referred to veterinary surgeons appear to be associated with fear and anxiety, including vocalization, restlessness, pacing, night waking, phobias and separation anxiety. A decline in self-hygiene, alterations in appetite and an altered responsiveness to stimuli (information processing) might also be signs of cognitive decline.

### Prevalence

The prevalence of CDS varies between studies. In some studies prevalence may be overestimated since all medical causes may not be entirely ruled out, while in other studies it may be underestimated since medical cases have been excluded that may have had concurrent CDS. However, the primary concern for inaccurate data is the lack of owner reporting. In one study, owners of dogs aged 11–16 years of age that had no underlying illness according to their medical records were interviewed by telephone and it was determined that 28% of 11–12-year-old dogs and 68% of 15–16-year-old dogs showed at least one sign of CDS (Neilson *et al.*, 2001). In a study of 124 dogs with signs of CDS, 22 were eliminated due to medical factors; of the remaining dogs, 42 had alterations in one category and 33 had signs in two or more categories, therefore 75 dogs (60.5%) had signs consistent with CDS (Osella *et al.*, 2007). In a study of cats presented to veterinary clinics for routine annual care, 154 owners of cats aged 11 and older were asked about signs consistent with cognitive dysfunction. After 19 cats with medical problems (which may have also had concurrent CDS) were eliminated from the study, 35% of the cats were diagnosed with CDS. This ranged from 28% of 95 cats in the 11–15 age group to 50% of 46 cats in the over-15 age group (Gunn-Moore *et al.*, 2007). The challenge is firstly to identify cases through history and questionnaires, and then to determine whether the problem has a cause (behavioural or medical) other than CDS.

### Behavioural biology

Arguably the most sensitive measure of the onset of cognitive decline in humans as well as pets would be the identification of early deficits in learning and memory. In fact, a diagnosis of canine CDS based solely on clinical signs is most commonly reported at 11 years and older, while laboratory studies have demonstrated impairment in memory tasks early as 6–8 years of age (Studzinski *et al.*, 2006). In the home environment, learning and memory decline might not be noticeable until a fairly late stage such as when there is a loss of name recognition, or a loss in housetraining or previously learned behaviours or commands. Changes might be identified at an earlier age in dogs trained to a higher level of performance such as agility, therapy (e.g. guide dogs for the blind) or working dogs (e.g. drug or explosive detection).

In the French behavioural literature the term confusional syndrome has been used to describe cognitive disorders such as disorientation, loss of previously learned behaviours and altered sleep/wake cycles. A depressed mood is also described, with signs of lethargy, changes in appetite, decreased activity and decreased interest in interactions with family members and other pets. In chronic states the pet becomes more anxious and fearful, which may be associated with displacement behaviours, alterations in appetite, alterations in sleep and increased following of the owners (Landsberg *et al.*, 2003). ARCAD denotes a scoring system for the evaluation of Age-related Cognitive and Affective Disorders, including both emotional parameters (such as eating, drinking, elimination behaviour and sleep) and cognitive parameters (such as learned behaviours and adaptive abilities) (Landsberg *et al.*, 2003).

### Ageing and its effect on the brain

With increasing age there is a reduction in brain mass (including cerebral and basal ganglia atrophy), an increase in ventricular size, meningeal calcification, demyelination, increasing amounts of lipofuscin and apoptic bodies, neuroaxonal degeneration and a reduction in neurons (Borras *et al.*, 1999). There is also an increase in diffuse beta amyloid plaques and perivascular infiltrates in dogs, cats and humans with CDS. In dogs and cats the plaques are diffuse; in humans amyloid distribution may progress to neuritic plaques and neurofibrillary tangles (NFT) (Cummings *et al.*, 1996ab). No evidence for NFT has been found in aged dogs or cats. However, staining for hyperphosphorylated tau has been demonstrated in cats, indicating a possible pre-tangle formation (Gunn-Moore *et al.*, 2007). Numerous vascular and perivascular changes have been identified in older dogs, including microhaemorrhage, or infarcts in periventricular vessels and arteriosclerosis of the non-lipid variety. With age, there may also be a depletion of catecholamine neurotransmitters and an increase in monoamine oxidase B (MAOB) activity as well as a decline in the cholinergic system (Milgram et al., 1993; Araujo et al., 2005b).

## Possible causes of clinical signs

### Beta amyloid
Studies have shown that beta amyloid is undetectable in young dogs and is most extensive in the oldest canines. In dogs, errors in discrimination, reversal and delayed non-matching-to-position (DNMP) testing are strongly associated with increased amounts of beta amyloid deposition (Cummings et al., 1996b; Colle et al., 2000). Although the exact role of beta amyloid accumulation in the development of CDS is yet to be determined, it is neurotoxic and can lead to compromised neuronal function, degeneration of synapses, cell loss and a depletion of neurotransmitters. In cats, an increase in the deposition of diffuse beta amyloid with increasing age has also been identified, but the relationship between senile plaque formation and clinical signs remains to be clarified (Gunn-Moore et al., 2007).

### Reactive oxygen species (ROS)
As mitochondria age, they produce relatively more free radicals and less energy (Head et al., 2002). Increased MAOB activity may also result in increased liberation of free radicals. Normally the body's antioxidant defences including enzymes such as superoxide dismutase, catalase, and glutathione peroxidase and free radical scavengers such as vitamins A, C and E eliminate free radicals. With increasing age, the net effect of increased production and decreased clearance leads to an increase in ROS which react with DNA, lipids and proteins, leading to cell damage, dysfunction, mutation, neoplasia and cell death. While an increase in free radical load has been demonstrated in the brains of ageing dogs, it is likely that similar changes occur in most mammalian species, including cats (Gunn-Moore et al., 2007). The brain is particularly susceptible to the toxicity of free radicals.

### Vascular insufficiency
There may also be a link between vascular insufficiency, decreased perfusion and the signs of brain ageing in both dogs and cats (Landsberg and Araujo, 2005; Gunn-Moore et al., 2007).

### Receptor function, neurotransmission and neuronal loss
In the brains of ageing dogs and cats, a depletion in neurotransmitters and receptor function as well as reduction in neurons, alterations of morphology and synaptic impairments may also contribute to clinical signs. In cats and dogs, dysfunctional cholinergic transmission and neuron loss have been documented (Borras et al., 1999; Araujo et al., 2005b; Gunn-Moore et al., 2007).

### Tau pathology
While NFT formation has not been documented in dogs or cats, staining for hyperphosphorylated tau has been demonstrated in neurons of cats with senile plaque development, providing evidence of possible pre-tangle formation in senior cats (Gunn-Moore et al., 2007). However, an association between tau hyperphosphorylation and clinical signs of CDS has yet to be documented.

## Treatment for CDS

### Prevention and acute management
The first step when dealing with cognitive dysfunction is to resolve or control any medical problems that might be leading to the signs. In fact, if medical problems are not effectively controlled or improved (e.g. arthritis, diabetes, cystitis) successful modification of the pet's behaviour is likely to be impractical. Although response to therapy may take some time, a more stimulating and predictable daily routine, reinforcing desirable behaviours and ceasing any form of punishment by the owner must be addressed immediately. In fact, studies have shown that continued enrichment in the form of training, play, exercise and novel toys can help to maintain cognitive function or slow cognitive decline (Milgram et al., 2004). It is also likely but not documented that the supplements and diets discussed below may have neuroprotective (preventive) effects.

Since medical problems may preclude the pet from engaging in previous types and levels of enrichment, owners should find alternative forms of social activities (e.g. short walks, tug toys, find-and-seek, reward training) and forms of object play (e.g. food manipulation toys, chew toys) that are within the pet's physical and mental capabilities. In addition, immediate alterations to environment may be required to address the needs of the owner and the pet adequately and to maintain a strong human–animal bond. For example, dogs may require more frequent trips outdoors, a dog walker or an indoor elimination area if they have medical conditions leading to polyuria or incontinence, while ramps and physical support devices may be required to help address mobility issues. For cats, more litterboxes or more frequent cleaning may be required to treat house soiling due to polyuria (see Chapter 11), while ramps, litterboxes with lower sides, larger litterboxes or relocation of litterboxes may be required for cats with mobility problems. Behavioural drugs such as benzodiazepines or buspirone and pheromone therapy (DAP® and Feliway®; see Chapter 21) may be useful in more immediately addressing anxiety and altered sleep/wake cycles while waiting for medical therapy, drugs for CDS and behaviour therapy to take effect.

### Long-term management
Medical therapy, environmental enrichment, behaviour modification, environmental modifications, cognitive drugs and perhaps concurrent use of drugs for specific behaviour signs can take from several weeks to several months to achieve maximal improvement. Even if the signs are not entirely controlled, ongoing mental enrichment and the use of cognitive drugs should be continued life long to help to maintain maximal cognitive function and to slow further decline.

Maintaining a predictable daily routine with sufficient daytime enrichment may help to reduce anxiety and maintain temporal orientation. Any changes to the pet's household or routine should be made gradually, to help the pet better adapt. As sensory acuity, sensory processing and cognitive function decline, adding new odour, tactile and sound cues might help the pet to navigate its environment more easily and maintain some degree of environmental familiarity.

### Drug therapy
Selegiline is a selective and irreversible inhibitor of MAOB in the dog (see Chapter 21). It has been shown to increase 2-phenylethylamine (PEA) in the dog brain (Milgram *et al.*, 2004). PEA is a neuromodulator that enhances dopamine and catecholamine function and may itself enhance cognitive function. Selegiline may also contribute to a decrease in free-radical load in the brain, by inhibiting MAOB, and increasing free-radical clearance by enhancing enzymes such as superoxide dismutase (SOD) (Carillo *et al.*, 1994).

Propentofylline is indicated for the treatment of dullness, lethargy and depressed demeanour in older dogs and may be particularly useful for increasing exercise tolerance. It may increase blood flow to the heart, skeletal muscles and brain. It inhibits platelet aggregation and thrombus formation and has a bronchodilator action equivalent to aminophylline.

Other treatment options that might be useful but are not licensed are modafinil and adrafinil and drugs that aid in cholinergic transmission (Siwak *et al.*, 2000; Araujo *et al.*, 2005b).

There are no drugs licensed for the treatment of cognitive dysfunction in cats, though there have been anecdotal reports of the successful use of some of the canine medications (including selegiline and propentofylline). The possibility of improving signs must be weighed against the potential risks.

For doses, see Figure 12.3.

### Nutritional and dietary therapy
A variety of studies have shown that high intake of fruits and vegetables and of vitamins E and C decreases the risk for cognitive decline (Sano *et al.*, 1997; Joseph *et al.*, 1998). A senior diet (Hill's Prescription Diet canine b/d, Hills Pet Nutrition, Topeka, Kansas) is supplemented with antioxidants (vitamins C and E, beta carotene, selenium, fruits and vegetables), mitochondrial cofactors (alpha-lipoic acid and l-carnitine) and essential fatty acids. Senior dogs with cognitive dysfunction that were fed this diet showed improved performance on a number of cognitive tasks when compared with other older dogs that were fed regular senior diet. Over 2 years, the control group (no enrichment, no supplemented diet) showed a dramatic decline in cognitive function, while those dogs in either the enriched diet group or an environmental enrichment group performed better than control (Araujo *et al.*, 2005a). The combined effect of the enriched diet plus the enriched environment provided the greatest improvement (Milgram *et al.*, 2004).

In a wide variety of other complementary therapies nutraceuticals, herbal extracts and vitamins have been formulated into combination products that are purported to have antioxidant and neuroprotective effects that may enhance cognition, slow cognitive decline and help to normalize neurotransmitter levels. These products may contain a mixture of herbal extracts, vitamins, phospholipids, fatty acids, antioxidants and mitochondrial cofactors that are believed to act in a synergistic or potentiating manner to slow the progression or improve the clinical signs associated with brain ageing but for many of these products data are weak or not available to document efficacy.

Several clinical trials have demonstrated improvements in clinical signs associated with CDS in dogs using dietary supplements containing phosphatidylserine (Heath *et al.*, 2007; Osella *et al.*, 2007). One of these products, Senilife® (CEVA Sante Animale), was also studied in laboratory testing of dogs. Performance accuracy was significantly improved in the treatment group compared with baseline (Araujo *et al.*, 2008). In addition, dogs receiving the supplement in the first portion of the study maintained their improved performance. Senilife, which is available in Italy and was recently introduced to the US market, contains phosphatidylserine, *Ginkgo biloba*, resveratrol, and vitamins E and B6. Phosphatidylserine is a membrane phospholipid that may facilitate signal transduction and has been shown to improve activity, social interactions, memory and learning in humans with cognitive decline. Phosphatidylserine may stimulate the release of acetylcholine and dopamine (Osella *et al.*, 2008). Vitamin B6 (pyridoxine) is a cofactor in the synthesis of neurotransmitters and may support phosphatidylserine in normalizing neurotransmitter levels. *Ginkgo biloba* may act as an MAO inhibitor and free radical scavenger and may enhance blood flow. It may also enhance dopaminergic, serotonergic and cholinergic transmission, and has been reported to improve cognitive function in humans. Vitamin E may further enhance the effects of *Ginkgo biloba* as well as neutralize free radicals. Resveratrol may protect against oxidative damage and reduce beta amyloid secretion (Miolo and Re, 2007).

| Drug name | Canine | Feline |
|---|---|---|
| Selegiline | 0.5–1 mg/kg orally q24h (mornings) | 0.5–1 mg/kg orally q24h (mornings) |
| Propentofylline | 5 mg/kg orally q12h | ¼ of 50 mg tablet q24h |
| SAMe | 10–20 mg/kg orally q24h | 100 mg orally q24h |
| Combination supplements and therapeutic diets | Follow veterinary advice and label directions | Follow veterinary advice and label directions |

**12.3** Drug doses for the treatment of cognitive dysfunction.

Another product (Activait, VetPlus Ltd, Lytham, UK) for brain ageing in dogs contains (in addition to phosphatidylserine and vitamin E) essential fatty acids, n-acetyl cysteine, CoQ10, vitamin C, glutathione, carnitine, alpha-lipoic acid and glutathione. The cat product is similar but has had the alpha-lipoic acid removed, since high levels may be toxic to cats. In one study cognitive signs were improved in senior dogs after treatment with this supplement (Heath et al., 2007).

S-adenosyl methionine or SAMe (Novifit, Virbac, Carros, France) has also recently been introduced as a treatment for cognitive dysfunction in dogs and cats (see Figure 12.3 for doses). SAMe plays a role in the treatment of liver disease and mood disorders, and in humans with Alzheimer's disease. SAMe may help to maintain cell membrane fluidity, receptor function and the synthesis of monoamine neurotransmitters such as noradrenaline (norepinephrine), dopamine and serotonin. It is also a precursor in the production of glutathione. In a recent placebo-controlled clinical trial of 36 dogs over 8 years of age with signs of cognitive dysfunction, greater improvement in activity and awareness was reported in the SAMe group after 8 weeks (Rème et al., 2008).

### Adjunctive therapy
In conjunction with drugs for cognitive dysfunction it might also be necessary to consider medications that address specific signs. For example, antidepressants and anxiolytics may be indicated for the pet that is anxious or night waking. Since selective serotonin reuptake inhibitors such as fluoxetine and the anxiolytic buspirone have little or no cardiovascular or anticholinergic effects, they might have less potential for side effects in the elderly. Although drug combinations may be useful, caution should be exercised against potential contraindications or side effects. For example, selegiline should not be used in combination with tricyclic antidepressants and selective serotonin reuptake inhibitors. Lorazepam, oxazepam and clonazepam have no active intermediate metabolite and might therefore be safer than other benzodiazepines in patients with compromised hepatic function. Natural therapies that might also be used in the senior pet for calming, reducing anxiety or inducing sleep include melatonin, valerian, aromatherapy and pheromones (see Chapter 21).

### Obstacles to treatment success
The success rate of treating behaviour problems in senior pets is greatly reduced as compared with younger animals. Even in the relatively healthy senior pet, studies have shown that learning new tasks is more difficult and that senior pets are less able to adapt to change. In many cases senior pets have concurrent medical conditions that contribute to the behavioural signs and these may be chronic or uncontrollable. Similarly medical problems that lead to sensory loss, a decline in mobility, pain or altered neurological function may make it impractical to alter the behaviour, to acquire new behaviours or to relearn the behaviours that have been 'lost'. Furthermore, due to the progressive nature of CDS and the ageing process itself, therapeutic agents that are initially successful may become less effective over time. Finally, when age, health, quality of life and finances are considered, some owners may be reluctant to undergo the necessary diagnostics or implement treatment.

## Prognosis

The prognosis will be variable, depending on cause. It is poor if there is a medical cause that cannot be sufficiently resolved. When medical problems can be controlled and the owner is compliant, a combination of behaviour modification, drugs or natural supplements and environmental modification can be effective. This is especially true when detection, diagnosis and treatment are early in the course of the disease so that cognitive decline might be improved or slowed and emerging undesirable behaviours can be more easily retrained. However, cognitive dysfunction is a progressive disease over time (Bain et al., 2001). CDS and senior behaviour problems are seldom the primary reason for death or euthanasia but they do play an important role in the final decision, since the behavioural signs become less treatable or tolerable as the health of the pet deteriorates and the quality of life declines for the pet and the owner.

## Follow-up

While a general rule of thumb would be a minimum of twice-annual visits for senior pets, pets with health and behaviour problems may need to be followed up at more frequent intervals. The veterinary surgeon should be aware of the time expected for a drug or behavioural plan to begin to show efficacy or side effects and should follow up accordingly. For example, cognitive supplements and associated behaviour therapy may take 1–2 months before determining full effect. In addition, owners should be informed to report any new changes in health or behaviour as soon as they develop.

## References and further reading

Adams B, Chan A, Callahan H et al. (2000) The canine as a model of human brain aging: recent developments. Progress in Neuro-psychopharmacology & Biological Psychiatry **24**, 675–692

Araujo JA, Landsberg GM, Milgram NW et al. (2008) Improvement of short-term memory performance in aged beagles by a nutraceutical supplement containing phosphatidylserine, Ginkgo biloba, vitamin E and pyridoxine. Canadian Veterinary Journal **19**, 379–385

Araujo JA, Studzinski CM, Head E et al. (2005a) Assessment of nutritional interventions for modification of age-associated cognitive decline using a canine model of human aging. AGE **27**, 27–37

Araujo JA, Studzinski CM, Head E et al. (2005b) Further evidence for the cholinergic hypothesis of aging and dementia from the canine model of aging. Progress in Neuro-psychopharmacology & Biological Psychiatry **29**, 411–422

Azkona G, Garcia-Belenguer S, Cacon G et al. (2009) Prevalence and risk factors of behavioural changes associated with age related cognitive impairment in geriatric dogs. Journal of Small Animal Practice **50**, 87–91

Bain MJ, Hart BL, Cliff KD et al. (2001) Predicting behavioral changes associated with age-related cognitive impairment in dogs. Journal of the American Veterinary Medical Association **218**, 1792–1795

Borras D, Ferrer I and Pumarola M (1999) Age related changes in the brain of the dog. Veterinary Pathology **36**, 202–211

Carillo MC, Ivy GO, Milgram NW et al. (1994) Deprenyl increases activity of superoxide dismutase in striatum of dog brain. *Life Sciences* **54**, 1483–1489

Catanzaro TE (1999) Care of aging pets. In: *Healthcare of the Well Pet*, ed. C Jevring and TE Catanzaro, pp. 49–65. WB Saunders, Philadelphia

Clark SP and Bennett D (2006) Feline osteoarthritis: a prospective study. *Journal of Small Animal Practice* **47**, 439–445

Colle M-A, Hauw J-J, Crespau F *et al.* (2000) Vascular and parenchymal beta-amyloid deposition in the aging dog: correlation with behavior. *Neurobiology of Aging* **21**, 695–704

Cummings BJ, Head E, Afagh AJ *et al.* (1996b) B-Amyloid accumulation correlates with cognitive dysfunction in the aged canine. *Neurobiology of Learning and Memory* **66**, 11–23

Cummings BJ, Satou T, Head E *et al.* (1996a) Diffuse plaques contain c-terminal AB42 and not AB40: evidence from cats and dogs. *Neurobiology of Aging* **17**, 4653–4659

Davies M (1996) *Canine and Feline Geriatrics*. Blackwell Science, Oxford

Denenberg S, Landsberg GM, Horwitz D *et al.* (2005) Comparison of cases referred to behaviorists in three different countries. In: *Current Issues and Research in Veterinary Behavioral Medicine*, ed. D Mills *et al.*, pp. 56–62. Purdue University Press, West Lafayette

Epstein M, Kuehn NF, Landsberg GM *et al.* (2005) AAHA Senior Care Guidelines for Dogs and Cats. *Journal of the American Animal Hospital Association* **41**, 81–91

Gunn-Moore D, Moffat K, Christie LA *et al.* (2007) Cognitive dysfunction and the neurobiology of ageing in cats. *Journal of Small Animal Practice* **48**, 546–553

Harvey CE (1988) Oral diseases of aging animals. In: *Proceedings of Symposium on Clinical Conditions of the Older Cat and Dog*, London, pp. 58–62

Head E, Liu J, Hagen TM *et al.* (2002) Oxidative damage increases with age in a canine model of human brain aging. *Journal of Neurochemistry* **82**, 75–381

Heath SE, Barabas S and Craze PG (2007) Nutritional supplementation in cases of canine cognitive dysfunction – a clinical trial. *Journal of Applied Animal Behaviour Science* **105**, 274–283

Hills Pet Nutrition (2000) *US Marketing Research Summary: Omnibus Study on Aging Pets*. Hill's Pet Nutrition, Inc, Topeka, Kansas

Horwitz D (2001) Dealing with common behavior problems in senior dogs. *Veterinary Medicine* **96**, 869–879

Joseph JA, Shukitt-Hale B, Denisova NA *et al.* (1998) Long-term dietary strawberry, spinach, or vitamin E supplementation retards the onset of age-related neuronal signal transduction and cognitive behavioral deficits. *Journal of Neuroscience* **18**, 8047–8055

Landsberg GM (1995) The most common behavior problems in older dogs. *Veterinary Medicine* **90** (suppl.), 16–24

Landsberg GM and Araujo JA (2005) Behavior problems in geriatric pets. *Veterinary Clinics of North America: Small Animal Practice* **35**, 675–698

Landsberg G, Hunthausen W and Ackerman L (2003) The effects of aging on behavior and senior pets. In: *Handbook of Behavior Problems of the Dog and Cat*, pp. 269–304. Elsevier Saunders, Edinburgh

Milgram NW, Head EA, Zicker SC *et al.* (2004) Long term treatment with antioxidants and a program of behavioral enrichment reduces age-dependant impairment in discrimination and reversal learning in beagle dogs. *Experimental Gerontology* **39**, 753–765

Milgram NW, Ivy GO, Head E *et al.* (1993) The effect of l-deprenyl on behavior, cognitive function, and biogenic amines in the dog. *Neurochemical Research* **18**, 1211–1219

Miolo A and Re G (2007) Emerging roles of polyphenols ginkgo biloba and resveratrol as neuroprotectors in brain aging of dogs and cats: a review. Poster. In: *Proceedings of the 6th International Veterinary Behaviour Meeting and ECVBM-CA*, Fondazione Iniziative Zooprofilattiche E Zootecniche, Brescia, Italy, pp. 129–130

Nielson JC, Hart BL, Cliff KD *et al.* (2001) Prevalence of behavioral changes associated with age-related cognitive impairment in dogs. *Journal of the American Veterinary Medical Association* **218**, 1787–1791

Osella CM, Re G, Badino P *et al.* (2008) Phosphatidylserine (PS) as a potential nutraceutical for canine brain aging: a review. *Journal of Veterinary Behavior* **3**, 41–51

Osella MC, Re G, Odore R *et al.* (2007) Canine cognitive dysfunction syndrome: prevalence, clinical signs and treatment with a neuroprotective nutraceutical. *Journal of Applied Animal Behaviour Science* **105**, 297–310

Rème CA, Dramard V, Kern L *et al.* (2008) Effect of *S*-adenosylmethionine tablets on the reduction of age-related mental decline in dogs: a double-blind placebo-controlled trial. *Veterinary Therapeutics* **9**, 69–82

Sano M, Ernesto C, Thomas R *et al.* (1997) A controlled trial of selegiline, alpha tocopherol, or both for the treatment for Alzheimer's disease. *New England Journal of Medicine* **336**, 1216–1222

Senanarong V, Cummings JL, Fairbanks L *et al.* (2004) Agitation in Alzheimer's disease is a manifestation of frontal lobe dysfunction. *Dementia in Geriatric Cognitive Disorders* **17**, 14–20

Siwak CT, Gruet P, Woehrle F *et al.* (2000) Comparison of the effects of adrafinil, propentofylline and nicergoline on behavior in aged dogs. *American Journal of Veterinary Research* **61**, 1410–1414

Stewart M (1999) Reasons for contemplating euthanasia. In: *Companion Animal Death – A Practical and Comprehensive Guide for Veterinary Practice*, pp. 63–65. Butterworth Heinemann, Oxford

Studzinski CM, Christie L-A, Araujo JA *et al.* (2006) Visuospatial function in the beagle dog: an early marker of cognitive decline in a model of human cognitive aging and dementia. *Neurobiology of Learning and Memory* **86**, 197–204

Tapp PD, Siwak CT, Gao FQ *et al.* (2004) Frontal lobe volume, function, and beta-amyloid pathology in a canine model of aging. *Journal of Neuroscience* **24**, 8205–8213

Watson D (1996) Longevity and diet. *Veterinary Record* **3**, 7

## Client handouts (bsavalibrary.com/behaviour_leaflets)

- Avoiding house soiling by cats
- Avoiding house soiling by dogs
- Canine behaviour questionnaire
- Cognitive dysfunction syndrome
- Environmental enrichment for cats in animal shelters
- Environmental enrichment for dogs in animal shelters
- Feline behaviour questionnaire
- Handling exercises for an aggressive cat

- Ladder of Aggression
- Litterbox training
- Muzzle training
- Playing with your dog – toys
- Playing with your kitten
- Request for information on problem behaviours
- Treating a noise fear using desensitization and counter-conditioning
- What your cat needs
- What your dog needs

# 13

# Stress in veterinary behavioural medicine

## Lorella Notari

## Introduction

Stress describes the phenomenon whereby stimuli threaten the optimal state of an organism which, as a consequence, responds (with a stress response) to try to re-establish the original state. As such, understanding stress is integral to all aspects of veterinary medicine. Stress stimuli (stressors), the system processing this information and stress responses are integrated into a complex system whose feedback contributes to the self-regulation of the organism and the effects of one part of the system should not be considered independently of the other. It is important to be able to identify what stress stimuli are, how they are processed and how animals can respond as a consequence of different stress stimuli.

Stress is important for adaptation and survival: problems arise when animals cannot perform adaptive responses or when these responses do not lead to the expected outcome. In such cases, self-regulation of the organism is impaired, with a number of physical and behavioural consequences.

The goal of this chapter is to give an overview of stress and what impact it can have on companion animal behaviour and welfare.

## The physiology of stress

Two main physiological systems constitute the main 'stress response pathways': the hypothalamus–pituitary–adrenal (HPA) axis and the sympathetic nervous system. These have evolved to deal efficiently with short-term stressors, which are more typical of the wild state. Unfortunately, captive animals (including companion animals) are often faced with chronic challenges for which the system is less well adapted and which can lead to malfunction and secondary physical and behavioural health problems.

### Sympathetic nervous system and stress
The activity of the autonomic nervous system is controlled by a central autonomic network of nuclei in the brain, from which signals are sent to both parasympathetic and sympathetic neurons. In response to stimulation along nerves of the sympathetic nervous system the adrenal medulla releases the catecholamines adrenaline (epinephrine) and noradrenaline (norepinephrine). Under stressful conditions, adrenaline results in increased heart rate, blood pressure and the hydrolysis of glycogen to glucose, increasing

energy availability for facing a challenge, all of which can be used to determine whether an animal is 'stressed' by an immediate challenge.

Effective behavioural strategies, both in animals and humans, require the capacity for selective response in a stable environment and rapid adaptive response to a changing environment. This means that animals, in order to adapt successfully, should be able to regulate their attention selectively and be flexible or focused in their responses, depending on the situation. Overly focused or overly labile attention are often the basis of behaviour disorders, and may present as either apparent hyperactivity and hyper-responsiveness at one extreme or apathy and non-responsiveness at the other. The locus coeruleus–noradrenaline system seems to play a central role in regulating the balance of the response in the appropriate way (Aston-Jones, 1999).

## Hypothalamus–pituitary–adrenal axis
The HPA axis (Figure 13.1) is essential for the control of neural, endocrine and immune responses to challenges. The pituitary gland is constantly controlled by hypothalamic secretions and by biochemical

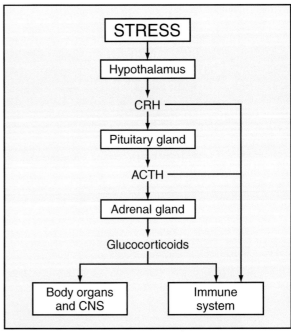

**13.1** Regulation of the hypothalamus–pituitary–adrenal axis. (ACTH, adrenocorticotropic hormone; CRH, corticotropin-releasing hormone.)

feedback messages from the periphery. Neurons in the hypothalamus produce corticotropin-releasing hormone/factor (CRH/CRF) and arginine vasopressin (AVP) to modulate corticotropin-producing cells in the pituitary gland and increase the synthesis and secretion of adrenocorticotropic hormone (ACTH).

CRH and its receptors are important for the production and secretion of ACTH under stressful conditions, but the maintenance of basal levels of ACTH production depends on AVP and its receptors. Under stressful conditions CRH stimulates the production of ACTH in the pituitary and this induces the release of glucocorticosteroids in the adrenal gland. Along with this adrenal secretion, there is secretion of prolactin and growth hormone in the pituitary in response to stress. All these hormones have an impact on the endocrine and the immune system, and have been used to assess the level of stress in animals in experimental situations. Cytokines act directly on pituitary cells and indirectly by controlling the release of hypothalamic factors; and the production of cytokines (and immunocompetence as a result) is also affected by stress.

The HPA axis and the locus coeruleus–central nervous system (CNS) network are not independent of one another: activation of one system tends to activate the other. For example, CRH activates the locus coeruleus in addition to its primary function of stimulating ACTH release. CRH is the principal stimulus for ACTH production and induces transcription of propiomelanocortin (POMC) mRNA, the ACTH precursor protein, but also a precursor of the endogenous opiate, beta-endorphin. Both beta-endorphin and ACTH are expressed in immune cells and contribute to immunoregulatory control. Under conditions of stress, the brain can stimulate immune cell functions by coordinated activation of the HPA axis and the sympathetic nervous system. A population of CRH parvocellular neurons project to extra-hypothalamic sites, including limbic nuclei (where they may affect emotional responses) and the brainstem. In some cases, CRH-containing parvocellular neurons can also express the inhibitory neurotransmitter gamma-amino-butyric acid (GABA) instead of AVP.

## Glucocorticoids and stress response regulation

ACTH stimulates the adrenal cortex to secrete glucocorticoids in a pulsatile fashion and peaks of glucocorticoids typically occur after 15–30 minutes of ACTH pulse, with variations during the day that follow a circadian rhythm. The HPA axis can have alternate periods of activation and inhibition and there is a refractory period when the HPA axis is no longer sensitive to activation by mild stressors. Therefore direct assessment and interpretation of glucocorticoid levels is often more complex than generally suggested.

Glucocorticoids exert negative feedback control in two distinct ways:

- Rapid feedback acts immediately after a rise in circulating glucocorticoids and lasts from 5 to 15 minutes; this rapid feedback inhibits the release and synthesis of ACTH in the hypothalamus

- Delayed feedback relies on the genomic action on glucocorticoid receptors in the brain. These receptors influence transcription of target genes, leading to a change in protein synthesis. Along with this genomic action, another is probably exerted at the level of the adenohypophysis by decreasing mRNA expression of the ACTH precursor protein POMC. Glucocorticoids can act centrally at the hypothalamus and higher centres (hippocampus in particular) with a negative feedback action in order to prevent a continued activation of the HPA axis.

CRH acts not just as a hormone-releasing factor but also as a neurotransmitter and several studies demonstrate that peptide hormones like CRH have functional targets in the brain that are unrelated to the neuroendocrine HPA circuit. However, both functions of CRH are activated by factors that disturb organismal homeostasis. Studies have revealed the presence of novel types of CRH receptor-selective agonists with a structure and functions similar to CRH; in the near future studies about the CRH peptide family and their receptors are likely to provide new therapies for stress-related problems (Smagin *et al.*, 2001; Heinrichs, 2005; Hsu, 2005).

## Impact of stress during the developmental period

Both genes and environment influence the fundamental neuroendocrinological processes involved in the stress response and the variation in susceptibility to stressors that occurs between individuals. Several studies have shown that environmental influences during the developmental period affect the neural and hormonal pathways controlling emotional responses and behaviour.

During the developmental period, as a consequence of external stimulation, the neuroendocrine system and the cascade of hormonal and neurotransmitter responses are shaped and the 'tone' of the stress-processing system is adjusted as a consequence. Thus the capacity to cope with environmental stress or social challenges depends on both innate and learned features of the individual and the stressful stimuli and situations that they have encountered early in life or even during pregnancy (Levine, 1966; Alonso *et al.*, 2000; Sanchez *et al.*, 2001; Fulford and Harbuz, 2005). Animals that have been deprived of normal maternal care and early social contact with conspecifics, human beings and other common social and environmental stimulations will be more prone to stress and to the development of non-adaptive coping strategies that often form the basis of behaviour problems (Caldji *et al.*, 1988; Francis *et al.*, 1999).

## What can be considered a stress stimulus?

Different kinds of stimuli can threaten an animal's homeostasis and provoke both the cascades of events described above. Stress stimuli can be physiological or psychological: the former involve physical challenges, the latter a reaction to an aversive stimulus without direct physical modification of the animal body.

## Physiological stressors

Physiological stressors challenge body integrity and physiological balance – a balance that has to be maintained around a relatively narrow range of parameters, such as a range of temperature, a range of extracellular sodium concentration or a range of blood glucose level. Any challenge to these balances is taken under homeostatic control. Stressors that directly challenge physiological balance produce responses in order to meet set points. It might be said that these kind of stressors are physiological stressors, because they directly challenge physiological parameters and their effects are managed through autonomic body receptor systems: viscerosensory pathways that activate subcortical autonomic circuits and directly affect stress-related motor neurons often without significant cortical contributions unless these systems fail to cope. Distress caused by hunger, thirst, or cold or hot temperatures are examples of physiological stressors; and blood glucose, body temperature and blood pressure are examples of physiological parameters that can be affected by them. These challenges activate the CRH-secreting neurons in the paraventricular nucleus and initiate a stress hormone cascade. Not just the neuroendocrine response but also an autonomic efferent projection is activated, in order to induce adaptive responses (cardiovascular, respiratory, thermoregulatory), including the sympatheticoadrenal system responses.

## Psychological stressors

Psychological stressors, also called emotional stressors, are processed through higher-order brain circuits and involve learned, emotional and cognitive processes. In the same way as physiological stressors, psychological stimuli such as social conflicts, inappropriate handling, fearful stimuli, individual subjective perceptions of an inability to cope and many others (Figure 13.2) also activate parvocellular neurosecretory motor neurons in the paraventricular nucleus (PVN). Visceral responses to psychological stressors also include cardiovascular, respiratory, gastrointestinal and thermoregulatory changes and are stressor specific.

Restraint
Inappropriate handling
Social conflicts with other animals or human beings
Unpredictable social environment (e.g. frequent change of social group members; children that disturb the animal when it sleeps or eats; inconsistent punishment)
View/presence of predators or social antagonists without possibility of avoiding them
Insufficient exercise and stimulation (both physical and mental)
Continuous exposure to disturbing or fearful environmental stimuli (e.g. cars, motorbikes, people)
Loud noises
Exposure to fearful natural events (e.g. thunderstorms, wind)

**13.2** Some examples of psychological stressors.

Change of status in a social context or hiding from a predator, for example, are psychological stressors that require different physical and behavioural coping responses. The former challenge requires a process that maintains stability through change and promotes adaptation and coping in a social environment. The latter may require an active (escape) or passive (immobility) coping strategy (Keay and Bandler, 2001). The subjective perception of physical distress or impairment is an important psychological stressor that provokes centrally mediated coordinated responses (including HPA-axis and autonomic activations). Although it may seem that psychological and physical stressors activate different pathways at a functional neuroanatomical level, stressors are often compound – both psychological and physical – and it is unwise to make an absolute distinction between these two types of stressors (Kovàks et al., 2005).

## Acute stressors

Different stress responses are also performed as a consequence of challenges of different intensity, duration and frequency of exposure. In the event of single exposure to a single intense challenge we can talk about acute stress. Animals are often subjected to stressful situations, such as fighting for mates or escaping from predators. The responses to these situations contribute to the process of adaptation to the environment and should be considered as normal.

When animals are kept in captivity or in different housing conditions, they might be subjected to short-term stressful situations such as transport, physical restraint, exposure to predators or social threat that they cannot escape from. If the normal behavioural responses to threatening situations cannot be performed for any reason, animals are likely to suffer from acute stress. Behavioural signs of acute stress that may be observed include:

- Cessation of or reduction in normal behaviours such as grooming and feeding
- The presence of somatic signs of fear and anxiety, such as spontaneous urination, defecation, vocalization and trembling, along with fear/anxiety postures.

These expressions are sufficient to state that the animal is not feeling well. Aggressive behaviour or immobility might be signs of acute stress as well. Some of the signs of acute stress that the veterinary surgeon needs to be aware of are given in Figure 13.3.

## Repeated stressors

Animals that are suffering from acute stress can rapidly regain a normal state when the negative stimuli and/or their predictors are removed, unless they perceive a repeated or prolonged sense of lack of control over the environment. Repeated stress (also called **chronic intermittent stress**) is a single exposure repeated over a prolonged time. Examples of repeated stressors are emotional stressors such as restraint or repeated exposure to social conflicts in an unstable social group.

| Dogs |
| --- |
| Urination and defecation/diarrhoea |
| Increased motor activity |
| Vocalizations |
| Salivation |
| Piloerection |
| Trembling |
| Polypnoea/panting |
| Looking away |
| Protrusion of the tongue |
| Muzzle licking |
| Yawning |
| Paw lifting (front paw held at 45 degrees) |
| Frequent shifting of body position |
| Low postures |

| Cats |
| --- |
| Urination, spraying and defecation/diarrhoea |
| Trembling |
| Might vocalize with hiss/spit on approach |
| Hiding, withdrawal to back of cage |
| Sitting on all four legs with head low |
| Eyes wide open |
| Pupils dilated |
| Polypnoea |
| Ears flattened |
| Whiskers back |
| Tail close to body |

**13.3** Behavioural and somatic signs of acute stress in dogs and cats.

When an animal is unable to reduce the subjective perceived risk for its safety and fitness through the avoidance or elimination of a challenge, other behavioural signs of stress are likely to appear. Along with behavioural signs of acute stress, signs of chronic stress are also likely to appear if stressors are not removed.

## Chronic stressors

Chronic stress is long-term exposure to a stress. In chronic stress the HPA axis can become dysregulated and several brain structures can be affected by excessive corticosteroid exposure, with a deterioration of learning and memory. In chronic stress conditions, noradrenaline stores in the locus coeruleus become exhausted and stress-induced depression can appear. Behavioural signs of chronic stress are different and might be less evident, or less problematic to an animal owner, compared with signs of acute stress.

Protracted lack of or insufficient exercise and mental stimulation, constant social threats without the possibility of avoiding them and continuous exposure to fearful stimulations can all be considered chronic stressors. The chronically stressed animal tends to become more passive, less explorative and less playful but might show abnormal behaviours. A decrease in the variety of the behavioural repertoire is a sign that might not be easily detected in dogs and cats until high levels of passivity are reached. Increased sleeping time, decreased appetite, the frequent appearance of displacement activities (often simple behaviours that appear to be out of context – see below) or stereotypic behaviours (see Chapter 20) are all signs of chronic stress. Some signs of chronic stress are listed in Figure 13.4.

| |
| --- |
| Decreased behavioural repertoire (less variation in behaviour) |
| Decreased exploratory behaviour |
| Reduced social behaviour and increased antagonistic behaviour |
| Displacement activities |
| Stereotypic behaviours |
| Passivity/apathy |
| Increased sleep, or disturbance to sleep patterns |
| Anorexia or binge eating |

**13.4** Behavioural and somatic signs of chronic stress.

## Stress as a risk factor for diseases and behavioural problems

The management of stress is integral to all aspects of veterinary medicine. Physical and psychological stressors that overtax the stress system cause elevated levels of circulating corticosteroids and the HPA axis feedback control can become dysregulated. This dysregulation can both contribute to the onset of stress-induced behaviour and increase the risk of physical and behavioural pathologies.

### Stress and the immune system

Longer-term responses to stressors are more typically linked to immunological changes. The link between the HPA axis and the immune system is demonstrated by the action of glucocorticoids which, via their potent anti-inflammatory action with important effects on the immune system, can exert an inhibitory effect on cell growth, proliferation and differentiation, on leucocyte activity, on the production of cytokines, on antibody formation and other immune cell modifications. Conversely, during an acute inflammatory episode, cytokine-mediated responses involve potent activation of the neuroendocrine stress axis. Cytokines can also indirectly stimulate the HPA axis, because they can evoke pain pathways that can activate somatosensory networks in the brain that in turn activate the HPA axis. During immune challenge, along with HPA activation that contributes to modulating the overreaction of the immune system during infections, there is a simultaneous production of immunoprotective factors by the pituitary gland. From an evolutionary point of view, stress-induced immunosuppression delays inflammatory pain until the danger may have passed. However, problems arise when the stress response is extremely intense and persistent.

### Infections, tumours and stress

The release of glucocorticoids, adrenaline and noradrenaline during stress can suppress immune factors that regulate the action of T-helper (Th) cells. Th cells are lymphocytes that, interacting with macrophages, block and destroy pathogens. Different types of Th cells secrete different types of cytokines that are in turn involved in the control of different immune responses: allergic responses, inflammatory responses, cytotoxic responses and the delayed hypersensitivity reaction. In particular, stress suppresses the production of the cytokine interleukin 12. Disorders such as respiratory diseases, toxoplasmosis, some bacterial infections and also cancer are likely to be worsened by stress.

In humans and in experimental animals, it has been shown that psychological stress increases the incidence of tumours. The increase of tumour-cell proliferation due to both suppression and reduced recruitment of antitumour immune cells has been related to an increase of beta-adrenergic and glucocorticoid actions. In experimental mice, the incidence of mammary tumours (experimentally infected with mammary tumour virus) increased from 7% to 92% as a result of handling stress. Stress also reduced the effectiveness of chemotherapy in these subjects (Riley, 1975; Gregory, 2004; Antoni *et al.*, 2006).

## Stress and the gastrointestinal system

Physical signs of acute stress are largely the manifestation of sympathetic activation. Profound salivation and vomiting, diarrhoea and also cardiovascular clinical signs have been related to acute stress of different origins. As a consequence of acute stress – for example, in response to a highly frightening event – an increase in gastrointestinal motility with nausea, vomiting and diarrhoea is likely to occur. During veterinary examinations it is possible to observe all these manifestations of acute stress, including profuse salivation. These effects are due not only to sympathetic nervous system activation, but also to the release of CRH. During chronic stress conditions various changes occur: gastric acid secretion increases, blood flow to the gut decreases, mucus secretion is impaired; and so the risk of damage due to gastric acid secretions increases, resulting in gastric ulcers. Corticosteroids contribute to the inhibition of prostaglandin synthesis and impair the repair of ulcers.

## Abnormal behaviours and coping strategies

Pets can be deprived of adequate stimulation and exercise and suffer because of chronic stress conditions; they can be forced to face social conflicts with other pets or with people, without being able to find successful coping strategies. Conflict situations in which the animal wants to do something but is not allowed to do it can generate stress responses manifest by repetitive out-of-context behaviours that are called **displacement activities**.

**Self-directed** and **environment-directed behaviours** can be the consequence of stress induced by social conflicts, frustration at the deprivation of possible access to highly motivating social or environmental resources or the possibility to perform some behaviours. Acral licking, flank sucking, tail biting in dogs, feather picking in birds and excessive grooming in cats are the most frequently described self-directed behaviours. Environment-directed behaviours such as coprophagia, pica, overeating and polydipsia have been described both in dogs and cats. These abnormal behaviours, with no apparent beneficial effects, can also be generated as a consequence of deprivation or exposure to aversive situations prolonged over time.

In extreme situations all the above described stressors (deprivation, conflicts, perpetrated threats) can lead to **stereotypic behaviour** (see Chapter 20). These are patterns of behaviour that appear to be obsessively repeated without an apparent goal. Stereotypic behaviours can continue to be performed even after the removal of stressors and some scientists consider them as 'scars' of certain forms of chronic suffering.

Preventing access to motivating stimuli in the environment can also generate **redirected behaviours**, in which the animal directs its actions towards stimuli that are not directly the cause of their current motivational state. For example, a cat that is prevented from catching a bird by the presence of a window pane can redirect the paw towards another object or living being and scratch it. Some aggressive behaviours (e.g. toward cats in the garden) can be redirected toward housemates in similar circumstances.

Other types of behaviour generated by stress are **ambivalent behaviours**, where the animal seems to approach and withdraw, or threaten and behave in a submissive way, alternating behavioural patterns with opposite meaning in the same situation and very closely in time. These kinds of inconsistent behaviour are generated by internal conflicts and might be quite difficult to interpret initially, until the cause of conflict is identified.

Stress can also be the cause of failure of normal biological functions, especially as a result of disruption of normal endocrinological processes, and so result in **abnormal parental behaviours** or **abnormal sexual behaviours**.

## Stress-related aggressive behaviours

Exaggerated defensive behaviours or exaggerated alarm responses, including apparently unpredictable aggression when handled, can be related to an undercurrent of stressful conditions. Impulsivity will increase and an animal that feels threatened or that is in pain may respond to a (perceived) threat with aggression, especially when escape or immobilization has proved to be ineffective, or appears inappropriate.

Being able to recognize signs of acute and chronic stress, along with the signs of physical pain, is of paramount importance because the overlapping of physical and psychological stressors can lead to HPA axis overload and dysregulation, and/or serious behavioural consequences. For example, handling an animal that is in pain can cause a stress response, and the animal may already be under physiological stress because of its physical condition. In this situation, its stress system may already be 'primed' and even minimal external perceived threat such as the touch of a human hand can result in acute-stress defensive responses. The risk of aggression in such a situation is very high. Continued exposure to both physical (pain) and psychological stressors (restraint and handling that the animal is motivated to avoid), are likely to prolong the stress response, with severe physical and behavioural consequences. Therefore veterinary surgeons should be able to recognize and differentiate signs of both pain and stress in order to prevent the onset of cycles such as the one described above.

There are many other examples of compounded stress conditions that can lead to aggressive reactions, such as occurs when there is a reduction in the available free space as a result of hospitalization or following the introduction of new individuals. In these situations attempts at handling and restraint can also induce aggressive responses.

## Depression, apathy and post-traumatic stress disorder

In contrast to stress-related aggression, consistent lowering of response to stimuli that elicit responses in normal situations might also be a sign of stress. This lack of response might be comparable to human depression and can be considered the consequence of a severe loss of adaptive abilities. When animals are repeatedly negatively stimulated without the possibility of avoiding the stressors, they can develop what some authors call 'learned helplessness' and others (using a more human emotional analogy) term 'despair'. These conditions appear very similar to human depression. While a lack of responsiveness may not be problematic to many owners, it is nonetheless an important welfare concern and so needs to be assessed by those responsible for the animal's welfare.

Post-traumatic stress disorder (PTSD) occurs in people who have been victims of severe traumas of different origins. These human patients present severe clinical signs (exaggerated startle responses, learning and memory impairments and social adaptation problems) and phobic reactions to cues that are related to the experienced trauma. Comparable effects have been observed in laboratory mice that were studied as models of human PTSD and it seems reasonable to suggest that similar disorders can affect companion animals as a consequence of severe stressful events (Garrick *et al.*, 2001), though they are not well documented at present.

## Stress and emotions

Emotional responses are coordinated by the limbic system in the brain, especially the central nucleus of the amygdala. The amygdala receives inputs from the thalamus and, indirectly, from cortical areas. The thalamus processes much of the sensory input that is transmitted to the amygdala through a single synaptic link, and therefore the response is often very rapid. The amygdala and other limbic structures can be activated by psychological stressors and emotional responses form an integral part of the stress response, giving it both qualitative and quantitative properties.

Appetitive stimuli generate pleasant emotional states (e.g. happiness, joy), while aversive stimuli generate unpleasant emotional states (fear, anger, sadness, despair). The two general behavioural expressions of these emotional states are: approach to the appetitive stimulus; and withdrawal (with or without hesitation) from the aversive one. Animals respond to appetitive and aversive stimulation on the basis of their individual features, the context and their previous experiences, and so a given response may be individual and context specific, with one stimulus being perceived as potentially aversive to one individual and appetitive to another. Past experiences help to organize the processing of the present situa-

tion and the response hierarchically. The response follows typical patterns of activation – from calm and controlled to high arousal with little feedback – which may range from attraction and pleasure to aversion and displeasure.

## Fear and anxiety

Arousal is generally greater in the presence of unpleasant stimulation than in the presence of positive, pleasant stimuli.

- Fear is an emotional state that represents the response to an immediate present challenge (a stressor), i.e. it is the reaction to a real and well defined adverse situation.
- Anxiety is the emotional anticipation of an adverse event, i.e. it is the anticipation of something unpleasant that may or may not be real.

The distinction between these two emotions might not be easy to make from a clinical perspective; and in human psychiatry different types of pathological fear are considered to be part of anxiety disorders (American Psychiatric Association, 2000). The terms emotionality, stress and anxiety tend to be used in similar contexts in a lot of literature and high levels of stressful arousal and emotional activation seem to have much in common.

The neural structures engaged in pleasant and unpleasant emotional responses seem to be different and the startle reflex seems to be exaggerated when animals are defensively motivated, since stress reduces impulse control, with important consequences for the onset of avoidance behaviours, including aggression (Falls and Davis, 1995; Tice *et al.*, 2001). When animals are presented with a stimulus that elicits fear, the concurrent emotional arousal is likely to dominate the behaviour that occurs around this time. Emotional responses can be seen as a predisposition to action – they represent a tactical response to contextual demands. In stressful conditions, emotional responses can be facilitated and the animal may become more impulsive, more prone to startle and (depending on the types of stressors, on individual features and context) more likely to perform the innate emotional responses of fight, flight or freeze (Lang *et al.*, 1998).

## Anger and frustration

A wider range of emotions can probably be attributed to different companion animals species based on their behavioural ecology and cognitive development, though scientific demonstration and acceptance is more limited. Anger, happiness, sadness, relief and frustration are potentially comparable internal states that may exist in a range of species, and more recently it has been suggested on the basis of experimental work that dogs may also demonstrate more complex social emotional responses akin to jealousy (Range *et al.*, 2009).

Simple observation, when an animal's emotional state might be inferred, runs the risk of inappropriately giving a human-like explanation (anthropomorphism) to the motivation of an emotional response, but this risk can be reduced by using a thorough knowledge of the ethological and psychological characteristics of the observed species. The issue of anthropomorphism is important, even though its application to understanding and predicting the behaviour of non-humans is a tool that many scientists admit to using and relying on (Serpell, 1996). For example, it is only by anthropomorphizing to a certain degree that we can infer, at least in a broad way, what a dog feels like when it is kept behind a door or a gate when it might be motivated to chase strangers. Behavioural and neuroendocrine changes in animals during frustrating situations are similar to human ones and it might be inferred that they are generated by similar emotional states, even if they are experienced differently at the subjective level. It can then be suggested that a dog that is prevented from having access to a resource that it expects to have (for example, a female, space or food) might feel frustrated or even angry (Verrier *et al.*, 1987); in such cases, aggressive behaviour might be an expression of the emotional response to the stressor that generates frustration.

## Effect of stress on learning and memory

Cognitive, emotional, mood-related and motivational processes take place in the brain in an integrated manner in order to produce adaptive behaviours in response to stressful stimuli. Glucocorticoids are the main players in response to stressors and exert their action on memory, learning and attention. Mineralocorticoid receptors (MRs) and glucocorticoid receptors (GRs) both mediate glucocorticoid effects in the brain areas that are crucial for memory, learning and emotions. MRs have an affinity for glucocorticoids that is tenfold higher than GRs. MRs are mainly expressed in the hippocampus, a brain region that is crucial for memory processes. Under baseline conditions they are primarily occupied, but during stress they become saturated and the occupation of GRs increases. GRs are distributed in different areas in the brain but are more abundant in hypothalamic CRH neurons and the pituitary. When MRs are predominantly activated, hippocampal neurons receive excitatory activation, while additional activation of GRs induces an impairment in hippocampal transmission. This means that when glucocorticoid levels are too low (and MRs are not sufficiently activated) or too high (GRs becomes predominantly activated), memory and learning may be impaired (De Kloet *et al.*, 1998, Prickaerts and Steckler, 2005), but this will depend on the events to be learned.

## Associative learning and stress

Stress can affect learning in many ways and it is well known that a stressful event is often very well remembered. In an acute stressful situation an animal can associate two stimuli or events after very few exposures, or even after a single exposure. This type of learning in relation to predictions of aversion is probably an evolutionary adaptation, since it is advantageous to learn very quickly about all the salient stimuli

that can predict life-threatening events. This form of associative learning should be acknowledged every time an animal that is in pain or very frightened must be handled: it might very quickly associate any contextual stimulus (including human hands) with a negative internal state and perform a defensive response that will probably be repeated in the future in the presence of similar stimuli.

## Stress, memory and cognition

Stressful experiences can also impair cognitive abilities, such as remembering the details of the event, including positive experience (Gamaro *et al.*, 1999). Several studies have also shown that stress induced in close association with a learning task (or induced by the learning task) can facilitate the memory consolidation of that situation. In such circumstances, stress becomes part of the situation that the animal has to remember (De Kloet *et al.*, 1999). For example, in rats it has been found that learning a task under stressful conditions enhanced the memory of that task, but performance did not improve when the intensity of the stressful stimulus was too high; i.e. mild stressors may improve the learning of memory tasks, while high-intensity stressors can have the opposite effect (Joels *et al.*, 2006).

Along with the context of the stressful experience, the effect of learning under stress is linked to the time of exposure to the stressors. As explained before, stress hormones can facilitate learning when presented at the same time as the learning task but the opposite effect can be noticed when a strong stressful stimulus is presented before or even a considerable time after the learning task; i.e. stress has different effects on learning, depending on the phase of the learning and memory processes.

All these effects of stress on learning should be considered during training and when avoidance responses need to be prevented: mild stress (leading to appropriate arousal) is crucial for focusing attention and promoting learning; intense stress is often the basis for the onset of emotionally dominated responses.

## Habituation and dishabituation

One of the first and most important learning abilities of animals is the ability to habituate to non-threatening neutral stimuli (see Chapter 5). Habituation is a form of non-associative learning and it is very important for maintaining a state of good welfare: through habituation, animals learn not to respond to non-threatening stimuli and situations. Novel stimuli can initially be perceived as stressors and animals respond with HPA axis activation. In the case of mild stressors, repeated activation is often associated with habituation and attenuation of the neurohormonal stress response, though physiological habituation often takes longer than the behavioural process.

Stress can influence the ability of animals to habituate to irrelevant stimuli in the environment and several studies have demonstrated that animals that are stressed can fail to habituate to non-harmful repeated environmental stimuli. Furthermore, stress conditions can lead to a reappearance of previously habituated responses (dishabituation). Classic examples of this involve mildly fearful responses: if habituation has occurred but the animal is under stressful management conditions, it might become dishabituated (see Chapter 5). This recovery of previously habituated responses can be observed in cases such as fear of noises, for example fireworks or thunderstorms (see Chapter 15), but also in case of habituation to social contacts (see Chapter 17) with humans or other animals and cause the onset of avoidance behaviours such as freezing, attempting to escape or aggressive behaviour when the animal previously appeared well habituated or socialized (Gamaro *et al.*, 1999; Garrick *et al.*, 2001; Poulton and Menzies, 2001; Mills, 2005).

## Stress-related psychogenic problems

There is a relationship between psychological distress, physiological stress reactions and somatic disorders: medical and behavioural disorders are not mutually exclusive. There are many areas of overlap between psychogenic problems, repetitive, compulsive, stereotyped behaviour (see Chapter 20) and self-injurious and medical problems. The definition of psychogenic disorders as mental or emotional rather than physiological in origin is a false dichotomy: there is no clear boundary between a stress response of psychological origin and one of physical origin. If an animal is physically damaged, there is likely to be a psychological component – if only because of the pain involved. Social conflicts, environmental disturbance or deprivation, physical pain and traumas are some of the stressors that can be related to the onset of physical problems or difficulty in recovery.

In the case of stress-related dermatological problems, the origin of skin damage may be a stress-induced self-directed behaviour and perpetration might be due to both physical (infection, ulceration) and behavioural stress-related issues. Acral licking, flank sucking, tail chasing in dogs and psychogenic alopecia and hyperaesthesia in cats are the most frequently recognized examples (Broom, 1989; Beerda *et al.*, 1997, 2000). Figure 13.5 shows a dog with acral lick lesions: restraint stress was the likely cause of the dermatological problem in this case.

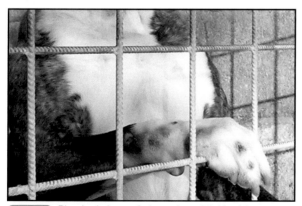

**13.5** Physical signs of stress (acral licking) in a rescue dog.

Pruritus is linked to very different physical and psychological variables and is correlated to stress at both a causal and consequential level (Paus *et al.*, 2006). Psychogenic vomiting is a condition that is considered stress-related in human psychiatry and has also been considered a possible differential diagnosis in companion animals in cases of vomiting of unknown origin (Muraoka *et al.*, 1990; Mills, 2000).

Feline lower urinary tract disease is frequently diagnosed in cats and is often accompanied by feline interstitial cystitis, a neurogenic inflammation where stress is believed to play an important role in both its onset and exacerbation: a cat with chronic urinary tract disease may become stressed for a number of reasons and this stress contributes to the perpetuation of the disease (Horwitz, 1997; Jones *et al.*, 1997; see also Chapter 11).

Compulsive water drinking, also called psychogenic polydipsia, has been described in both animals and humans and can also be a sign of stress. In humans, primary polydipsia may result from a defect in the thirst centre (dipsogenic polydipsia) or may be associated with mental illness (psychogenic polydipsia). In dogs, primary polydipsia has been described both as a psychological disorder and as a behavioural problem (Olenick, 1999; Vonderen *et al.*, 1999).

Polyphagia can also be related to stress, since high levels of glucocorticoids produce increased appetite. When food intake is excessive, while physical medical causes are being evaluated the significance of stress should also be considered. Pica, an eating disorder that some authors consider a compulsive disorder, has been described in dogs and cats (Bowen, 2002; Broom and Fraser, 2007).

Stress should not just be considered as a direct cause of physical problems, but also the reason for the perpetuation of many organic diseases. In virtually any veterinary case, it is worth investigating in order to optimize case management and safeguard patient welfare.

## Management of stressed animals during veterinary visits

Veterinary visits are often stressful for pets but the distress can be more severe for sensitive subjects (see Chapter 2). Pain, fear of humans, unfamiliar contexts and restraint stress are elements that can contribute to the onset of severe stress responses. Crucial elements for reducing stress are the predictability of events and the reduction of intensity and length of stress stimulation.

Gentle handling, protection from loud noises and voices, preventive analgesia and, when required, sedation or anaesthesia can reduce the intensity of stressors. It is also very helpful to increase the predictability of events by instructing owners to train their pet at home, so that responses are on cue. A pet habituated to being handled by its owners in a way that is similar to that undertaken during veterinary visits will be calmer when clinically examined. In the same way, if the pet is trained in a positive way (using treats, for example) to wear a muzzle, it will be less stressed during visits if a muzzle is required. In pets that are prone to stress as a consequence of handling, owners should be trained to work with their animals at home to counteract this. These concepts are summarized in Figure 13.6.

---

- Avoid painful or invasive procedures during the first visit of a puppy or kitten and try to establish a positive association with the clinical environment from the outset
- Keep the waiting time in the waiting room short in the case of fearful or poorly socialized animals
- Gentle handling
- Fearful or poorly socialized animals and those in great pain should be attended to in the quietest room available
- Minimize the length of the visit in the case of fearful or poorly socialized animals
- Consider preventive analgesia, sedation or anaesthesia for animals that are in pain or very stressed
- Instruct owners on how to handle their pet in order to avoid excessive physical restraint and the possibility of escape
- Prescribe muzzle training for dogs
- Instruct owners to pre-train clinical procedures at home (e.g. being put on a table; lifting tail and paws; inspecting mouth, ears and belly) using treats or other appropriate rewards to establish positive associations
- Use pheromone diffusers in the waiting and consulting rooms (see Chapter 21)

---

**13.6** Preventing and reducing stress during veterinary visits.

## Conclusion

When an animal is under stress, many physiological modifications take place in order to 'prepare' its body to cope with the challenge. Physiological and behavioural responses have the goal of addressing the challenge and therefore they are adaptive, increasing survival chances and fitness. The boundary between normal and adaptive responses and a state of poor welfare is difficult to define; but the stress system can become dysregulated when the stress is prolonged and intense and normal behavioural responses such as escape or avoiding the stressor are prevented or do not lead to the expected outcomes, so that the motivational state of an animal is constantly challenged. In this situation the physical and psychological health of the animal is at risk. Fearful stimuli, social conflicts and deprivation of the possibility to satisfy basic physical and behavioural needs (see Chapters 3 and 4) create conditions and motivational states that cause prolonged activation of the stress system. The interplay between body and mind is a sort of feedback loop: psychological distress can lead to physical diseases; and an animal that is in physical pain will by definition 'feel' its pain and so suffer psychological distress. The two kinds of stress, although often separated by clinicians, are an integral risk factor in all aspects of veterinary medicine: physical stress can cause behavioural disturbance; and psychological stress can cause severe physical problems. A stressed animal will be more prone to react impulsively, to fear normal stimuli and to try to defend itself without cognitively elaborating the specific context.

The ability of the veterinary surgeon to recognize signs of physical pain and of stress is of paramount importance in order to prevent and manage the onset and multiple consequences of stress.

## References and further reading

Alonso SJ, Damas C and Navarro E (2000) Behavioural despair in mice after prenatal stress. *Journal of Physiology and Biochemistry* **56**, 77–82

American Psychiatric Association (2000) *Diagnostic and Statistical Manual of Mental Disorders, 4th edn*, pp. 429–484. APA, Washington DC

Antoni MH, Lutgendorf SK, Cole SW *et al.* (2006) The influence of bio-behavioural factors on tumour biology: Pathways and mechanisms. *Nature Reviews Cancer* **6**, 240–248

Aston-Jones G, Rajkowski J and Cohen J (1999) Role of locus ceruleus in attention and behavioral flexibility. *Biological Psychiatry* **46**, 1309–1320

Beerda B, Schlider MBH, van Hoff JARAM and de Vries HW (1997) Manifestation of chronic and acute stress in dogs. *Applied Animal Behaviour Science* **52**, 307–319

Beerda B, Schlider MBH, van Hoff JARAM *et al.* (2000) Behavioural and hormonal indicators of enduring environmental stress in dogs. *Animal Welfare* **9**, 49–62

Bowen J (2002) Miscellaneous behaviour problems. In: *BSAVA Manual of Canine and Feline Behavioural Medicine*, ed. DF Horwitz, DS Mills and S Heath, pp. 119–127. BSAVA Publications, Gloucester

Broom DM (1989) Psychological problems of companion animals. In: *The Welfare of Companion Animals: Proceedings of the BVA Animal Welfare Foundation*, pp. 46–51. British Veterinary Association, London

Broom DM and Fraser AF (2007) *Domestic Animal Behavior and Welfare, 4th edn*, pp. 40–51, 58–69. CAB International, Cambridge, Massachusetts

Caldji C, Annenbau B, Sharma S *et al.* (1988) Maternal care during infancy regulates the development of neural systems mediating the expression of fearfulness in the rat. In: *Proceedings of the National Academy of Sciences of the United States of America* **95**, 5335–5340

De Kloet ER, Oitzl MS and Joels M (1999) Stress and cognition: are corticosteroids good or bad guys? *Trends in Neuroscience* **22**, 422–426

De Kloet ER, Vreugdenhil E, Oitsl MS and Joels M (1998) Brain corticosteroid receptor balance in health and disease. *Endocrine Reviews* **19**, 269–301

Falls WA and Davis M (1995) Lesions of the central nucleus of the amygdala block conditioned excitation, but not conditioned inhibition of fear as measured with the fear-potentiated strale effect. *Behavioural Neuroscience* **109**, 379–387

Francis DD, Caldji C, Champagne F *et al.* (1999) The role of corticotrophin-releasing factor-norepinephrine systems in mediating the effects of early experience on the development of behavioral and endocrine responses to stress: norepinephrine: new vistas for an old neurotransmitter. *Biological Psychiatry* **46**, 1153–1166

Fulford AJ and Harbuz MS (2005) An introduction to the HPA axis. In: *Handbook of Stress and the Brain*, ed. T Stekler, NH Kalin and JMHM Reul, pp. 43–65. Elsevier, Amsterdam

Gamaro GD, Michalowsky MB, Catelli DH *et al.* (1999) Effect of repeated restraint stress on memory in different tasks. *Brazilian Journal of Medical and Biological Research* **32**, 341–347

Garrick T, Morrow N, Shalev AY and Eth S (2001) Stress-induced enhancement of auditory startle: an animal model of posttraumatic stress disorder. *Psychiatry* **64**, 346–354

Gregory NG (2004) *Physiology and Behaviour of Animal Suffering*. Blackwell Science, Oxford

Harris G (1948) Neural control of the pituitary gland. *Physiology Review* **28**, 139–179

Heinrichs SC (2005) Behavioural consequences of altered corticotrophin-releasing factor activation in the brain: a functionalist view of affective neuroscience. In: *Handbook of Stress and the Brain*, ed. T Stekler, NH Kalin and JMHM Reul, pp. 155–177. Elsevier, Amsterdam

Horwitz DF (1997) Behavioral and environmental factors associated with elimination behavior problems in cats: a retrospective study. *Applied Animal Behaviour Science* **52**, 129–137

Hsu SY (2005) Novel CRH family peptides and their receptors: an evolutionary analysis. In: *Handbook of Stress and the Brain*, ed. T Stekler, NH Kalin and JMHM Reul, pp. 115–131. Elsevier, Amsterdam

Joels M, Pu Z, Wiegert O *et al.* (2006) Learning under stress: how does it work? *Trends in Cognitive Science* **10**, 152–158

Jones BR, Sanson RL, Morris RS (1997) Elucidating the risk factors on feline lower urinary tract disease. *New Zealand Veterinary Journal* **45**, 100–108

Keay AK and Bandler R (2001) Parallel circuits mediating distinct emotional coping reactions to different types of stress. *Neuroscience &*

*Biobehavioral Reviews* **25**, 669–678

Kovàks KJ, Miklòs IH and Bali B (2005) Psychological and physiological stressors. In: *Handbook of Stress and the Brain*, ed. T Stekler, NH Kalin and JMHM Reul, pp. 775–792. Elsevier, Amsterdam

Lang PJ, Bradley MM and Cuthbert BN (1998) Emotion motivation and anxiety: brain mechanisms and psychophysiology. *Biological Psychiatry* **44**, 1248–1263

Levine S (1966) Hormone influences on brain organization in infant rats. *Science* **152**, 1585–1592

Mills DS (2000) Animal behavior case of the month. *Journal of the American Veterinary Medical Association* **216**, 1225–1226

Mills DS (2005) Management of noise fears and phobias in pets. *In Practice* **27**, 248–255

Muraoka M, Mine K, Matsumoto K *et al.* (1990) Psychogenic vomiting: the relation between patterns of vomiting and psychiatric diagnoses. *Gut* **31**, 526–528

Olenick CL (1999) Congenital renal dysplasia and psychogenic polydipsia in a Bernese mountain dog. *Canine Veterinary Journal,* **40**, 425–426

Paus R, Schmelz M, Bíró T and Steinhoff M (2006) Frontiers in pruritus research: scratching the brain for more effective itch therapy. *Journal of Clinical Investigation* **116**, 1174–1186

Poulton R and Menzies RG (2001) Fear born *and* bred: toward a more inclusive theory of fear acquisition. *Behaviour Research and Therapy* **40**, 197–208

Prickaerts J and Steckler T (2005) Effects of glucocorticoids on emotion and cognitive processes in animals. In: *Handbook of Stress and the Brain*, ed. T Stekler, NH Kalin and JMHM Reul, pp. 359–385. Elsevier, Amsterdam

Range F, Horn L, Viranyi Z and Huber L (2009) The absence of reward induces inequity aversion in dogs. *Proceedings of the National Academy of Science* **106**, 340–345

Riley V (1975) Mouse mammary tumors: alteration of incidence as apparent function of stress. *Science* **189**, 465–467

Sanchez MM, Ladd CO and Plotsky PM (2001) Early adverse experience as developmental risk factor for later psychopathology: evidence from rodents and primate models. *Developmental Psychopathology* **13**, 419–449

Serpell J (1996) *In the Company of Animals. A Study of Human–Animal Relationship*. Cambridge University Press, New York

Smagin GN, Heinrichs SC and Dunn AJ (2001) The role of CRH in behavioral response to stress. *Peptides* **22**, 713–724

Tice DM, Bratslavsky E and Baumeister RF (2001) Emotional distress regulation takes precedence over impulse control: if you feel bad, do it! *Journal of Personality and Social Psychology* **80**, 53–67

Verrier L, Hagestad EL and Lown B (1987) Delayed myocardial ischemia induced by anger. *Circulation* **75**, 249–254

Vonderen IK, Kooistra HS, Sprang E and Rijnberk A (1999) Disturbed vasopressin release in four dogs with so-called primary polydipsia. *Journal of Veterinary Internal Medicine* **13**, 419–425

## Client handouts (bsavalibrary.com/behaviour_leaflets)

- Adopting a rescue dog: the pros and cons
- Avoiding aggression in cats
- Avoiding house soiling by cats
- Avoiding urine marking by cats
- Environmental enrichment for cats in animal shelters
- Environmental enrichment for dogs in animal shelters
- Handling exercises for an aggressive cat
- Handling exercises for puppies and kittens
- Headcollar training
- Introducing a new cat into the household
- Muzzle training
- Noise fear score sheet
- 'Nothing in Life is Free'

- Playing with your dog – toys
- Playing with your kitten
- Puppy socialization: getting used to new people
- Questionnaire to assess separation anxiety
- Redirected aggression in dogs
- Request for information on problem behaviours
- Taking your cat in the car
- The newly adopted rescue dog: preventing problems
- Treating a fear of car journeys using desensitization and counter-conditioning
- What your cat needs
- What your dog needs
- Your puppy's first year

# 14

# Separation-related problems in dogs and cats

## Debra F. Horwitz

## Introduction

A range of separation-related behaviour problems (including destruction, vocalization and elimination) may occur in the partial or complete absence of a pet's owner. These problems can have different underlying motivations, relating to factors such as fear, anxiety, over-attachment and lack of appropriate stimulation, and require different treatment interventions. In some situations the presenting signs may not be due to distress and these will be discussed in the differential diagnosis section.

Because domestic dogs include the human family within their social group, they become bonded to family members and in some cases this attachment can be the source of separation-related problem behaviours. When separated from social group members, dogs (and perhaps cats) may experience distress and engage in problem behaviours as a consequence. This response is often referred to as **separation anxiety**, and should be considered a subset of separation-related problem behaviours. When dogs experience separation anxiety they commonly engage in behaviours that may include anorexia, drooling, attempts at escape and behavioural depression, as well as destruction, vocalization and elimination of urine or stools (McCrave, 1991).

Separation distress disorders in cats are not as well documented as those in dogs. Recent research has suggested that cats do form social bonds and therefore may be at risk for separation distress responses (Turner, 2000; Edwards et al., 2007). Other behaviour practitioners have suggested that owner-absent house soiling and over-grooming behaviours may be signs of separation distress in the companion cat (Schwartz, 2002). Because very little is available to substantiate the diagnosis and treatment of separation-related problems in cats beyond the application of the principles used in dogs (but see Schwartz, 2002), this chapter will primarily deal with separation-related problems in dogs.

Separation anxiety is a common behavioural diagnosis in dogs, with 20–40% of dogs presented to behavioural referral clinics being diagnosed with the problem. Separation anxiety appears to increase in the behaviour patient population as dogs age (Chapman and Voith, 1990; Landsberg and Ruehl, 1997). The criteria for diagnosis may differ from country to country; for example, the French school emphasizes 'hyperattachment' as crucial to diagnosis,

defining hyperattachment as resulting from persistence of the primary attachment bond to the mother in young dogs, which leads to separation anxiety (Landsberg et al., 2003). Others suggest that adoption from animal shelters may be associated with separation anxiety in dogs (McCrave, 1991). It is recognized that severe stress can precipitate hyperattachment; this later-onset condition may therefore relate to a form of secondary hyperattachment.

Regardless of how the disorder is classified, separation anxiety and unwanted behaviours that occur in the absence of the owner for other reasons can have profound implications for the human–animal bond and pet welfare. Animals experiencing separation distress and the related behaviours seem quite anxious. They can do considerable damage to themselves in attempting to escape from confinement or the home. Constant anxiety can lower resistance and result in disease. Destruction and elimination in the home, whether anxiety based or not, are quite frustrating to owners and may contribute to pet relinquishment to animal shelters or euthanasia. Salman et al. (2000) reported that house soiling was the most frequently listed behavioural reason for both dogs and cats to be relinquished; for dogs, destruction was also frequently recorded as a reason for relinquishment. Both house soiling and destruction may be signs of separation anxiety, a very treatable condition.

Possible risk factors for the development of separation anxiety in dogs have been identified. In one study of Labrador Retrievers and Border Collies, breeders and owners were interviewed about dogs at several age intervals (Bradshaw et al., 2002). Collected data included interactions with people over various time intervals to establish a social referencing score, and a separation score. Data were also collected from a random selection of dog owners walking their dogs in three locations in the UK to determine whether the dogs experienced any signs of separation-related behaviours. Such behaviours were reported in about 50% in each group. Puppies with extensive social referencing (puppy experience with people outside the regular family, strangers and children) at 3 months of age were more predisposed to show separation-related problems between 6 and 9 months of age; but those that received the most social referencing between 6 and 9 months were the least likely to develop the behaviours. The data from the random dog owners did not show an increase in separation-related behaviours in dogs from a rescue centre, nor in those that had been rehomed. Flannigan and Dodman (2001) found that dogs from homes with a single adult human were 2.5 times more likely to show separation-related behaviours than those from a multiple-owner home. Certain behaviours that might have been indicative of hyperattachment, such as extreme following, departure cue anxiety and excessive greeting, were also associated with separation anxiety in this study, while spoiling behaviours and the presence of other pets in the home were not.

## Evaluation of the patient

### Presenting signs and history

As a starting point, basic information such as age of the pet, recent and past medical and health examinations and current medications should be obtained. Because medical problems can contribute to separation-related problems (for example, by increasing anxiety, or incomplete dental eruption encouraging chewing, or age-related physical and cognitive factors resulting in a loss of housetraining), a good physical examination and any related laboratory testing or imaging should be performed.

Attempts should be made to determine the duration of the problem behaviour. Some animals will have shown separation-related problems (destruction, elimination, etc., with or without anxiety) since puppyhood, while for others the onset may be associated with changes in the household, such as different work hours, moving, or change in household composition (Simpson, 2000). Mild separation distress may have been present for some time but signs have increased and become more prevalent with age. In some situations separation distress may be related to a separation after a period of intense togetherness, such as when the owner vacations at home or with the dog. An association with this type of schedule change and the signs of destruction, vocalization and/or elimination is highly suggestive of separation distress disorder. For some dogs, it may not be possible to establish the inciting incident or trigger. For others, the duration of the behaviour may or may not be helpful in diagnosis (for example, ongoing destruction may only indicate outside stimulation), while knowing the age of the animal may help in differentiating motivations for the problem behaviours (old-age onset may signal medical or cognitive changes).

Separation distress responses often have four major components and exploring these can help with diagnosis.

- Dogs with separation distress may show anxiety-based responses when the owner is home.
- They often show anxious responses as the owner begins their departure routine and as they depart.
- Most dogs will continue the distress response after the owner has left.
- Finally, some dogs will have other anxiety or behavioural disorders concurrently that may or may not be part of the separation distress problem.

If animals do not show these signs, other causes for the owner-absent behaviour not related to distress need to be explored.

### Exploring pet–owner relationship and interactions

The behavioural history should include all facets of pet–owner interactions, including a summary of how they interact throughout a 24-hour time period. Information on feeding, toileting routine, training and play time together and how long the pet is alone on a daily basis should be obtained, since lack of outdoor access or exercise may explain soiling or destructive behaviour. Some studies have indicated that following behaviours and those indicating hyperattachment may be contributory to these disorders and so questions should attempt to find out whether these situations occur. These might include:

- Does your dog follow you excessively, need to be close to you or keep you in sight?
- Do you need to be present for your dog to eat or will your pet eat a treat as you prepare to depart?
- Does your pet have multiple attention-seeking behaviours and seem to need constant interaction?

Answers to such questions can impart useful information on the pet–owner relationship. However, animals may show distress when left home alone without showing any signs of over-attachment to the owner and this may indicate a fear-related distress response.

### Exploring behaviour as owner prepares to depart

In cases of separation anxiety a pet will usually show behavioural changes prior to owner departure and these should be explored. Typical questions might include:

- What does your pet do as you prepare to depart?
- As you get closer to the end of your departure routine, how does your pet behave?

As the owner departs, or once the owner has departed, a distress response may begin. It is pertinent to ask whether the dog vocalizes (bark, whine or howl), scratches at the door or confinement area, or attempts to block departure. Dogs that are experiencing separation distress problems for other reasons may not show distinctive signs at owner departure.

It is also useful to ascertain whether the animal is placed in some type of confinement, such as a crate or locked room. For some dogs confinement itself can provoke anxiety and the signs noted are related to confinement, not owner departure.

Determining which departures seem to elicit the problem behaviour and quantifying the presentation may be useful later on to evaluate response to therapeutic interventions. Extensive variation is possible in what each patient perceives as triggers or underlying motivation for the distress response.

- Some dogs will tolerate regular daily work departures and only show separation distress on unscheduled departures that are not related to work.
- In other cases the problem occurs on all work-related departures but not any other, such as when the owner is dressed in casual clothing and merely runs out briefly for an errand.
- Some dogs engage in the problem behaviours every time the owner leaves, regardless of how long they will be gone, time of day, day of the week or any other signal.
- Some dogs only show signs if they are totally alone and will be fine if any person is present.
- Others are only distressed if a particular attachment figure leaves the home, even if other people remain there.
- Some dogs are distressed when crated, but fine if left out in the home.

This may suggest differing underlying motivations or attachments between the dog and family members. Identification of these factors may be significant and useful for treatment recommendations and evaluation.

## Exploring owner-absent behaviours

It should be determined what the dog does when the owner is absent. Does the dog vocalize, or eliminate urine or stool, or is the dog destructive? Other signs include over-grooming, dermatological lesions, intestinal distress and immobility.

The most common distress behaviours seen in dogs showing separation anxiety are: destruction; house soiling; vocalization; motor activity (circling, trembling, shaking); gastrointestinal signs; and self-trauma.

- Some studies have revealed that destructive behaviours often target either windows and doors or owner possessions, or both, and this may relate to differences in motivation such as attempts to escape from confinement versus distress associated with an attachment.
- When confined, some dogs may move the crates they are confined in or can be injured in their attempts to escape confinement (Simpson, 2000) and it is not always clear whether this is a response to being alone or to being crated.
- On occasion, dogs will actively attempt to prevent owner departure, even using aggression (McCrave, 1991; Horwitz and Neilson, 2007a).
- Indoor elimination may occur even though the owner, prior to departure, has witnessed outdoor access and elimination.
- Vocalization occurs frequently and commonly consists of whining, howling and high-pitched barking (Lund and Jorgensen, 1997). High-pitched vocalizations are associated with distress and are distinct from those made in territorial defence, play or other activities.
- Motor activity may include pacing, circling or trembling prior to departure and continue once the owner is gone.

- Gastrointestinal signs may consist of inappetence, vomiting or diarrhoea (Simpson, 2000).
- Self-trauma may be manifest as acral lick granulomas or injury due to attempts to escape confinement (Simpson, 2000).

Videotapes made when the pet is home alone may aid or verify diagnosis.

The time sequence of the behaviour is important for establishing the diagnosis. For most dogs with separation anxiety, as compared with other separation-related problem behaviours, the behaviour occurs within 5–30 minutes after owner departure (Borchelt and Voith, 1982). A typical question might be: 'What is the shortest amount of time you have been gone and returned to find the problem behaviour (elimination, destruction etc.)?' Some dogs with separation anxiety may engage in problem behaviour shortly after the owner departs and become aroused again later in the day (Lund and Jorgensen, 1997). In addition, dogs with separation anxiety often act extremely excited upon owner return, with jumping, running and vocalization activities that last for quite some time. On the other hand, dogs with fear responses to events that occur when the owner is gone (storms, loud noises, territorial incursions into the territory) may show a more variable pattern of expression of owner-absent problem behaviours. When this becomes evident, more exploration is needed to come to a diagnosis.

## Exploring other areas of pet behaviour

Dogs with separation-related problems may also show distress due to other concurrent anxieties, fears or phobias; or, conversely, the distress response may not be separation anxiety but rather a distress response due to something else. Dogs that are fearful may experience the fearful stimulus when left alone and engage in fear-motivated behaviours when separated from the owner that might resemble separation anxiety but are in fact related to both the fear of the stimulus and the anxiety about being alone, rather than an inability to cope with being alone due to over-attachment to the owner or lack of owner presence. Therefore questions should target pet responses to loud noises, thunder and lightning, fireworks and other outdoor stimuli.

Other areas of pet–owner behaviour should not be neglected in separation anxiety cases; underlying anxiety can contribute to other behavioural disorders (Overall, 1996).

- The owner should be asked about any aggressive behaviour related to food, possessions, body handling, removal of objects from the dog and discipline.
- The behaviour of the dog with visitors, in the garden, territorial displays and behaviour with children should all be examined and explored as possible areas that need attention. Dogs that routinely exhibit territorial displays while their owners are home may also do so when the owner is absent.

- Questions regarding reliability of outdoor elimination may help to differentiate separation anxiety from a house soiling problem.
- Enquiring about destructive episodes while the owner is otherwise occupied in the home may indicate problems other than separation anxiety, such as lack of appropriate outlets for play and exploration, outdoor stimuli that cause arousal and other motivations.
- Owners of elderly dogs should also be asked about signs of cognitive decline: loss of housetraining, changes in sleep/wake cycle, changes in social interactions and disorientation and confusion (see Chapter 12).

## Evaluation of client attitudes, beliefs and behaviour

Common owner misconceptions that may hinder obtaining good historical information include the perception that the dog is being 'spiteful', 'knows that it did something wrong', or is 'ungrateful' or 'mean'. In many cases the owners are punishing the dog when they return and find the result of unwanted behaviours while they had been absent, and this is not productive. There can be multiple explanations for the expressions of vocalization, elimination and destruction in the absence of the owner and all possibilities must be explored, ruled out and explained to the owner (see Figure 14.1 and the client questionnaire).

If the problem is deemed to be separation anxiety, some owners may not realize that the behaviour is the result of anxiety, not spite, and fail to see the need for treatment. Therefore it is imperative that owners understand what separation anxiety is: a distress response specifically related to being separated from social group members. Explaining this early in the consultation process will aid in the exchange of accurate unbiased information and a willingness to treat the pet. Unless this takes place and reprimands cease, not only will the dog remain distressed when the owner leaves, but also it may be anxious when the owner returns. If the problem is not separation anxiety, but another separation-related behavioural problem, this too must be explained to the owner so that they understand what is going on with their pet.

## Differential diagnosis

A definitive diagnosis of which separation distress problem is presented should be based on several key findings in the behavioural history (a history of attachment or not, other fears and phobias noted, territorial responses, etc.) and the exclusion of alternative behavioural and medical diagnoses. The history should have established evidence of elimination, vocalization, destruction and the other signs noted above and in Figure 14.2. The behavioural history should have established which behaviours take place in the absence of the owner and at what frequency. Differential diagnoses (Figure 14.3) for the typical separation-related problem behaviours seen are as follows.

## Destruction

Destruction can occur as an element of play or exploratory behaviour in young or active animals without appropriate exercise (Simpson, 2000). It can also occur in the course of territorial displays at windows and doors, or during phobic episodes related

| Questions | Interpretation |
|---|---|
| Does your dog:<br>• Follow you excessively?<br>• Need always to be close to you?<br>• Need to keep you in sight? | A yes response to any of these may indicate hyperattachment and possible separation anxiety |
| What does your dog do as you prepare to depart? | Signs of agitation, whining, panting and pacing may indicate an anxiety about departure |
| Does your dog vocalize (bark, whine or howl), scratch at the door or confinement area, or attempt to block your departure as you leave? | Any of these behaviours may indicate separation anxiety |
| Does your dog vocalize, or house soil or cause damage while you are gone? | An irregular occurrence may be due to an outside stimulus, but a daily occurrence may indicate anxiety |
| Does your dog ever go to the toilet in the house while you are at home? | Dogs that eliminate when the owners are both home and away usually do not have separation anxiety – but may have a house soiling problem (see Chapter 10) |
| Is your dog ever destructive (e.g. chewing blinds, scratching at carpet, chewing furniture) while you are home? | Destructive behaviour when the owner is both home and away often indicates other problems such as inappropriate outlets for exercise and activity |
| Does your dog vocalize at external stimuli when you are at home? | Dogs that vocalize at external stimuli when the owner is home may also do so when alone |
| What is the shortest amount of time you have been gone and returned to find the problem behaviour (soiling, destruction, etc.)? | Extremely short departures that elicit the problem behaviour may indicate separation anxiety |
| What departure triggers elicit the distress behaviour? | Understanding the triggers will help the formulation of a treatment plan |

**14.1** Questions to ask clients and the rationale behind them. A sample client questionnaire is available from bsavalibrary.com/behaviour_leaflets.

Evidence of strong attachment to caregivers (following behaviour, attention-seeking behaviours), though not present in all cases

Behaviour occurs in the absence (or perceived absence) of the attachment person(s)

Behaviour occurs shortly after departure (usually within 30 minutes)

One or more of the following problem behaviours occurs during owner absence (these require the additional disorder to be treated):
- Destruction (which for separation anxiety is usually focused on exits)
- Vocalization
- Elimination of urine and/or stool
- Hypersalivation
- Inappetence
- Behavioural depression (immobility)
- Gastrointestinal signs
- Self-trauma
- Excessive or unusual motor activity

Excessive excitement and activity upon owner return

Other fear or anxiety conditions in addition, such as noise or storm reactions, may mimic separation anxiety when the latter is not present

**14.2** Criteria necessary for a diagnosis of separation anxiety in dogs (not all may be present in each case).

| Behaviour | Possible cause |
|---|---|
| Destruction (Figure 14.4) | Playful behaviours<br>Over-activity<br>Lack of appropriate exercise and stimulation<br>Thunderstorm or noise sensitivity<br>Territorial behaviours<br>Fearful stimuli<br>Separation anxiety (with or without hyper-attachment) |
| Vocalization | Outside stimuli<br>Social facilitation with other dogs<br>Territorial displays<br>Play<br>Fears or phobic responses<br>Separation anxiety (with or without hyper-attachment) |
| House soiling | Inadequate housetraining<br>Lack of opportunity or lack of access to the elimination location<br>Fear<br>Excitement<br>Submissive urination<br>Urine marking<br>Faecal incontinence<br>Medical causes of increased urination or defecation<br>Parasites<br>Cognitive dysfunction<br>Separation anxiety (with or without hyper-attachment) |
| Self-trauma and licking behaviours | Primary dermatological conditions<br>Allergies<br>Neuritis<br>Separation anxiety (with or without hyper-attachment) |

**14.3** Differential diagnosis for behaviour problems expressed when a dog is separated from its owner (separation-related behaviour problem).

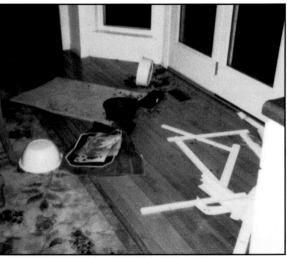

**14.4** Destruction and disruption is commonly seen with separation anxiety.

to noises or storms. Young teething animals may be destructive and so might animals with other dental problems. For these explanations to be likely, the problem behaviour will often occur while the owner is present as well as when the owner is absent. However, in some cases there is the possibility that fear responses causing these behaviours are only seen in the owner's absence – for example owner inhibition of territorial responses results in these behaviours being more commonly displayed when the owner is not there. Destruction can also occur due to an anxious response to confinement when a dog is crated or closely confined. Dogs experiencing this issue will usually have problems being confined when the owner is home as well (see Chapter 8).

## Vocalization
Vocalization in dogs is common and may be due to outside stimuli, social facilitation with other dogs, territorial displays or play (Horwitz and Neilson, 2007). Again, in these circumstances the behaviours are commonly present when the owner is home. When unsure of the motivation for vocalization, audio tapes often help to determine the inciting cause: the veterinary surgeon should listen for other background noises and the tone, pitch and frequency of the vocalization. See Chapter 8 for further information on the management of excessive vocalization due to external arousal, including play and territorial responses.

## Elimination
Elimination in the owner's absence can occur due to poor housetraining, medical abnormalities of the urinary tract or intestinal tract, endocrine dysfunction causing increased water consumption, excitement or submissive urination, urine marking, fear and cognitive dysfunction.

- Medical problems would most likely result in elimination while the owner was present as well as when they were absent and might be accompanied by straining, blood, increased frequency of elimination, diarrhoea or constipation. Urinalysis, faecal examination, blood chemistry screening and possibly imaging studies are indicated when medical causes of house soiling are suspected.

- Excitement and submissive urination (see Chapter 10) would occur at other times as well (and rarely when the owner is absent) and with other people.
- Lack of appropriate housetraining or poor access to elimination locations may be difficult to distinguish from separation anxiety if the owner does not observe the animal eliminate outside or does not search the home for soiling on a daily basis. When the timing of the elimination is not clear, daily diaries of elimination times and locations may be helpful as will videotaping the pet when the owner departs.
- Dogs suffering from cognitive dysfunction often show other signs of cognitive decline such as confusion, disorientation and changes in their sleep/wake cycle (see Chapter 12).

## Other fears or anxieties

Separation anxiety can be co-morbid with other anxiety conditions or may be a differential diagnosis for another anxiety condition. Fear and anxiety of new and novel situations, fear of strangers, aggression, compulsive behaviours and aggression between housemates may all occur in conjunction with separation anxiety (Overall, 1998) or with separation-related behaviour problems. When an extremely fearful dog encounters fear-inducing stimuli while the owner is absent, it may engage in behaviours (especially destruction) that may mimic separation anxiety. These types of response may be seen with any number of stimulus variables (for example, external noises, the postman, the rubbish collector, storms and fireworks) and may be separate from separation anxiety or part of the complex of behaviour problems exhibited by the patient. This may result in the owner being unaware that separation anxiety exists where the dog is not particularly destructive on a daily basis, but much worse when the fear-inducing event is present so that the behaviour becomes much more noticeable. However, for treatment to be successful for either condition, all the underlying fears and anxieties must be identified and treated. When multiple diagnoses coexist, it becomes necessary to triage treatment to make best use of the owner's time and resources.

Although aggression may be present, often the destruction of property takes precedence for the owner. It is important for the veterinary surgeon to help the owner in treating the most pressing problems while at the same time ensuring safety if aggressive behaviour is also present.

## Early or late onset of distress responses

Animals showing early onset of vocalization, elimination indoors and destruction in the absence of the owner may be particularly difficult to diagnose. Owners may assume that the signs noted are associated with the young age, lack of training or activity. Videotaping the animal when it is alone will help to verify that it is distressed and not just occupying its time. Late-onset clinical signs may be puzzling if the dog had not shown these signs before. These may be dogs with other existing fears or anxieties or dogs that are cognitively impaired, resulting in loss of learned responses such as housetraining, or emotional disturbances such as increased anxiety when left alone. These need to be differentiated as they require different treatments. Video or audio tapes are useful in those situations as well.

## Behavioural biology of separation anxiety

Separation anxiety is not necessarily maladaptive: young animals will vocalize to be reunited with their mother; and other animals may vocalize to be reunited with their herd or pack. In the companion animal, the repetition of this behaviour can be problematic and the tendency to show these responses may be influenced by the individual temperament of the patient (for example, temperamentally anxious individuals may not be able to cope with a range of anxious situations, separation of the owner just being the one instance that causes a problem from the owner's perspective). Separation anxiety may have an inherited predisposition and be related to the selective breeding that has created dogs that are extremely socially oriented toward humans and socially dependent upon them.

Some research suggests that early onset may be related to early experiences, such as lack of proper detachment from the dam (Serpell and Jagoe, 1995). While some schools of thought consider hyper-attachment to people an integral part of the diagnosis, experimental studies have yet to find a significant difference in the degree of attachment to owners between dogs diagnosed with separation anxiety and those dogs without signs of separation anxiety, although the former may have an attachment to their owner that is inappropriate (Parthasarathy and Crowell-Davis, 2006). A diagnosis should not be made solely on the basis of signs of attachment between the owner and the patient.

Later onset may be related to changes in the social environment or may even be a learned behaviour in which the dog predicts that certain situations signal a long-term absence of the owner. Other animals seem to experience distress because something upsetting has occurred when they were home alone, though normally they would not be upset if the owner were not present. These dogs often also experience noise or storm phobias and sensitivities and often need different treatment interventions. In some cases the patient may then generalize their anxiety to all departures, not just those in which the stimuli occur (Overall *et al.*, 2001).

Finally, older animals often show increased anxiety and separation distress responses, perhaps due to ageing and cognitive decline (Landsberg and Ruehl, 1997), which may be described differently in some countries, e.g. involutive depression. Due to their impairment, older animals with other cognitive signs may not respond as well to treatment. Animals experiencing other sensitivities may be difficult to control if the stimulus cannot be avoided or the animal desensitized to it.

## Contribution of underlying medical disorders

The contribution of underlying medical disorders should not be underestimated.

- Animals suffering from chronic medical conditions may be anxious (see Chapter 13).
- Chronic dermatological and intestinal disorders may lower the animal's threshold for anxiety responses.
- Metabolic disorders that affect mental condition (Cushing's disease, thyroid disorders, Addison's disease) may also change how the pet perceives being left at home alone if hormonal levels have altered perception of the environment.
- The additional owner attention that often accompanies caring for a chronically ill animal may alter the pet–owner relationship, resulting in greater dependence on the owner, which becomes problematic when the animal is expected to be more independent.
- Behaviour may also be influenced by some medications, such as corticosteroids (increase in water consumption), diuretics (increased need to eliminate) and medication to stop urine leakage (phenylpropanolamine causing excitability in susceptible individuals).
- Medical disorders that alter water intake or urine or stool output may result in house soiling not related to distress.

## Treatment of separation-related behaviour problems

Behaviour problems related to owner absence that are primarily due to conditions other than social distress are covered in other chapters: for control problems see Chapter 8; for housetraining see Chapter 10; for sound sensitivities see Chapter 15; and for special considerations in the older animal see Chapter 12.

## Acute management protocols

### Separation anxiety

Environmental management can make living with a dog with separation anxiety easier until the dog has learned how to be home alone. This might include increased opportunities for play and exercise, especially with the owner, tailored to individual pet needs since often increased exercise can make pets calmer (Simpson, 2000).

Obviously, the best acute management protocol is whenever possible not to leave the pet home alone while it is learning new associations. Each anxiety-producing departure reinforces stress responses as well as potentially continuing the ongoing soiling and destruction that upsets the owners. Options include 'day care' boarding situations, keeping the pet at work, or arranging a pet sitter or a friend to be with the dog.

In cases where departure cues seem to be a potent trigger for distress, mixing up or eliminating those cues may decrease anxiety. This could mean packing the car the night before, or dressing in casual clothes and changing at work, or masking the departure with noises like the washing machine or dishwasher while the dog is busy in another location with a stuffed chew toy.

For some animals, gradual conditioning to a confinement area such as a crate or room can help with the anxiety associated with owner departure, but may not show results immediately. Also, some animals are especially stressed if confined in small areas such as crates and their distress might diminish if given a larger area. While it is tempting to suggest confinement to stop the soiling or destruction, veterinary surgeons should be very cautious about recommending crating for anxious animals. If the animal is not used to being in a small confined location the distress might actually increase and the animal may severely injure itself in attempts to escape. A diagnosis should always be established before treatment recommendations are given.

Medication is another possibility, but in the absence of additional behavioural training it is unlikely to be useful in the long term; it will be covered later in this chapter. Pheromones might calm some pets but again cannot be relied upon as a sole intervention.

Some animals may benefit from the presentation of owner objects or clothing as comfort signals, but in this author's experience these have not been particularly helpful in very distressed patients.

### Other causes of separation distress responses

For dogs that are experiencing a fear-based response when at home alone, acute strategies will vary according to the stimuli that cause the fear. For fear of noises, some dogs may benefit from closed shutters, background noises and other attempts to block out the offending stimulus. For other noise sensitivities, see Chapter 15 for treatment options. For dogs that will not be confined, allowing more space may be useful.

## Long-term treatment strategies

Treatment of separation anxiety typically involves environmental, behavioural and pharmacological interventions. Psychopharmacological and pheromone intervention have been shown to be a useful adjunct to behaviour modification techniques for separation anxiety. Because dogs with separation anxiety are already anxious, punishment is contraindicated and owners must be instructed to stop all punishment for behaviours that occur in their absence.

Dividing the behaviour into the four problem areas mentioned earlier will allow treatment to target specific areas (Figure 14.5).

Treatment routines for separation anxiety include:

- Changing the pet–owner relationship
- Teaching the pet to settle and relax on command
- Decreasing the predictive value of pre-departure cues
- Counter-conditioning and response substitution to pre-departure cues
- Changing the leaving and return routine
- Graduated planned departures.

A **client handout** is provided.

| Target area | Treatment aims |
|---|---|
| For anxiety-based behaviour that occurs when the owner is home | Treatment should focus on changing the pet–owner interactions: <br>• Making the dog more secure and independent <br>• Teaching the dog to settle and relax in a safe place |
| To diminish the anxiety associated with preparations for departure and the eventual departure | Treatment modalities must address these specific triggers: <br>• Diminish the predictive value of departure cues by uncoupling them from departure |
| For anxiety that remains when the owner is gone | Treatment must teach the pet how to be calm when at home alone: <br>• Short training departures specifically designed to diminish anxiety must be implemented |
| Any other coexisting anxieties and sensitivities | These must also be addressed as they are likely to contribute to the distress response: <br>• Noise sensitivities must be treated separately <br>• Barrier frustration or fear of confinement must be treated separately |

**14.5** Treatment target areas for separation distress responses.

## Changing the pet–owner interaction

***Making the dog more independent:*** Many dogs with separation anxiety show signs of strong attachment to one or more persons in the home. This is usually manifest by following behaviours, attention-seeking behaviours and pestering the owner (Simpson, 2000; Horwitz and Neilson, 2007a). This behaviour may occur toward some family members but not all. By changing the way the pet relates to family members, the dog may become more independent, secure and less anxious when left alone.

Owners are instructed to ignore attention-seeking behaviours such as pawing, leaning, barking and nudging and only attend to the dog when it is calm and quiet. Although they must ignore the dog when it solicits attention, they can initiate attention when the dog is calm and quiet. They should clearly signal to the dog when attention will be given and when it will be denied. Limiting periods of non-attention to 5 minutes initially can help to ease gradually into the therapy. The signalling can be accomplished by, for example, the owner placing a towel on their lap: when the towel is present the dog will not receive attention; when the towel is removed the owner will interact with the pet, but will initiate the interaction.

The owner is only to ignore the attention-seeking behaviours, not the pet itself. They should be encouraged to spend pleasurable time with the pet, for example in the form of increased exercise, walks, teaching tricks, attending a training class or grooming session.

Owners are also encouraged to teach dogs to sit or down-stay away from them and off the furniture rather than always in close physical contact. Podberscek *et al.* (1999) emphasized changing the way owners relate to their pets to help to ameliorate separation distress responses. The behaviour changes include: no longer allowing the dog to sit on their lap or furniture; not allowing the dog to sleep in the bedroom; no gratuitous titbits; all interaction to be at the owner's initiative; not allowing following; and having times of enforced separation whilst the owners are home. This is facilitated by teaching the dog how to settle, relax and be calm in certain safe or confined locations when the owner is home. If the dog can learn how to be calm away from the owner when they are home, this seems to help the dog to remain calm when they are gone. This is not an obedience exercise, rather it is an exercise in relaxation so that the owner can cue the dog to relax with verbal and/or hand direction. The pet is slowly conditioned to remain in a safe location that is not associated with owner departure. This usually takes several weeks and requires patience and persistence so that the safe/confinement area is always associated with pleasant things.

These treatment recommendations are not easily implemented by pet owners and to encourage them to comply it must be explained how attention-seeking behaviour and attention from the owner may contribute to the anxiety condition in their pet. In essence the aim is to minimize the contrast between 'owner home' and 'owner gone', as far as receiving attention is concerned, to help to decrease anxiety when the pet is alone.

***Creating predictable and structured interactions:*** Engaging the pet and owner in a routine of regular training can also be beneficial to the pet–owner relationship. The terms often used include 'Nothing in Life is Free' (Voith and Borchelt, 1996; see **client handout**) and 'Learn to Earn' (Campbell, 1999). The programme simply requires the owner to request that the pet perform a task such as 'sit' prior to receiving something it wants. This means that before they let out the dog, before they feed it, before they pet it, put on the lead and so on, the dog must perform a task. The resulting structure often helps some owners to feel more in control and makes life more predictable for the pet, which can reduce anxiety.

## Changing anxiety-based behaviour associated with departure

***Changing the predictive value of pre-departure cues:*** Often dogs with separation anxiety have learned that certain owner activities predict departure and become anxious when these are presented. Extinction (the elimination of a learned response through the removal of the learned predictive association between events) is commonly used in the treatment of separation anxiety in dogs to help decrease the response to pre-departure cues (see Chapter 5). The behavioural history should have identified departure triggers (things the owner does prior to departure that elicit the beginning of the anxiety behaviours) and the predictive value of these as cues to departure needs to be diminished.

The owner should be instructed to go through portions of their leaving routine that would normally predict departure. This can include picking up their keys, putting on a coat or shoes and walking toward the door. These actions may make the dog anxious and it might get up and follow them. They are to ignore the dog and most importantly *not* leave the house; instead, they remove any outerwear, put back keys, purses and briefcases and sit down again. They perform this exercise two to five times daily, only initiating the process when the dog is relaxed and not anxious. The goal is to disassociate the cues from actual departure, so that they are no longer predictive of departure and do not lead to an anxious response. As the owner repeatedly presents these stimuli without significant associations, they should become less important and easier for the dog to ignore.

However, if done incorrectly some dogs may become more anxious rather than less so. Therefore it is important for owners to watch and judge the reaction of their pet. Presenting the departure cues too frequently or presenting too many cues all at once may lead to an increase in anxiety. With some pets it may only be possible to pick up the keys and take two steps and then put them down before the dog gets much too anxious. It is also important to stress to owners that the dog must be calm between presentations of the departure cues or else anxiety may heighten and the separation distress increase.

When the dog's response to the departure cues has been extinguished, there should be little or no response (the dog may get up, but not look anxious or follow them) when they are performed.

*Counter-conditioning:* Counter-conditioning (also called response substitution) is another technique used to decrease the response of the dog to departure cues. The dog is taught to sit-and-stay or down-and-stay in the vicinity of the exit door, since these behaviours are incompatible with (or counter to) the problem behaviour of pacing around anxiously. At first, the owner only steps a short distance from the dog, then returns and rewards the dog (food rewards and praise are used initially). Gradually the owner increases the time and the distance from the dog. Eventually the owner can add in opening and closing the door without leaving. In this way the dog learns that the owner approaching and opening the door can be pleasant and associated with something other than owner departure. Finally the owner may step outside the door and quickly return. As the dog learns the task, the owner may stay outside the door for a few seconds longer and then return. If a dog gets extremely excited by food rewards, they may need to be phased out in the course of learning this task.

Alternatively classical or respondent counter-conditioning (see Chapter 5) may be used. This involves giving the dog a tasty titbit to consume, such as a toy stuffed with food, as the owner prepares to depart. Eating often decreases anxiety in dogs, perhaps allowing the owner to depart without the dog becoming anxiously aroused.

*Changing departure and return pet–owner interactions:* The goal is for the dog to remain calm as the owner prepares to depart. To facilitate this, owners are instructed to change the way that they interact with the dog prior to departure and when they return. The owner should ignore the dog for 15–30 minutes prior to departure and again on return by avoiding playing, talking or interacting with their dog during this time (Horwitz, 1998; Simpson, 2000). Naturally, they can allow the dog outside to eliminate as necessary, but should do so in a detached manner.

### Diminishing anxiety about being 'home alone'

*Planned training departures:* The final commonly used behavioural technique used in the treatment of separation anxiety involves planned training departures. These are started after the dog's response to departure cues has been extinguished and/or the dog has learned to sit and stay by the exit door or can settle and relax in their 'safe' location.

Using short departures, the aim is to desensitize the dog to the owner leaving and being gone. Three changes help to distinguish these training departures from regular departures:

- The time away will be carefully controlled with the initial departures being *very* short
- Before they depart the owner will place the dog in its relaxation location
- As the owner departs they leave a new and consistent 'safety cue' (Simpson, 2000) or signal (discriminatory stimulus) for the dog.

This training involves classical conditioning in which a neutral stimulus (the new cue) is paired with a conditioned stimulus (short/manageable departure) and gets a conditioned response (relaxed behaviour) (see Chapter 5).

The goal is to have the dog associate the owner departure, the new signal and good behaviour with each other so that it learns how to cope when left alone. To be effective, this departure must have all the characteristics of the real departures: if the owner drives, they take car keys; if the departure is work related, they take a briefcase; if they always leave in their car, they must drive away.

- The initial departure will be very short (1–5 minutes or less) so that the dog does not engage in any separation-related behaviours (for some dogs, the initial departures may only be seconds if the dog is not able to remain calm for long after the owner departs).
- The owner leaves the dog a new cue or signal, such as the radio or television or a spray of air freshener, to aid the dog in distinguishing this departure from a real or work departure. The new safety cue is *only* used on a planned

departure, *never* when the owner must be gone for long periods of time (work-related departures, for example).

- If possible, the dog should be left in a novel location – perhaps where the owner would like to leave the dog if it did not engage in separation anxiety behaviours or where they have practised the counter-conditioning and relaxation.
- As always, they must keep departures and returns low key. The message they are trying to communicate is: 'the owner is only gone for a short time, they are coming back and I can cope'.
- The length of the departure is *slowly increased* by 3–5-minute intervals, with short departures interspersed with longer ones. The increase must be irregular, not a steady progression. If done in a steady progression of increasing time, it may be possible for the dog to identify the pattern and anxiety will not decrease.
- If the dog is destructive or engaged in any separation-related behaviour during a planned training departure, then the owner was gone too long or the dog was not ready for the training situation and the next departure must be shorter.
- To help to assess behaviour, audio or video taping can be used, and responses recorded to identify contexts that seem to elicit distress.

Initial departures must be short enough not to elicit separation distress. When desensitization is done incorrectly, sensitization can occur and the problem behaviour may worsen. Usually, once a dog can be left on a planned departure for 2 hours, it can be left for longer times. The safety cue or signal (discriminatory stimulus) can be gradually phased out, or can be used for as long as the owner feels it is necessary. Most importantly, the owner cannot quickly go from a 20-minute planned departure to a 3-hour one. This can elicit separation-related distress and may render the safety cue at best useless and at worst a signal of prolonged departure that the dog cannot cope with.

During training, owners should be encouraged to keep diaries to assess progress and treatment success. The journals should include length of departure, time of day and pet response to departure and return.

Graduated planned departures are laborious and time consuming and owners should be warned about this at the outset. It can take quite some time for the pet to associate the safety signal and owner return and become calm on all departures. Therefore it is very important to set up a situation where the dog will succeed, by keeping initial departures very short and making sure the pet's inappropriate response to pre-departure cues has been extinguished and that it can settle and relax in a safe location prior to beginning a programme of planned training departures.

Because these are often difficult for owners to work into their schedule, they can be done prior to work departures (a very short 1–3-minute planned departure) provided that the owner can stay home long enough after completion for the dog to become calm. They also can be done in the evening and on weekends.

In some cases the dog is only attached to one person and they are the only one who needs to participate in this phase of treatment. Usually, however, various family members leave last and all should participate in graduated planned departures if possible.

The history should have identified what areas seem to trigger the most profound pet responses: preparations for departure or hyperattachment issues with the owner. Because most pet owners have limited time to work on problems, it may be useful to identify which of these appears to predominate and make that area the initial focus of treatment (independence versus extinction of departure cue reaction).

### Addressing other concurrent fears and anxieties
As mentioned earlier, many dogs suffer from multiple anxiety conditions. All must be identified and treated to facilitate improvement of the separation distress responses. See Chapter 12 for behaviour problems in the senior pet, Chapters 15 and 16 for sound and situational sensitivities and Chapter 20 for repetitive and compulsive behaviours.

### Pheromones
Dog appeasing pheromone (DAP®, CEVA Animal Health) is a synthetic version of the intermammary appeasing pheromone that has been identified in the lactating bitch and may be useful in reducing anxiety associated with owner departure (see Chapter 21). The pheromone is available as a diffuser that plugs into the wall or as an impregnated collar, both of which remain active for 30 days. One study comparing the efficacy of a DAP® diffuser *versus* clomipramine for the treatment of separation distress in dogs showing signs of hyper-attachment found no significant difference with respect to owner global assessment scores and there were no significant differences between the two groups in individual signs (Gaultier *et al.*, 2005), although the sample sizes were too small to evaluate equivalence scientifically.

Pheromones (see Chapter 21) can be a useful adjunct to therapy since most of the medications discussed below may take several weeks to achieve therapeutic effect, and behaviour modification plans also take time to change behaviour. More immediate actions may be needed on a short-term basis and pheromones can be used in conjunction with medication regimes.

### Pharmacological intervention
Pharmacological intervention (see Chapter 21) has been used for some time to aid in the treatment of separation anxiety in dogs (Voith and Borchelt, 1996; Horwitz, 1998; Simpson, 2000). Not all cases need medication, but many will benefit from its addition by perhaps showing a more rapid response to behavioural therapy. However, results with drug therapy may not be seen for 14–30 days or even longer, so the owner must be committed to prolonged usage.

Animals that might be put on these medications should have a physical examination and a minimum database of a biochemical screen, complete blood count (CBC) and urinalysis (see Chapter 21). Owners should be informed of potential side effects and in some cases the extra-label nature of the usage, and release forms should be signed.

Currently there are two medications specifically authorized for use in dogs for the treatment of separation anxiety: clomipramine hydrochloride (Clomicalm®, Novartis Animal Health) and fluoxetine (Reconcile®, Elanco Animal Health). Selegiline is licensed more broadly in Europe and the UK (but not the USA and Canada) for emotional disorders in dogs, which might include separation anxiety.

Medications that are used in the treatment of separation anxiety often have a delay in the onset of action and this should be considered when using pharamacological therapy in separation-related behaviour problems. Clomipramine and fluoxetine may take 2–4 weeks or longer for a behavioural effect to be noted and selegiline may take as long as 6 weeks to take effect in some cases. In the meantime the owner may need immediate help with the separation anxiety signs. In some cases low doses of benzodiazepines may be appropriate to aid in calming the dog until behavioural therapy takes hold.

### Clomipramine and fluoxetine

Several studies have been done to ascertain the efficacy of clomipramine as an adjunct in the treatment of separation anxiety in dogs, with varying results. In a prospective randomized double-blinded placebo-controlled trial (King *et al.*, 2000) for use of clomipramine in separation anxiety there were three groups of dogs: two dosage groups and one placebo. Results indicate that more dogs were rated as improved in their scores for destruction, defecation and urination, when compared with dogs receiving placebo. All dogs received a standard behaviour modification protocol. A smaller similar study (Podberscek *et al.*, 1999) that used a more detailed behavioural plan found no difference between groups and concluded that behavioural therapy was highly effective on its own.

The recommended dose of clomipramine for treatment of separation anxiety is 2–4 mg/kg total daily dose, either as one dose or divided twice daily (see Clomicalm package insert for contraindications). The most common adverse reactions are vomiting, diarrhoea and lethargy. Caution is advised in using clomipramine with other central nervous system (CNS)-active drugs, including general anaesthetics, neuroleptics and anticholinergic and sympathomimetic drugs. See Chapter 21 for additional information on medication.

In a large multi-centered double-blind placebo-controlled study (Simpson *et al.*, 2007) fluoxetine was dosed at 1–2 mg/kg once daily and dogs in both groups received a behaviour modification plan. At the conclusion of the study after 8 weeks, 73% of the dogs treated with medication and behaviour modification showed improvement in overall severity scores, compared with 51% of the dogs treated with placebo and behaviour modification. Of the treated dogs, 42% showed improvement within the first week. In this study, the frequency of adverse events was generally similar for fluoxetine- and placebo-treated dogs. The most common adverse events reported following fluoxetine treatment were lethargy and vomiting. Seizures occurred in three fluoxetine-treated and one placebo dog, therefore fluoxetine is not recommended in dogs known to suffer from a seizure disorder.

Neither clomipramine nor fluoxetine should be given in combination with monoamine oxidase inhibitors (selegiline or amitraz) or within 14 days prior to or after treatment with a monoamine oxidase inhibitor. Fluoxetine and clomipramine should not be used concurrently, due to the risk of producing serotonin syndrome. When either is used in a treatment programme, the medication must be given daily and may take 2–4 weeks to see some effect. Patients may need several months of treatment for sustained improvement to be noted. In some cases, withdrawal of medication may result in the return of clinical signs (King *et al.*, 2004).

### Benzodiazepines

Benzodiazepines have often been suggested for providing immediate relief or short-term control. Benzodiazepines such as alprazolam (0.02–0.1 mg/kg orally q6–8h) (Horwitz and Neilson, 2007) can be dispensed on an as-needed basis shortly before departures. Benzodiazepines may inhibit learning, usually require frequent dosing and may cause dependence and a rebound anxiety when discontinued.

### Selegiline

In Europe, selegiline is approved for use in dogs for the treatment of behavioural disorders. It has been used in fear-motivated separation-related behaviour problems where the dog has experienced something fearful in the absence of the owner and consequently associates being alone with being afraid. The commonly used dosage is 0.5 mg/kg once a day.

## Prognosis

Separation anxiety often responds well to behavioural therapy. At times some cases can be difficult for the following reasons:

- Drug therapy alone is rarely curative for most behavioural disorders
- Realistically, drug therapy can be expected to decrease the anxiety associated with owner departure. It also may have some effect on the behaviour of the pet when the owner is home and may decrease attention-seeking behaviours. However, the drug alone will not change behaviour in the long term
- If the pet is not taught how to remain at home alone, and if the predictability of the anxiety-producing cues is not extinguished, very little improvement might occur. In fact, some dogs may become worse
- Owners are used to veterinary pharmacological treatments resulting in a fairly rapid response from their pet. This does not occur with behavioural drugs
- The ongoing destruction, vocalization and elimination continue to strain the human–animal bond.

To counter these problems, emphasis on extinction, changing the pet–owner interactions, changing the leaving and returning routines and teaching relaxation are important. These are the first treatments that should be implemented and studies have indicated that pets improve with these simple changes (King *et al.*, 2000; Simpson *et al.*, 2007).

Owners must be counselled that the aim is to desensitize the dog, but there is a fine line between desensitization and making the dog more sensitive. Therefore it is extremely important to set aside time for regular follow-ups with owners of dogs with separation anxiety. When extinction or planned graduated departures are continued despite increasing pet anxiety, the dog may become even more sensitive to owner departure and the problem behaviours will escalate. Finally, there can be a delay in the onset of action of medication and the medication must be given daily, not on an as-needed basis.

The treatment outcomes of 52 dogs diagnosed with separation anxiety were examined by Takeuchi *et al.* (2000). The authors contacted owners of dogs diagnosed with separation anxiety between 6 and 24 months after the behavioural examination and questioned them about outcome of treatment, compliance with treatment instructions and perception of the effectiveness of each instruction. Owners who had been given more than five instructions were less likely to have dogs that were improved when compared with those given fewer than five instructions. Owners complied with instructions that involved little time, such as eliminating punishment, giving chew toys on departure and increasing exercise. Fewer owners were willing to uncouple departure cues from departure. However, the degree of owner compliance was not related to outcome in this study. It was unclear whether owners with more than five instructions were confused or reluctant to comply, or that these dogs exhibited more severe signs of separation anxiety. It may be that ability and willingness to follow discharge instructions has an enormous impact on prognosis and problem resolution.

## Follow-up

Continued information and feedback are needed to see if the owners are properly administering the behavioural treatment plan. Initially follow-up should be on a weekly basis for the first several weeks. What is being sought is a change in the dog's response to pre-departure activities and increasing pet independence. If no response to these treatments is seen and medication or pheromones has not been started, a discussion on adding them into the plan is appropriate.

Owner diaries can help in assessing progress and are often essential to monitor progress. In them owners can keep track of actual departures, pet reactions and training sessions.

Often what the owner wants, especially in cases of destructiveness, is complete resolution of the problem behaviour. Most likely what will first occur is a decrease in the frequency and/or severity of target behaviours. When the animal no longer responds with anxiety to departure cues, can settle and relax on command, and is more independent, graduated planned departures may be added if needed. It is important to speak with the owner after one or two practice departures to determine whether they are being done properly and the dog is relaxed rather than more anxious.

Drug therapy is usually employed for at least 3 months and perhaps more if the case is particularly difficult. Medication should be continued for 1 month beyond problem resolution. Once the problem is resolved, medication can be withdrawn. It is possible to stop medication abruptly, especially with fluoxetine due to residual effects of the active metabolite, but this author does not usually do so. Often the dosage of medication is slowly decreased by 25% a week and the patient is observed for increase in the target problem behaviours. This enables either staying at the lower dose while waiting to see if the behaviour stabilizes, or returning to the previously effective dose. During this time weekly to semi-weekly follow-up is advised so that adjustments can be made before problem behaviours return or escalate.

## Prevention of the problem

Strong data-based evidence is lacking on what types of early interventions may prevent separation anxiety. Teaching the pet how to be calm and settled away from the owner is likely to be useful. Keeping departures and returns low key may also be helpful. Teaching the dog how to be left at home alone slowly over time may have some value. Hopefully future research will help to establish other preventive tools.

## References and further reading

Borchelt PL and Voith VL (1982) Diagnosis and treatment of separation-related behaviour problems in dogs. *Veterinary Clinics of North America: Small Animal Practice* **12**, 625–635

Bradshaw JWS, McPherson JA, Casey RA and Larter IS (2002) Aetiology of separation-related behaviour in domestic dogs. *Veterinary Record* **151**, 43–46

Campbell WE (1999) *Behavior Problems in Dogs, 3rd revised edn.* Behavior RX Systems, Grants Pass, Oregon

Chapman BL and Voith VL (1990) Behavioral problems in old dogs: 26 cases. *Journal of the American Veterinary Medical Association* **196**, 944–946

Denenberg S, Landsberg GM and Horwitz D (2005) A comparison of cases referred to behaviorists in three different countries. In: *Current Issues and Research in Veterinary Behavioral Medicine*, ed. D Mills, E Levine, GM Landsberg *et al*, pp. 56–62. Purdue University Press, West Lafayette, Indiana

Edwards C , Heiblum M , Tejeda A and Galindo F (2007) Experimental evaluation of attachment behaviors in owned cats. *Journal of Veterinary Behavior: Clinical Applications and Research* **2**, 119–125

Flannigan G and Dodman NH (2001) Risk factors and behaviors associated with separation anxiety in dogs. *Journal of the American Veterinary Medical Association* **219**, 460–466

Gaultier E, Bonnafous L, Bougrat L *et al.* (2005) Comparison of the efficacy of a synthetic dog-appeasing pheromone with clomipramine for the treatment of separation-related disorders in dogs. *Veterinary Record* **156**, 533–538

Horwitz DF (1998) Diagnosis and treatment of separation-related disorders. *Veterinary International* **10**, 26–34

Horwitz DF and Neilson JC (2007b) *Blackwell's Five Minute Veterinary Consult Clinical Companion Canine and Feline Behavior.* Blackwell Publishing, Ames, Iowa

Houpt KA, Honig SU and Reisner IR (1996) Breaking the human–animal companion bond. *Journal of the American Veterinary Medical Association* **208,** 1653–1658

King JN, Overall KL, Appleby BS *et al.* (2004) Results of a follow-up investigation to a clinical trial testing the efficacy of clomipramine in the treatment of separation anxiety. *Applied Animal Behaviour Sciience* **89,** 233–242

King JN, Simpson BS, Overall KL *et al.* (2000) Treatment of separation anxiety in dogs with clomipramine: results from a prospective, randomised, double-blind, placebo-controlled, parallel-group multicenter clinical trial. *Applied Animal Behaviour Science* **67,** 255–275

Landsberg G and Ruehl W (1997) Geriatric behavioral problems. *Veterinary Clinics of North America: Small Animal Practice* **27,** 1537–1559

Landsberg G, Hunthausen W and Ackerman L (2003) The European approach to behaviour counselling. In: *Handbook of Behaviour Problems 2nd edn,* ed. G Landsberg, W Hunthausen and L Ackerman, pp. 455–482. Saunders, Philadelphia

Lund DJ and Jorgensen MC (1997) Separation anxiety in pet dogs: behaviour patterns and time course of activity. *Proceedings, 1st International Conference on Veterinary Behavioural Medicine,* pp. 133–142.

McCrave EA (1991) Diagnostic criteria for separation anxiety in the dog. *Veterinary Clinics of North America: Small Animal Practice* **21,** 247–255

Miller DD, Staats SR, Partlo C and Rada K (1996) Factors associated with the decision to surrender a pet to an animal shelter. *Journal of the American Veterinary Medical Association* **209,** 738–742

Mugford RA (1995) Canine behavioural therapy. In: *The Domestic Dog: Its Evolution, Behaviour and Interactions with People,* ed. J Serpell, pp. 139–152. Cambridge University Press, Cambridge

Overall KL (1996) Anxiety-related disorder very correctable with proper diagnosis, treatment and follow-up. *DVM Magazine* 8S–10S

Overall KL (1998) Animal behavior case of the month. *Journal of the American Veterinary Medical Association* **213,** 34–36

Overall KL, Dunham AE and Frank D (2001) Frequency of nonspecific clinical signs in dogs with separation anxiety, thunderstorm phobia, and noise phobia, alone or in combination. *Journal of the American Veterinary Medical Association* **219,** 467–473

Parthasarathy V and Crowell-Davis SL (2006) Relationship between attachment to owners and separation anxiety in pet dogs. *Journal of Veterinary Behavior* **1,** 109–120

Patronek GJ, Glickman LT, Beck AM *et al.* (1996) Risk factors for relinquishment of dogs to an animal shelter. *Journal of the American Veterinary Medical Association* **209,** 572–581

Podberscek AL, Hsu Y and Serpell JA (1999) Evaluation of clomipramine as an adjunct to behavioural therapy in the treatment of separation-related problems in dogs. *Veterinary Record* **145,** 365–369

Salman MoD, Hutchinson J, Ruch-Gallie R *et al.* (2000) Behavioral reasons for relinquishment of dogs and cats to 12 shelters. *Journal of Applied Animal Welfare Science* **3,** 93–106

Schwartz B and Robbins SJ (1995) *Psychology of Learning and Behavior.* WW Norton, New York

Schwartz S (2002) Separation anxiety syndrome in cats: 136 cases (1991–2000). *Journal of the American Veterinary Medical Association* **220,** 1028–1033

Serpell J and Jagoe JA (1995) Early experience and the development of behaviour. In: *The Domestic Dog: Its Evolution, Behaviour and Interactions with People,* ed. J Serpell, pp. 79–102. Cambridge University Press, Cambridge

Simpson BS (2000) Canine separation anxiety. *Compendium on Continuing Education for the Practicing Veterinarian* **22,** 328–339

Simpson BS, Landsberg GM, Reisner IR *et al.* (2007) Effects of Reconcile (fluoxetine) chewable tablets plus behavior management for canine separation anxiety. *Veterinary Therapeutics* **8,** 18–31

Takeuchi Y, Houpt KA and Scarlett JM (2000) Evaluation of treatments for separation anxiety in dogs. *Journal of the American Veterinary Medical Association* **217,** 342–345

Turner DC (2000) The human–cat relationship. In: *The Domestic Cat, 2nd edn,* ed. DC Turner and P Bateson, pp. 193–206. Cambridge University Press, Cambridge

Voith VL and Borchelt PL (1996) Separation anxiety in dogs. In: *Readings in Companion Animal Behavior,* ed. VL Voith and PL Borchelt, pp. 124–139. Veterinary Learning Systems, Trenton, New Jersey

## Client handouts (bsavalibrary.com/behaviour_leaflets)

- Adopting a rescue dog: the pros and cons
- Avoiding house soiling by dogs
- Canine behaviour questionnaire
- Cognitive dysfunction syndrome
- Down–stay mat exercises
- Headcollar training
- How to find a good trainer
- Noise fear score sheet
- 'Nothing in Life is Free'
- Questionnaire to assess separation anxiety

- Sit–stay exercises
- Teaching your dog to go to a place on command
- The newly adopted rescue dog: preventing problems
- Treating a noise fear using desensitization and counter-conditioning
- Treating separation anxiety in dogs
- What your dog needs
- Your puppy's first year

# 15

# Sound sensitivities

## Emily D. Levine

## Introduction

Noise sensitivity is a commonly reported behavioural problem in dogs. It is occasionally reported in cats, though this should not be taken to mean that it is uncommon in cats since they tend not to display behaviours that are problematic to owners (e.g. they run away and hide) and so will be presented less frequently.

The most commonly reported noises to which dogs are sensitive are thunder, fireworks, engine noises and gunshots. Very little is known about how these fears are acquired and so treatment plans may not be as efficacious, because different acquisitional or developmental mechanisms may require different treatment modalities or have different prognoses.

Although previous traumatic experience with a loud noise has been reported as a risk factor for canine noise aversions, 60% of owners report that their dogs have not had a traumatic experience with noises. This indicates that other mechanisms are involved in noise fear acquisition. Other possible mechanisms as reported in human literature include social facilitation, lack of habituation, sensitization and stress-induced dishabituation. These concepts are explained later in the chapter.

Throughout this chapter, noise sensitivity will be used as a general descriptive term to include noise anxieties, noise fears and noise phobias. It is important to note that these are not the same problem, since anxiety, fears and phobias have different characteristics (Figure 15.1). However, overlap is common, particularly with the expression of fear and anxiety. While the term phobia is used for many noise sensitivities,

| Term | Definition |
|------|-----------|
| Anxiety response | Anticipation of a danger or threat. Its sources may or may not be identifiable. Anxious behaviour can be displayed in the absence of an eliciting stimulus |
| Fear response | Normal whole-body response to a perceived threatening stimulus that has physiological, emotional and behavioural components. It is associated with specific stimuli. If the animal has no control over the situation, fear may turn into anxiety |
| Phobia | A fear response that is persistent, maladaptive and out of proportion to the situation/stimulus |

**15.1** Definitions.

there may be many more cases where noise fear or noise anxiety is a more appropriate diagnosis.

Ultimately an understanding of the interplay amongst the behavioural functions and neurophysiology of audition, behavioural responses to aversive stimuli, genetics and the environment in which a dog was raised and lives are necessary to understanding noise sensitivities and in making the most accurate diagnosis and the most efficacious treatment plan.

## Behavioural functions and neurophysiology of the auditory system

Hearing serves vital functions in an animal's survival. The ability to hear allows sounds to be detected and location of the origin to be determined. Ideally and of utmost importance, the animal should be able to identify the origin of the sound (Carlson, 2004). These basic functions of hearing allow the animal to communicate with conspecifics, to reproduce and, pertinent to noise sensitivity problems, to identify sounds potentially associated with environmental and social dangers. If there is a danger signal or an unknown signal that may represent a danger and the animal has located its origin, the animal can make decisions about how to get away safely from that source. Hearing may help to inform the speed of assessment and decision making in relation to potential danger, with certain audible features (e.g. very loud noises) resulting in an immediate response before higher cognitive functions assess the degree of danger more precisely.

The ears of dogs are an important start of the auditory process. The pinnae help to funnel the sound into the ear canal, where the cell receptors within the inner ear (organ of Corti) send auditory information to the brain. Once a sound is heard, it is transmitted via neuronal impulses to the sensory thalamus; from there, there is parallel processing to the amygdala and to the auditory cortex (Figure 15.2).

The amygdala is stimulated in the auditory pathway as described above, but it is also stimulated when an animal feels frightened, stressed, or anxious. It is the amygdala's involvement in this manner along with the body's other stress-induced responses (see Chapter 13) that can contribute to the clinical problem of noise sensitivity in dogs. Whilst initially responding aversely to certain noises may not be abnormal, the lack of habituation to these noises does appear to be

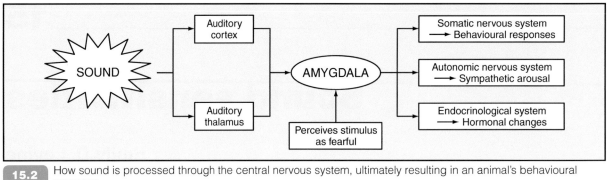

**15.2** How sound is processed through the central nervous system, ultimately resulting in an animal's behavioural response.

abnormal. Because learning not to be fearful of a stimulus is an active process, the difficulty in adapting to noises may be the result of a malfunctioning prefrontal cortex, a stressful living environment, genetics and/or other factors.

Given the universality of the noises that most commonly induce sensitivities (thunder, fireworks, guns, engine noises), it should be considered that there are characteristic of those noises that may help to explain an animal's initial response to them even if it is the animal's individual genetics, learning capabilities and environment that assist in the maintenance of the noise sensitivities.

## Sound characteristics

Sounds are audible variations in air pressure.

- The **frequency** of a sound, measured in hertz (Hz), is the number of cycles per second. Tone or **pitch** is related to frequency. Dogs are able to detect frequencies of 40,000–50,000 Hz, whereas people can only detect up to 20,000 Hz. Dogs are most sensitive at frequencies of 500–16,000 Hz, whereas in humans it is within the range of 2,000–4,000 Hz (Heffner, 1983; Ducan Luce, 1993).
- The **intensity** of a sound is its loudness, measured in decibels (dB); this relates to the height (**amplitude**) of the sound waves or the volume of medium being vibrated. For humans, noises above 70 dB are perceived as loud, above 100 dB as very loud and above 120–140 as painful (Howald and Angus, 2001). Noises above 85 dB can harm human hearing. Dogs exposed to a noise at 95 dB exhibit a variety of stress-related behaviours such as shaking, paw lifting, increased heart rate and lip licking (Beerda et al., 1997).
- The **impulsivity** of a sound relates to the rise time. Impulsive sounds consist of short bursts rather than sustained tones. If a sound registers as impulsive (for example, a balloon popping) it can actually appear 'louder' than a sound of similar intensity that is not impulsive, due to a lack of accommodation of the hearing apparatus.

Animals will generally react to a noise with an orientating response and many will engage in this response upon first hearing a sound, with the brain becoming more alert while the body becomes quieter. During the few seconds of an orientating response, the heart rate may be decreased (Leeds and Wagner, 2008a). For any noise that is being evaluated, the brain may be looking for a pattern so that the animal can identify its source; and the ultrasonic spectra of a noise appear to be particularly important in its localization. It has been postulated that, if a noise evokes an immediate defensive response, habituation to that particular noise may be very slow or nonexistent, as opposed to other noises that simply evoke an orientating response (Tuber *et al.*, 1982). If this is true, it would explain why certain noises in particular seem to affect animals, as their characteristics would invoke a defensive response in predisposed animals as opposed to simply an orientating response. When one looks at the more common noises to which dogs react (Figure 15.3), it is not surprising that their reaction is aversive. These sounds have high decibels, can reach pain thresholds for people, lack a pattern, in some cases may not feature much ultrasound or other cues to localization, and are impulsive – all noise characteristics that biologically would incite a defensive or startled response.

| Sound | Loudness |
|---|---|
| Gunshots | 130 dB |
| Fireworks | 70–110 dB |
| Thunder | 120 dBA |
| Engine noise | 90 dBA |

**15.3** Common sounds to which dogs show noise sensitivity.

## Acquisition or development of fears

Although little research has been done in dogs with respect to how noise sensitivities develop, several theories on fear development are proposed based on the human literature. These theories are divided into associative processes and non-associative processes.

- **Associative** processes include traumatic experiences with loud noises and social facilitation.
- **Non-associative** processes include sensitization, lack of habituation, and disinhibition via chronic stress.

A questionnaire designed to examine the possibility of these potential mechanisms of fear acquisition in dogs (Iimura, 2007) was made available via the worldwide web. Information was gathered for 3403 dogs, of which 2468 were fearful of noises. The majority of respondents were from the United States and the UK.

## Associative processes

### Pavlovian conditioning (traumatic experience)

Early research on the acquisition of fears in humans supported the theory that fear can be elicited by Pavlovian conditioning. In studies of social phobias and agoraphobias, it was reported that more than 50% of patients reported that their fear stemmed from a direct traumatic experience (Ost and Hugdahl, 1981, 1983). In dogs, there have been several reports of owners stating that their dog's noise aversions developed after a traumatic experience (Hothersall and Tuber, 1979; Estelles et al., 2005). Iimura (2007) found that 33.4% (523 out of 1566) of noise-sensitive dogs were reported to have had a traumatic experience associated with a loud noise. In fearful dogs the most frequent traumatic experiences related to fireworks (35%), followed by storms (24.7%) and gunfire (8%). When evaluating the behavioural differences between dogs that had noise fears due to a traumatic experience *versus* those that did not have a traumatic experience, it was found that dogs with traumatic experiences were more likely to tremble, look around the whole time, pant, be destructive, run around and be jumpy to noises. Dogs with traumatic experiences were less likely to bark. The proportion of fearful dogs with traumatic experiences was highest for dogs > 2–3 years of age (59.6%) and for those > 3–4 years of age (57.4%). There was no difference with breed, sex, age obtained, or source of pet acquisition.

### Social transmission

Fear transmission via social learning or the influence of others has been observed in humans and monkeys (Rachman, 1977; Cook and Mineka, 1989). Some studies have suggested that dogs may be more likely to express a certain behaviour in the presence of another animal exhibiting that same behaviour (Juarbe-Diaz, 1997). Estelles et al. (2005) reported that several owners believed that their dogs had learned to be fearful from their other dogs. It has also been suggested that dogs may become fearful of noises if their owners exhibit fear of noises. In Iimura's recent study of multi-dog homes in which there were several noise-sensitive dogs living in a home, only 4.2% of households reported that one dog's fear behaviours stopped when another fearful dog was no longer in sight (Iimura, 2007); when comparing the behaviours of fearful dogs living with other fearful dogs to those of fearful dogs living with non-fearful dogs, no differences were found in the fearful dogs. There was no association between the presence of a fearful human family member and the presence of noise fear problem in dogs. This was similar to findings by Dreschel and Granger (2005), who found that the owner's behaviour did not influence the dog's behaviour. At present there is little evidence to support social factors in either the acquisition or transmission of noise sensitivities in dogs.

## Non-associative processes

### Lack of habituation to noises early in life

In people, it has been found that those with a fear of heights had less experience in their childhood of engaging in activities associated with heights, such as climbing trees and playing on swings (Poulton et al., 2001). The proposed theory or assumption was that children who do not (or cannot) habituate to certain stimuli such as height could develop a fear of the relevant stimuli in later life. For dogs, exposure to various stimuli in the first few months of life plays an important role in their behaviour in later life. The most important developmental period for habituation and acceptance of new stimuli is within the first 3–6 months (O'Farrell, 1992; Overall, 1997; Houpt, 1998). If dogs have little contact with stimuli during these times, fear of the respective stimuli can be developed later in life (Fuller and Clark, 1966b; Fuller, 1967). In studies where animals were isolated for the first 4 months of life, extreme fear response to novelty developed.

It is interesting to note that, where extreme fear responses developed, the behaviours that were shown seemed to depend on breed. Beagles in the Fuller study were very withdrawn, whereas the terriers were more likely to be very reactive. In another study where a fearful strain of pointers was bred, extreme fear responses were demonstrated at 3 months of age and attempts to socialize them were not successful (Murphree et al., 1967; Murphree and Newton, 1971). In the Iimura (2007) study, subgroups of dogs whose life history was known for the first 6 months of life for both fearful (n = 1547) and non-fearful dogs (n = 740) were analysed and it was found that non-fearful dogs were more likely to have been exposed to engine sounds, door bangs and loud voices early in life, suggesting that early experience may be important.

### Sensitization

Sensitization occurs when a stimulus is repeated and the animal's response gets more intense with each presentation of the stimulus. As a result of sensitization, an animal may develop a fear of that particular stimulus. Iimura (2007) found that the sensitization process was more likely to occur with thunderstorms than for other noises. This may be because the nature of storm noises is such that they maintain a high level of arousal and so reduce the potential for habituation. Iimura (2007) also found that dogs who were possibly sensitized were more likely to show behavioural signs associated with autonomic arousal, such as panting, pacing, looking around the whole time and being more restless. Dogs whose fears were more acute were more likely to show behavioural signs associated with overt fear strategies of avoidance, such as hiding, cowering and being jumpy to noises more frequently.

### Stress-induced dishabituation

In humans, fears can appear following a stressful but non-contingent event despite not having fear of that stimulus prior to a period of stress. Chronic stress can affect auditory perception of warning signals and may impair emotional and cognitive behaviours, affecting the ability to adapt to the environment (Daginno-Subiabre *et al.*, 2005). It may be that the neurophysiological changes that occur with stress lead to stress-related learning impairments and an increase in fear responses (Shors, 2006). Therefore if a dog suddenly shows fear of noises that previously induced no fear-related behaviours, it is important to examine the quality of life of that dog to correct potential stressors in the home (see Chapter 3). Lack of an adequate environment or management of a dog can lead to a state of chronic stress (Beerda *et al.*, 1997). When evaluating behaviours that may be associated with chronic stress, such as gastrointestinal upset, pica and flank sucking, it has been found that noise-sensitive dogs have significantly more signs of chronic stress than non-sensitive dogs (Iimura, 2007).

## Internal factors

Genetics appears to play a role in noise sensitivities, as some dogs may be more likely to react to noises if they have a fearful temperament (Goddard and Beilharz, 1985; Willis, 1995; Sheppard and Mills, 2002). Hormones may also play a role in the development of noise sensitivities. Performing early-age gonadectomies in both female and male dogs has been associated with noise fears (Spain *et al.*, 2004) and a report from the American Kennel Club found that neutered females were more likely to be fearful of noises.

The role of thyroid hormone in noise fears is not fully understood. Some animals with noise fears have low or borderline thyroid hormone levels and respond to treatment well, but it is not clear if low thyroid levels are the cause of the problem or a reflection of it.

## Diagnosis

Diagnosis of noise sensitivities is generally straightforward. A behavioural history should be taken, to determine the noises to which the dog is sensitive and which behaviours the dog exhibits during the noise event. The author uses a score sheet (see client handout) to denote a numerical fear score (from 1 to 5) for purposes of gaining a baseline value from which to measure improvement once treatment is implemented.

There is also a place for a numerical **global** score rated from 0 to 10, with 0 being no fear at all to 10 being the most intense fear possible. The reason for this global score is that a straightforward numerical score based on individual specific behaviours may not capture some of the more subtle aspects of fear, anxiety or phobic responses (Mills *et al.*, 2006). This second measurement is used to capture aspects missed when just asking about individual behaviours. The reason it is important to use a numerical system to measure success of a treatment plan is that there may be some behaviour signs, such as house soiling, that the owner finds so problematic that they may report no improvement even if many of the other signs

resolve or decrease. This may lead to abandoning a treatment plan that is working but may require just minor adjustments (Crowell-Davis *et al.*, 2003). By using a numerical score and being able to show the numbers decreasing to the owner, it may be possible to increase satisfaction with the treatment plan and hence encourage further compliance.

During the history taking it is important to determine how long it takes the dog to calm down after the noise event is over. In addition, it is important to know how many aversive noises the dog is exposed to on a daily or weekly basis. If a dog's behaviour occurs only during the noise event and it recovers quickly without any signs of anxiety, fear or phobia in between noise events, the dog may not be as likely to need medication or may need a different class of medication compared to dogs that exhibit a more chronic anxiety. However, if a dog does recover quickly and shows no signs of anxiety in between noise events but those noise events are frequent (for example, in firework or thunderstorm seasons), chronic intermittent stress can occur and may require a treatment plan similar to that for a dog with generalized chronic anxiety (Ladewig, 2000). It is important to identify any co-morbid diagnosis such as generalized anxiety, separation anxiety and aggression, as this will influence the treatment plan (Overall *et al.*, 2001).

### Recording behaviours during a noise event
Ideally the client will be able to videotape their dog during a noise event so that the veterinary surgeon can view the behaviours. If this is not possible, many dogs will react to noise CD recordings in an examination room. Even if their responses are not as intense at home, it gives the veterinary surgeon an opportunity to see some of the behaviours and the owner can confirm whether that response is mild, moderate or severe compared with the home environment.

An important reason to play the CD in the examination room is to see whether the dog will react aversively to the noise recording, so that it can be determined whether using a recording will be a valid treatment option. Where the dog does not have a full-blown response to the CD, owners often assume that the recording will not be a useful method of treatment and may report that using CDs did not work because the dog did not react as intensely as it would to a real event. For treatment purposes, intense responses are not the goal and so owners need to be informed that even a milder reaction to the CD warrants the use of a noise recording as part of the treatment plan.

Using a CD in the examination room is not a good way to measure improvement, however. Two studies have shown that, despite improvement at home where the training was performed, the dogs did not show improvement compared with baseline when exposed to the noise recording in the clinic after treatment (Crowell-Davis *et al.*, 2003; Levine *et al.*, 2007).

### Physiological assessment
Although there are no standard physiological measurements used in diagnosing fear sensitivities, it is important to note that various findings have

been found in dogs that were scared of certain noises. For example, dogs that were scared of gunshots had higher heart rates, higher haematocrit levels and higher levels of plasma cortisol, progesterone, vasopressin and beta-endorphins compared with dogs that were not fearful of gunshots (Hydbring-Sandberg *et al.*, 2004). Dogs that were fearful of thunderstorms had higher levels of cortisol when listening to thunder recordings than dogs that were not fearful (Dreschel and Granger, 2005).

One method of assessing heart rate while dogs are reacting to fearful noises is to attach a portable exercise heart rate monitor to the dog and note the heart rate with the recording watch. If the heart rate is a measurable response for that particular dog, this tool may be used while implementing behaviour modifications for noise fears, in particular desensitization and counter-conditioning to a noise recording. This gives the owner another simple guideline with which to judge when the dog is calm, as some dogs may appear overtly calm to the owner but their heart rate may be high. This is important because physiological and behavioural habituation do not necessarily occur at the same rate.

### Pseudo-fears

Owners should be informed of the potential for pseudo-fears to develop. This occurs when dogs realize that if they seek out the owner they get rewarded. The attention-seeking behaviours become learned and possibly associated with other noises. In these cases, the dog is not truly anxious or fearful. It can be challenging to distinguish such pseudo-fearful dogs and, during the behavioural history, it is important for the veterinary surgeon to help the client to distinguish between an attention-seeking dog and an anxious dog that benefits from owner contact. If it is too difficult to tease these behaviours apart and the owner cannot videotape the dog during a noisy episode when they are not present, they should be advised not to reward the behaviours but to focus on other treatment strategies that will help the dog to cope with its anxiety without needing the owner's reassurance.

### Treatment strategies

Clinicians should always aim to treat fears and phobias rather than manage them, as these conditions have an impact on welfare and can become severe. Treatment for noise sensitivities falls into several categories (Figure 15.4). Treatment should include evidence-based therapies.

### Medications

Prior to administering any medication, a physical examination and blood work are recommended (ideally a complete blood count, chemistry and free T4). See also Chapter 21 for pharmacology and pheromone treatments.

### Benzodiazepines

Benzodiazepines work by facilitating gamma-aminobutyric acid (GABA) in the central nervous system, in

| Category | Examples |
|---|---|
| Medications | Benzodiazepines<br>Selective serotonin reuptake inhibitors<br>Tricyclic antidepressants<br>Monoamine oxidase inhibitors<br>Atypical antidepressants |
| Behaviour modifications | Desensitization and counter-conditioning using a noise recording |
| Pheromone therapy | Dog appeasing pheromone |
| Environmental modifications | Shades for windows<br>Safe haven<br>'Storm defender'<br>Ear plugs<br>White noise machine |
| Massage and touch therapy | TTouch<br>Stroking<br>Anxiety wrap |
| Music therapy | throughadogsear.com |
| Herbal remedies | |
| Alternative interventions | Homeopathy<br>Bach flower remedies |

**15.4** Categories of treatment.

particular by binding GABA$_A$ receptors. The highest density of specific binding sites in the brain is in the cerebral cortex, the cerebellum and the limbic system (Crowell-Davis and Murray, 2006). The limbic system is the 'emotional centre' of the brain and this is one of the reasons benzodiazepines are a good medication choice for noise aversions: they have anxiolytic and antipanic properties that take effect relatively rapidly and can last for several hours. For maximum efficacy it is advised that the animal be given the medication 1 hour prior to the noise event (e.g. a storm).

Because it is not always possible to time things perfectly, the author commonly advises owners to start medicating the animal hours before a storm and re-dose every 4–12 hours, depending upon which benzodiazepine is selected. For example, if a storm is predicted with a 50% or greater chance to occur in late afternoon, the owner can start medication in the early or mid afternoon and re-dose according to instructions. Many owners are concerned about giving medication unnecessarily (e.g. when the storm does not occur), but it is better for the animal to have taken the medication and no storm to occur than for a storm to occur and the dog experience another anxious, fear, or phobic cycle.

The reason for early dosing is simply that benzodiazepines appear to be less efficacious when given after a storm has already started and the animal has already shown aversion signs. If one benzodiazepine does not work well, it is worth trying others as the dog may respond well to some but not to others. Dosages for some of the more common benzodiazepines used are given in Figure 15.5.

For elderly patients, or for patients whose liver function is compromised, oxazepam may be the safest option as it has no active metabolites. Owners should be informed of potential side effects such as an increase in appetite, sedation, ataxia and muscle

| Medication | Dosage |
|---|---|
| Alprazolam | 0.02–0.1 mg/kg q4h |
| Clonazepam | 0.1–0.5 mg/kg q8–12h |
| Clorazepate | 0.5–2.0 mg/kg q4–24h |
| Diazepam | 0.5–2.0 mg/kg q4h |
| Lorazepam | 0.02–0.5 mg/kg q8–12h |
| Oxazepam | 0.04–0.5 mg/kg q12–24h |

**15.5** Dosages for benzodiazepines for noise sensitivity in the dog.

relaxation. Some dogs may experience an increase in anxiety or a paradoxical excitement reaction; therefore, it is advised that owners give a test dose on a day when there are no storms to ensure that the latter two side effects do not occur. Although some benzodiazepines are intended to have longer-lasting effects than others, in the author's experience each dog's metabolism is so variable that each medication should be evaluated for its duration of effect in each individual patient.

For dogs with no co-morbid diagnoses, who recover very quickly (within 30 minutes) after a noise event and who are not exposed to aversive noises on a very regular basis, benzodiazepines may be the only medication needed for treatment. It is highly advisable for owners to complement this medication with behavioural and environmental modifications, so as not to have to use medication in the long term. The importance of implementing behaviour modifications must be emphasized: one study found that owners using medications were less likely to implement behaviour modifications (Estelles *et al.*, 2005).

### Selective serotonin reuptake inhibitors (SSRIs) and tricyclic antidepressants (TCAs)

Both TCAs and SSRIs work by inhibiting the reuptake of serotonin, which allows the molecules to work for a longer period of time, thereby increasing serotonergic transmission. Ultimately there is a down-regulation of serotonin receptors.

There are differences between the classes of medications and with each individual medication (see Chapter 21). Dosages for some of the more commonly used TCAs and SSRIs used for noise sensitivities are given in Figure 15.6.

| Group | Medication | Dosage |
|---|---|---|
| Selective serotonin reuptake inhibitors | Fluoxetine | 0.5–2.0 mg/kg q24h |
| | Paroxetine | 0.5–1.5 mg/kg q24h |
| | Sertraline | 1–3 mg/kg q24h |
| Tricyclic antidepressants | Amitriptyline | 1–3 mg/kg q12h |
| | Clomipramine | 2–4 mg/kg q12h |
| | Imipramine | 0.5–2.0 mg/kg q8–12h |

**15.6** Dosages for commonly used TCAs and SSRIs in the management of noise sensitivities in dogs.

Ideally one would start with a low end of the dose and titrate up as needed. For any titration, it is advisable to wait for 4 weeks before evaluating the medication's efficacy, as the therapeutic effects can take several weeks whereas some of the more common side effects (see Chapter 21) can occur sooner. Some dogs may respond better to one medication than another, so it may be necessary to try several medications within these classes.

Because it can take several weeks for therapeutic effects to be seen, it is advised that these medications be started at least 6 weeks prior to a noise season (firework season, thunderstorm season). The animal can then be weaned off the SSRI or TCA after the noise season has ended, unless there are other behavioural issues that require the use of year-round medication. It is not uncommon to have to 'cocktail' a TCA or an SSRI (which are given daily) with a benzodiazepine (which is given only on the days when storms are predicted) if the TCA or SSRI alone is not sufficient. One study found that using clomipramine, alprazolam and behaviour modifications with noise recordings resulted in 30 of 32 dogs showing improvement with storm phobias (Crowell-Davis *et al.*, 2003).

For dogs with phobias, generalized anxiety, co-morbid diagnoses and exposure to intense noise events on a regular basis, using a daily medication such as a TCA or SSRI along with a benzodiazepine is advised. Combination of TCAs and SSRIs is not recommended due to the possibility of serotonin syndrome which can be fatal.

### Monoamine oxidase inhibitors (MAOIs)

MAOIs inhibit the enzyme monoamine oxidase, which is responsible for the degradation of various compounds, including dopamine, noradrenaline (norepinephrine), adrenaline (epinephrine) and serotonin. MAOIs enhance the activity of catecholamines via other mechanisms as well. Selegiline may be a good option for dogs that exhibit freezing behaviours during noise events.

It is important to note that MAOIs should not be used in conjunction with TCAs or SSRIs. If an animal has been on a TCA or SSRI , there should be a 5-week washout period prior to starting an MAOI. Selegiline is licensed for use in dogs in Europe for emotional disorders and in North America for the treatment of cognitive dysfunction and Cushing's disease, and is given in the morning at 0.5–1.0 mg/kg q24h.

### Trazadone

Trazadone is an atypical antidepressant that has mixed serotonergic agonist/antagonist properties. It is becoming a more commonly used adjunctive treatment for various anxiety disorders in dogs, including storm phobias. It has been used in conjunction with TCAs, SSRIs and benzodiazepines.

According to a retrospective study of anxiety cases, trazadone can be used safely and efficaciously (Gruen and Sherman, 2008; Figure 15.7). Because of its serotonergic effects it is advised that clients be made aware of early signs of serotonin syndrome,

| Dog's weight | Initial dose | Target dose |
| --- | --- | --- |
| Up to 10 kg | 25 mg | 50 mg |
| 11–20 kg | 50 mg | 100 mg |
| 21–40 kg | 100 mg | 200 mg |
| > 41 kg | 100 mg | 100–300 mg |

**15.7** Dosages for trazadone for treatment of dogs with noise sensitivity. (Data from Gruen and Sherman, 2008.)

which can manifest in a variety of ways. Some of the manifestations include hypertension, hyperthermia, restlessness, tremors, seizures and altered mental states (Simpson and Papich, 2003). Trazadone was historically reported to cause diarrhoea, but this was not found to be a significant side effect in the retrospective study by Gruen and Sherman (2008). More studies are needed and it is advised that the dose be started low and titrated up as necessary.

## Behaviour modification

### Desensitization and counter-conditioning (DSCC) to a noise recording
DSCC using noise recordings was first reported in the 1970s and has since become the standard treatment, though only a couple of studies have examined its efficacy. Crowell-Davis et al. (2003) found that using DSCC with noise recording along with medication improved dogs' reactions to thunderstorms; and Levine et al. (2007) found that DSCC with noise recordings plus the use of dog appeasing pheromone (DAP®) improved dogs' responses to fireworks. A retrospective study showed that the combination of CD recording with DAP® had better results than either of those treatment modalities alone (Estelles et al., 2005). Iimura (2007) found that the dogs who did respond to noise recordings were less likely to show cowering, hiding and panting behaviours and that neutered dogs were less likely to respond than entire males. Levine et al. (2007) found that the actual noise recording did not influence efficacy as much as the quality of instructions that accompanied the recording; therefore, instruction on how to use noise recordings appears to be of utmost importance to maximize success (see **client handout**).

The same study found that, during an 8-week period of DSCC using a noise recording, most improvement that was seen to the recording itself seemed to occur during the first month, but continued improvement was seen during the second month of training. For dogs that underwent treatment with a noise recording and DAP® for firework fears, the improvement in their overall fear levels was sustained for 1 year after treatment (Levine and Mills, 2008).

## Dog appeasing pheromone
Pheromones can help to reduce noise sensitivities in dogs in conjunction with other treatment modalities or when used by themselves (Sheppard and Mills, 2003; Estelles et al., 2005; Levine et al., 2007; Levine and

Mills, 2008). The concept behind pheromonatherapy is simply to have a chemical cue in the environment that biologically signals to the animal to be calm (see Chapter 21).

Pheromone products come in diffusers, sprays and collars. Which one(s) to use ultimately depends on the environment in which the dog is when exposed to the noise fear, the size of the house and whether windows are kept open.

- For very large homes or those where windows and doors are kept open, the diffuser may be less efficacious than other forms. One diffuser effectively covers up to 650 square feet (60.4 m²) in a single non-airconditioned space.
- The spray is useful to help localize the calming cue to specific areas (e.g. on the safe-haven towel or on a dog's bed).
- When a dog wears a DAP® collar, the dog will still be exposed to the pheromone if it is more mobile. The collar lasts about 1 month and should be removed prior to giving the dog a bath and replaced when the dog is dry. If the collar is too expensive for an owner to use for intermittent storms, they can repeatedly spray a bandana instead.

An owner may opt to use more than one delivery system at a time. It has also been reported that DAP® may be less efficacious in dogs that exhibit destructive behaviours, but may be particularly useful if the complaint focuses on vocalization and elimination behaviour (Gaultier et al., 2005).

## Environmental modifications
For certain noise sensitivities an owner can make changes in the environment to help their dog. For example:

- With noises such as thunder and fireworks where light may be an associated factor, owners can pull the blinds or curtains on the window
- In addition, for noise sensitivity to storms, some dogs may be reacting to ionic changes in the atmosphere and may benefit from a storm defender, which has a thin metal lining inside the soft material that purportedly helps repel ionic charges. A pilot study showed encouraging results but more work is needed to evaluate the efficacy of this product (Cottam et al., 2005). There is anecdotal evidence that the storm defender can be helpful for some dogs, especially those that choose to hide in bathrooms or behind plumbing
- Although there are no soundproof dog enclosures, ear plugs are a way of decreasing the noise stimuli. The dog may need to be taught how to wear these calmly by using DSCC techniques (see Chapter 5)
- Placing the dog in a windowless space and playing either white noise (fan) or music can also help to block both the sound and visual aspects of the stimulus.

## Ancillary aids

### Massage therapy
When an owner creates a safe haven, one of the calming techniques that can be used is massage therapy. Linda Tellington Jones developed TTouch as a technique that has been used now in many species (see Chapter 22). The owner can be instructed to try this for 1 week to see if it is a form of touch that their dog finds calming and relaxing. If it is, the owner should be instructed to associate a word with the touch such as 'relax' or 'chill' as they are massaging their dog. The reason for associating a word with this activity is simply to classically condition a calm physiological state with a word, so that during a noise event the owner can use a word to help to calm their dog without actually having to massage it at that time.

For dogs that do not appear to like TTouch, long gentle strokes appear to induce a low heart rate and should be tried next.

Dogs in a down position have lower heart rates than dogs in a sit position and so massages should ideally be done with the dog in a down position. This is another situation where a polar heart rate monitor may be useful so that the owner can pinpoint which type of petting or massage relaxes their dog the most.

### Music therapy
Different styles of music have been shown to affect an animal's behaviour. For example, heavy metal music causes more behavioural arousal and agitation in dogs, whereas classical music causes more relaxed and calm behaviours (Wells et al., 2002). There is some evidence that music may provoke a neurological response in dogs similar to that in people and that the music that humans respond to most calmly is also the music that dogs respond to most calmly (Leeds and Wagner, 2008b). There are various aspects of music that can influence behaviour, such as resonance, entrainment and pattern identification (harmonic complexity). High frequencies tend to arouse, whereas low frequencies tend to derouse. Fast rhythms excite an individual, whereas slow rhythms will calm an individual. Compositions vary in harmonic complexity: the less complex a composition, the more relaxed the individual. Leeds and Wagner (2008b) showed that compositions that had slower tempos and less complex arrangements, along with solo instruments, had a greater calming effect than more complex harmonic and orchestral music, and they have now developed music CDs designed for calming purposes.

### Complementary therapy
Only one placebo-controlled study evaluating the effect of a homeopathic remedy on dogs with a fear of fireworks has been published and it revealed that there was no difference between dogs receiving placebo versus a homeopathic remedy (Cracknell and Mills, 2008), although both groups significantly improved during the study. More studies are needed to further evaluate the efficacy of various homeopathic remedies.

The author is not aware of any studies on herbal remedies with respect to noise sensitivities, though licensed products are available in some countries. There is some evidence that lavender and chamomile can help to induce calm behaviours in shelter dogs (Graham et al., 2005) but there seem to be no studies looking specifically at noise fears. Chapter 22 looks more closely at complementary therapies.

### Anxiety wrap
The anxiety wrap involves binding the animal in a tight cloth. Anecdotal reports show some encouraging results. The wrap is intended to help to calm animals but the mechanism by which this works is not yet known, though biofeedback is one possible explanation. It is advised that, if this is recommended, the owner be present for safety purposes, to ensure that the wrap does not get caught on anything.

### Diet
There is a complex relationship between insulin, glucose and other hormones and their effects on neurotransmitters. Although more research is needed in this area, some studies highlight possible beneficial effects on mood by altering the protein levels in the dog's diet (DiNapoli and Dodman, 2000).

Tryptophan is the dietary precursor to serotonin and tryptophan availability in most commercial dog foods is low in comparison with other amino acids that compete preferentially for uptake; therefore there is less opportunity for it to cross the blood–brain barrier and be converted into serotonin. In order to increase tryptophan levels relative to other amino acids, one can feed a low-protein diet (less than or equal to 18%). Unfortunately, the labels of many dog foods are unreliable indicators of available tryptophan. Alternatively, prescription diets specifically made for dogs with liver or kidney disease and which cannot handle high levels of protein can also be used.

Other research has shown that insulin production is stimulated by increasing carbohydrates, which can help increase serotonin levels. An owner can try feeding a low-protein, carbohydrate-heavy food such as pasta between 30 minutes and 3 hours after the main protein meal (see Chapter 22).

### Nutraceuticals
Zylkene (alpha-casozepine) has been studied in animals with anxiety disorders. Although it may theoretically be useful in conditions like noise sensitivity (Beata et al., 2007), there are no published studies on this indication. The dose of Zylkene is typically 15 mg/kg orally once a day.

## Other important information for owners

- Owners often comment that their dog is 'stupid' or 'dumb' or make other derogatory comments about the dog's intelligence because the dog is fearful during noise events. It is important to inform them that their dog has no control over its fears and that there are biological underpinnings for such behaviours.

- Owners are often advised to ignore any fearful or anxious behaviour during noise events in order to avoid reinforcing the dog's fear. For some dogs, attention from the owner may reinforce its anxiety, but many owners are simply unable to ignore their dog. An alternative recommendation for those who cannot or will not ignore their dog would be specifically to avoid cuddling, stroking and saying 'it's okay' but to replace those activities with being jolly and encouraging the dog to play a game or do some obedience exercises. This allows the owner not to feel guilty about ignoring their dog yet encourages interactions that would not be conducive to reinforcing anxiety.
- Punishment is never an acceptable option for dogs that are showing noise aversions, as it exacerbates the fear state.
- It is important during puppy visits to educate owners what to watch for during noise events so that they can report early signs of noise sensitivity to their veterinary surgeon.
- Inquiring about behavioural responses to noise during annual check-ups is advised. Many people fail to mention the problem when their dog simply chooses to hide or pant a little, but it is not uncommon for the behaviour to escalate from year to year. The earlier these issues are treated, theoretically the easier they will be to resolve. In addition, for the dog's own welfare, any signs of anxiety or fear should be addressed regardless of its concern to the owner.

## Prognosis

The prognosis is generally quite good if owners can commit to and follow a DSCC programme and if the animal will respond to recordings. Estelles *et al.* (2005) found that neither the duration nor the severity of the problem predicted outcome, although greater improvement was noted by owners of dogs with more than one noise sensitivity.

## Prevention

Until more research is done on the acquisition and development of noise aversion, the following are some basic recommendations to help to prevent the problem.

- When purchasing a dog, owners should enquire about the behavioural responses to noises by the dam, the sire and previous offspring.
- Owners should be advised to abstain from early-age gondadectomy unless indicated for good reason.
- Owners should be advised to expose their puppies to various noises, starting as young as 3 months. They should make sure that these noise exposures are not intense at first and are associated with positive things such as treats and playing games, as simply exposing puppies to noises may not be sufficient. In particular, young

dogs should be exposed to engine noises when they are actually able to see cars, so that they associate the engine noise with a source, as opposed to just playing a noise CD.
- During puppy appointments, owners should be asked to report any noise aversion to their veterinary surgeon as soon as the behaviour is seen. Enquiries should be made at annual check-ups about the dog's reaction to noise events.

## References and further reading

Beata C, Beaumont-Graff E, Diaz C *et al.* (2007) Effects of alpha casozepine (Zylkene) versus selegiline hydrochloride (Seligan, Anipryl) on anxiety disorders in dogs. *Journal of Veterinary Behavior* **2**, 175–183

Beaver BV (1999) *Canine Behavior: A Guide for Veterinarians.* WB Saunders, Philadelphia

Beerda B, Schilder BH, VanHoof JARAM and de Vries HW (1997) Manifestations of chronic and acute stress in dogs. *Applied Animal Behaviour Science* **52**, 307–319

Blackwell E, Casey R and Bradshaw J (2005) *Firework Fears and Phobias in the Domestic Dog.* Royal Society for the Prevention of Cruelty to Animals, Horsham

Carlson NR (2004) *Physiology of Behavior.* Pearson Education, New York

Cook M and Mineka S (1989) Observational conditioning of fear to fear related vs fear irrelevant stimuli in rhesus monkeys. *Journal of Abnormal Psychology* **98**, 448–459

Cottam N, Dodman N, and Critzer T (2005) Use of a cape (The Storm Defender) in the treatment of canine storm phobia. In: *Current Issues and Research in Veterinary Behavioural Medicine,* ed. D Mills *et al.*, pp. 165–167. Purdue University Press, West Lafayette, Indiana

Cracknell NR and Mills DS (2008) A double-blind placebo-controlled study into the efficacy of a homeopathic remedy for fear of firework noises in the dog (*Canis familiaris*). *The Veterinary Journal* **177**, 80–88

Crowell-Davis SL and Murray T (2006) *Veterinary Psychopharmocology.* Blackwell, Ames, Iowa

Crowell-Davis SL, Seibert LM, Sung W *et al.* (2003) Use of clomipramine, alprazolam, and behavior modification for treatment of storm phobia in dogs. *Journal of the American Veterinary Medical Association* **222**, 744–749

Daginno-Subiabre A, Terreros G, Carmona-Fontaine C *et al.* (2005) Chronic stress impairs acoustic conditioning more than visual conditioning in rats: morphological and behavioural evidence. *Neuroscience* **135**, 1067–1074

DeNapoli J, Dodman N, Shuster L *et al.* (2000) Effect of dietary protein content and tryptophan supplementation on dominance aggression, territorial aggression and hyperactivity in dogs. *Journal of the American Veterinary Medical Association* **217**, 504–508

Dreschel NA and Granger DA (2005) Physiological and behavioral reactivity to stress in thunderstorm-phobic dogs and their caregivers. *Applied Animal Behaviour Science* **95**, 153–168

Ducan Luce R (1993) *Sound and Hearing: a Conceptual Introduction.* Lawrence Erlbaum Associates, Mahwah, New Jersey

Estelles G, Mills D, Coleshaw PH and Shorthouse C (2005) A retrospective analysis of relationships with severity of signs of fear of fireworks and treatment outcome in 99 cases. In: *Current Issues and Research in Veterinary Behavioural Medicine,* ed. D Mills *et al.*, pp. 161–164. Purdue University Press, West Lafayette, Indiana

Fuller JL (1967) Experiential deprivation and later behavior. *Science* **158**, 1645–1652

Fuller JL and Clark LD (1966a) Genetic and treatment factors modifying the postisolation syndrome in dogs. *Journal of Comparative Physiology and Psychology* **61**, 251–257

Fuller JL and Clark LD (1966b) Effects of rearing with specific stimulation upon postisolation behavior in dogs. *Journal of Comparative Physiology and Psychology* **61**, 258–263

Gaultier E, Bonnafous L, Bougrat L *et al.* (2005) Comparison of the efficacy of a synthetic dog appeasing pheromone with clomipramine for the treatment of separation-related disorders in dogs. *The Veterinary Record* **156**, 533–538

Goddard ME and Beilharz RG (1985) A multivariate analysis of the genetics of fearfulness in potential guide dogs. *Behavior Genetics* **15**, 69–89

Graham L, Wells DL and Hepper PG (2005) The influence of olfactory stimulation on the behaviour of dogs housed in a rescue shelter. *Applied Animal Behaviour Science* **91**, 143–153

Gruen ME and Sherman BL (2008) Use of Trazadone as an adjunctive treatment for canine anxiety disorders: 56 cases. *Journal of the American Veterinary Medical Association* **223**, 1902–1907

Heffner HE (1983) Hearing in large and small dogs: absolute thresholds and size of the tympanic membrane. *Behavioral Neuroscience* **97**,

310–318

Hothersall D and Tuber DS (1979) Fears in companion dogs: characteristics and treatment. In: *Psychopathology in Animals Research and Clinical Implications*, ed. JD Keehn, pp. 239–255. Academic Press, New York

Houpt KA (1998) *Domestic Animal Behavior for Veterinarians and Animal Scientists, 3rd edn*. Iowa State Press, Ames, Iowa

Howald DM and Angus J (2001) *Acoustics and Psychoacoustics, 2nd edn*. Focal Press, Oxford

Hydbring-Sandberg E, von Walter LW, Hoglund K *et al.* (2004) Physiologic reactions to fear provocation in dogs. *Journal of Endocrinology* **180**, 439–448

Iimura K (2007) The nature of noise fears in domestic dogs. MPhil thesis, University of Lincoln

Juarbe-Diaz SV (1997) Social dynamics and behavior problems in multiple-dog households. *Veterinary Clinics of North America: Small Animal Practice* **27**, 497–514

Ladewig J (2000) Chronic intermittent stress: a model for the study of long-term stressors. In: *The Biology of Animal Stress, 1st edn*, ed. GP Moberg and JA Mench, pp. 159–169. CABI Publishing, New York

Landsberg GM, Hunthausen W and Ackerman L (1997) Fears and phobias. In: *Handbook of Behavior Problems of the Dog and Cat*, p. 227. Saunders, Oxford

Leeds J and Wagner S (2008a) The effect of sound on inhabitants of your home. In: *Through a Dog's Ear*, pp. 29–35. Sounds True Inc, Louisville, Colorado

Leeds J and Wagner S (2008b) Why music affects you and your canine companion In: *Through a Dog's Ear*, pp. 67–76. Sounds True Inc, Louisville, Colorado

Levine ED and Mills DS (2008) Long term follow up of the efficacy of a behavioral treatment programme for dogs with firework fears. *The Veterinary Record* **162**, 657–659

Levine ED, Ramos D and Mills DS (2007) A prospective study of two self help CD based desensitization and counter-conditioning programmes with the use of Dog Appeasing Pheromone (DAP) for the treatment of firework fears in dogs (*Canis familiaris*). *Applied Animal Behaviour Science* **105**, 311–329

Mills DS, Ramos D, Estelles MG and Hargrave C (2006) A triple blind placebo controlled investigation into the assessment of the effect of the dog appeasing pheromone (DAP) on anxiety related behavior of problem dogs in the veterinary clinic. *Applied Animal Behaviour Science* **98**, 114–126

Murphree OD, Dykman RD and Peters JE (1967) Genetically determined abnormal behavior in dogs: results of behavioral tests. *Conditioned Reflex* **2**, 199–205

Murphree OD and Newton JE (1971) Cross breeding and special handling of genetically nervous dogs. *Conditioned Reflex* **6**, 129–136

Neilson JC, Eckstein RA and Hart BL (1997) effects of castration on problem behaviors in male dogs with reference to age and duration of behavior. *Journal of the American Veterinary Medical Association* **211**, 180–182

O'Farrell V (1992) *Manual of Canine Behaviour*. BSAVA Publications, Cheltenham

Ost LG and Hugdahl K (1981) Acquisition of phobias and anxiety response patterns in clinical patients. *Behaviour Research and Therapy* **19**, 439

Ost LG and Hugdahl K (1983) Acquisition of agoraphobia, mode of onset and anxiety response patterns. *Behaviour Research and Therapy* **21**, 623–632

Overall KL (1997) *Clinical Behavioral Medicine For Small Animals*. Mosby Year Inc., St. Louis, Missouri

Overall KL, Dunham AE and Frank D (2001) Frequency of non specific clinical signs in dogs with separation anxiety, thunderstorm phobia, and noise phobia, alone or in combination. *Journal of the American Veterinary Medical Association* **219**, 467–473

Poulton R, Waldie, KE, Menzies RG *et al.* (2001) Failure to overcome 'innate' fear: a developmental test of the non associative model of fear acquisition. *Behaviour Research and Therapy* **39**, 29–43

Rachman S (1977) The conditioning theory of fear acquisition: a critical examination. *Behaviour Research and Therapy* **15**, 375–387

RSPCA (undated) BANG! Keep the noise down: loud fireworks frighten animals. Royal Society for the Prevention of Cruelty to Animals, Horsham

Sheppard G and Mills DS (2002) The development of a psychometric scale for the evaluation of the emotional predispositions of pet dogs. *International Journal of Comparative Psychology* **15**, 201–222

Sheppard G and Mills DS (2003) Evaluation of a dog-appeasing pheromone as a potential treatment for dogs fearful of fireworks. *The Veterinary Record* **152**, 432–436

Shors TJ (2006) Stressful experience and learning across the lifespan. *Annual Review of Psychology* **57**, 55–85

Simpson B and Papich M (2003) Pharmacological management in veterinary behavioral medicine. *Veterinary Clinics of North America: Small Animal Practice* **33**, 365–404

Spain CV, Scarlett JM and Houpt KA (2004) Long term risks and benefits of early age gonadectomy in dogs. *Journal of the American Veterinary Medical Association* **224**, 380–387

The Bearded Collie Foundation for Health (2002) *Fear of Sounds in Bearded Collies*. Available from www.beaconforhealth.org/Newsletter_Sept_2002.pdf

Tuber DS, Hothersall D and Peters MF (1982) Treatment of fears and phobias in dogs. *Veterinary Clinics of North America: Small Animal Practice* **12**, 607–623

Wells DL, Graham L and Hepper PG (2002) The influence of auditory stimulation on the behaviour of dogs housed in a rescue shelter. *Animal Welfare* **11**, 385–393

Willis MB (1995) Genetic aspects of dog behavior with particular reference to working ability. In: *The Domestic Dog: Its Evolution, Behaviour and Interactions with People*, ed. J Serpell, pp. 51–64. Cambridge University Press, Cambridge

## Client handouts (bsavalibrary.com/behaviour_leaflets)

- Adopting a rescue dog: the pros and cons
- Canine behaviour questionnaire
- Cognitive dysfunction syndrome
- Down–stay mat exercises
- Headcollar training
- How to find a good trainer
- Noise fear score sheet
- Playing with your dog–toys
- Questionnaire to assess separation anxiety
- Sit–stay exercises
- Teaching your dog to go to a place on command
- Treating a noise fear using desensitization and counter-conditioning

# 16

# Situational sensitivities

## Clara Palestrini

## Introduction

In the field of veterinary behavioural medicine, aversion responses, particularly fear of places or particular objects, play an important part in the development of a large variety of behavioural 'problems' in domestic cats and dogs. It is therefore essential to understand the processes underlying aversion responses in household pets, in order to understand better why specific behaviours occur in certain circumstances and the most effective methods for managing and preventing them.

Clinically, the distinction between anxiety and fear is often difficult since there is a common tendency to use these terms as if they were interchangeable. However, although both fear and anxiety are emotional responses sharing the same behavioural and physiological mechanisms, their different meanings should be clarified (see also Chapter 13).

## Definitions

### Anxiety

The term anxiety is used when an animal anticipates a negative outcome. Anxiety is an emotional (apprehensive) response occurring prior to a stimulus/situation that the animal perceives as probable and dangerous. Thus, when anxious, the animal exhibits a somatic and behavioural response to a situation or stimuli that *might* occur. The term anxiety may be used within the context of either a widespread and generalized state of apprehension or the specific anticipation of danger. It is a response to signs of potential danger or, more generally, to a novel event.

Behavioural and physiological responses accompanying anxiety prepare an individual to react appropriately, for instance by displaying defensive or offensive behaviour (Livesey, 1986). If anxiety responses are inappropriate, the individual's ability to adapt to environmental conditions will be substantially compromised (Ohl *et al.*, 2008). In humans, pathological anxiety is characterized by excessive anxiousness and worry occurring for at least 6 months. The extent of the similarities between the human and the animal condition is not yet known and a lot of work is needed to validate the diagnosis of pathological anxiety in animals; it is, for example, not yet possible to obtain evidence about 'apprehensive expectations' in animals. In an attempt to characterize anxiety, which appears to lack adaptive value and severely

interferes with the normal (i.e. adaptive) interaction of the sufferer with its physical and social environment, Ohl *et al.* (2008) proposed the following definition of pathological anxiety in animals:

> *'Pathological anxiety is a persistent, uncontrollable, excessive, inappropriate and generalized dysfunctional and aversive emotion, triggering physiological and behavioural responses lacking adaptive value. Pathological anxiety related behaviour is a response to the exaggerated anticipation or perception of threats, which is incommensurate with the actual situation.'*

### Fear

Fear is an adaptive emotional response to an existing stimulus/situation that the animal perceives as potentially dangerous. In fear, the emotional response starts when the animal perceives the presence of the stimulus considered to be potentially dangerous. Fear allows an animal to avoid situations and activities that may be dangerous, thus increasing its chances of survival.

### Phobia

A sudden, excessive and profound fear is classified as a phobia. The intensity of a phobic response is greater than that of a fear response. The phobic clinical signs also persist when the stimulus is removed or disappears and eventually the phobic reaction may emerge in the absence of the triggering stimuli. It is important to note that whereas fears may be adaptive responses, phobias are not. By definition, phobias interfere with normal functioning (Overall, 1997). Phobias develop quickly, with little change in their presentation. It has been postulated that once a phobic event has been experienced, any event associated with it or the memory of it is sufficient to generate the response. Usually the origin of such an event was traumatic. Phobic situations are avoided where possible or, if unavoidable, are endured with intense anxiety and distress.

Although the term phobia is often used in common language to mean a severe fear, this is not how it should be used within a medical context. There are multiple forms of responses to phobias. The most common include startle and fear reactions to sudden or loud noises (traffic, dropped objects) and fearful reactions to some types of people or situations. Phobias, anxiety and fears seem to be related at the neurochemical level (Overall *et al.*, 2001).

## Inappropriate fear responses

Although a specific fear response may be of little consequence either because the trigger stimulus can be easily avoided or because the intensity of the fear response is relatively mild, other fears may significantly interfere with the human–animal relationship. For example, a fear of the veterinary clinic may impact on the health care of the pet, or a fearful animal may inflict injury upon itself or others if fear triggers escape behaviour, which can include defensive aggression.

Specific aversive experiences may be associated with the development of intense fear, particularly if the experience was intense. However, although many fear-related reactions may be explained in terms of conditioned processes (e.g. a past negative experience causes the fearful response), not all fearful reactions develop in this manner (Poulton et al., 1998). In some cases inadequate or inappropriate exposure to specific stimuli (such as locations, objects, people or animals) during developmental phases may lead to a development of fearful responses in relation to these in later life (see Chapters 6 and 7). During development, animals may be exposed to a variety of stimuli in a non-threatening context, which affects not only their specific response to these stimuli but also their general response to novelty. The importance of exposure of young puppies to a wide variety of environmental stimuli has been well demonstrated, and it would seem that quality of exposure rather than quantity is of the essence (Wolfle, 1990). However, chronic stress later in life may result in the loss of this learning and the emergence of a fear response to stimuli to which the animal was previously habituated (see Chapter 13).

Living in a group and having the ability to adapt to a variety of environments requires a degree of emotional stability that is possible only through habituation and the disappearance of fear responses to certain stimuli. Conversely, lack of early stimulation may lead to poor learning capacity, possibly related to a general lack of ability to habituate to novel environments (Dehasse, 1994). Fears may also be transmitted as a result of social learning, from one individual to another, but the extent to which this occurs in even a social species like the dog is unknown.

Reversion to fear and avoidance is possible if a puppy is environmentally deprived of experience relevant to the life it will encounter and be expected to cope with later. Animals with limited exposure tend to become more inhibited by or fearful to a range of stimuli and this can give rise to many behaviour problems later.

As mentioned above, fear is an adaptive response, essential for survival, in that it allows an animal to avoid potentially dangerous situations. Many fears are largely innate and species specific; there is often no need, for example, to teach a cat to fear a dog (Berton et al., 1998). Other fears require learning: a single contact with a hot surface is normally sufficient to engender in an animal a sense of fear towards it. However, fear is not the most appropriate or adaptive response in all situations (Bear et al., 2001). Avoidance responses may become a problem, both when a behavioural response towards a stimulus is inappropriate in the human environment (such as running away or aggression) and when the animal is unable to perform an appropriate behavioural response to resolve the situation.

The typical features of situational sensitivities are inappropriate fear responses when no stressor is present, when it is not potentially dangerous (Bear et al., 2001), and/or when the intensity or duration of the response becomes excessive (Sheppard and Mills, 2003). In these cases the behavioural response may be described as 'abnormal', because the behavioural pattern being exhibited is not adaptive and may be ineffective at removing the individual from the fearful situation. The fear response in these animals may not only start automatically when coming into direct contact with the triggering stimuli, an unknown/novel situation, or the precursors of the above, but may also become generalized to similar stimuli and situations, aggravating the problem. However, any response that takes a form that interferes with the owner's expectations or quality of life may be more likely to be considered a problem, whether it is normal or not and whether it is associated with aversion or positive emotional states. For example, the dog that becomes over-excited in a positive way when meeting another dog or people is often inappropriately managed by owners, leading to a more complex problem (see Chapter 5). Control problems are dealt with in Chapter 8, and this chapter will focus on those problems that have their origins in fear and avoidance.

## Evaluation of the patient

### Presenting signs and history

To understand whether an animal is trying to avoid a certain place or object, it is important to know how the animal behaves when exposed to the fear-inducing stimulus. Useful initial steps are a description of the posture and behaviours exhibited by the animal in that context (rather than accepting the owner's interpretation at face value) and finding out how often this happens and whether or not the stimulus could be avoided.

Clients often report the obvious signs (e.g. elimination, apparent aggression, vocalization) but not so often do they recognize the more subtle clinical signs, such as a decrease in activity levels, salivation, slight whining or pacing, which can be so important in managing the case. A detailed history collected while observing the dog or by asking owners to videotape the dog's behaviour at home can help in pinpointing the exact behaviours exhibited, their order and whether they truly are indicative of a state of fear or anxiety.

A critical part of the historical evaluation is determining the trigger or triggers of the fearful behaviour and the threshold of the fearful response. This information is important, because it helps the veterinary surgeon to establish the treatment programme and monitor progress. Attempting to grade the response over aspects of stimulus presentation will be useful when attempting to set up treatment plans.

Obtaining information with regard to the initial appearance of the problem and its duration may help in formulating the prognosis and aid owners in their understanding of the reasons behind the development of the problem.

### Determining and describing the fear

Fearful animals may display a wide range of signs, not all of which necessarily present every time and which may be exhibited with differing intensity and frequency according to the individual.

When an animal experiences a stressful situation, physiological changes occur, aimed at preparing the animal's response to the perceived danger (see Chapter 13). Heart rate accelerates with a consequent increase in cardiac output, breathing becomes faster, pupils dilate and the acuity of its senses increases. The animal may also empty its bladder and bowels.

From a behavioural viewpoint, the most frequently observed signs of fear are avoidance, immobility, flight and aggressive behaviours. An animal's fearful posture depends on the behaviour the animal is about to exhibit, but, in general, the body is lowered, the tail is down or tucked under the body, the ears are pinned back against the head and the eyes are wide (Figures 16.1 and 16.2).

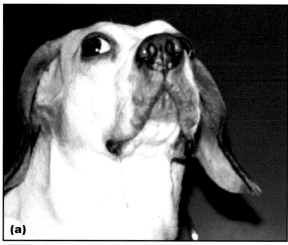

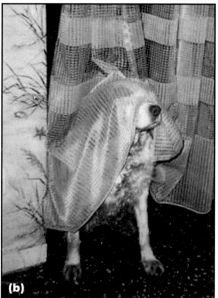

(b)

**16.2** Fear in dogs. **(a)** A fearful dog: salivation, ears pinned back against the head, and eyes wide. (Courtesy of D. Frank.) **(b)** A fearful dog exhibiting hiding posture.

Behavioural signs of fear (Figure 16.3) may include increased vigilance, reactivity, motor activity (pacing) and environmental exploration. In sociable individuals (cats or dogs) there may also be excessive demands for human attention and reassurance. Equally a fearful animal may show behavioural inhibition, shyness,

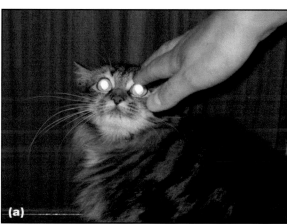

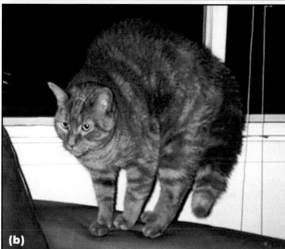

**16.1** Fear in cats. **(a)** Fearful cat showing a typical defensive withdrawal posture. If the threatening stimulus is not withdrawn, the cat will often flee (given the opportunity). **(b)** When startled, cats may adopt an aggressive posture. (Photograph: courtesy of D. Frank.)

| Panting |
| Dilated pupils |
| Hypervigilance |
| Elimination of urine/faeces |
| Flattened posture |
| Hyperactivity/pacing |
| Attention seeking |
| Shyness |
| Avoidance |
| Flight/freeze |
| Trembling |
| Aggression |
| Lip licking, swallowing, salivation |
| Vocalization |
| Piloerection |

**16.3** Behavioural signs of fear.

avoidance, reduction of locomotor activity (freezing), hiding (see Figure 16.2b) and running away, aggressive manifestations or displacement behaviours such as self-grooming. Other noticeable signs of fear are licking of lips, yawning, swallowing, salivation, diarrhoea, vomiting, panting, piloerection (see Figure 16.1b), shaking and vocalizing (normally whining but also repeated barking or howling).

In extreme cases animals can show a state of panic: they are insensitive to pain and social stimuli and their reaction is immediate and extreme. In these cases, the flight behaviour can be so violent that dogs may go to such extremes as breaking their own nails and teeth and jumping out of windows regardless of the height. Both cats and dogs can also show extreme aggression when in a state of panic and escape is not possible. The owner should either leave the animal alone (as long as it is not putting itself or others at risk of injury) or they can sit and stay quietly by it. Quiet association may provide some security without accidentally reinforcing the behaviour. Owners should allow their pet to hide if that is the animal's choice. When panicking the animal is unable to pay attention to the owner and in these situations pharmacological therapy might be a useful adjunct to behaviour techniques.

The time taken for the animal to return to normal after exposure can be a useful measure for monitoring treatment progress.

### Other associated changes in behaviour

Apart from the signs described above, a persistent state of anxiety or fear may lead to changes in the animal's main behavioural patterns (Figure 16.4).

| |
|---|
| Changes in feeding habits (loss of or increased appetite; pica) |
| Changes in habits and social relationships (toward both humans and other animals) |
| Elimination and marking behaviour (soiling in the house, scratching furniture, head rubbing) |
| Changes in sleep patterns (increased or decreased duration) |
| Changes in grooming behaviour (reduced frequency) |
| Frequent displacement activities |
| Onset of compulsive behaviours |

**16.4** General changes in behaviour in a chronically stressed animal.

When an animal lives in a constant state of distress, there may be changes in the intensity, frequency or social context of the feeding habits. These can range from a significant decrease to a total absence of feeding (anorexia), or the opposite, i.e. excessive food intake. In some cases it may involve the development of pica, i.e. the ingestion of inedible substances.

Under stressful conditions, changes may occur not only in the type and level of activity which the animal normally exhibits but also in the location in which they are manifested. In general, there is a decrease in exploratory and play behaviour and a greater tendency to use hiding places. Interactions with the owner and with other household pets may also change. In some cases aggressive behaviours

may be exhibited. Problems of elimination in the household environment and of territory marking (particularly with urine, by head rubbing or by scratching in cats) may be due to anxiety and fear (Houpt, 1991; Frank and Dehasse, 2003). An increase or decrease in sleep time and/or an overall change in sleeping habits, such as using hiding places instead of the usual sleeping areas, often occurs in fearful or anxious subjects.

There may be either an increase or a decrease in grooming behaviours. An excessive increase in grooming behaviours may lead to compulsive behaviours such as biting or pulling out fur (see Chapter 20). In some cases displacement behaviours may involve auto-grooming. This behaviour seems to indicate a motivational conflict when the animal encounters the feared stimulus, in that the animal has a desire to avoid the stimulus but is unable to do so. If these changes in behaviour occur in the older animal, it is important to assess whether or not there is a concomitant cognitive decline, which may precipitate emotional disturbance (see Chapter 12).

### Fear and aggression

Both fear and anxiety play a significant role in aggression (see Chapters 17 to 19). Fear is involved in the development and expression of aggression between animals of the same family and toward the owner or animals outside the family unit. Most dogs and cats taken to behavioural veterinary clinics for problems related to aggression appear to be motivated by either anxiety or fear.

Normally if the threat is very close and the animal has no chance of escaping, it will first exhibit threatening behaviours, only later followed by overt attack. The purpose of defensive threatening behaviours is to show a willingness to attack if the threat continues, mostly expressed through characteristic postures, such as piloerection (Eibl-Eisfeldt and Sutterin, 1990), and vocalizations (Blanchard et al., 1998). Attack is the last resort in the defensive strategy (Blanchard et al., 1998; Shuhama et al., 2007). If the aggressive reaction successfully deters the fear-inducing stimulus from approaching closer, the animal will learn that this particular reaction works and it may thus generalize it to similar situations and manifest the behaviour at the early stages of exposure to the fear-related stimulus.

### Client attitudes, beliefs and behaviours

Owners often consider their pet to be difficult or 'naughty' and need to understand that the motivation behind the behaviour is fear. To increase the owner's desire to collaborate in the treatment process, it is essential that they understand the motives behind the undesired behaviour and the logic of the treatment process.

The owner's response to the fearful animal may influence its subsequent reactions to the triggering stimuli, potentially worsening the problem. Attempts by the owner to reassure the animal often have the opposite effect by reinforcing its manifestation of fear and the behaviour it is performing at the time. In general, people have the tendency to comfort pets showing fearful behaviours, but this may increase the manifestation of the behaviour through involuntary reinforcement.

Punishment may further increase the animal's fear and thus lead to an escalation of the fearful and aggressive response without improving the animal's emotional state. The use of punishment alone is never adequate to modify behaviour.

## Risk evaluation

Fear has an adaptive function since it is linked to the perception of danger and the related behavioural reactions are meant to avoid such events. Unfortunately, owners of fearfully aggressive dogs and cats often attempt to correct or prevent the behaviour using punishment. As a result fear and its associated aggressive reaction are increased, placing owner and pet in a potentially more dangerous situation. Furthermore, if the punishing actions of the owner are insufficient to control the undesired behaviour, not only can the relationship between pet and owner be seriously compromised by this action on the owner's part, but also fear may develop even when it was initially absent, potentially resulting in ambivalent behavioural signals and a more complicated problem. Finally, punishment may only serve to diminish the outward manifestations of the fearful response, such as growling and snarling, making increased aggressive responses appear unpredictable and therefore more dangerous and putting others at risk.

During treatment, control of access to the stimulus is essential or the risk of escalation of the problem behaviour increases. If uncontrolled access to the stimulus occurs after treatment is instituted, the treatment may be hampered and the animal may relapse.

## Diagnosis

The diagnosis of fear of people and animals, objects or specific places is based on several key findings in the behavioural history and the evaluation of possible other behavioural and medical diagnoses. It includes the following criteria:

- A specific trigger or triggers can be identified
- Exposure to the trigger(s) reliably evokes a fear response
- The animal exhibits behavioural signs of fear (see Figure 16.3) when exposed to the fear-inducing stimuli
- The animal exhibits somatic manifestation of fear (e.g. increased breathing, pupils dilated)
- The animal exhibits changes in its main behavioural patterns (see Figure 16.4).

There are numerous situations that may cause fear reactions in cats and dogs. Examples of fear-inducing stimuli include objects, people in general or a specific category (e.g. men or children), other animals (conspecifics, members of a different species, or both), car traffic, types of floor such as tiling or floor grates, thunderstorms or strong and sudden noises, specific places such as the veterinary clinic or the groomer's, or car journeys.

## Diagnostic categories and underlying possible motivations

### Fear of people and animals

Inadequate or inappropriate exposure to certain areas or objects may induce a fear reaction. With cats in particular, the arrival of a new cat, social interactions with cats or other animals in the same home, the presence of a neighbour's cat and the arrival of a child or a new person may all induce fear reactions that can result in either active or passive aggressive behaviours, scratching, marking (with urine or by rubbing against objects or people) or pica.

### Fear of things

Car traffic, metal gratings, stairs, thunderstorms and strong sudden noises are amongst the most common fear-inducing stimuli. There are various sounds that dogs seem to be particularly sensitive to, the more common ones being thunder, fireworks and gunshots (see Chapter 15). Fear of walking on certain floors is also a frequently observed problem, particularly in certain breeds such as collies.

### Fear of places

***The veterinary clinic:*** An animal's fear and anxiety upon entering the veterinary clinic and the correlated problems are a well known welfare issue. Fear of the clinic may have a strong impact on the animal's health: the owner may forgo routine checkups and vaccinations to avoid stressing the animal; and veterinary surgeons may have difficulties in guaranteeing appropriate care of a very fearful animal. A study on the behaviour of dogs at the veterinary clinic showed that 60% manifested anxiety, 18% showed signs of fear-induced aggression, 5% showed defensive behaviour and only 17% exhibited friendly, non-fearful behaviours (Stanford, 1981).

Veterinary clinics are often a novel environment for the animal and may be associated with previous negative experiences, which, together with restraint during the visit or the perception of having no way out of the situation, may result in fear that can be displayed in forms of aggression. This can make some pets very difficult and dangerous to treat, which may in turn influence the quality of the veterinary surgeon's evaluation and the subsequent treatment, further diminishing the animal's welfare (Figure 16.5).

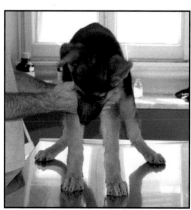

**16.5**

A fearful dog during a clinical examination. (Courtesy of D. Groppetti.)

It would thus be best if cats and dogs could have positive experiences of the veterinary clinic and owners encouraged to make the experience as pleasant as possible, praising the pet and feeding small pieces of treats prior to a necessary visit (see Chapter 2). This will help to reduce the possibility of developing a fearful association with the clinic, even if on subsequent occasions the visit may not be as pleasant. The use of pheromones seems to help reduce the signs of anxiety in dogs with the less aversive aspects of a visit (see Chapter 21). However, there is no evidence that it reduces aggressive reaction during the clinical examination (Mills *et al.*, 2006) and so it is not a substitute for good management. If the first experience at the clinic is unpleasant, it is more likely that the animal will demonstrate a fearful reaction to this location. Strategies for preventing this problem are dealt with in more detail in Chapter 2.

***Fear of car journeys:*** Most owners at some point have to take their pet on a car journey. Reactions differ: some animals may calmly adapt to the situation, whilst others may manifest a host of difficult behaviours, such as destructiveness, vocalizations, escape attempts, avoidance, excessive salivation, vomiting, panting, trembling and inability to relax. A fearful response needs to be distinguished from over-excitability and over-reactivity to passing stimuli, or motion sickness, or anticipation of what lies ahead, such as a walk or a visit to the veterinary clinic. Most dogs with travel problems fall into the primary categories of excitable, fearful, nervous, anxious or suffering from motion sickness.

Effective treatment depends on an accurate assessment of the case, because different problems will require different treatments (Gandia Estellés and Mills, 2006). For example, if a pet has a fear of the car, the owner should be questioned as to any history of car sickness. If the pet experiences nausea every time it rides in the car, it will be necessary to treat the underlying nausea in addition to drawing up a behavioural modification programme to address the associated fear of the car. One study suggests that the use of pheromones may be effective in helping to control signs related to sympathetic arousal in dogs with travel-related problems (Gandia Estellés and Mills, 2006).

***Fear of new places:*** Being taken to a boarding facility or moving house may be a highly stressful event. Changes in the physical environment may induce high levels of fear and anxiety in cats (Frank and Dehasse, 2003). Any aversive experience in a new environment may result in avoidance of that place in future. In fact, emotional states act as discriminative stimuli in learning (see Chapter 5). It is the emotional response associated with an external stimulus that determines whether that particular stimulus is associated with a positive or negative outcome and hence directs the behavioural response (Young, 1959). Negative emotional responses also become conditioned to previously unimportant stimuli through classical conditioning, and to an animal's own actions through operant conditioning. Hence, a fear response is a highly adaptive mechanism for ensuring that an animal learns that certain stimuli predict something unpleasant and so, as a consequence of this learning, the stimuli are avoided. For example, a dog that has gone out at night and been frightened by a loud noise or fireworks may well refuse to go out at night again, because this action is associated with a negative emotion.

### Concurrent and contributing problems

It is always critical to exclude other contributing disorders that need to be diagnosed and treated. A complete physical and neurological examination should always be carried out as well as routine blood work (complete blood count, chemistry panel and thyroid panel); more specialized tests, based on the observed clinical signs, should also be performed as necessary. For example, an animal showing a fear of stairs or certain types of flooring may have musculoskeletal problems causing difficulty or pain in movement that is not apparent on the level surface. Similarly, a dog exhibiting avoidance of the car may feel nauseous every time it goes on a car journey.

It is extremely important to evaluate each case individually, since the type and efficacy of the treatment will depend on correct and complete diagnosis of the problem.

## Behavioural biology of the condition

### Causes of aversion responses

Aversion may have different causes and often such causes result from a combination of risk factors within the individual. The threshold that may trigger an avoidance response may vary between species, between breeds and between individuals as well as with the properties of the stimulus. There may be one or more triggering stimuli, and these may be more or less specific.

The behavioural response of a specific individual to aversive stimuli may be influenced by a number of factors, including but not exclusively:

- Species-specific and breed-typical behaviours
- Experience during development
- Previous learning about the success or otherwise of the animal's own behavioural strategies in similar situations
- Individual differences in reactivity.

### Species-specific and breed-typical responses

An individual's behavioural response to an external event is influenced by predetermined genetic factors pertaining to that species and/or breed. These species-specific or breed-typical responses essentially are models of synaptic connections which form the underlying basis of the behaviours an animal will learn during its life. The responses have been modified during evolution, emerging as the most adaptive behaviours for successful reproduction in a given environment.

The genetically predetermined synaptic blueprint in the brain equips the individual with the best tools for survival and reproductive success. Each species is genetically predisposed to differ compared with others in the extent to which it is frightened by certain kinds of stimuli, objects or situations, despite having had no direct experience with them; and this may apply at the breed level too. For example, the traditional gundog breeds appear less predisposed to sensitivity to noise. Thus, not only are stimuli that in an animal's evolutionary history were indicative of potentially dangerous situations more likely to trigger a fear response, compared with stimuli that had no such predictive value, but also aversion to other stimuli may be bred out to a certain extent.

The genetic predisposition to display avoidance behaviours in specific contexts may be more obvious in social species such as dogs, compared to cats, since the behaviour may also have a communicative value that contributes to survival. Thus cats may be more subtle in their expression of aversion. Cats also tend to avoid drawing attention to themselves more generally when scared or anxious and tend to hide quietly, which often means that their aversion responses may go unnoticed by an owner or not be reported as a 'problem'.

### Experiences during development

Experiences during development can affect the adult animal's fear responses. Traumatic events or inappropriate exposure to environmental stimuli, including places, people and objects, may result in decreased capacity to adapt to new environments and thus an increased probability of a fear response when encountering such stimuli. For example, if a puppy is deprived of environmental experiences that it is predicted will be part of its adult life, when such events do occur an avoidance or fear reaction may follow. In some cases aggressive reactions may emerge, since these are often a manifestation of fear (see Chapters 6 and 7) .

During neonatal cerebral development, when there is greater neuronal plasticity (Hovda *et al.*, 1996), individuals learn to accept and recognize aspects of their social and physical environment as 'normal'; but if an animal is exposed to novel stimuli after this period it is normal for it to respond fearfully (McCune, 1995). In other words during this delicate postpartum phase the animal is creating the neuronal substrate capable of supporting all the stimuli that will be considered 'normal' in its lifetime. It is thus essential that the puppy or kitten is introduced to conspecifics, heterospecifics and their surrounding environment to allow the supporting structure that is being built to become fully compatible with the reality of the animal's adult life. However, even this is not a guarantee of success, since stress later in life may result in dishabituation and avoidance of stimuli previously accepted (see Chapter 13).

### Previously learned experiences

An individual's behavioural response is influenced by a series of learned experiences occurring during their lifetime. Specific unpleasant experiences may be associated with the development of intense fear, particularly if the experience was intensely negative. As already noted, emotional states act as discriminative stimuli in learning. It is the emotional response associated with an external stimulus that determines whether that specific stimulus is associated with a positive or negative outcome and that elicits the behavioural response (Young, 1959).

Positive emotion acts as an internal reinforcer through the rapid neurochemical processes associated with its production (Gallagher and Holland, 1994). An animal will be more inclined to repeat a specific action in a particular context if the performance of that action was associated with a subjectively positive state of being. For example, if a dog that is fearful of humans approaching the house discovers that the postman leaves when it barks, it will re-enact this same behaviour whenever a person approaches the house. Similarly, aversive emotional responses will encourage the avoidance of certain stimuli, and certain actions will not be repeated because they precede negative, unpleasant or harmful outcomes. A cat emerging from a cat-flap and immediately being attacked by the neighbour's cat will, understandably, refuse to use the cat-flap again, because this action is associated with a negative emotion.

In this context, an important aspect to consider is a process called 'latent inhibition' (see Chapter 5). Positive association with a specific stimulus safeguards against the development of a subsequent negative one with the same stimulus. Thus, by making sure that puppies and kittens experience positive associations with as many social and physical stimuli as possible, we can safeguard them from the subsequent development of fear responses to such stimuli. Once an association is made between a stimulus and a positive emotion, it is less likely that the animal will subsequently associate the stimulus with a negative emotion, especially compared with a situation in which no such positive association had been previously established.

### Reactivity

There are noticeable differences between individuals with regard to their reactivity to an aversive event and the responses correlated to fear are easily conditioned by sensory and motor activity. These differences have a strong impact on the probability that an individual, presented with a specific event, will develop a learned fear response. Individual differences also go some way to explaining the breed and bloodline predispositions to particular kinds of clinical problems. The ease with which fearful responses are learned is linked to reactivity and individual sensitivity to stress. These differences in terms of reactivity tend to predispose certain individuals to the development of behavioural problems related to fear. For example, studies on pointer dogs established proof of heritability of nervous behaviour (Thomas *et al.*, 1972); and 'noise-sensitive' and 'noise-insensitive/stable' lines of dogs have long been recognized in many working and hunting breeds (Willis, 1989). If some dogs have extreme sensitivity for specific tones or frequencies, they may be more sensitive to certain noises. Temperament may also be an important risk factor in cats.

## Treatment

For the treatment to be successful it is essential to keep it within the owner's range of possibilities in terms of both time and commitment load, and it must not require overly strict or unnatural rules for the owner–animal relationship. Behavioural protocols should be as simple as possible, easily integrated into the owner's daily routine, clarifying owner–animal communication and keeping to the application of the basic learning principles (see Chapter 5). The suggested behavioural modification protocol for situational sensitivities relating to aversion includes a combination of the following four basic strategies (Figure 16.6):

- Education and modification of the owner's behaviour
- Changes to the pet's environment
- Changing the pet's behaviour
- Pharmacological therapy.

| Education and modification of the client's behaviour |
|---|
| Keep it within the owner's capacity |
| It must not require overly strict or unnatural rules |
| Ability to read and interpret pet's body language correctly |
| Avoid client's involuntary reinforcement of the problem |
| No punishment of the animal |
| Avoid eliciting the fearful response |

| Changes to the patient's environment |
|---|
| Control access with fences, baby gates, pens, etc. in the domestic environment |
| Use harnesses, headcollars, leads and muzzles during walks |
| Use pheromones to reduce anxiety |

| Changes of the patient's behaviour |
|---|
| Correct and improve human–animal communication |
| Always praise the appropriate behaviour |
| Prevent, ignore and interrupt undesirable or inappropriate behaviours |
| Desensitization and counter-conditioning |

| Pharmacological intervention combined with behavioural modification |
|---|
| Explain to the client that drugs do not teach the animal what is the correct response |
| Responses to the treatment may vary from one animal to the next |
| There may be side effects |
| A complete blood count is essential prior to prescribing a particular product |
| Drug treatment must be administered for several months |
| Relapses are possible |
| It may be necessary to modify the dosage or change the drug |

**16.6** Considerations during treatment for situational sensitivities.

## Acute management protocols

### Client education

Client education can help to change the pet–owner dynamics and thus modify the pet's behaviour. Fear-related responses are characterized by a manifestation of non-specific clinical signs when the animal perceives or anticipates the stimuli. The ability to anticipate the triggering stimulus is an important aspect in the treatment of fear-related disorders and it is very important to help owners to recognize the early behavioural manifestations of the animal's problem to allow for early and efficacious treatment (see Ladder of Aggression in Chapter 2).

The owner's ability to read their pet's body language correctly allows them to act appropriately and prevent the development of undesired behaviours and situations. Once the owner understands their animal's needs and body language and their own influence on its behaviour, they will be less upset or worried about their pet and, being more aware of the reasons behind its behaviour, they should be more willing to cooperate in the behavioural modification programme. In addition, to limit further learning and intensification of the behaviour, the owner must be advised to avoid situations known to evoke the undesirable response.

### Environmental modification

In some cases it may be necessary to change the pet's environment to avoid contact with fear-inducing stimuli. Fences, baby gates and pens in the domestic environment and harnesses, headcollars, leads and muzzles during walks can decrease or prevent the manifestation of undesired behaviours and avoid potentially dangerous situations, such as in the case of the pet that is uneasy around young children. In many fearful animals the use of a headcollar seems to induce a state of relaxation and thus may be used during behavioural modification.

Some studies (Gandia Estellés and Mills, 2006; Mills *et al.*, 2006) exist to support the use of pheromonal products to reduce situational anxieties.

Environmental modification is particularly important for cats where fear may be caused by the arrival of a new person, cat or other animal (see Chapters 4 and 7).

Aggression is dealt with in Chapters 17 to 19 and assessment of the risk of this must form part of the recommendations to the client.

## Long-term management protocols

### Behavioural modification

To change an animal's aversion implies changing their perception of the stimulus so that it is no longer associated with a negative emotion. It also implies changing the consequences of the animal's response so that the inappropriate behaviour is no longer successful, but rather the appropriate and alternative behaviour achieves the desired outcome.

The identification of all fear-inducing stimuli is the key to successful treatment, even if this is not always possible (Levine *et al.*, 2007). The aim of the treatment is to substitute the fear response towards the triggering stimuli with a more acceptable and relaxed response.

The first step is to achieve a calm and relaxed response when the stimuli are in sight of the subject. It is important for the owner to recognize this particular state in the animal and reinforce it. This first step is very important, since it will increase the probability of success when a fear-inducing stimulus is presented.

The behavioural modification programme consists of teaching the animal to exhibit desirable behaviours, reinforcing them each time they are manifested, and pre-empting, ignoring or interrupting the inappropriate behaviours. This is achieved first of all by establishing a successful method of communication between the animal and its owner.

***Correcting human–animal communication:*** The goal of this intervention is to create a consistent and predictable relationship between the owner and the pet. With dogs this can be obtained by asking the animal to sit or undertake some other action before every interaction with the owner, e.g. to ask for food, play, attention or going out (see Chapter 5 and client handouts). The owner will be asked to reinforce the dog not only each time it obeys a command but also when it chooses to exhibit certain calm behaviours spontaneously. The aim is to achieve a clear form of communication, calming the dog by letting it know what happens next. This has little to do with controlling or exhibiting the owner's 'power' over the animal but rather it is a way of providing consistency and strengthening the bond between the owner and animal.

Although cats can also be trained to exhibit behaviours on command and be reinforced for relaxed behaviours, it is more common to use this method with dogs. Cat owners can be taught to identify relaxed and calm postures and behaviours in their pets and to reinforce these behaviours using food, toys or petting. Adding a secondary reinforcement such as clicker or a bell associated with the desired behaviour may also help.

Owners must be taught to recognize and praise their pet when it carries out the appropriate behaviours as requested and also when they are exhibited spontaneously (particularly if the animal shows calm and relaxed postures in a context in which it normally exhibits fearful ones). It is essential that the animal knows what is expected (by asking it to exhibit a particular behaviour) rather than being scolded for doing the wrong things. Rewarding the appropriate behaviour rather than focusing on correcting the wrong one will be more productive. The aim is to increase the probability, frequency and intensity of the desired behaviours.

***Ignoring and interrupting inappropriate behaviours:*** Interacting with the pet once the behaviour has started to occur may inadvertently reinforce the behaviour that the owner wants to stop. Ignoring the behaviour, on the other hand, minimizes the risk of reinforcing it, thus initiating the extinction process (see Chapter 5). Ignoring means giving no attention, even eye contact, to the pet at this time. An alternative strategy involves encouraging owners to show an intense interest in something else, rather than just ignore the pet, as this gives them something to do and also provides an alternative focus for the animal. For example, the owner might be encouraged to show a lot of interest in the animal's toys but not directly encourage the animal to engage with them. If the animal then chooses to play rather than hide, the owner can reinforce this response.

When behaviours cannot be ignored, it is best to interrupt them. It is important to interrupt the behaviour at the earliest possible stage, refocus the pet and reward an appropriate response. For example, an owner may be asked to recall their dog if the problem situation is likely and instruct it to sit or lie, i.e. to exhibit a behaviour that is incompatible with the manifestation of a fearful response and that encourages the dog to focus on the owner. The dog is then praised for exhibiting the correct behaviour. Interruptions must occur calmly; yelling, scolding and grabbing the dog only serve to increase emotional arousal in the situation and do not help it to learn a new response. Owners should be advised to refrain from any physical force and verbal reprimands for fearful behaviour. Punishment will not resolve the problem and might increase the fear and induce an aggressive response.

***Desensitization and counter-conditioning:*** Desensitization and counter-conditioning (DSCC) are the most utilized methods in the treatment of fearful responses. Once the owner has instilled the occurrence of calm and relaxed behaviours in the absence of the fear-inducing stimulus, a gradual desensitization programme to the triggering stimulus needs to be carried out. Desensitization requires a gradual and controlled exposure to the stimulus so as to extinguish the manifestation of fearful behaviours (see Chapter 5). The stimulus and response gradient established during history taking will be useful, taking into account its intensity and distance from the patient. During the course of controlled exposure it is important that the stimulus is presented below the threshold at which the fearful behaviour is manifested; however, some sort of response, such as pricking the ears, is necessary in order to confirm that the animal has noticed the stimulus and to determine progress.

The counter-conditioning phase represents the reinforcing component of the programme. The relatively neutral response to the triggering stimulus is replaced with a positive emotional state. This is achieved by reinforcing the animal when, with the triggering stimulus present, it manifests a calm and controlled behaviour instead of the fear response. Thus the animal is conditioned to experience a positive feeling in direct competition with the previous feelings of fear.

Especially in cats, play behaviour can be encouraged by providing and encouraging chase of appropriate items. Toys that bounce, flutter or move in such a way as to entice the cat to play can be useful in these cases (see Chapters 4 and 7).

It is quite possible that the animal will be unable to pay attention to the owner if it is overly reactive or fearful, which usually means that the stimulus intensity was too great. In these cases it is important to remove the animal from the fear-inducing situation, without drawing attention to the events, as quickly as possible. When the animal shows even the slightest fear response, it must be removed from the situation and the intensity of the stimulus must be reduced to below the fear threshold. Each time an animal is given the possibility of manifesting an inappropriate behaviour it learns from it and thus is more likely to repeat that same behaviour.

In some cases it is impossible to avoid the fear-inducing situation, either because of the intensity of the animal's response or because the triggering situation is unavoidable. In these instances it may be necessary to use a pharmacological approach to reduce the fear response. In the editors' experience, some animals may benefit from pheromonal products.

## Managing specific contextual fears

Fear of the veterinary clinic is one of the most frequently reported problems. A number of methods to control this situation have traditionally been adopted, including containment strategies such as the use of kennels, leads and muzzles, and chemical restraint such as sedation. These methods are not without risk and potential side effects. Furthermore, these strategies do not help the animal to overcome its fear and in some cases they can have the reverse effect and actually reinforce the fear response.

A gentle approach and handling of the animal during visits to the clinic may help to prevent the occurrence of such situations (see also Chapter 2 for advice on best management practice in the clinic). Specific behavioural modification programmes may, in the long run, aid in overcoming the fear response associated with clinics. These programmes generally involve multiple and controlled visits to the clinic, starting with visits involving no direct manipulation and only positive reinforcement of calm behaviours, followed by simulations of visits when the fear response is no longer present, with the aim of desensitizing the animal to the visit (see **client handout**). While the use of pheromone products in the clinic has been reported to be useful in producing desirable change in the case of more severe problems (Mills *et al.*, 2006), this does not reflect the author's experience in practice.

A similar procedure can be adopted with car journeys (see **client handout**). To begin with, the behaviour being reinforced is a spontaneous approach to the car, followed by jumping into the car but with the door open and engine cut off. If the relaxed behaviours continue, short trips associated with pleasant outcomes should follow, until longer trips can be carried out without the animal manifesting fear responses.

Setbacks may occur if the animal is suddenly in need of medical attention or must unavoidably be taken on a car journey.

## Pharmacological intervention

The decision to prescribe a drug for the treatment of a situational fear or anxiety should be based on a number of factors, including:

- The severity and type of problem
- The owner's urgency to resolve it
- Familiarity with relevant psychotropic drugs
- The capacity of the owner to follow the behaviour modification programme appropriately.

If in doubt, the veterinary surgeon should seek specialist veterinary behavioural advice and/or consider referral.

The aim of pharmacological treatment is to reduce the fear response and the animal's reactivity towards the fear-inducing stimulus without sedation and without interfering with its learning ability, but rather to help to facilitate the learning necessary for long-term behavioural modification. It is always important to explain to the owner that drugs do not teach the animal what the correct response is; rather, they create a window of opportunity for learning to take place by reducing the animal's reaction to the stimulus and allowing a faster recovery from it.

It is equally important to let the owner know that:

- The drug treatment may need to be administered for several months
- Relapses are possible
- The response to the treatment may vary from one animal to the next
- It may therefore be necessary to modify the dosage and perhaps even change the drug.

Many drugs used in behavioural medicine are not registered veterinary products and so information in terms of long-term effects is relatively unknown. It is important to be cautious when deciding to administer a drug and to obtain written consent from the owner. A complete blood count (CBC) is an essential prerequisite to prescribing a particular product, in order to safeguard against hidden medical complications. Dosages for some of the medications that may be beneficial in the treatment of fear are listed in Figure 16.7.

| Drug class | Drug | Dosage for dogs | Dosage for cats |
|---|---|---|---|
| Tricyclic antidepressants (TCAs) | Amitriptyline | 1–2 mg/kg q12h | 0.5–1 mg/kg q12–24h |
| | Clomipramine | 1–3 mg/kg q12h | 0.5 mg/kg q24h |
| Selective serotonin reuptake inhibitors (SSRIs) | Fluoxetine | 1–2 mg/kg q24h | 0.5–1 mg/kg q24h |
| | Fluvoxamine | 1–2 mg/kg q24h | 0.25–0.5 mg/kg q24h |
| | Paroxetine | 0.5–2 mg/kg q24h | 0.25–0.5 mg/kg q24h |
| | Sertraline | 1–3 mg/kg q24h | 0.5–1.5 mg/kg q24h [a] |
| Monoamine oxidase inhibitors (MAOIs) | Selegiline | 0.5–1 mg/kg q24h | 0.5–1 mg/kg q24h |

**16.7** Recommended pharmacological therapy in the treatment of fear. [a] From Crowell-Davis and Murray (2006) (continued) ▶

| Drug class | Drug | Dosage for dogs | Dosage for cats |
|---|---|---|---|
| Benzodiazepines (BZs) | Alprazolam | 0.01–0.1mg/kg q8–12h | 0.125–0.25 mg/cat q24h |
| | Clorazepate | 0.55–2.2 mg/kg q4–24h | 0.02–0.4mg/kg q12–24h |
| | Diazepam | 0.55–2.2 mg/kg q6–24h | 0.2–0.4mg/kg q12–24h |
| Azapirones | Buspirone | 0.5–2 mg/kg q8–12h | 0.5–1 mg/kg q12h |

**16.7** (continued) Recommended pharmacological therapy in the treatment of fear. [a] From Crowell-Davis and Murray (2006)

*Tricyclic antidepressants (TCAs):* TCAs variously block serotonin and noradrenaline (norepinephrine) reuptake. The most widely utilized drugs to aid treatment of these problems are amitriptyline and clomipramine. TCAs should be used on a daily basis regardless of the potential for exposure to the trigger stimuli. The therapeutic effects often appear only in the second to fourth week of treatment. They are normally tolerated well by cats and dogs but they can have a sedative effect, particularly during the first week, as well as producing dry mouth, urinary/faecal retention and, for animals predisposed to this condition, cardiac conduction disturbances (Crowell-Davis and Murray, 2006). It is important to assess the animal's cardiac status before prescribing these drugs.

*Selective serotonin reuptake inhibitors (SSRIs):* SSRIs act to block the reuptake of serotonin at the 5-HT subtype receptors. The most utilized in veterinary behavioural medicine are fluoxetine, paroxetine, sertraline and fluvoxamine. SSRIs should be used on a daily basis regardless of the risk of exposure to trigger stimuli. Changes should be noted within the first 3–4 weeks. Cats administered SSRIs must be carefully monitored for water and food consumption, weight changes and faeces/urine retention. Serotonin is closely associated with the modulation of a wide range of behaviour thresholds and so it can have a particular role in problems relating to impulsiveness. Side effects in pets may include gastrointestinal irritation, sedation, insomnia and irritability. The gastrointestinal problems may involve anorexia, appetite loss, nausea or diarrhoea. The side effects can be avoided by starting with a low dosage during the first week and gradually increasing it over time.

*Monoamine oxidase inhibitors (MAOIs):* MAOIs (e.g. selegiline) may be used successfully alongside behaviour therapy for the treatment of these problems. MAOIs act as irreversible inhibitors of monoamine oxidase (MAO), an enzyme that catabolizes intracellular monoamine neurotransmitters (noradrenaline, adrenaline (epinephrine), dopamine, tyramine and serotonin). MAOIs should be used on a daily basis regardless of the risk of exposure to the trigger stimuli. It may take several weeks for the drug to take effect. They must not be combined with SSRIs, TCAs, opioids or any other MAOI and a 2–4-week washout period between the use of these drugs is recommended. Side effects are mild and normally disappear spontaneously; they usually manifest as gastrointestinal signs (Crowell-Davis and Murray, 2006).

*Benzodiazepines (BZs):* Benzodiazepines activate the corresponding receptors in the central nervous system, thereby facilitating GABA, an inhibitory neurotransmitter. All the BZs share the same mechanism, but differences in their pharmacokinetic properties and clinical behaviour may dictate their specific use. At low dosage BZs act as mild sedatives, facilitating daytime activity by tempering excitement; at moderate dosages they act as anti-anxiety agents, facilitating social interaction in a more proactive manner; and at high dosages they act as hypnotics, facilitating sleep.

BZs (alprazolam, diazepam, clorazepate) should not be used with animals exhibiting fear-related aggression, since the drugs may facilitate uninhibited behaviour and subsequently more serious aggression (Overall, 1997; Crowell-Davis and Murray, 2006).

Unlike the preceding drugs, BZs can be used either on a routine or on a 'when needed' basis, since action onset is rapid (within an hour or two). The frequency of dosing, sedative side effects, tolerance, drug dependence and their potentially erroneous use by clients have made these drugs less popular for use in the long term, although the rapid effects make them ideal for use in the short term. Since BZs can be combined with most serotonin-enhancing drugs, they can be used in the short term to address immediate needs until the serotonin-enhancing medication has a chance to take full effect.

*Azapirones:* The only azapirone in much veterinary clinical use is buspirone, whose chief mode of activity is thought to be as a partial serotonin-1$\alpha$ agonist. It is used to treat generalized anxiety and to balance states of high arousal (Crowell-Davis and Murray, 2006). It may decrease aggressive behaviour between cats when administered to the most fearful cat. It is a slow-acting drug, taking between 1 and 3 weeks. Side effects are generally mild and mostly related to gastrointestinal problems and irritability.

*Phenothiazines:* Phenothiazines (such as acepromazine) are generally not recommended for use in this condition, with the possible exception of travel problems associated with nausea. They act poorly as anxiolytics and so an animal's response to these drugs may be highly variable. The sedative effect seems to suppress behavioural responses but without allowing the animal to overcome its underlying fear (Voith and Borchelt, 1996; Sheppard and Mills, 2003; Crowell-Davis and Murray, 2006).

## Additional therapies

Other interventions include the use of synthetic pheromones (see Chapter 21). A number of studies have investigated the use of pheromones in the treatment of conditions with an underlying stress component in cats and dogs, suggesting that the common mode of action of these substances is in fact to reduce the level of anxiety.

## Prognosis

The prognosis of a particular case depends on numerous factors, including the intensity of the fear and the duration of the problem. It should be expected that fears that have been manifested for a long time are normally harder to treat. Owners capable of recognizing early signs of anxiety and the desirable behaviours displayed by their pet are much more likely to be successful than owners who expect pharmacological treatment alone to be sufficient.

## Follow-up

In the week following the first visit, the owner should be contacted so that any questions they may have can be answered and the response to date can be assessed. Subsequently, owners should be encouraged to keep in regular contact by phone in order to discuss any specific issue that arises.

If it is difficult for the owner to control the presence of the triggering stimuli, it may be advisable to use pharmacological treatment in conjunction with the behavioural programme. If pharmacological treatment is not initially suggested, it may be added at a later date, perhaps as an incentive after the first month of therapy.

## Prevention of the problem

Although many fear-related reactions may be explained in terms of conditioned processes (e.g. a past negative experience causes the fearful response), not all fearful reactions develop in this manner. In some cases inadequate or inappropriate exposure to specific stimuli, such as locations, objects, people or animals during the developmental phases may lead to the development of fearful responses in relation to these in later life.

To avoid such an occurrence, owners should expose young animals to as many stimuli as possible within the capacity of the individual during the sensitive socialization stage of development, i.e. when animals are well suited to accept novelty. Ideally exposure to these should be gradual so as to allow the animal to habituate and become used to the novel stimuli. In some cases rewards may be required to build positive associations (see Chapters 3 and 4). Thus fearful behaviours can be prevented with frequent exposure to people, animals and a wide range of environments in a controlled, positive way during the early months of the pet's life (Landsberg *et al.*, 2003).

Reducing general stress in later life will also reduce the risk of dishabituation and prevent problems developing later in life as a result of this phenomenon (see Chapter 13).

## Conclusion

It is essential to understand the normal processes underlying the fear response in pets, in order to explain why in certain circumstances specific behaviours emerge and what the best methods are to resolve these. Preventive advice depends on an understanding of the normal species-typical developmental processes in dogs and cats. One of the most fundamental roles of a veterinary surgeon is as an educator, i.e. to teach owners the importance of allowing their pets the opportunity to form positive associations with their environment so as to inhibit negative ones as far as possible.

## References and further reading

Appleby D, Bradshaw JWS and Casey R (2002) Relationship between aggressive and avoidance behavior by dogs and their experience in the first six months of life. *The Veterinary Record* **150**, 434–438

Archer J (1976) The organization of aggression and fear in vertebrates. In: *Perspectives in Ethology, Vol. 2*, ed. PPG Bateson and PH Klopfer, pp. 231–298. Plenum Press, New York

Bear MF, Connors BW and Paradiso MA (2001) *Neuroscience: Exploring the Brain*. Lippincott Williams and Wilkins, Baltimore, Maryland

Beaver B (1999) Canine behavior of sensory and neural origin. In: *Canine Behavior: A Guide for Veterinarians*, ed. B Beaver, pp. 43–105. WB Saunders, Philadelphia

Berton F, Vogel E and Belzung C (1998) Modulation of mice anxiety in response to cat odor as a consequence of predators diet. *Physiology and Behavior* **65**, 247–254

Blanchard RJ, Hebert MA, Ferrari P *et al.* (1998) Defensive behaviours in wild and laboratory (Swiss) mice: the Mouse Defense Test Battery. *Physiology and Behavior* **65**, 561–569

Crowell-Davis S and Murray T (2006) *Veterinary Psychopharmacology*. Blackwell Publishing, Ames, Iowa

Dehasse J (1994) Sensory, emotional and social development of the young dog. *Bulletin of Veterinary Clinical Ethology* **2**, 6–29

Eibl-Eibesfeldt I and Sutterlin C (1990) Fear, defense and aggression in animals and men: some ethological perspectives. In: *Fear and Defense*, ed. PF Brain and S Parmigiani, pp. 381–408. Harwood Academic, London

Frank D and Dehasse J (2003) Differential diagnosis and management of human-directed aggression in cats. *Veterinary Clinics of North America: Small Animal Practice* **33**, 269–286

Fox MW (1978) Behavior, develoment and psychopathology of cardiac activity. In: *The Dog. Its Domestication and Behavior*. Garland STPM Press, New York

Gallagher M and Holland PC (1994) The amygdala complex: multiple roles in associative learning and attention. *Proceedings of the National Academy of Sciences USA* **91**, 11771–11776

Gandia Estellés M and Mills DS (2006) Signs of travel-related problems in dogs and their response to treatment with dog-appeasing pheromone. *The Veterinary Record* **159**, 143–148

Gross JJ (1999) Emotion regulation: past, present, future. *Cognition and Emotion* **13**, 551–573

Houpt KA (1991) House soiling: treatment of a common feline problem. *Veterinary Medicine* **86**, 1000–1006

Hovda DA, Villabianca JR, Chugani HT *et al.* (1996) Cerebral metabolism following neonatal or adult hemineocortication in cats. 1. Effects on glucose metabolism using [C-14]2-deoxy-D-glucose autoradiography. *Journal of Cerebral Blood Flow and Metabolism* **16**, 134–146

Hydbring-Sandberg E, von Walter LW, Höglund K *et al.* (2004) Physiological reactions to fear provocation in dogs. *Journal of Endocrinology* **180**, 439–448

King T, Hemsworth PH and Coleman GJ (2003) Fear of novel and startling stimuli in domestic dogs. *Applied Animal Behaviour Science* **82**, 45–64

Landsberg GM, Hunthausen W and Ackerman L (2003) *Handbook of Behaviour Problems of the Cat and Dog, 2nd edn*, pp. 314–315. Butterworth Heinemann, Oxford

Levine ED, Ramos D and Mills DS (2007) A prospective study of two self-help CD based desensitization and counter-conditioning programmes with the use of Dog Appeasing Pheromone for the treatment of firework fears in dogs (*Canis familiaris*). *Applied Animal Behaviour Science* **105**, 311–329

Lindsay SR (2001) Etiology and assessment of behavior problems. In: *Handbook of Applied Dog Behavior and Training, Vol. 2*, pp. 147–159. Iowa State University Press, Ames, Iowa

Livesey PJ (1986) *Learning and Emotion: A Biological Synthesis.* Lawrence Erlbaum Associates, Hillsdale, New Jersey

McCune S (1995) The impact of paternity and early socialisation on the development of cats' behaviour to people and novel objects. *Applied Animal Behaviour Science* **45**, 109–124

Mills DS, Ramos D, Estelles MG and Hargrave C (2006) A triple blind placebo-controlled investigation into the assessment of the effect of Dog Appeasing Pheromone (DAP) on anxiety related behavior of problem dogs in the veterinary clinic. *Applied Animal Behaviour Science* **98**, 114–126

Ohl F, Arndt SS, van der Staay FJ (2008) Pathological anxiety in animals. *Veterinary Journal* **175**, 18–26

Overall KL (1997) *Clinical Behavioral Medicine for Small Animals.* Mosby Year Book, St Louis

Overall KL, Dunham AE and Frank D (2001) Frequency of nonspecific clinical signs in dogs with separation anxiety, thunderstorm phobia, and noise phobia, alone or in combination. *Journal of the American Veterinary Medical Association* **219**, 467–472

Poulton R, Davies S, Menzies RG *et al.* (1998) Evidence of a non-associative model of the acquisition of fear of heights. *Behaviour and Research Therapy* **36**, 537–544

Scott JP and Fuller M (1965) *Genetic and Social Behavior of the Dog.* University of Chicago Press, Chicago

Sheppard G and Mills DS (2003) Evaluation of dog-appeasing pheromone as a potential treatment for dogs fearful of fireworks. *The Veterinary Record* **152**, 432–436

Shuhama R, Del-Ben CM, Loureiro SR *et al.* (2007) Animal defense strategies and anxiety disorders. *Annals of the Brazilian Academy of Sciences* **79**, 97–109

Shull-Selcer E and Stagg W (1991) Advances in the understanding and treatment of noise phobias. In: *Veterinary Clinics of North America: Small Animal Practice* **21**, 353–367.

Stanford TL (1981) Behaviour of dogs entering a veterinary clinic. *Applied Animal Ethology* **7**, 271–279

Thomas KJ, Murphee OD and Newton JEO (1972) Effect of person and environment on heart rates in two strains of pointer dogs. *Conditional Reflex* **7**, 74–81

Tuber DS, Hotersall D and Peters MF (1982) Treatment of fears and phobias in dogs. *Veterinary Clinics of North America: Small Animal Practice* **12**, 607–623

Voith VL and Borchelt PL (1996) Separation anxiety in dogs. In: *Readings in Companion Animal Behaviour*, ed. PL Borchelt. Veterinary Learning Systems, Trenton, New Jersey

Willis MB (1989) *Genetics of the Dog.* Howell Book House, New York

Wolfle TL (1990) Policy, program and people: the three P's to wellbeing. In: *Canine Research Environment*, ed. JA Mench and L Krulisch, pp. 41–47. Scientist Center for Animal Welfare, Bethesda, Maryland

Young PT (1959) The role of affective processes in learning and motivation. *Psychological Review* **66**, 104–125

## Client handouts (bsavalibrary.com/behaviour_leaflets)

- Adopting a rescue dog: the pros and cons
- Canine behaviour profile
- Canine behaviour questionnaire
- Cognitive dysfunction syndrome
- Down–stay mat exercises
- Headcollar training
- Introducing a new cat into the household
- Muzzle training
- 'Nothing in Life is Free'
- Playing with your dog – toys

- Request for information on problem behaviours
- Sit–stay exercises
- Teaching your dog to go to a place on command
- Treating a fear of car journeys using desensitization and counter-conditioning
- Treating a fear of the veterinary clinic using desensitization and counter-conditioning
- What your dog needs

# 17

# Aggression toward familiar people and animals

## Tiny De Keuster and Hildegard Jung

## Introduction

Dogs can provide love, companionship and acceptance for all family members, particularly young children. Children who have pets engage more in social interactions and empathy (Poresky, 1996) and having a good relationship with a dog can help a child to overcome grief and sadness (Triebenbacher, 1998). However, dog bites to humans represent an important public health problem: for example, it is estimated that 1.5% of the US population (Gilchrist *et al.*, 2008) and more than 1% of the UK population (NHS Statistics, 2008) are affected annually, and the proportion appears to be increasing. The majority of bites happen in familiar surroundings and it is estimated that more than half go unreported (Bernardo *et al.*, 2002; Kahn *et al.*, 2004). In addition, owning pets may represent potential hazards through the zoonotic transmission of disease (Bender and Minicucci, 2007). Veterinary surgeons have a crucial role in providing information and practical advice on living safely with a pet dog, retaining the benefits and minimizing the risks of cohabitation.

Treating problems of aggression toward family members can be considered as one of the most challenging problems. The veterinary surgeon is confronted not only with the risk of injury to the family, but also with the emotional consequences of the pet's behaviour: doubts, anger, grief, disappointment about their beloved pet turning against them. The primary aim of veterinary intervention should be to prevent aggression occurring in the first place.

## Evaluation of the patient

The way the term aggression is (mis)used in the media may enhance the perception that aggression is about ill-intentioned and violent behaviour. For this reason, where a family member is involved, owners may tell the veterinary surgeon that the dog was just 'nipping' or giving 'a love bite'. It is important for the veterinary surgeon to be sensitive to suggestions of aggression and potentially a proactive approach to the problem may be warranted.

The goals in evaluating the presenting case should be:

- To check correspondence between owner observations and owner interpretations
- To encourage owners to give their accounts in full

- To avoid any judgement about the dog's behaviour or character
- To evaluate the physical health of the animal
- To keep people and other animals safe.

## Managing initial presentations

### The direct request for help

Any request for help with an aggressive animal must be taken seriously. While aggressive behaviour is reported to be the most frequent reason for referral to a behaviourist, it remains unclear how often owners report their pet's aggressive behaviour to their veterinary surgeon. A Canadian study found that 15% of dogs had bitten someone, but none of the bites had been a reason for consulting the veterinary surgeon (Guy *et al.*, 2001). It is important to stay within the level of competence, and the option of referral should be considered at all times.

### The casual comment during a routine health check

Dog owners may talk informally to the veterinary surgeon during a routine health check, mentioning a growl or a bite without any specific detail, and may just want to check whether there is a problem or may hope to receive assurance. For example, they may say: 'By the way, yesterday Bobby growled at my daughter a few times, but I don't think it meant anything. I don't think there's anything to worry about, because he is such a loving pet and has never done this before.' In this situation it is easy to miss an opportunity to follow up a potential problem because of a lack of time in the typical consultation, the ambiguous information provided by the owner (just a few growls, otherwise he behaves as a beloved pet), or being misled by the dog's good behaviour during the clinical examination. It is equally important to realize that actions like judging the dog ('Oh, that's not very good'), or offering quick solutions ('He needs to be properly trained') without proper investigation, may stop the owner from revealing important details. An owner's remark about a pet otherwise not being 'aggressive' should prompt a thorough clinical examination in order to exclude underlying physical disease (painful processes, sensory impairment, etc). A client-centred approach, taking a collaborative role, is the best way to manage these situations. This means engaging with the owners, showing empathy and encouraging them to tell the full story, with steering questions to help (see History taking, below).

**Proactive investigation of risk**

Even when a pet has bitten a family member, or another pet in the household, the owner may not necessarily take the lead and request a behavioural evaluation. Owners need to appreciate that aggressive behaviour includes not only bites but also threats and snapping. Routine assessment for these signs should be the norm and prompt a more complete behavioural investigation. To encourage owners to come forward with potentially important information, it may be useful to show them the Ladder of Aggression (Figure 17.1; see Chapter 2 for full explanation) and explain that a growl, snap and bite are the strategies representing the highest steps on the ladder, meaning that the dog feels stressed and threatened and uses them as the ultimate strategy. The veterinary surgeon should explain to the owner that it is better to manage these potential problems early on if possible.

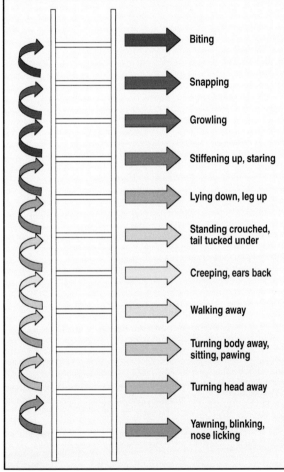

**17.1** The canine Ladder of Aggression: how a dog reacts to stress or threat. Concept developed by Kendal Shepherd.

**The emergency phone call**

Owners may contact the practice with an immediate request for help and advice on damage control, especially after an incident. Good communication at this time is an important skill. Questions should be short and clear, and aimed at understanding: what has happened; with whom; in what context (where and how); and where the dog is now. Safety is paramount and the following advice should be given to the owner:

1. Be calm.
2. Do not shout at the dog or at the victim.
3. Do not punish the dog (because of the risk of further escalation or renewed arousal).
4. Put the dog in a safe location and provide safety for the victim. If this is not possible, summon emergency help.
5. Seek medical assistance for the victim.
6. Make an appointment for clinical examination of the dog and/or referral to a veterinary behaviour specialist as soon as possible.

**Making the appointment**

The degree of emergency may be influenced by several factors: what has happened; who the victim is; how severe the injuries are; and to what extent the owner can secure the situation until the time of appointment. If the owner feels unsafe for themselves or for others, the option of immediately placing the dog in a secure kennel or hospital shelter might be considered in order to protect the safety of the family.

In all cases relating to aggression, it is advisable to establish a safety protocol for clinic staff concerning the planning of the appointment. It is essential to inform all staff about the imminent appointment and the safety measures to take, *before* the dog arrives.

Safety precautions should also be taken in preparation for the clinical examination. To minimize the risk, the context of the aggression should be initially investigated to provide facts about how the dog reacts to stimuli or actions such as eye contact, standing up, approaching the dog, reaching out for the dog, or any other form of physical contact. If it is concluded that any of the manipulations required during a clinical examination may trigger aggression (a threat or a bite), the use of a muzzle is indicated before starting the examination. It is advisable to ask whether the owner is capable of putting the muzzle in place themselves; if not, advice on muzzle training can be given in advance of the consultation, if it is safe to do so (see **client handout**).

In order to obtain information that is as complete as possible, any adults who witnessed the bite should be invited to the appointment. If a child has been bitten, parents will quite often not have seen it happen and the context of the bite remains unclear. The victim's feelings and safety should always be addressed. In case of doubt, talking to the victim without the dog being present may be a preferred first step.

Legally, responsibility for the safety of others extends to the waiting room. It is therefore necessary to have the owner's agreement that they will keep the dog on a short lead at all times. Where a dog has injured a family member, it is preferable to schedule the appointment when there are no other adults or children in the waiting room and the owners should be asked to muzzle the dog before entering the clinic if possible.

**History taking**

In most cases the professional will not have the chance to witness the accident or have a video recording of the event, so investigation depends on the ability to investigate the owner's observations through skilful history taking.

Aggressive behaviour can be described in terms of individual behavioural elements such as growling, baring teeth, biting, snapping, body postures and vocalizations. Each of these elements can be exhibited in a range of functionally distinct behaviour patterns, including agonistic behaviour, predation and play (Beaver, 1999). While any of these three behavioural patterns may potentially cause harm to an individual, they arise from differing motivational states with different goals. It is therefore important to recognize the differences between them (Figure 17.2; see also Figure 17.27).

In addition, the incident that led to the appointment may not necessarily be the worst that has happened.

It is necessary to investigate whether aggressive responses are only presented in this context and with this stimulus, or whether the animal presents aggressive reactions in other situations. However, owners might have no idea how their dog responds in some situations (e.g. when a child approaches), because they have always avoided such situations. It is important to distinguish between known experience and anticipated response.

When taking the history, it is important to resist the temptation to comment on what happened and instead to focus on professional behavioural questioning in order to obtain a full history. Open-ended questions invite owners to tell their stories (Figure 17.3). They

| Element | Agonistic behaviour | Play | Predation |
|---|---|---|---|
| Goal | Threat aversion<br>Conflict resolution | Development of social and predatory skills<br>No conflict | Killing prey; feeding<br>No conflict |
| Associated emotional valence | Negative<br>Unpleasant | Positive<br>Pleasant | Positive<br>Pleasant |
| Behavioural precedents | Threat or frustration related | Enticement, including approach and avoidance | Stalking |
| **Arousal** | | | |
| Growling | Yes | Yes | No |
| Barking | Yes/no | Yes/no | No |
| Sympathetic nervous system | High | Variable | Low generally |
| **Visual signals** | | | |
| Play-bow | No | Yes | No |
| Threatening body postures | Yes | No | No |
| Baring of teeth | Yes | Yes | No |
| Snapping | Yes | Possibly | No |
| Staring | Yes | Yes | Yes |
| Stalking | Rarely | Possibly | Yes |
| Biting | Possibly | Possibly | Yes |

**17.2** Differences in aggressive elements of agonistic behaviour, aggressive play and predation.

| **Event: *Dog takes a nap on his dog bed; 3-year-old Emma approaches and wants to hug him; dog snaps at child's face, leaving a mark*** | | |
|---|---|---|
| Exploring content of aggression | Question (open-ended questions) | Example answer |
| What | *Please tell me what happened.* | Our dog has bitten 3-year-old Emma in the face. |
| Detail of injury | *How deep is the injury?* | Well, a tooth went through the skin of her upper cheek. They had to do four stitches. |
| Where | *Please describe how it happened.* | My dog was having a nap on his bed and somehow Emma was bitten. |
| How | *What did you see just before it happened?* | I saw Emma running around and playing and then she must have gone near the dog's resting place. |
| Threatening signals | *And what happened next?* | Well, I heard him growl twice, I'm pretty sure about that. |
| Explore how far owner intervened | *And how did you react?* | I told him off immediately and said loudly 'Stop growling!' |
| Explore dog's reaction | *What happened then?* | Then he bit her in the face. |
| Explore owner's reactions | *What did you do next?* | I took Emma away and punished my dog for being naughty. |
| Explore other contexts | *In what other situation(s) do you observe your dog growling?* | My dog growls at me when I try to clean his feet. He growls at my husband when he punishes him. |

**17.3** Examples of open-ended questions.

cannot be answered with a 'no' or 'yes' or 'three times in the last week'. While closed questions focus on the questioner's agenda and thus place the owner in a passive and less engaged role, open questions allow spontaneous and unguided responses, which help to build rapport and trust. Closed questions usually begin with 'Did you … (punish your dog after he attacked you)?', whereas open questions usually begin with the phrase: 'Tell me about … (what happened after your dog attacked you) – please describe what you observed.'

By asking the owner to describe the incident and other contexts where aggression has been observed, a few things may quickly become apparent. Taking the example in Figure 17.3:

- The veterinary surgeon may be able to conclude from the answers that the incident was due to aggression associated with negative emotional arousal, and not to play or predation behaviour
- The dog emitted warning signals prior to the bite, such as growls or signs of unease (see Ladder of Aggression, Figure 17.1)
- The owner did not understand the meaning of the behaviour or preceding signs and reacted inappropriately, e.g. with punishment
- The bite resulted from inappropriate intervention when the animal was highly aroused or frustrated (redirected aggression), in which case the focus should be on managing the frustration and teaching owners how to intervene without risking injury (see **client handout** on redirected aggression)

- Further contexts are evident (cleaning feet, punishment) when aggression has happened
- This case requires specialist intervention, an option that should be considered at all times in the evaluation of these cases.

It is important to distinguish:

- Negative emotional behaviour from aggressive behaviour that is not associated with a negative emotional state (e.g. play and predatory behaviour)
- Incidents that arise as a result of inappropriate intervention (e.g. when a dog is highly aroused and someone intervenes, resulting in a redirected bite) from those that arise from a dog's insecurity in a social situation (which is the focus of this chapter), since the former is relatively straightforward to recognize and is covered in the section on teaching owners how to interact safely with their pet at the end of this chapter
- Aggression that has been largely conditioned as a result of inappropriate attempts at control and punishment in response to other individuals. In these cases the individuals may be familiar but are not part of the dog's normal social group. This is covered in Chapter 5.

To clarify these distinctions it is necessary to explore the daily routine of the client and their pet specifically (Figure 17.4), in order to make sure that all the household contexts that might give rise to aggression have been covered, and to obtain an overview of the day-to-day interactions between the

| Behaviour | Questions | Considerations |
|---|---|---|
| Feeding | What (daily food, extras, bones)?<br>How, when, where, by whom?<br>Stealing food: Y/N; when, from whom?<br>Guarding food: Y/N; when, where?<br>Pica: Y/N<br>How solved: by whom, punishment? | Aggressive signalling (specify context)<br>Predatory patterns |
| Drinking | Amount: normal/excessive<br>How, when, where, by whom? | Aggressive signalling (specify context) |
| Self-grooming | Frequency: normal/excessive<br>Lesions?<br>Owner's reaction (specify)<br>Punishment: Y/N; How, when, where, by whom? | Anxious personality<br>Aggressive signalling (specify context) |
| Elimination | Housetrained: Y/N; how, when, where, by whom?<br>House soiling: Y/N; when, what, where, when?<br>Urine marking: Y/N; when, what, where, when?<br>Owner's reaction (specify)<br>Punishment: Y/N; how, when, where, by whom? | Aggressive signalling (specify context)<br>Anxiety disorders |
| Sleeping | Where (dog bed, owner's bed, other)?<br>Amount of sleep (night/day): how long, with whom? | Aggressive signalling (specify context)<br>Restlessness, anxiety |
| Exploratory | Sequence (normal/inhibited/overactive); specify context; specify owner's reaction<br>Quality: normal/oral/sucking/pica; specify context; specify owner's reaction<br>Spatial orientation, e.g.:<br>• star-shaped, focused on owner (indicative of anxiety/attachment)<br>• disorientation (specify context; see cognitive dysfunction syndrome in Chapter 12)<br>Owner's reaction (specify)<br>Punishment: Y/N; how, when, where, by whom? | Anxiety<br>Aggressive signalling (specify context)<br>Prelude to predatory behaviour<br>Prelude to play-biting |

**17.4** Example of questions exploring daily routine for a dog that growls and bites while interacting with familiar people or pets. (continues) ▶

| Behaviour | Questions | Considerations |
|---|---|---|
| Sexual | Mounting: people/conspecific/other species/inanimate objects?<br>Owner's reaction (specify)<br>Punishment: Y/N; how, when, where, by whom? | Anxiety, frustration<br>Aggressive signalling (specify context)<br>Play-bite related |
| Play | Excessive/appropriate/lack?<br>With whom: family members/conspecifics /other family pets?<br>Describe play session: who initiates, who stops session?<br>Bite inhibition: Y/N (specify context)<br>Specify problems; specify owner's reaction<br>Punishment: Y/N; how, when, where, by whom? | Play-bite<br>Aggressive signalling (specify context)<br>Anxiety |

**17.4** (continued) Example of questions exploring daily routine for a dog that growls and bites while interacting with familiar people or pets.

family and the dog(s) and the owner's expectations of how a dog should behave. It is worth emphasizing that aggression may arise in any of these contexts as a result of a physical condition; a medical examination should therefore always precede the behavioural interpretation of the signs.

Ideally, the owner will provide clear facts about the animal's problem, but in reality the messages provided by owners will be a mixture of fact (the problem) and interpretation (the owner's view on the problem). In addition, messages might be coloured by the way the problem makes the owner feel (unhappy, angry, frightened, disappointed) or how the problem influences family life (disagreement, guilt, blame, conflict) (Miller and Rollnick, 1991). Examples of different interpretations of the same event that might be expressed are shown in Figure 17.5. The aim is to encourage the owner to express things objectively, but not to 'put words into their mouth' or assume the objective from the subjective (Figure 17.6).

**Event: *Dog takes a nap on his dog bed; 3-year-old Emma approaches and wants to hug him; dog snaps at child's face, leaving a mark (see also Figure 17.3)***

| Type of communication in describing event | Examples of description of event |
|---|---|
| Client objectively describes what happened | Our dog Brutus has snapped at Emma, our 3-year-old daughter, and wounded her in the face. It happened like this: Brutus was having a nap on his dog bed while Emma approached to hug him. He snapped at her, leaving a small mark on her face. |
| Client describes his view on the problem | I think Brutus must have been jealous of Emma approaching his dog bed. Or Emma must have done something naughty to him and therefore he snapped at her. |
| Client describes how it made him feel (angry, guilty, unhappy, frightened, despair) | I don't understand what happened. Brutus is such a lovely dog and we treat him with so much love, and now he does this to my little Emma! I feel angry and very disappointed about him. |
| Client describes what happened, mixed with how the situation influences family dynamics | My husband thinks we should euthanize the dog, because he has 'attacked' our daughter Emma. I think it was just a little misunderstanding, but my husband is convinced that a dog who once has tasted blood is 'lost' and should be euthanized. |

**17.5** Examples of interpretation of an event – the subjective evaluations are important elements to consider in the management of the problem.

**Event: *Dog takes a nap on his dog bed; 3-year-old Emma approaches and wants to hug him; dog snaps at child's face, leaving a mark (see also Figures 17.3 and 17.5)***

| Exploring context of aggression | Open-ended questions | Example answer |
|---|---|---|
| Explore action | *Please tell me what happened.* | I think our dog is jealous of our 3-year-old daughter and therefore he snapped at her. |
| | When owner responds by interpreting the event, change the way of questioning:<br>*Please describe what you witnessed.* | Brutus was having a nap on his dog bed while 3-year-old Emma approached to hug him. He snapped at her, leaving a small puncture mark on her face. |
| Explore owner reaction | *What happened next?* | Well, I told him off and punished him for being naughty, and then he bit my finger – as you can see I have two stitches. |
| Empathize and explore dog's reaction | *It's good that you sought medical advice on the bite. How did your dog react after he had bitten you?* | He had this guilty look on his face, so I assume he knew he'd done wrong! First with Emma and then with me! |
| | When owner responds by interpreting the event, change the way of questioning:<br>*Please describe to me what you mean by guilty look?* | Well, he lay down in his basket, with his leg lifted up, his ear backwards, and licking his lips. He looked at me with big black eyes, which made me feel frightened. |

**17.6** Example of how the consultation may be guided to obtain the necessary information in relation to an incident. (continues) ▶

| Event: *Dog takes a nap on his dog bed; 3-year-old Emma approaches and wants to hug him; dog snaps at child's face, leaving a mark (see also Figures 17.3 and 17.5)* | | |
|---|---|---|
| **Exploring context of aggression** | **Open-ended questions** | **Example answer** |
| Explore other contexts | *Which other situations can you describe where your dog growled or snapped or behaved with the signs you can see on this ladder?* (Show the Ladder of Aggression and ask owner to use colours and words on the Ladder) | Brutus does the red one [growl] when any of the family approaches his food bowl or when he's chewing a bone. He normally does the yellow one [leaving] when my 3-year-old wants to cuddle him while he's lying in his basket – he goes hiding under the table. So when Emma follows him to cuddle, he does the orange-red one, he growls at her. |
| Explore owner's reaction to these contexts | *How do you and your husband handle these situations? What do you both do?* | I am used to telling Brutus off and raising my finger to show him he has done wrong. The problem is that my husband thinks I am too strict and that growling is normal, so he then cuddles the dog to make friends again. |

**17.6** (continued) Example of how the consultation may be guided to obtain the necessary information in relation to an incident.

## Client attitudes, beliefs and behaviour

It is particularly important that the attitudes, beliefs and behaviour of a client are evaluated with sensitivity. Owners are likely to be very distressed by events and their conflicting loyalties and potentially confused and/or defensive as a consequence, but it is also important to address misconceptions. In contrast to the belief that the ability to talk to people or to communicate effectively is an inherent attribute, studies in human medicine confirm that communication skills can be learned and applied effectively (Miller and Rollnick, 1991; Cornell and Kopcha, 2007). Figure 17.7 gives some examples of these skills in a veterinary context.

### Typical owner misconceptions

Owner misconceptions need to be identified and addressed in order to manage the risk of the situation. Typical misconceptions include:

- If I train my dog, he won't bite – it's really an obedience problem
- My dog won't bite (again) – it was a one-off event that could happen to anyone
- My dog felt jealous – overcomplicating the problem with anthropomorphism
- Punishment reduces aggression – I must be dominant to my dog.

*'If I train my dog, he won't bite':* Owners may assume that an obedient dog will not bite (Figure 17.8). Training is also generally promoted as a positive strategy to reduce the incidence of bites. However, a study of child-directed canine aggression showed that in 66% of cases where a dog had bitten a child, the dog had previously attended obedience classes (Reisner *et al.*, 2007).

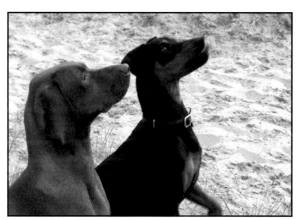

**17.8** Training alone is not sufficient to reduce dog bites. A dog may be obedient but still anxious and so a potential risk. Note the nose licking and paw lifting apparent in this obediently sitting dog. (Courtesy of M. Laureys.)

| Example: *The owner has told the veterinary surgeon: 'My dog is such a nice companion, but since he has bitten my child I feel confused. I really don't want to euthanize my dog.'* | | |
|---|---|---|
| **Type of communication** | **Meaning** | **Importance** |
| Empathetic approach (providing understanding for the owner's situation) | Seeing the world through the owner's eyes Sharing in the owner's experiences | Understands owner's perspective Lets the owner know you are listening Emphasizes the owner's positive statements to diffuse resistance |
| Appropriate, empathetic response | 'I understand that you came to see me in order to find out if you can work out a safe solution for keeping your dog while preserving the safety of your child.' | This response will improve the chances of obtaining sensitive information |
| Inappropriate 'judgmental' response | 'Of course you're confused, because you're living with a potential time-bomb with that dog!' | This response might induce resistance or 'block' the owner's request for help |

**17.7** Client communication skills.

***'My dog won't bite (again)':*** Wilson *et al.* (2003) found that most parents were unaware of the possible dangers that accompany owning a dog. Even though 20% of the dog-owning households in the study reported that their child had been bitten by the family dog, nearly all of the parents allowed their children to play unsupervised with their dog at least some of the time. In addition, the majority of parents believed that their dog would not bite if their child interrupted their dog while it was eating or sleeping, when it was guarding a toy or possession, when it was challenged, or when it was excited. In reality, these are all situations that might be considered high risk, as to the dog they represent potentially threatening behaviour. Hence parents need to become more knowledgeable about potentially dangerous child–dog interactions and the influence of the behaviour of the potential victim on normal responses by a dog.

***'My dog felt jealous':*** Dog owners may have difficulties in understanding the reason for their dog's aggressive behaviour, and will often tend to use anthropomorphism and complex human-like explanations rather than recognizing that the dog may have felt threatened. Owners have less difficulty understanding the connection between a painful condition (e.g. ear infection) and reacting aggressively when handled at non-painful times, even though the dog is normally friendly. However, aggression in either context can be a response to perceived threat. The veterinary surgeon should be supportive and try to understand the owner's viewpoint. The Ladder of Aggression can be useful in helping the owner to understand that the dog was reacting to a stressful situation. By going through all the day-to-day situations where the dog displayed signs relating to the lower end of the ladder, owners can be guided to appreciate how their pet is often uneasy in a wider range of situations which perhaps come together in certain circumstances to produce a more overt response (see Figure 17.23).

***'Punishment reduces aggression':*** Owners may have been advised by someone who 'knows about dogs' that their dog wants to be 'vicious or dominant' or that they are 'guilty' of being 'too soft' and not having educated their dog about who is the boss. Owners often take this advice seriously, because it appears intuitively reasonable and is often supported by misrepresentations of dog and/or wolf social structure.

They are therefore told to start to punish the dog physically in order to reduce aggression. However, there is no evidence that dogs are motivated by dominance; rather, aggressive encounters with familiar individuals are context-specific and reinforced by learning. Stable social groups are, by definition, characterized by peaceful interactions between individuals rather than by violence.

An investigation of trigger factors for bites in children found that 59% of bites happened as a consequence of discipline measures (Reisner *et al.*, 2007). Physical punishment and harsh training methods may induce fear, anxiety and aggressive reactions in the dog and should therefore be avoided. Punishment may also suppress lower level aggressive indicators (growling, snarling) and thus make the more serious aggressive responses seem unpredictable.

## Risk evaluation

Even if aggressive behaviour does not result in injury, it may have other serious ramifications. It may permanently disrupt the bond and trust that owners feel with their pet; and this may ultimately lead to euthanasia or the relinquishment of the pet to a shelter. In one US study, 40% of dog owners cited behavioural problems as one of the reasons for surrender, and of these 40% cited 'aggressive behaviour' (Salman *et al.*, 1998). However, the problem does not relate only to the dog, but also to its environment. Therefore risk assessment requires consideration of:

- The ability to control the environmental triggers for the behaviour as identified from the history (e.g. if the dog was provoked by a screaming child nearby, can this realistically be controlled in a household with several young children?)
- The physical and behavioural characteristics of the dog that alter either the risk associated with the severity of any bite, or the risk of recurrence. Figure 17.9 outlines factors that should guide an assessment of risk of severe injury should the problem recur. Figure 17.11 lists the dog-related factors that inform an assessment of the risk of recurrence. The chance that a dog who has bitten in the past in a specific context in response to specific stimuli will bite again is increased when the same situation recurs. However, it cannot be concluded that the risk for a bite in a different context (the presence of adults) is necessarily also elevated.

| Factors | Detail | High risk for injury to victim |
|---|---|---|
| *Dog-related* | | |
| Size, weight, strength | Large, heavy, muscular | Higher potential to cause physical harm to victim (e.g. jumping against/on), independent of biting behaviour |
| Bite inhibition/ control | Lack of bite inhibition | Higher potential to cause injury to humans, especially children, during excitement, play and other forms of arousal |
| Thresholds for arousal and biting | Lower thresholds | A dog with a lower threshold for arousal, linked to a lowered threshold for aggression, biting, mouthing and play-biting, represents a higher risk of injury to all humans, especially children. Hence, dogs with lack of self-control and dogs suffering from anxiety represent high risks |

**17.9** Dog- and victim-related bite factors to consider in evaluating the injury risk should an aggressive incident recur. (continues) ▶

| Factors | Detail | High risk for injury to victim |
|---|---|---|
| **Victim-related** | | |
| Human target of injury | Young age | Children are bitten seriously twice as often as other age groups. Young children (average 5 years) are at especially high risk. Child age and bite severity are inversely correlated |
| Location of injury | Head, neck, facial injuries | Child age is significantly and inversely related to the number of facial injuries (see Figure 17.10). More frequently associated with: hospitalization; post-traumatic stress disorder; fatality |
| Severity of injury | Small puncture *versus* laceration *versus* lesion with tissue loss | Injuries that break skin should be considered higher risk. Risk from type in ascending order: haematoma; tooth through the skin; deep tissue loss |
| Number of bites | More than one | Multiple bites represent higher risk for the victim. Multiple bites represent poor behavioural sequence (no stop signal after the first bite), thus higher risk situation |

**17.9** (continued) Dog- and victim-related bite factors to consider in evaluating the injury risk should an aggressive incident recur.

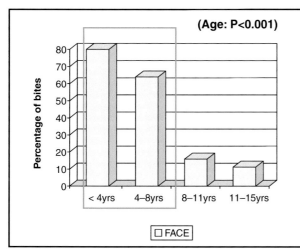
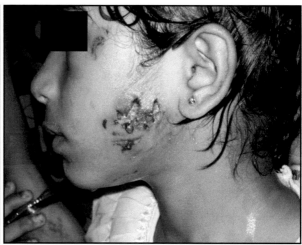

**17.10** In a survey of children presented at emergency departments for dog bites, facial injuries were more common in younger children. The photo shows a bite on the face of a young girl. (Data from Kahn *et al.* (2003); photograph courtesy of R. Butcher.)

| Dog risk factor | Detail | High risk of recurrence |
|---|---|---|
| Type of aggression | Offensive | Dog shows aggression toward victim without 'apparent' previous action/interaction of the victim |
| Context of aggression | Unclear | Owner unable to list context where aggression happens |
| | Undefined | No witness ('We don't know how it happened') |
| | Many contexts | All contexts are possible ('It could happen at any time') |
| Triggering stimuli | Unclear | Owner unable to identify the eliciting stimulus of aggression |
| | Undefined | No witness ('We don't know exactly what the victim did') |
| | Multiple | All stimuli may trigger a bite ('It could happen at any time') |
| Kind of triggering stimuli | Benign | Gazing, eye contact, looking at, passing by, approaching, bending towards, reaching out. Touching, petting, handling, hugging, kissing. Stepping over, walking by, sitting beside, lying beside, lifting up, holding |
| Reaction towards triggering stimuli | Inconsistent | Dog sometimes responds in an aggressive way and at other times in a non-aggressive way |
| Warning signals prior to bite | Absent or Present but not observed | Dog bites without detectable warning stimulus or dog warns and bites at the same time. Victim has no chance to escape the bite |
| Historical information | Known bite history with context/trigger | Risk of recurrence in this context or with this trigger is high(er) |

**17.11** Dog behavioural context features associated with an aggressive incident that alter the general risk of recurrence. See main text for details of other factors to consider in evaluating the specific risk, including a recurrence of the eliciting behaviour of potential victims.

## Diagnosis

The term aggression is descriptive and not diagnostic; it should be interpreted as a general sign of a more complicated condition. It indicates merely that a behaviour has taken place that someone believes might have resulted in harm and does not indicate a cause.

In the first instance it is necessary to distinguish between aggressive behaviour associated with predation, play and some form of mental challenge (e.g. threat or frustration). Beyond this, there is no consensus between scientists on how aggression should be classified. Some authors classify aggression by its target (e.g. owner-directed, child-directed, stranger-directed, dog-directed), others by its context (food-related, territorial, fear-related), or supposed function (dominance, hierarchical). This causes inevitable confusion for practitioners reading handbooks on canine behaviour. Yet, by looking at the aforementioned list of popular subtypes of what is called 'aggression' (as opposed to play or predation), it is important to recognize that they all share a common element of underlying motivation: they all reflect responses to an aversive situation and so indicate that the dog's welfare is being compromised, and are associated with a negative '**affect**' (or emotion).

### Clinical diagnosis

In order to infer the underlying motivation, correct information is required about the contexts that have triggered the aggression and about the human–dog relationship and the family dynamics involved (other pets and people living in the family who influence the dog's behaviour). While diagnosing a physical disease is commonly based on laboratory and clinical evidence, behavioural diagnoses should be considered more as a working hypothesis to be checked and rechecked.

In this chapter an essential *functional* distinction is made first between **predation** and **play** (both being non-affective behaviours) and **affective aggression** (behaviours associated with a negative emotional state) toward familiar individuals who form part of the animal's normal social contacts (see Figures 17.2 and 17.27). Affective aggression is then subdivided on a *contextual* basis to highlight the difference in risk associated with different contexts. This facilitates the creation of more specific treatment measures for management of the response to potential threat in the particular contexts described.

This chapter does not consider in detail redirected aggression (see **client handout**) and learned/conditioned affective aggression arising from inappropriate and often unintentional owner training (see Chapter 5). It should be stressed that the presenting complaint may extend beyond a single context, with more than one clinical and/or behavioural condition contributing to the problem (e.g. aggression over resources as a result of anxiety and sensory impairment). It is therefore important to investigate all contexts where all levels of aggression take place.

## Predation behaviour toward familiar pets and people

### Target

Targets may be normal prey species or any species to which the dog has not been properly socialized. Particular groups at risk are: infants or young children; smaller dogs; cats; and prey species kept as pets (e.g. rats, rabbits; Figure 17.12).

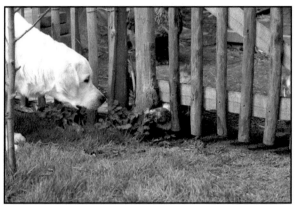

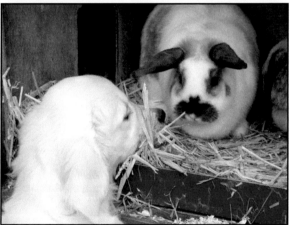

**17.12** Early exposure to prey species helps to prevent predatory behaviour later in life and may even encourage social behaviour toward these individuals. (Courtesy of H. Blancke.)

### Context

This behaviour is typically triggered by the appearance or movements of the perceived 'prey'. The behaviour might be encouraged by learning as a result of availability, access and outcome.

### Motivation

Predation describes behaviours associated with catching and killing another animal for consumption. It may involve all the steps of hunting: watching, stalking, chasing, attack and biting, characteristic of the breed. Predatory behaviour should be considered a normal canine trait, but may be inhibited or enhanced in some breeds through decades of selection.

### Emotion

Predation involves no threatening behaviour toward the victim. It is assumed that prey killing is associated with positive emotions (positive mood changes) in the build-up to and execution of the kill.

### Contributing/triggering factors

- Selective breeding for specific aspects of predation may intensify different elements of these responses (e.g. terriers may be more prone to aggressive chasing; herding breeds may be more prone to chasing and rounding up).
- Early exposure to prey species, without eliciting hunting behaviour, will encourage social behaviour and inhibit prey chasing. Lack of exposure to children at an early age may increase the risk that a dog may see children as prey.
- Because predation is a behaviour that is mentally rewarding, it should be assumed that hunting experience may encourage future predation.
- Unsupervised access to potential prey (infants, toddlers, pets) may also increase the risk.

### Differential diagnosis

- Play: this may look similar to predation, but elements such as the play-bow, interrupted sequencing of the behaviour, or high arousal are typically apparent.
- Attention-seeking: a learned process reinforced by the owner.
- Affective aggression: aggressive signalling, conflict or potential perceived threat is typically apparent.

### Risks

Most owners tolerate some form of predation (e.g. dogs catching mice, rats, squirrels) and may only seek assistance when the target becomes more socially unacceptable. Predation toward familiar people and pets should always be seen as high-risk behaviour even though it is not 'aggression' in the functional social sense.

### Management

- Identify all at-risk contexts (e.g. arousal by children playing in the garden).
- Check how access to these contexts can be prevented in both the short and long term.
- Predation needs lifelong safety management through restraint and segregation (e.g. on the lead around sheep).
- No behavioural modification techniques should be considered curative, but an effective recall is essential in case of accidental access. This needs extensive training and professional support, given the seriousness of any failure.

## Play-biting, play 'aggression'

### Target

A wide range of individuals can be targets, including children of all ages, adolescents, adults, other dogs in the household or familiar animals of any species (Figures 17.13 and 17.14).

### Context

The behaviour is triggered by the movements of the target and stimuli that induce playful arousal. Play is typically preceded by a play-bow and vocalization, including barking and a distinct type of panting noise

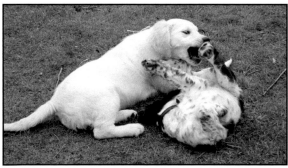

**17.13** Biting during play is normal for puppies as they learn to use their mouths. Unless managed appropriately, however, the behaviour can extend into adulthood and cause significant injury to other animals or to people. (Courtesy of H. Blancke.)

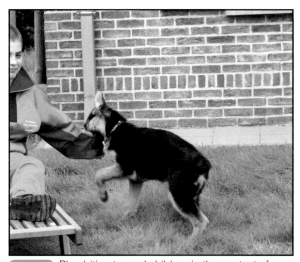

**17.14** Play-biting toward children in the context of chasing or teasing games that result in high arousal can cause injuries, even when a young dog is involved, and so needs to be addressed. (Courtesy of O. Van Den Broecke.)

and possibly growling but without the same tension in the body. Nipping may be used as an enticement to play and will typically be followed by a playful 'run away'. Play often consists of rapidly interchanging partial behaviour sequences, relating to diverse functional systems, and will usually involve an element of reciprocity. The gait of the dog during play is typically rounded and gambolling, rather than stealthy and/or tightly controlled.

### Motivation

Play-biting is sometimes referred to as play 'aggression' but should be seen as a normal dog–dog interaction. Over-exuberant use of the mouth is normally self-limiting as partners will refuse to continue to play if hurt. Play-bites (of puppies) toward humans follow the same learning process, and should be self-limiting if owners consistently refuse to continue play if hurt. At the same time, play and other pro-social behaviours may turn into affective aggression for a number of reasons:

- When humans misinterpret play-biting and punish the puppy or young dog each time it is aroused and play-bites. The physical intervention may have the opposite effect: increasing arousal and escalating the biting behaviour, resulting in more punishment and the potential for a more serious conflict between owner and dog

- The owner issues a very physical response (pulling the lead, pulling on a choke chain) when their dog in fact is aroused and potentially interested in showing play behaviour (mistaken for aggression by the owner) toward another dog, which then may induce a self-fulfilling prophecy: a conspecific turns into a cue predicting aversive behaviour from the owner (see Chapter 5)
- In addition some individuals may not have appropriate play skills and provoke attack from other dogs who feel threatened by their behaviour (see Chapter 3). In these situations play may quickly turn into aggression and treatment will need to focus on developing appropriate social interactive and play skills as well as handling aggressive arousal.

### Emotion

Play and play-biting are associated with positive emotional consequences. Play-biting is not linked to a threat or an aversive experience, but is self-reinforcing. It is therefore unlikely simply to go away of its own accord.

### Contributing/triggering factors

A lack of 'education' on how to play properly at an early age (e.g. by encouraging a puppy to mouth people as part of a game (see Figure 17.14), in the expectation that the puppy will 'grow out of it') can lead to poor play skills and poor bite inhibition (see Chapter 6 for further preventive information). Inappropriate responses by owners when the dog does bite, such as giving it a meal to get it to calm down or becoming more boisterous in response to any mouthing or as a dog gets more excited, may reinforce the behaviour and increase the chance of biting in future. Play should be well structured and rules applied consistently to prevent frustration and a possible bite as a result. Also, if there is an imbalance between the dog's exercise requirements, diet and living environment (e.g. if a dog from a working line is kept in an apartment), then the animal may become over-exuberant in its interactions with others.

### Differential diagnosis

- A trained bite: the owner may inadvertently be rewarding the behaviour (see above), or the dog may have been trained to bite and unintentionally signalled to do so. The signals used to control the behaviour should be identifiable together with owner reinforcement.
- Attention-seeking behaviour: the dog has learned to bite to get attention and this may be reinforced by the owner's response.
- Hyperactive/hyper-reactive (i.e. an overreaction triggered by minor stimuli): the dog will normally have a history of sensitivity.
- Affective aggression: aggressive signalling, conflict or a perceived potential threat trigger should be apparent.

### Risks

- Play-biting may be accompanied by other exuberant play behaviours such as jumping, mouthing and body slamming.
- Play-biting may become a particular problem when it is directed toward people (especially children) and when the dog lacks bite control (every time the dog plays, people have 'bite' marks).
- Cats can often be observed to 'stop' the behaviour by stopping all action, but with small potential prey animals exuberant and wild play may end up with involuntary 'deadly' injuries.

### Management

- Identify contextual risks (e.g. arousal from children playing in the garden).
- Check how the risks from these contexts can be minimized in the short and long term, for example by segregating children and the dog in order to prevent accidents.
- Reinforce more controlled play (see Chapter 8).
- Avoid inadvertent reinforcement of the behaviour (stop all actions when dog's behaviour is excessive).
- Explain the pitfalls of physical punishment, which is likely to increase arousal, may provoke affective aggression and potentially reinforces the behaviour through providing attention; the latter is also a problem with verbal punishment ('Don't do that!').

## Affective aggression in differing contexts

### Aggression related to resources

Resources might include food, bones, toys, objects, resting places, doorways, human attention or puppies.

***Target:*** Competitive disputes over resources (including a bitch's own puppies) may occur with family members of all ages, but tend to occur with children (Figure 17.15) more than adolescents, with adults being least frequently involved. The disputes may also occur with other familiar animals in the home, including other dogs and certain pets, such as less fearful cats.

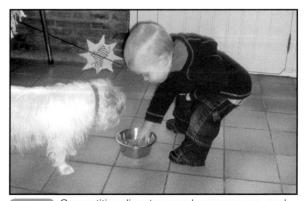

**17.15** Competitive disputes over key resources, such as a food bowl, tend to occur most with children. Clear protocols for managing children as well as dogs are required to prevent aggressive incidents. (Courtesy of M. Verbocht.)

**Context:** The situation is normally characterized by aggressive signalling (growling, lip lifting, teeth showing, staring, threatening posture(s), snapping, biting) around resources, or situations associated with resources. In practice, it is often 'defensive', i.e. the dog responds to the action of another, which is perceived by the dog (correctly or incorrectly) as a potential threat. Resource-related aggression can develop out of very subtle responses (see Ladder of Aggression) to a continued low-grade 'offensive' threat (the dog responds to subtle predicting cues of a 'planned' action). The problem may become particularly apparent when routines are changed, e.g. when the dog is no longer allowed on the furniture or into a room following the arrival of a baby.

**Motivation:** Competitive aggression in a social context is evoked by conflict: a perceived threat over resources. There is no evidence that dogs are motivated or driven by a desire to be 'top dog', although some may be more competitive than others. The perceived value of the resource may differ between individuals and, importantly, some dogs will only respond with aggression in the context of a highly palatable food item or valued toy, while others may present the behaviour in the context of apparently (to humans) relatively neutral objects such as cardboard boxes, towels, or an empty food bowl, or in response to actions like giving attention to one dog of the household (attention is the resource in this case).

**Emotion:** The dog feels threatened and potentially frustrated and so the underlying emotion is negative. The choice of strategy (whether or not escalating into a bite) will depend on many factors, including actual mood state, perception of the situation, and previous learning experiences (aggressive episodes) and their outcomes. Explicit food-related aggression may exist independently of a wider range of fear-related or 'other' owner-directed aggressive behaviours (Reisner, 2003). Dogs displaying aggression over resources should be screened for signs of generalized anxiety independent of the target.

**Contributing/triggering factors:**

- Competitive aggression over resources is not necessarily learned and may begin at an early age. It should be a cause for concern if seen in puppies or juvenile dogs, even in the absence of biting (Reisner *et al.*, 2007).
- The presence of young children in the home, who may not appreciate the dog's normal 'rights' and behave less consistently around dogs, should be seen as a risk factor.
- Changes to the dog's routine, so that access to previous rewards is denied or reduced, increase the risk of a dispute and cause frustration, both of which may result in aggression.
- Disease processes may alter the threshold towards aggressive behaviour (see Chapter 1).
- Owner misinterpretations ('He is trying to be dominant/bossy!', hence the misnomer 'dominance aggression') and owner

misconceptions ('I need to be able to disturb my dog at any time to be leader of the pack'), which often lead to miscommunication (verbal and physical punishment), are likely to aggravate the problem by intensifying the negative emotional load on the dog. Even if this behaviour by the owner suppresses the behaviour in the short term, it will disrupt the social relationship and could result in a catastrophic conflict at a later date in another context.

**Differential diagnosis:**

- An underlying physical problem leading to sensory impairment, irritability or the lowering of threshold towards aggressive behaviour (e.g. hypothyroidism, Cushing's disease, pseudo-pregnancy, brain neoplasia, chronic pain).
- Iatrogenic as a result of medication (e.g. acepromazine, metoclopramide, ketamine).
- A generalized mood disturbance (e.g. fearfulness) or generalized anxiety disorder.
- A conditioned response (e.g. as a result of teasing, punishment or other inappropriate owner intervention).

**Risk to humans:** It is estimated that nearly two-thirds of dog bites to children happen in the context of resource guarding. The prognosis for treatment depends on the ability to control major risk factors including: young children in the home; owner compliance; and underlying physical causes.

**Management:**

- Identify contextual risks (e.g. list significant resources, their location, use, as well as bite risk factors described above) (Figure 17.16).
- Check how risks from these contexts can be minimized in the short and long term, for example by segregating children and the dog in order to prevent accidents, such as access to a bitch's puppies.
- Explain the pitfalls of physical and verbal punishment, which is likely to increase negative emotional arousal and potentially provoke more intense aggression.
- Behavioural modification techniques for desensitization and counter-conditioning (see

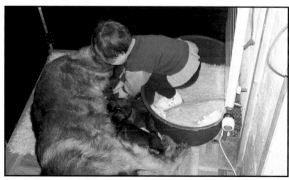

**17.16** Two-thirds of dog bites in children happen in the context of conflict over resources. (Courtesy of B. Proesmans.)

Chapter 5) for stressful interactions need to be applied (starting at the lower end of the Ladder of Aggression).

- The instigation of new routines, based on consistent interaction, will help to reduce anxiety and threat perception and increase acceptance of all sorts of interactions.
- Chronic generalized anxiety may need to be treated with long-term psychotherapeutic interventions (see Chapter 21).

### Aggression related to 'benign' interactions

**Target:** Problems may occur with family members of all ages, but tend to occur with children more than adolescents, with adults least frequently involved. They may also occur with other familiar animals in the home, including other dogs and certain pets, such as less fearful cats.

**Context:** Aggressive signalling occurs in the context of benign interactions. These include: gazing, eye contact, looking at, talking to, passing by, approaching, reaching out a hand or foot, bending towards, touching, petting (Figure 17.17), kissing, hugging, handling and lifting up. The response is often 'defensive', i.e. the dog responds to the action of another, which is perceived (possibly incorrectly by the dog) as a potential threat. The response can involve growling, lip lifting, teeth showing, staring, threatening posture(s), snapping, biting or a mixture of these. In cases where the benign trigger or the interaction becomes 'unidentifiable' and the dog bites without apparent stimulus, the aggression has been called idiopathic aggression.

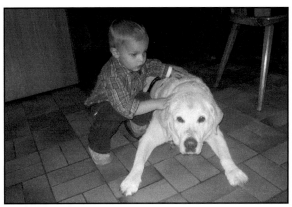

**17.17** Dogs that react aggressively in the context of benign interactions should be screened for underlying physical disorders, including an anxiety disorder. (Courtesy of H. Jung.)

**Motivation:** A dog that reacts with aggression following a benign interaction perceives the 'benign' interaction as a threat or something to be avoided. Dogs that bite following benign triggers often have an underlying physical disease, are in pain or have a fear/anxiety disorder.

**Emotion:** Dogs that bite following benign triggers are often in a predominantly negative emotional state, hence the low threshold for the response. The animal

feels threatened and will often respond with one or more overtly aggressive behaviours, but at other times frequently shows other behaviours lower down the Ladder of Aggression, such as hiding (Figure 17.18). The choice of strategy (whether or not escalating into a bite) will depend on the actual context (moment, target, interaction, previous experience) and the severity of any underlying physical disease or painful processes. These dogs should always be screened for anxiety.

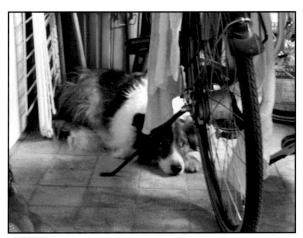

**17.18** Hiding should be recognized as a strategy used in response to a stressful situation. When the triggering stimulus is benign, the dog should be screened for underlying emotional disorders such as anxiety. (Courtesy of M. Van De Velde.)

### Contributing/triggering factors:

- Underlying physical disease, pain or sensory impairment will exacerbate the problem (see Chapter 1).
- Chronic anxiety will make the dog more irritable (this problem may be referred to as irritable aggression).
- There may be a genetic predisposition, with possible lines within the Cocker Spaniel, Springer Spaniel, Bernese Mountain Dog and Golden Retriever being particularly prone to express the problem (sometime referred to as 'rage' or 'impulsive aggression'), but it may occur in any breed.
- Lack of experience at an early age increases the risk that an animal will become temperamentally anxious.
- Learning and previous experience may play an important role. For example, it is possible that there is an association between the benign stimuli (being touched) and earlier harmful aversive stimuli (pain, discomfort, feeling fearful, anxious).
- Owner misinterpretations and misconceptions, as for aggression related to resources above.
- Irritability – dogs (like people) sometimes want and need to be left alone and it is important for people to recognize this and give the dog some space at this time; they should not force themselves on the dog just because they want to.
- The presence of young children in the home should be seen as a serious risk factor.

### Differential diagnosis:

- An underlying physical problem leading to sensory impairment, irritability or the lowering of threshold towards aggressive behaviour (e.g. hypothyroidism, Cushing's disease, pseudopregnancy, brain neoplasia) or a direct response to pain (see Chapter 1).
- Iatrogenic as a result of medication (as for resources).
- A generalized mood disturbance (as for resources).
- A conditioned response (as for resources).

**Risk to humans:** According to Reisner *et al.* (2007), 18% of bites on children followed a benign interaction with their dog. Among these biting dogs, 50% suffered from a medical condition and 77% had signs of anxiety. This stresses the importance of exploring underlying physical and emotional conditions responsible for aggression. Aggression following benign interactions should always be considered as a high-risk situation for a family.

### Management:

- Underlying physical disease needs to be treated.
- Chronic generalized anxiety may need to be treated with long-term therapeutic intervention (see Chapter 21).
- It is important to review daily family–dog interactions and clearly identify with the owner moments of 'risk' and assess these (see Figure 17.4).
- Owners should be informed of the inappropriateness and risks associated with punishment (e.g. escalation).

- The importance of physical safety barriers (e.g. muzzles) at times when preventing interactions is impossible must be recognized by the client.
- In order to minimize risk, owners need to be trained to become skilled observers of their dog's behaviour and to evaluate the risk of specific contexts.
- Behavioural modification techniques for desensitization and counter-conditioning to the type of interactions triggering the response.
- The instigation of new routines, based on consistent interaction (as for resources).

### Aggression related to aversive painful and non-painful interactions

**Target:** Any person or another animal may provoke a direct protective (i.e. self-preservation) response, but children may be at greatest risk, since they may be less aware of the consequences of their actions (Figure 17.19).

**Context:** Aggressive signalling occurs in the context of aversive interactions. This may also be referred to as 'irritable aggression'. Examples of painful interactions include touching an injury or trauma, painful manipulation after surgery, hitting, kicking, physical punishment, application of electric current during training or choke restraints, accidental injury, or falling on the dog. Non-painful aversive interactions include pulling, pushing, grabbing by the collar and other attempts at physical restraint. The response is 'defensive', i.e. the dog is responding to a perceived threat from another, or being frustrated (e.g. being pulled away from something it wishes to gain access to).

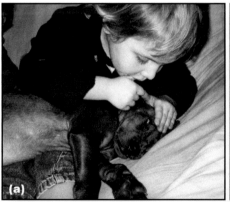
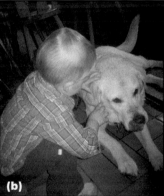
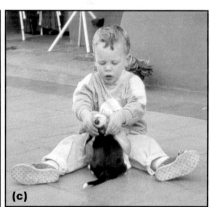
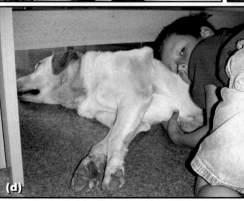
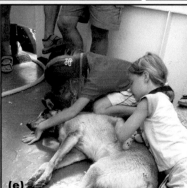

**17.19** Young children may unintentionally perform aversive (painful or non-painful) actions that can provoke an aggressive response. (a,e Courtesy of I. De Cock.)

The response can involve a single element or sequence of the following: growling, lip lifting, teeth showing, staring, threatening posture(s), snapping, biting or a mixture of these.

*Motivation:* A dog who reacts with aggression following an aversive interaction is normally trying to protect or free itself from the situation. Protectiveness will be accentuated if the animal is scared, has some underlying physical disease (especially if it is in pain) and/or is suffering from generalized anxiety.

*Emotion:* The dog will feel threatened and potentially frustrated by the interaction and so the underlying emotion is negative. The exact response (whether or not escalating into a bite) will depend on several factors, including the actual context and the physical and behavioural health of the individual.

*Contributing/triggering factors:*

- Underlying physical disease, pain or sensory impairment will exacerbate the problem (see Chapter 1).
- Chronic anxiety will make the dog more irritable.
- Previous experience may alter the likelihood of the problem, with a learned association between benign stimuli and earlier harmful aversive stimuli (pain, discomfort, feeling fearful, anxious) increasing the risk.
- Owner misinterpretations and misconceptions (as for resources).
- Young children may unintentionally undertake aversive actions (Montagner *et al.*, 1988) and so the presence of young children in the home should be seen as a major risk factor.

*Differential diagnosis:*

- An underlying physical problem leading to sensory impairment, irritability or the lowering of threshold towards aggressive behaviour (e.g. hypothyroidism, Cushing's disease, pseudo-pregnancy, brain neoplasia) or a direct response to pain (see Chapter 1).
- Iatrogenic as a result of medication (as for resources).
- A generalized mood disturbance (as for resources).
- A conditioned response (as for resources).

*Risk to humans:* According to one report (Reisner *et al.*, 2007), 18% of bites on children followed an aversive potentially painful interaction such as falling over, stepping over, hitting or punishing the dog. Another study found that 80% of all child interactions towards the dog were initiated by the child (see Figures 17.19 and 17.20) and that young children tended to redirect aggression received at the nursery or at school towards either other children in the household or the family dog. In this way the child may cross over the boundaries of safe conduct with the family dog (Montagner *et al.*, 1988). Assistance from a child psychologist may therefore be useful if these circumstances are suspected.

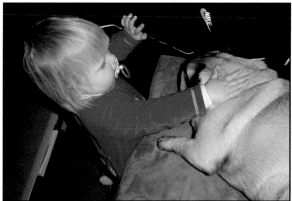

**17.20** Eighty percent of all child interactions with a dog are reportedly initiated by the child, putting the child at greater risk. (Courtesy of W. and S. van Hecke.)

*Management:*

- Underlying physical disease needs to be treated.
- Chronic generalized anxiety may need to be treated with long-term therapeutic intervention (see Chapter 21).
- Aversive family member–dog interactions need to be identified and assessed.
- Explain how aggression is a normal response to aversion and why this therefore needs to be prevented in all family members.
- Owners should be informed of the inappropriateness and risks associated with punishment (escalation, etc.).
- The importance of physical safety barriers (e.g. muzzles and segregation) must be recognized by the owner.
- In order to minimize risk, owners need to be trained to become skilled observers of their dog's behaviour and to evaluate the risk of specific contexts.
- Behavioural modification techniques for desensitization and counter-conditioning to the triggers of aggression.
- The instigation of new routines, based on consistent interaction, will help to reduce anxiety and increase acceptance, reducing the risk of aggression.

### Intra-specific aggression between dogs in the household

*Target:* In general, male dogs show more intra-specific aggression than bitches but, in practice, females are more often presented for interdog aggression toward other dogs within the same household when compared with male–male pairs or female–male pairs (Bamberger and Houpt, 2006; Mertens, 2006). Aggression between bitches within the same house can be much more physical and is believed by some to have a higher risk of being fatal than inter-male disputes in the home.

*Context:* Threatening or fighting is usually reported between two (or more) dogs in the same household. The dogs may be otherwise 'normal' in their behaviour and 'fights' may be just skirmishes or exchange of threats when priority of access is unclear or disputed (Figure 17.21). It is worth noting that consistent access to a resource, without challenge from others (i.e. as a result of their deference), results in the observation of a hierarchy between individuals. There is no evidence that hierarchical position *per se* is a motivational factor in dogs, but it may be the consequence of more competitive and less deferential behavioural tendencies. Social dominance arises primarily from the deference of others, rather than the assertive acts of a specific individual; otherwise there would be no predictability to social stability (with a consequent loss of some of its key benefits) and a serious risk of injury to members of the social group. Individuals may dispute priority of access in a previously stable social group when they assess that they can obtain the resource at a low cost, for example if the other individual is sick or ageing (especially if they are young and in their prime) or if they have allies, such as the owner, to assist them. Therefore the co-occurrence of medical conditions is an important contextual variable in many of these circumstances. Dogs who suffer from behavioural disorders (chronic anxiety, social fear) or those with inadequate socialization may respond incorrectly to the signals from another dog, resulting in aggression from either party.

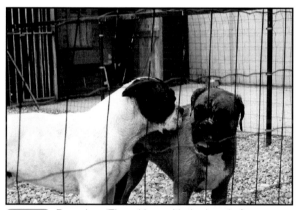

**17.21** Dogs in a 'T' position, with the head of one over the shoulders of the other. Acceptance of this head position is a sign of social deference that reduces the risk of aggression. However, the gesture may not be tolerated and so may also trigger an aggressive episode.

**Motivation:** These interactions are usually competitive and the consequence of a perceived threat to individually important resources, perceived threat during benign interactions, or perceived threat following direct or indirect challenges, or aversive interactions. The importance of underlying physical disease and anxiety in these situations should not be underestimated.

**Emotion:** Such conflicts involve a negative emotional state. Individuals may start an exchange with one or more of the behaviours illustrated on the Ladder of Aggression. The choice of strategy (whether or not to escalate the exchange to a bite) will depend on the actual context (moment, target, interaction, previous experience) and the co-occurrence of an underlying

behavioural disorder or physical disease. Both dogs should therefore be screened for anxiety and physical ailments.

***Contributing/triggering factors:***

- Competition will often be triggered over resources with a high value to one or both dogs: food, toys, owner attention, access to preferred areas, etc.
- When there is a clear disparity between individuals, the risk of a dispute is reduced; conversely, it is increased when there is similarity between the dogs in gender, age and size.
- Medical or behavioural conditions in one or more dogs may be significant contributors to the problem, as will any other factors affecting resource-holding potential, such as ageing or sensory impairment.
- Many cases of dog–dog aggression in the same home appear when a younger animal reaches sexual or social maturity. Female–female conflict may occur or escalate during oestrus. In male dogs, competition over a female may be a trigger.
- Owner misconceptions and incorrect interventions (e.g. providing inadvertent support to the dispute through the inappropriate use of punishment, rather than clarity in the rules for access) may trigger escalation (Figure 17.22).

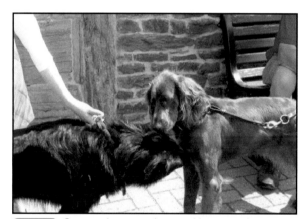

**17.22** Owner misconceptions and inappropriate intervention (e.g. jerking a dog back as it investigates another or exchanges social gestures) may trigger an unnecessary aggressive incident during an otherwise normal social encounter between familiar dogs.

***Differential diagnosis:***

- Normal (controlled and limited) canine signalling within a stable hierarchy.
- An underlying physical problem leading to sensory impairment, irritability or the lowering of threshold towards aggressive behaviour (e.g. hypothyroidism, Cushing's disease, pseudo-pregnancy, brain neoplasia) or a direct response to pain (see Chapter 1).
- A generalized mood disturbance (e.g. fearfulness) or generalized anxiety disorder.
- Play-biting.
- Predation.
- Other forms of affective aggression described above.

***Risk to humans:*** Adults and children may be injured while trying to separate their dogs during fighting as the dog redirects its aggression to the stimulus that is frustrating its behaviour (see above).

***Management:***

- Underlying physical disease needs to be treated.
- Chronic generalized anxiety may need to be treated with long-term therapeutic intervention (see Chapter 21).
- The range and extent of dog–dog interactions need to be identified and evaluated for their risk.
- The risks following human intervention towards the dogs need to be identified and evaluated.
- The role of humans (and access to them) in starting fights needs to be identified and managed. On the basis of this a decision can be made on whether or not it is advisable to separate dogs when people are about or when the dogs are unsupervised.
- In order to minimize risk, owners need to be trained to become skilled observers of their dogs' behaviour and to evaluate the risk of specific contexts, with particular emphasis on the avoidance of triggering situations that may lead to conflicts and how to provide consistent rules that support the natural ranking of precedence between the dogs.
- Ovariohysterectomy should be considered for bitches that fight only during oestrus, but the neutering of male dogs is not known to be effective.
- Owners should be informed of the inappropriateness and risks associated with punishment (e.g. escalation).
- The importance of physical safety barriers (e.g. muzzles) at times of potential risky interaction must be accepted by the owner.
- Behavioural modification techniques for desensitization and counter-conditioning (as in the contexts described previously).
- Instigate new routines, based on consistent interaction between dogs (e.g. using a headcollar and basket muzzle), to increase deferent behaviour and reduce the risk of aggression.
- The prognosis is best if fights have a low frequency, are predictable to the owners (triggers identifiable) and if no physical injuries have been inflicted (Mertens, 2006), but the prognosis is generally worse for females than for males.

## Treatment of aggression

### Evaluation of owner's understanding and expectations

The offer of treatment requires a proper risk assessment as a precondition, and this must be clearly communicated to the owner. As well as explaining the meaning of the behavioural signs relating to the emotional disturbance, the veterinary surgeon needs to check how far the owners understand the rationale and are able to change their perception of their dog being 'dominant' into 'My dog was displaying aggression because he felt threatened when I approached the food bowl'. This step change is more likely to happen when the owner is able to understand that emotional reactions such as 'feeling threatened' may be triggered by very benign events such as being looked at, passed by, approached, touched and so on.

Ultimately it is the owner's decision as to whether to try to resolve the problem, but the veterinary surgeon should be able to offer an informed opinion. Even though owners may openly ask for help, some may have decided already to euthanize their animal and their request for a behavioural examination may be an attempt to ease their conscience. The role of the veterinary surgeon should not be to argue with the client in these circumstances. It is for the client to decide whether the residual risk is acceptable, and then the veterinary surgeon's role to help to minimize this risk.

Management is perhaps a preferable term to treatment, since aggression is a normal behaviour and so cannot be cured, only managed and the risks reduced. The specific management exercises required in different circumstances have been given in the diagnosis section above. The sections below illustrate some of the general principles and methods involving the behavioural modification in more detail.

### Reducing risk through use of muzzles and headcollars

Muzzle training is an essential requirement for all aggressive dogs, as is gaining good control such as through the appropriate use of a headcollar. However a headcollar is not a substitute for a muzzle. Details on how to use these aids effectively are given in the **client handouts**.

### Desensitization and counter-conditioning

The main behavioural exercise for reducing reactivity focuses on desensitizing the dog to the triggers of aggression and training a more appropriate response. The principles of this technique are given in Chapter 5 and an illustrated example of the measures required to facilitate this efficiently in relation to aggression is provided in Figure 17.23. Before starting a programme intended to lower the chance of stressful interactions between a family member and the dog, it is necessary to perform:

- A physical examination – to identify and address any underlying painful conditions that may contribute to the problem
- A behavioural examination – to identify any underlying emotional disorder that may need pharmacological treatment
- A careful contextual evaluation of the problem, listing:
  - All contexts where the aggression has happened
  - All interactions that have triggered aggression
  - All interactions that trigger a stress reaction in the dog.

The writing of a safe and sound management protocol requires owners to understand fully the 'meaning' of the behaviours presented, so that the owner becomes a 'partner' in writing the protocol, rather than the veterinary surgeon 'dictating' what owners 'should' do. For all cases of 'affective aggression', underlying physical disease should be excluded or addressed where necessary. Educating owners as 'specialist observers' concerning their own dog contributes to better communication and a more realistic assessment of success, pitfalls and risk management over time. In addition, protocols need to be checked and *rechecked at each follow-up visit.*

| Actions of owner that trigger a response | Reaction of Bino | Reaction of owners | Evaluation of owner's interpretation |
|---|---|---|---|
| 1. Cleaning Bino's ears<br>2. Brushing Bino's head<br>3. Cleaning Bino's feet | Biting<br><br>Snapping | 1. We punish him verbally<br>2. Verbal punishment<br>3. We go and put gloves on | ☹<br>☹<br>☹ |
| 4. Pulling Bino out from underneath furniture<br>5. Verbal punishing when he jumps with his dirty feet on white carpet<br><br>Never seen stiffened posture | Growling<br><br>Stiffening up, staring<br><br>Lying down, leg up | 4. We shout, than he snaps<br><br>5. We shout and Bino growls more | ☹<br><br>☹ |
| 6. When Bino gets punished | Standing crouched, tail tucked under | 6. We think he feels guilty | ☺ |
| 7. When we shout at Bino | Creeping, ears back | 7. We think he feels guilty | ☺ |
| 8. When there is a thunderstorm<br><br>9. When we call him to clean his ears | Walking away<br><br>Turning body away, sitting, pawing | 8. We think of buying a sounds CD and playing it all the time to get him used to the noise<br>9. We chase him and then he bites (see above) | ☹<br><br><br>☹ |
| 10. When we hug him, pet him or talk gently to him<br><br>11. When he is sleepy, happens a lot when we brush his coat | Turning head away<br><br>Yawning, blinking, nose licking | 10. We think he is upset with us (won't look at us any more!)<br><br>11. We think he is bored | ☺<br><br><br>☺ |

## DIAGNOSIS AND TREATMENT

| Procedure | Diagnosis | Treatment |
|---|---|---|
| Physical examination | Bino suffers from a bilateral painful **ear infection.** Aetiological diagnosis (allergic/infectious, etc.) | Treatment will involve daily administration of eardrops or medication. In the first week, owner may need veterinary surgeon or nurse to insert eardrops until pain relief is achieved<br>Owner to start muzzle training so that eardrops can be administered without being bitten |
| Behavioural examination | Bino suffers from **thunderstorm phobia** | Treatment of thunderstorm phobia required. Exposure to loud noises would risk deterioration of the condition (see Chapter 15) |
| | Bino shows signs of **anxiety**, anticipating situations that are potentially harmful, when owner:<br>• Calls him for cleaning ears<br>• Punishes him<br>and also in related uneventful (benign) situations when:<br>• Cleaning feet<br>• Hugging him<br>• Talking gently to him | Treatment of anxiety may involve use of pharmacological agents (e.g. selective serotonin reuptake inhibitors) |

**17.23** Example of the processes involved in the development of an individualized programme facilitating desensitization and counter-conditioning to stressful interactions. Bino is a neutered male 7-year-old Shih Tsu, who has bitten his owner during a physical interaction. (continues) ▶

---

**ADVICE TO BINO'S OWNER**

- **Protocol to reduce stress:**
  - Stop all actions 1 to 7, since they are triggering a reactive response in the dog (red and orange in the Ladder)
  - Address no. 8 (thunderstorm) specifically
  - Reinterpret no. 9: leaving means 'I want to go away and hide because I feel frightened'
  - Evaluate actions 10 and 11 in a way that does not cause risk.
- **Desensitization:**
  - Owners will need to focus on controlled and graduated exposure to those stimuli that trigger the behavioural reactions at the lower end of the Ladder (green, yellow), since they reflect a lower stress response and do not induce overt aggression.
- **Counter-conditioning:**
  - Combine owner actions in the green level with rewards (check with owners which ones Bino likes); for example:
    - Call him gently (instead of shouting) and reward
    - When brushing his coat, stop and reward relaxed response
    - Repeat exercise several times a day and reward
    - Determine which rewards have the best effect
    - Make sure that the only thing that Bino gets from the owner is positive attention and reward.
- **Important: avoid red-level activities:**
  - Avoid chasing Bino when he leaves
  - Avoid cleaning his feet – no cleaning right now
  - Avoid pulling him out from underneath objects – leave him alone
  - Avoid punishment, including shouting.

**17.23** (continued) Example of the processes involved in the development of an individualized programme facilitating desensitization and counter-conditioning to stressful interactions. Bino is a neutered male 7-year-old Shih Tsu, who has bitten his owner during a physical interaction.

---

## Prognosis and follow-up

The prognosis for treatment, should it be considered desirable, depends on the assessment of several factors, some of which are indicated in Figure 17.24. Follow-up should take place in the short term (2 weeks), when owner compliance and response to therapy should be checked.

## Prevention

### Traditional advice

For many decades, dog-bite prevention advice has been published in medical and veterinary literature reflecting mainly preventive strategies *versus* risk factors found in hospital-based dog-bite studies (Love and Overall, 2001). This advice includes:

- Avoid certain breeds as family dogs (large breeds, working breeds, 'dangerous' breeds)
- Avoid having a male dog as a pet
- Neuter the pet
- Train the pet (this will reduce the dog's overall anxiety, but will not prevent aggression)
- Children should never be left unsupervised with a pet dog
- Educate children about the dog's body language
- When approaching a dog, let him first sniff the back of the hand, but do not suddenly pull the hand away upwards
- Do not pat dogs on the head; always pat them under the chin, or between the front legs
- Do not play rough games; be quiet around dogs.

Even though these suggestions appear 'sound', they do not appear to have reduced the number of bites within the home over time (Love and Overall, 2001; Shuler *et al.*, 2008).

| Detail | High risk |
|---|---|
| ***Human-related factors*** | |
| Family composition | Presence of young children (< 7 years) gives substantially poorer prognosis for likelihood of successful treatment |
| Relationships between family members | Disagreement between family members relating to awareness of problem, goals of therapy and understanding of safety provide a higher risk for poor prognosis |
| No awareness of problem | Holding on to beliefs, misconceptions, lack of awareness of problem, lack of understanding of safety protocols provide higher risk for poor prognosis |
| Control of dog only by physical restraint | Owners for whom the only way to control the dog is by physical restraint/power/force pose a higher risk for recurrent bites and higher risk for poor prognosis overall |
| Quality/spatial factors of home environment | Limitations to human–dog cohabitation in terms of space, resources and level of social welfare may increase risk of recurrence (Shuler *et al.*, 2008) and indicate poor prognosis |
| ***Dog-related factors*** | |
| Number of forms of aggression | The more types of aggression presented, the poorer the prognosis |
| Number of situations that trigger aggression | The more situations and contexts that may trigger aggression in the dog, the higher the risk of the situations and the poorer the prognosis |
| Number of co-morbid problems | The more physical and behavioural conditions that are co-morbid, the more difficult will be prevention and the higher the risk of the situation, and the poorer the prognosis |

**17.24** Prognostic factors.

Recent medical papers have even suggested that families with young children should avoid having dogs at all (Schalamon *et al.*, 2006; Besser, 2007). Banning dogs from households with children is not only impractical, it should also be considered highly undesirable: it denies children specific opportunities with regard to their general development and prevents them from learning to 'read' dogs, which may increase their risk of injury later in life.

## Dogs and children

According to research, young children score badly in discriminating dog body language. They mainly look at the dog's face in order to make their decisions. In addition, they do not necessarily understand the dog's intentions: they will often confuse a fearful dog with a friendly one (Lakestani *et al.*, 2005). To add to the confusion, there is commonly a mistaken belief by many parents that a wagging tail indicates a safe situation for their child. The focus needs to be on teaching parents and children how to recognize and assess situations that appear to trigger dog bites in a household situation.

### The role of safety rules

Safety rules have been applied for many decades in an attempt to prevent dog bites to children, but no data are available to support their effectiveness. Evidence from research concerning in-home injuries in young children suggests that the children's *knowledge* of safety rules does not reduce their risk-taking behaviours. Reduction of injuries is instead related to the children's *compliance* with these rules and to the extent of parental supervision (Morrongiello *et al.*, 2001; Zeedyk *et al.*, 2001).

### The role of the parent

The role of the parent appears obvious: parents are responsible for the safe cohabitation of their child and the family dog. There are no data on efficient parental supervision for dogs with children, but Morrongiello *et al.* (2001) indicated that physical proximity was the only aspect of parental supervisory behaviour that served a protective function: parents who remained close to their children had children who engaged in less risk taking. Parental factors relevant to child injury included parental protectiveness and beliefs about child supervision.

### Child–dog interactions

Extrapolating from the published guidelines in human medicine, it would seem that dog-bite prevention objectives should differentiate between child and dog behaviours at different ages (Love and Overall, 2001; Bond and Hauf, 2004). Therefore a new generation of programmes is being developed (see also Chapter 2 for advice on safe interactions between children and puppies). For example, the Blue Dog© dog-bite prevention tool for families with young children includes an interactive CD and parental guide that educates parents and children about the safest way to interact with their dog in a household setting

(De Keuster *et al.*, 2005; Meints and de Keuster, in press); it is intended as a prevention tool to be incorporated as part of a bigger prevention programme in veterinary practices, human healthcare practices, schools and canine rescue centres (Figure 17.25).

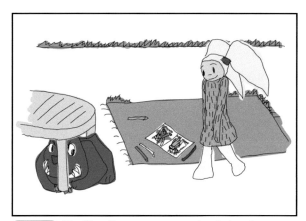

**17.25** The Blue Dog programme aims to teach young children through interactive animated sequences about appropriate and inappropriate behaviour around dogs in different circumstances.

Children aged 7–9 years are better able to understand and comply with safety rules when trained in a cognitive way (Limbourg, 1994). In the German multidisciplinary prevention programme 'Is he going to bite?' (Jung, 2007), school children engage in 'risk situations' by means of role play. The goal of the training is to engage the children in prevention and to understand risk situations from the dog's angle. This age group has more tendency to 'test' a dog or a 'situation' and to engage actively in risk situations by breaking safety rules (Hubacher, 2001). In this way it is assumed that interactive demonstration with a trained dog – who is able to bark or growl on command without presenting a real risk – may be more effective for children of this age.

## Teaching owners how to interact safely with their pet

There are four steps in teaching owners how to interact safely with their pet:

- Investigate (summarize risk situations)
- Diagnose (define the dog's motivation)
- Differentiate (triggering/contributing factors)
- Implement (provide safety protocols).

### Investigation

It should be stressed that it is not possible to give owners advice that is applicable to *all* situations. In each case the veterinary surgeon needs to investigate the underlying cause of the aggression, as well as take into account risk factors relating to the dog, the humans and the context of the incident. Figure 17.26 gives four contextual examples based on the owner's complaint. Safety protocols for each example are considered later.

| Context | Response towards adults | Response towards other human age groups | Response towards other animals in family |
|---|---|---|---|
| **Example 1**<br>*The male owner tried to clean the dog's ear (the dog was sitting on the sofa)* | Dog growled; when the owner reprimanded him, the dog bit the owner's finger | None – their 5-year-old child has never cleaned the dog's ears | None – this family has no other animals |
| **Example 2**<br>*Dog was chewing rawhide and owner wanted to take it away* | Dog lifted his lips, growled and showed his teeth | None – the family has no children at home | Last week the other family dog was bitten on the ear when passing nearby |
| **Example 3**<br>*Dog and child playing in garden* | Dog growls, jumps and tears clothing | Dog has bitten 4-year-old child on the arm | None – this family has no other animals |
| **Example 4**<br>*The dog (4 years old) was playing with a young kitten in the kitchen and killed it* | No complaints | No problems with the children identifiable | None – this family has no other animals. This was their first kitten |

**17.26** Examples of aggressive scenarios involving familiar individuals, more fully defined by contextual elaboration to include available information relating to dog's responses to known social stimuli.

## Diagnosis

In order to provide guidance, it is crucial to have a clear motivational diagnosis, i.e. understanding of the motivation of the dog. Findings should be checked against the behavioural history and the elements in Figure 17.27 (see also Figure 17.2).

## Differentiation

In addition to the diagnosis, it is necessary to investigate factors that may lower the threshold of an aggressive response:

- Physical problem (disease, pain, sensory impairment)
- Emotional disturbance (e.g. generalized anxiety)
- Genetic predisposition (e.g. Golden Cocker Spaniel, Bernese Mountain Dog)
- Early life experiences (e.g. sensorial deprivation)
- Education (e.g. punishment)
- Human factors (e.g. miscommunication, victim behaviour)
- Sociocultural environment (e.g. housing conditions).

| Context | Triggers | Emotion | Motivations | Features | Potential victim |
|---|---|---|---|---|---|
| **Affective aggression** | | | | | |
| Resources | Frustration or threat related to food, toys, objects, resting places, human attention, puppies | Negative: frustration/conflicting/anxiety over perceived threat over resources | Defensive response Response following frustration Offensive threat: dog responds to subtle predicting cues of a planned action | See Ladder of Aggression (Figure 17.1) | Family members; children more often involved Familiar pets (dogs, cats) |
| Benign interactions | Gaze, eye contact talking, passing by, approaching, reaching out, bending towards, touching, petting, kissing, hugging, handling, lifting up | Negative: dog perceives a benign interaction as a threat or something to be avoided | | | |
| Aversive painful interactions (irritable aggression) | Approach or touch, manipulation, physical punishment or threat of punishment, e.g. application of choke restraint | Negative: anxiety or fear in relation to pain or potentially painful interaction | Defensive: dog is responding to a perceived threat | | |
| Aversive non-painful interactions | Pulling, pushing, grabbing by collar, attempts at physical restraint | | | | |
| **Play-biting** | | | | | |
| Social interaction | Heightened arousal during social exchange, blowing on the dog | Positive | Enticement to respond, exuberance; self-reinforcing | May be preceded by play-bow or breathy exhalation Movement often associated with gambolling/rounded gait Barking Nipping and running away Rapidly changing behavioural sequences | Family members; children more often involved Familiar pets (dogs, cats) |

**17.27** Differentiating affective aggression, play and predation behaviour toward familiar individuals. (continues) ▶

| Context | Triggers | Emotion | Motivations | Features | Potential victim |
|---|---|---|---|---|---|
| *Predation* | | | | | |
| Hunting | Moving prey Learnt from previous successful encounters | Positive: anticipation leading to excitement | Feeding | Watching, pouncing/stalking, chasing, attack, biting, killing | Prey species kept as pets Species to which dog has not been properly socialized Cats Infants and young children |

**17.27** (continued) Differentiating affective aggression, play and predation behaviour toward familiar individuals.

## Implementation of safety protocols

### Prevention of aggression in the context of interactions

Consider Example 1 from Figure 17.26:

---

**Context:** The male owner tried to clean the dog's ear (the dog was sitting on the sofa)

**Response towards adult owner:** Dog growled; when the owner reprimanded him, the dog bit the owner's finger

**Response towards family children:** None – their 5-year-old child has never cleaned the dog's ears

**Response towards other household dogs:** None – this family has no other animals

---

Before giving safety advice, the veterinary surgeon should investigate the dog's responses toward each family member and *for each context*.

- Investigate the actions and the context(s) in which the dog responds with aggression and also the actions and context(s) in which the dog responds at the lower end of the Ladder of Aggression. It is important to note that the steps on the ladder represent the possible strategies a dog could use to avoid a threat, but they do not necessarily represent the chronological way in which a dog will react to that threat, because behaviour is influenced by learning from previous experience, the owner's reaction and so on.
- Discover whether the dog is feeling threatened by only one trigger (e.g. painful interaction) in one context (e.g. ear cleaning) by one family member (e.g. male owner) or whether the dog shows threat aversion in other contexts (e.g. benign interactions).
- Be aware of different behavioural responses in the dog toward different family members or age groups. Ensure that questions take into account the actions of all family members living in the home and also include familiar visitors (e.g. grandparents, dog sitters or babysitters).
- In families with young children, some of the questions may remain unanswered (e.g. no information on the dog's behaviour when the 5-year-old child cleaned the ears, or on verbal punishment, because these events never happened).
- Investigate the owner's reactions for each context. This will clarify to what extent the owner's reactions have been influencing the dog's behaviour. Verbal or physical punishment might appear 'safe and sound' to the owner because it stopped the unwanted behaviour (e.g. the dog walked away and growled). However, the dog may learn that walking away does not solve its problem and in the future might change its strategy (e.g. by snapping or biting immediately).
- The interview with the owner will clarify how the dog is reacting in each different context with humans. Cross-check the owner's descriptions about the dog's behaviour with observations made during the consultation (they should be consistent).

By learning about all risk situations (rather than only the one that was first described by the owner as being the problem), the veterinary surgeon will be able to provide more valid safety advice (Figure 17.28).

| Interaction | Risk context | Behaviour toward adults | Behaviour toward young children |
|---|---|---|---|
| Painful | Cleaning dog's ears on sofa, kitchen table | Bite | – |
| Aversive non-painful | Pulling or pushing dog from sofa | Growling | Snapping |
| | Verbal punishment when dog growls at children | Lying down with leg raised | – |
| Benign | Hugging dog when it lies on sofa or in bed | Ears back, turning head away | Growling |
| | Petting dog when it lies on sofa or sleeps in basket | Nose licking | Growling |
| | Approaching dog on sofa | Nose licking | Growling |
| | Approaching dog on carpet | Blinking | Walking away |

**17.28** Example risk situations identified in Example 1 in Figure 17.26. In this case no one has ever tried to take anything away from the dog directly.

The examples noted in Figure 17.28 reveal important points in terms of the prevention of accidents:

- Aggressive responses in one dog can include more than one category of aggression. For example, this dog reacts aggressively in the context of:
  - Aversive painful stimuli (ears)
  - Aversive non-painful stimuli (pushing, pulling)
  - Benign stimuli (petting, approaching).
- A dog's response to a human action may be different when the context changes (e.g. being approached by adult or by child: sofa *versus* carpet)
- A dog's response for a given context and a given action may be completely different with different family members (e.g. in the context of the sofa: being approached by adult *versus* being approached by child)
- When providing safety advice to families, all of the categories should be addressed (even though not necessarily all of them are owner complaints).

### Safety protocol: aggression in painful interactions

***Stop all painful interactions:*** Provide adequate treatment for the painful process. In cases of painful processes that need daily treatment, provide emergency help for the client (e.g. treatment in veterinary clinic) until the healing process has progressed to an appropriate stage.

***Check if the dog reacts to cues for painful interactions:*** Even after any painful condition has healed, it is useful to check whether the dog is showing signs of stress or avoidance behaviour when presented with previous cues for the painful interaction. Addressing this and installing a desensitization and counter-conditioning (DSCC) protocol will lower the dog's stress and lower the chances of aggressive responses in such situations later on. For example, in the case of putting eardrops in the dog's ear, start by breaking down the act into the different steps and note the dog's reactions at each step (Figure 17.29).

***Check what the dog finds most motivating:*** Rank these motivators from highest to lowest (lower-value rewards can then be used in easier situations and higher-value rewards in more difficult situations). Food may be used as a reward for this exercise. When the dog anticipates a (food) reward, the 'mood' of the dog is usually positive and not anxious or aggressive.

***DSCC protocol: start with an action in the 'safe zone':***

> **WARNING**
> **Applying DSCC protocols for dogs suffering from an emotional disorder might require extra safety measures, such as muzzling and psychopharmacological intervention, in order to prevent accidents.**

| Action | Dog's response | Step in DSCC procedure |
|---|---|---|
| Observing the bottle of eardrops | Relaxed | 1 |
| Owner holding bottle in his hand | Blinking, lip licking | 2 |
| Owner approaching with bottle in his hand | Ears back, turning head away | 3 |
| Owner touching dog's head | Turning body away | 4 |
| Owner touching dog's ear | Lying down, leg up | 5 |
| Owner lifting earflap | Growling | 6 |
| Bottle making contact with ear | Snapping | 7 |
| Owner holding eardropper in ear canal | Biting | 8 |
| Owner instilling eardrops in ear canal | Biting | 9 |
| Owner withdrawing eardropper from ear canal | Biting | 10 |

**17.29** Breakdown of the reactions of the dog in Example 1, Figure 17.26, to ear cleaning; as used in the construction of a desensitization and counter-conditioning protocol.

Start at step 1 (out of 10) and check if the dog is happy to see the bottle (see Figure 17.29) and take a food reward. Repeat this exercise and keep observing the dog's responses. The owner should only move to the next step if the dog shows relaxed behaviour (no sign of stress response; see Ladder of Aggression) consistently to the step.

### Safety protocol: aggression in non-painful aversive interactions

***Stop all aversive interactions:***

- Educate owners about the meaning of aggression in the context of aversive interactions.
- Check existing links with painful aversive interactions in the same contexts (e.g. painful interactions on sofa).
- Address the risk of recurrence and escalation.
- Stress the vulnerability of age groups (e.g. risk of facial bites in children).
- Inform parents that safe behaviours in young children (< 6 years) do not correlate with the knowledge of safety rules, but are significantly correlated with active parental supervision (teaching the children in an interactive way to make safe choices).
- Use appropriate techniques in order to change owner's perception from 'punishment is a good way to tell my dog off' to ' my dog feels stressed when someone pushes or pulls him off the sofa'.

***Encourage new behaviours for each of the contexts:*** In order to provide a safer environment it is crucial to guide owners and encourage new and non-stressful interactions from the owner towards the dog (Figure 17.30). The veterinary surgeon should ensure that the owners:

- Have understood the meaning of the new behaviours they will have to exercise
- Have understood that they act as an example, and that the children will copy
- Are comfortable with these new behaviours and will repeat them spontaneously
- Keep a record of the change in behaviour with their dog.

### Prevention of aggression in the context of resource guarding
Consider Example 2 from Figure 17.26:

---

**Context:** Dog was chewing rawhide and owner wanted to take it away

**Response towards adult owner:** Dog lifted his lips, growled and showed his teeth

**Response towards family children:** None – the family has no children at home

**Response towards other household dogs:** Last week the other family dog was bitten on the ear when passing nearby

---

***List resources that are linked to conflict contexts:*** Define which resources have been observed to be triggers for conflicts. In this example:

- The resources that triggered a conflict between the two dogs are rawhide and human attention
- The resources that triggered a conflict between owner and dog 1 are rawhide and sofa
- No conflicts over resources have been observed between owner and dog 2.

***List those resources and define location and relative value:*** In order to provide a safety protocol in cases of aggression relating to resources, the relative value of each resource needs to be assessed for each dog (Figure 17.31). It is then possible to identify:

- Which resources are of high importance to both dogs
- Which resources are of high importance to only one dog
- Which ones are of high importance to both owner and dog(s).

***List context(s) of conflict:*** Besides knowing the 'relative value' of each resource to the family dog(s), it is equally important to understand the chronological chain of events and the exact way in which events have followed each other. Here it will be crucial to check the dog's responses to each of the situations as well as the owner's interventions and the consequences. Assessing the different interactions that resulted in conflict and aggression will give information about the duration, the intensity and the change over time of the specific conflict context(s).

| Context | Behaviour of family members | Dog's response | Checks |
|---|---|---|---|
| Dog on sofa | **Previous** | | |
| | Pulling or pushing dog off sofa | Growling (adults) Snapping (children) | Check to what extent owner has understood consequences of their previous habit of pulling, pushing and verbal punishment and are willing to change |
| | Verbal punishment when dog growls at children | Lying down with leg raised | |
| | **New** | | |
| | Calling dog with friendly voice Rewarding dog for coming off sofa Parents give example to children to call dog instead of approaching it Parents exercise this with children on daily basis | Check whether dog is responding in relaxed way | Check whether dog is rewarded in correct way for behaviour Advise owners how to react when dog does not obey (try to motivate dog) Check to what extent owner is complying and has stopped their previous habit of pulling, pushing and verbal punishment Ask owner to keep diary of progress and difficulties encountered |

**17.30** Example of changes to be implemented in a family's behaviour towards an aggressive dog, with anticipated responses and necessary checks.

| Resource | Location/context | Value for dog 1 | Value for dog 2 |
|---|---|---|---|
| Rawhide | Spread around the house (e.g. in basket, on carpet) | Extremely high | Extremely high |
| Dog toys | Spread around the house | Ball > tug | Ball > tug |
| Objects | Objects belonging to owner, lying on table | All objects that can be stolen have high value | Not interested |
| Resting place | Sofa | Extremely high | Prefers to lie on floor |
| | Basket | Not interested | Not interested |
| Human attention | When owner is sitting on sofa | Extremely high | Extremely high |

**17.31** Relative resource values identified for two different dogs within a home, during investigation of a case (Example 2, Figure 17.26).

The example in Figure 17.32 illustrates the escalation of conflict over 'one' resource, a rawhide. In order to provide a safety protocol for this family, all other situations with conflict over the other resources will equally need to be analysed and appropriately addressed.

***Check how risk contexts can be minimized in the short term:*** Short-term management consists of avoiding the contexts in which possible competition over resources may develop. This might be by placing physical barriers between the resource and the dog. For example:

- Rawhide: stop giving rawhide; make sure rawhide is not lying around in the house or in the dog's basket; kennel the dog when having rawhide
- Toys: avoid having highly valued toys lying around everywhere; put toys in a closed box and control access.

However, short-term measures such as physical safety barriers to separate the dog from highly valued resources have to be carefully managed in the presence of small children. Young children (< 6 years) might not understand the reasoning behind these rules and break them (by opening doors, gates, kennels and boxes).

***Check how risk can be managed in the long term:*** In order to manage risk over resource-related aggression in the long term, a protocol using owner understanding and compliance as well as a protocol for DSCC is advisable.

- **Check the owner's aims (and consider how realistic they are):** in cases where the conflict over a highly valued resource has been going on for a long time and with owner punishment, chances of creating a relaxed situation might have become non-existent. In other cases owners might have quite unrealistic expectations, such as 'my dogs are one big family and therefore should share the nice things with each other'.
- **Check the extent to which owners understand consistency:** especially in cases about conflict over resources, the owner's understanding and compliance about being consistent towards the dog will influence the outcome of the behavioural management. For example, a protocol to encourage a dog to rest in its basket instead of on the sofa (because the sofa is a location of resource conflict) might have little chance of success with an owner who likes his dog to be on the sofa 'once in a while'.
- **Check the owner's understanding of the dog's behaviour:** conflict over resources has been shown to be a major risk context for dog bites to humans (both adults and children). In order to gain long-term improvement the owner's understanding of the concept of 'threat aversion' needs to be clarified, as well the risk of escalation by physical punishment.
- **Design a DSCC protocol for teaching the animal new behaviours:** teach the animal the 'drop' command on the basis of reward:
  1. Search for a small highly valued reward (e.g. pieces of meat).
  2. Make sure the dog is very relaxed when rewarded.
  3. List the resources from high value to the lowest.
  4. Start the exercise with the lowest valued resource.
  5. Ask the dog to drop the object.
  6. Reward the dog immediately (within half a second).
- **Check the progress of the situation:** make sure that the owner keeps a written record of progress. When no improvement is observable, recheck the diagnosis and involvement of medical factors or emotional disorders.

| Description of risk context | Response of older dog |
|---|---|
| The older dog chews on two pieces of rawhide. While he lies in his basket, the younger dog passes nearby, staring | The older dog growls at the younger dog |
| *At this point the owner intervenes*<br>• The owner is convinced that dogs should not steal from each other and that the older dog has no reason to growl at the young dog<br>• The owner verbally punishes the older dog and takes away his rawhide in order to give it back to the young dog | |
| The young dog is now chewing the rawhide | The older dog approaches, growls and bites the young dog's ear (no lesion); he takes back the rawhide and walks to his basket to chew on both rawhides |
| *The owner intervenes*<br>• The owner is convinced that dogs should not bite each other<br>• The owner feels that the young one is the victim and the old one is guilty<br>• The owner approaches the older dog's basket and wants to take away the rawhide | |
| The owner's action has now become a risk context | The older dog growls and protects his rawhide with both paws |
| *The owner intervenes*<br>• The owner is quite angry and starts to shout<br>• The owner tries to take away the rawhide with force | |
| The owner's interventions have triggered an escalation of the context | The old dog stiffens, stares and growls at the owner, showing his teeth |

**17.32** Example of conflict situations relating to a rawhide chew. The family has two dogs: an older one (4 years) and a younger one (1 year). Both dogs are chewing on rawhides; the older one steals the younger one's rawhide, goes to his basket and chews on both.

### Implementing a safety protocol to prevent play-biting

Consider Example 3 in Figure 17.26:

| |
|---|
| **Context:** Dog and child playing in garden |
| **Response towards adult owner:** Dog growls, jumps and tears clothing |
| **Response towards family children:** Dog has bitten 4-year-old child on the arm |
| **Response towards other household dogs:** None – this family has no other animals |

Play-biting is not about conflict. Play-bites are about exaggerated play which may result in nipping, biting and actually injuring humans, especially children. Before establishing a safety protocol some important points need to be addressed:

### Differentiate underlying cause(s) of overexcitement and nipping:

- Exclude the existence of a behavioural disorder (e.g. hyperactivity: lack of motor control in all situations).
- Exclude iatrogenic factors (e.g. psychotropic drugs such as diazepam may trigger disinhibition, overexcitement and biting).
- Check environmental factors (e.g. lack of physical exercise for a working dog).
- Check factors such as reinforcement by the owner (the dog only gets attention when jumping and nipping).
- Check the extent to which owner behaviour (e.g. physical punishment) has changed the animal's motivation (e.g. from happily jumping to conflict-related biting due to aversive stimuli).
- Check the extent to which the nipping and biting are related to frustration and consist of redirected behaviour (e.g. dog jumps in excitement to chase a cat and is restrained by the owner).

### Investigate all contexts of play-biting:
To start with, it is necessary to investigate all contexts of play-biting as well as contexts that may induce arousal and exaggerated play (see examples in Figure 17.33). As a general rule, the context of a play-bite will be 'high arousal', which might be:

- Actions (running, jumping), movement (waving arms, waving objects), vocal (shouting) or the play itself (ball game, tug of war game)
- Anticipation of actions, e.g. visual contact with the object that precedes the action (the ball) or opening the closet where the play object (ball) is stored
- Social arousal (visitors coming to the house, meeting people on the street)
- Anticipation of the social arousal (doorbell rings, indicating that there is a visitor).

Whenever dogs become excited and start play-biting in a non-aroused situation (e.g. the family is sitting quietly on the sofa, the child is quietly sitting and playing), the underlying reason for the behavioural response will need to be clarified. The clinician will need to differentiate whether the dog:

- Lacks appropriate exercise
- Suffers from a behavioural regulatory disorder (lack of self-control)
- Behaves in this way as the consequence of reinforced attention seeking.

It needs to be stressed that these cases will not be helped by the standard protocol for prevention of play-bites, but will need a correct diagnosis first.

### Check how play-bite contexts can be minimized in the short term:
Short-term management consists of avoiding the contexts in which the behaviour may develop:

- Avoid contexts relating to the dog's arousal (e.g. arrange with neighbour how their dogs can get to know each other and be more relaxed when seeing each other, or be permanently separated visually)
- Place physical barriers between the dog and potential victims (e.g. confine the dog when a child is playing in the garden)
- Stop punishment in order to avoid further escalation of the behaviour (e.g. teach the owner to call the dog and reward it instead of pulling it by the collar).

Even though these measures may appear safe and sound in the short term, they will not necessarily address the dog's problem (over-excitement, lack of bite control) and may become a source of conflict (e.g. pushing or pulling the dog behind a safety gate may induce aggression due to aversive interactions). It should also be stressed that physical measures, such as safety barriers separating dog and potential victim, will need to be carefully managed in the presence of small children. Young children might not necessarily understand the reasoning behind these rules and may break them.

| Context | Trigger(s) | Victim and injury |
|---|---|---|
| Dog and 4-year-old child playing in garden | Child running or cycling | Child nipped on arms and legs several times |
| Owner gardening; dog running around | Neighbour's dog at garden fence barking. Owner shouts at neighbour's dog; own dog nips owner's arm | Owner has several haematomas on arms |
| Owner sitting on sofa; dog starts nipping at clothes while growling | Owner moving arm around | Male owner has hole in jumper and blue bite marks |

**17.33** Example of evaluation of contexts for play-biting.

***Check how play-biting contexts can be minimized in the long term:*** Long-term solutions consist of a good level of owner compliance combined with encouraging new behaviours in the dog (rewarding controlled play). In families with small children the combination of the physical barriers mentioned earlier will be needed in addition until the dog has reached a good level of controlling its play behaviour.

***The basic idea of the behaviour modification DSCC:***

1. Identify the exciting triggers:
   a. List them in order of importance
   b. List them in order of controllability (e.g. cat in the garden)
   c. List levels of intensity of the triggers in terms of item, distance, intensity.
2. Start the exercises at the lowest level of trigger – the level where the dog is playing but still in control of itself (i.e. there is no play-biting).
3. Teach the owner to reward the dog each time it behaves in a relaxed manner and controls itself:
   a. Explain the importance of the kind of reward (preferably food rather than ball game)
   b. Inform owners about the importance of timing (initial rewards should be less than 1 second after the event – clicker training may help (see Chapter 5))
   c. Encourage owners to have realistic aims and to make the exercise easy at the start (some owners might want to practise relax + sit + pawing + lying down)
   d. Do not start the next step until the dog is capable of behaving calmly on several occasions for the same intensity and distance of trigger.
4. In addition, and because not all triggers of arousal can be controlled, the owner should be taught to ignore the dog when it behaves in an excited way:
   a. Inform owners what ignoring means (no eye contact, no talking, no action)
   b. Explain that dogs are capable of reading human gaze and body language
   c. Insist that consistency is the key (explain that intermittently rewarding the excitement might equal the charm of gambling and encourage the dog to go on being excited).
5. Check the progress of the situation.
6. Make sure the owner keeps a written record of the progress.
7. When no improvement is observable, recheck the diagnosis (e.g. hyperactivity).

## Implementing a safety protocol to prevent predation behaviour

Consider Example 4 in Figure 17.26:

> **Context:** The dog (4 years old) was playing with a young kitten in the kitchen and killed it
> **Response towards adult owner:** No complaints
> **Response towards family children:** No problems with the children identifiable
> **Response towards other household dogs:** None – this family has no other animals. This was their first kitten

Predation is a normal behavioural trait and is not about conflict. Predation is a behaviour that is triggered by the movement of the 'perceived' prey and is aimed at catching and killing the prey.

The risk this behaviour represents for society will be dependent on the predated species and the familiarity of it. Dogs killing wild-living mice, rats, rabbits or roaming cats may be seen as good hunters, while dogs killing family pets will be presented for having 'serious' problem behaviour. Predation (or attempted predation) of dogs and predation of humans (infants, small children) present an ethical issue as well as a serious responsibility to the veterinary surgeon in charge. Therefore these cases might benefit from being referred to specialists in the field.

***Differentiate contributing factors:***

- Selective breeding for specific aspects of hunting (e.g. stalking, chasing, chasing and round-up).
- Lack of social contacts in the early developmental phase of life might represent a higher risk (e.g. lack of socialization to children).
- Hunting experience should be seen as a positive learning experience and might lower the threshold for predation.
- Unsupervised access to prey species might increase the risk.

Even though the owner has no children at home and the clinical issue is about predating one species (e.g. a kitten that arrived the day before), the veterinary surgeon will need to check all contexts and species that are potential victims of predation. The history-taking should check whether the behaviour is about predation (as opposed to play-biting or aggression) and whether the behaviour is also directed at: different age groups of the same species (adult cats); dogs (small); other animal species; children.

***Safety protocol:*** Predation cannot be 'cured', and can only be attempted to be put under control. The efficacy of safety protocols to prevent predation will depend on the extent of external (human) control over the dog's behaviour.

- Check the extent to which the owner has control over the dog (without using physical force).
- In a safe environment (e.g. where the prey species is running behind a fence), check the owner's ability to command the recall and the dog's attitude to obeying the command.

Physical barriers (e.g. fences, muzzles) will prevent the dog from catching/killing the prey. However, when barriers are used in order to establish the safety of the children in the family, owners should be warned of the relative value of these (e.g. dogs might jump over, barriers accidently left open).

Electric collars are quite popular in hunting communities for stopping a dog from touching the prey (Christiansen *et al.*, 2001). The historic rationale behind the use of these collars is the emission of a painful electric stimulus (shock) that stops the dog from acting any further; this mode of use has been subject to considerable criticism based on its potential negative impact on the welfare of the animal and the human–animal relationship. However, they are now being advocated by some as part of a training programme which combines interruption (rather than punishment) of the behaviour using a lower level current, with a reward for recall. Because the collars have a preceding signal (audible beep), the dog may learn to anticipate and stop its action at the sound signal. Research in this context is lacking. However, this training method requires some considerable skill to perfect and it is easy for owners to abuse the system and resort to using the devices for punishment. Accordingly, many trainers (including the authors) do not recommend their use and support the use of alternative lower risk humane training methods; this is also the view of the BSAVA.

## Conclusion

Dog bites pose a serious problem to humans, and the incidence appears to be increasing. This suggests that current preventive interventions are inadequate. The causes of bites are multifactorial, and more research is needed on the epidemiology of bites to help to identify the most appropriate prevention strategies. It is clear, however, that this will require coordination and agreement of all major stakeholders, and that education will be the key – and perhaps the greatest challenge.

## References and further reading

Alves MCGP, Matos MR, Reichmann ML et al. (2005) Estimation of the dog and cat population in the state of Sao Paulo. Revista de Saúde Pública 39, 891–897

AVMA (2000) A community approach to dog bite prevention. Journal of the American Veterinary Medical Association 218, 1732–1749

Bamberger M and Houpt K (2006) Signalment factors, comorbidity, and trends in behavior diagnoses in dogs: 1644 cases (1991–2001). Journal of the American Veterinary Medical Association 229, 1591–1601

Bateman S (2007) Communication in the veterinary emergency setting. Veterinary Clinics of North America: Small Animal Practice 37, 109–121

Beaver B (1993) Profiles of dogs presented for aggression. Journal of the American Animal Hospital Association 29, 564–569

Beaver B (1999) Canine Behavior: A Guide for Veterinarians. WB Saunders, Philadelphia

Bender J and Minicucci L (2007) Diseases pets and people share. Minnesota Medicine 90, 43–47

Bernardo LM, Gardner RN, O'Dair J et al. (2002) The DOG BITES Program: documentation of growls and bites in the emergency setting. Journal of Emergency Nursing 28, 536–541

Besser R (2007) Dog attacks: it's time for doctors to bite back. British Medical Journal 334, 425

Bond L and Hauf CA (2004) Taking stock and putting stock in primary prevention: characteristics of effective programs. Journal of Primary Prevention 24, 199–221

Christiansen F, Bakken M and Braastadt B (2001) Behavioural changes and aversive conditioning in hunting dogs by the second year confrontation with domestic sheep. Applied Animal Behaviour Science 72, 131–143

Cornell K and Kopcha M (2007) Client–veterinarian communication: skills for client centred dialogue and shared decision making. Veterinary Clinics of North America: Small Animal Practice 37, 37–47

De Keuster T, Moons C and De Cock I (2005) Dog bite prevention – how a Blue Dog can help. European Journal of Companion Animal Practice 15, 137–139

Gilchrist J, Sacks JJ, White D and Kresnow M-J (2008) Dog bites: still a problem? Injury Prevention 14, 296–301

Guy N, Luescher A, Dohoo S et al. (2001) Risk factors for dog bites to owners in a general veterinary caseload. Applied Animal Behaviour Science 74, 29–42

Hart BL, Hart LA and Bain MJ (2006) Canine and Feline Behavior Therapy, 2nd edn. Blackwell Publishing, Ames, Iowa

Herron M, Shofer FS and Reisner IR (2009) Survey of the use and outcome of confrontational and non-confrontational training methods in client-owned dogs showing undesired behaviors. Applied Animal Behaviour Science 117, 47–54

Horisberger U (2002) Medizinisch versorgte Hubdebissverletzungen in der Schweiz: Opfer – Hunde – Unfallsituationen. Bern, Veterinarian med. Fakultät, Diss.

Horwitz D and Neilson J (2007) Blackwell's Five-Minute Veterinary Consult, Clinical Companion: Canine and Feline Behavior. Blackwell Publishing, Ames, Iowa

Hubacher M (2001) Unfälle und Unfallprävention im Kindesalter. Schweiz Medicine Forum 24, 631–635

Jung H (2007) Das Deutschland-Projekt „Beißt der?" – Arbeit mit 6-8jährigen Kindern und traumatisierten oder ängstlichen Menschen, DVG-Congress Berlin

Kahn A, Bauche P, Lamoureux J et al. (2003) Child victims of dog bites treated in emergency departments. European Journal of Pediatrics 162, 254–258

Kahn A, Robert E, Piette D et al. (2004) Prevalence of dog bites in children. A telephone survey. European Journal of Pediatrics 163, 424

Lakestani N, Waran N, Verga M and Phillips C (2005) Dog bites in children. European Journal of Companion Animal Practice 2, 133–135

Landsberg G, Hunthausen W and Ackermann L (2003) Handbook of Behavior Problems of the Dog and Cat, 2nd edn. Elsevier Saunders, Philadelphia

Limbourg M (1994) Ursachen und Vermeidung von Unfällen im Kindesalter. In: Sicher Leben: Bericht über die 1. Tagung Kindersicherheit: Was wirkt?, pp. 46–58. Universität GH Essen 1994 in Wien, 1995, Wien

Love M and Overall K (2001) How anticipating relationships between dogs and children can help prevent disasters. Journal of the American Veterinary Medical Association 219, 446–451

Meints K and De Keuster T (in press) Don't kiss a sleeping dog: the first assessment of 'The Blue Dog' bite prevention program. Journal of Pediatric Psychology

Mertens P (2006) Reproductive and sexual behavioural problems in dogs. Theriogenology 66, 606–609

Miller W and Rollnick S (1991) Motivational interviewing: preparing people for change. Guilford Press, New York

Montagner H, Millot JL, Filiatre JC et al. (1988) Recent data on the interaction between a child and its family pet. Bulletin of the Academy of National Medicine 172, 951–955

Morrongiello BA, Midgett C and Shields R (2001) Don't run with scissors: young children's knowledge of home safety rules. Journal of Pediatric Psychology 26, 105–115

NHS Statistics (2008) http://news.bbc.co.uk/1/hi/health/7264620.stm

Overall K (1997) Clinical Behavioural Medicine for Small Animals. Mosby–Yearbook, Inc, St Louis, Missouri

Overall K and Love M (2001) Dog bites to humans: demography, epidemiology, injury and risk. Journal of the American Veterinary Medical Association 218, 1923–1934

Ozanne-Smith J, Ashby K and Stathakis V (2001) Dog bite and injury prevention – analysis, critical review and research agenda. Injury Prevention 7, 321–326

Pageat P (1998) Pathologie du Comportement du Chien. Du Point Vétérinaire, Maisons Alfort, France

Poresky RH (1996) Companion animals and other factors affecting young children's development. Anthrozoos 9, 159–168

Reisner IR (1997) Assessment, management, and prognosis of canine dominance-related aggression. Veterinary Clinics of North America: Small Animal Practice 27, 479–495

Reisner IR (2003) Differential diagnosis and management of human-directed aggression in dogs. Veterinary Clinics of North America: Small Animal Practice 33, 303–320

Reisner IR, Shofer F and Nance M (2007) Behavioral assessment of child-directed canine aggression. Injury Prevention 13, 348–351

Salman M, New J, Scarlett J et al. (1998) Human and animal factors related to relinquishment of dogs and cats in 12 selected animal shelters in the United States. Journal of Applied Animal Welfare Science 1, 207–226

Schalamon J, Ainoedhofer H, Singer G et al. (2006) Analysis of dog bites in children who are younger than 17 years. Pediatrics 117, 374–379

Schilder M and van der Borg J (2004) Training dogs with help of the shock collar: short and long term behavioural effects. Applied Animal Behaviour Science 85, 319–334

Shuler C, DeBess E, Lapidus J and Hedberg K (2008) Canine and human factors related to dog bite injuries. *Journal of the American Veterinary Medical Association* **232**, 542–546

Triebenbacher SL (1998) Pets as transitional objects: their role in children's emotional development. *Psychological Reports* **82**, 191–200

Westgarth C, Pinchbeck, GL, Bradshaw JWS *et al.* (2008) Dog-human and dog-dog interactions of 260 dog-owning households in a community in Cheshire. *The Veterinary Record* **162**, 436–442

Wilson F, Dwyer F and Bennett P (2003) Prevention of dog bites: evaluation of a brief intervention program for preschool children. *Journal of Community Psychology* **I31**, 75–86

Zeedyk MS, Wallace L, Carcary B *et al.* (2001) Children and road safety: increasing knowledge does not improve behaviour. *British Journal of Educational Psychology* **71**, 573–594

## Client handouts (bsavalibrary.com/behaviour_leaflets)

- Canine behaviour questionnaire
- Cognitive dysfunction syndrome
- Down–stay mat exercises
- Handling exercises for puppies and kittens
- Headcollar training
- How to find a good trainer
- Ladder of Aggression
- 'Leave it' exercises
- Muzzle training
- 'Nothing in Life is Free'

- Puppy socialization: getting used to new people
- Recall exercises
- Redirected aggression in dogs
- Request for information on problem behaviours
- Sit–stay exercises
- Teaching your dog to go to a placed on command
- What your dog needs
- Your puppy's first year

# 18

# Aggression toward unfamiliar people and animals

## Melissa Bain

## Introduction

Aggression is a very common problem in companion dogs. It can roughly be separated into two types: directed toward *familiar* people or animals (see Chapter 17); and directed toward *unfamiliar* people or animals. One study found that only 11% of veterinary surgeons strongly agreed with a statement that it was their responsibility to initiate discussion of behaviour problems (Patronek and Dodman, 1999). This same study concluded that approximately 224,000 dogs and cats were euthanized by veterinary practitioners in the United States for problem behaviours. While this study did not limit its scope to canine aggression, it could be assumed that a good percentage of those dogs were euthanized because of aggression problems.

Given the number of dogs that display aggression, it should surprise no one that close to 70% of dogs that present to veterinary behaviourists have a diagnosis of aggression (Landsberg, 1991; Beaver, 1994; Patronek *et al.*, 1996). It should be noted that a variety of terms are used to describe the diagnosis of aggression but, regardless of the terminology they use, veterinary behaviourists have the same general understanding. This chapter uses a motivational basis for the classification of aggression and looks at differences in treatment relating to which species is the target of the aggression.

## Societal effects of aggression

The significance of canine aggression can be evaluated from its effect on the human–animal bond, as well as its effect on public safety. One study has shown that dogs relinquished to shelters have a higher incidence of aggression compared with dogs remaining in homes (Segurson *et al.*, 2005). Compared with client-owned dogs, significantly more dogs relinquished to shelters were reported to have owner-directed aggression, stranger-directed aggression, dog-directed aggression or fear, stranger-directed fear, non-social fear and separation-related behaviours. Another study reported that approximately 41% of dogs adopted from a shelter demonstrated aggressive behaviour once in the new home; this was further broken down to 52% of dogs demonstrating aggression toward unfamiliar people based on territoriality and 16.7% of dogs demonstrating aggression toward

unfamiliar dogs (Christensen *et al.*, 2007). A study by Hsu and Serpell (2003) concluded that close to 40% of dogs displayed aggression toward unfamiliar people and 25% displayed fear or aggression toward unfamiliar dogs.

Aggression can also be roughly broken down into defensive versus offensive threats. The motivations of a defensive threat are generally based on fear and/or anxiety, but the motivations for an offensive threat are sometimes not as clear. A dog demonstrating an offensive threat may indeed be confident in the given situation. Conversely, it may be fearful but has learned that an offensive threat, such as chasing a person or dog away, is more effective than demonstrating a fearful body posture.

## Risk factors

There are many identified risk factors for aggression, either dog-related or human-related.

### Breed

Certain breeds rank higher in different behavioural categories, such as territorial defence, watchdog barking, aggression toward other dogs and snapping at children (Hart and Miller, 1985). Dogs that rank higher for 'territorial defence' include those breeds historically bred for this behaviour, such as Rottweiler, Chow Chow and German Shepherd Dog, compared with breeds such as Pug and Bichon Frise, which are in the lowest ranks. However, these are generalizations and there are large variations between individuals within breeds.

### Gender

Gender plays a role as well, and males tend to be over-represented. Castration is usually recommended as part of a treatment plan, but while the aggression may be decreased, it will not be eliminated by castration. It is important to note that there is no correlation between age of castration, or experience prior to castration, and the outcome of decreased aggression post castration (Neilson *et al.*, 1997).

### Management

How the dog is housed, managed and trained also has an effect on its behaviour toward unfamiliar people and dogs. Dogs that are not properly socialized to people or other dogs during their primary socialization period (between approximately 3 and 14 weeks of age) may be more likely to be fearful of or aggressive toward others, or may signal inappropriately to their conspecifics. Sacks *et al.* (1996) identified that 22% of the 109 reported fatal attacks on people involved an unrestrained dog not on its owner's property, 18% involved a restrained dog on its owner's property and 59% involved an unrestrained dog on its owner's property. The breed most commonly involved was the Pit Bull Terrier (24), followed by Rottweiler (16) and German Shepherd Dog (10). This may reflect a potential breed disposition toward more severe attacks, but also may reflect a size discrimination in dogs fatally attacking a person, or differences in the management of these animals.

## The behavioural biology of aggression

Aggression is considered by some to be 'abnormal'. While it is certainly socially unacceptable in human society, many manifestations are likely to be normal given the dog's background, what it has learned previously, genetic predisposition, and how it is managed and housed.

An important biological relationship exists between aggressive behaviour and the brain neurotransmitter serotonin. One study demonstrated that low serotonin levels in cerebrospinal fluid were correlated with severe aggression in Springer Spaniels (Reisner *et al.*, 1996). A study looking at serum serotonin and lipid levels in aggressive dogs found that aggressive dogs had serotonin levels lower than non-aggressive dogs (Cakiroglu *et al.*, 2007). In another study, dogs receiving tryptophan-supplemented low-protein diets had a lower behavioural score of territorial aggression than those receiving a low-protein diet without supplementation (DeNapoli *et al.*, 2000). It would seem this relationship relates especially to the role of serotonin on impulse control, with more impulsive or reactive dogs more likely to show aggression when challenged, while others are more self-controlled in their behaviour.

Properly done, early environmental exposure and socialization during the dog's primary socialization period (3–14 weeks) may serve to inoculate the dog against potential fear and the tendency to show aggression at a later stage in its life (see Chapter 6). Appleby *et al.* (2002) found that dogs that were not raised in a home environment as a puppy but rather in, say, a kennel, garage, barn or shed, and those that had a lack of experience of urban environments between 3 and 6 months of age, were both significantly more likely to show aggression and avoidance behaviour toward unfamiliar people. Aggression during a veterinary examination was more likely in dogs raised in a kennel after birth. There was no significant association with environment for aggression toward familiar people, or toward dogs.

## Evaluation of the patient

Developing a behavioural diagnosis is based largely on obtaining an accurate history from the owner and observing the behaviour of the dog (and owner) during the consultation. The other arm of behavioural diagnosis is the elimination of medical problems that could contribute to the aggression.

## Presenting signs and history

The owner may not be presenting the dog specifically for aggression, but may approach for help in a more circuitous manner (see Chapter 17). The ability to take a complete history is very important, and using a more open-ended manner of asking questions helps to gather more complete information from owners. Owners must be able to confide adequately some potentially damaging information regarding their dog's aggression. The skills and pitfalls of history taking in canine aggression cases are covered in Chapter 17. Essential areas of questioning are summarized as follows:

- What is the medical history?
- What are the household demographics?
- What is the role of the dog in the household?
- To whom or what is the dog aggressive (e.g. visitors, passers-by, dogs in the park)?
- Where is the dog aggressive?
- When is the dog aggressive?
- With which owner is the dog most aggressive?
- What are the specific triggers of aggression?
- What does the owner do?
- How does the dog respond?
- What is the severity, intensity, frequency and predictability of the aggression?
- What are the owner's goals?

The veterinary surgeon must remain non-judgemental, not only by asking open questions in a neutral tone, but also by being aware of non-verbal communication, since people are more likely to believe non-verbal communication when compared with the concurrent verbal communication.

When taking a history and evaluating a dog for aggression, care must be taken to do so safely for all people and animals in the room. Since these consultations are generally longer than a traditional veterinary visit, a place for all people to sit is important. It is preferable to have no examination table dividing the space, both for facilitating communication as well as for safety. The veterinary surgeon and staff should position themselves so that the dog does not feel cornered and also so that they can safely leave the room without passing a potentially aggressive dog. Care must be taken not to trigger the dog to display aggression (for example, by staring intently at the dog) although owners will often ask for this as part of the consultation. One study was equivocal in the benefits of performing a behavioural 'test' in the examination room and did not show a strong correlation between the results of the test for aggression and what the owner supplied in the history (Kroll *et al.*, 2004). However, the behaviours that are observed can help to support the diagnosis. Watching the dog carefully from the time it comes into the veterinary clinic to the time it leaves gives a lot of information as to its motivation and underlying temperament.

Even though only one aspect of the problem behaviours of the dog is the primary focus, other problems (physical and behavioural) need to be identified and addressed or else the treatment plan may be less effective. For example, a dog that is diagnosed with territorial aggression and separation anxiety may show barking as a sign. Barking when the owners are absent needs to be evaluated to determine whether it is due to the dog panicking, or whether it is due to the dog barking at passers-by. The choice of medication, if any, also needs to be tempered by taking all diagnoses into consideration.

## Client attitudes, beliefs and behaviours

Interaction between the owner and the dog can provide information regarding the owner's attachment to the dog. Is the owner constantly correcting the dog for various misbehaviours? Or are they comforting the dog when it looks fearful? Understanding these non-verbal communications helps when developing the diagnosis, prognosis and treatment plan. Special note should be made of any interactions that change the behaviour of the dog. Does the dog show fear when the owner pulls sharply on the lead, or does it redirect aggression toward the owner? Does petting from its owner actually calm the dog down, or does it attempt to move away from its owner? It is also important to note any differences in the dog's behaviour toward different family members.

Owners may come in with a 'diagnosis' determined by watching a television show or going on to the Internet. It is essential to obtain objective information and not simply accept what they say (see Chapter 17). It is also worth noting that they may have exacerbated the problem by experimenting with potentially harmful training techniques.

## Risk evaluation

Part of the entire evaluation is to determine what risks are present when considering other dogs and people, as well as considering that particular dog. The subject of risk assessment has been dealt with extensively in Chapter 17, but Figure 18.1 summarizes some of the key general points to be considered.

---

**Risk to people and other dogs**

- Physical injury – redirected aggression to family members if not recognized; by being physically pulled down when attempting to stop a dog fight
- Emotional injury – stress in avoiding situations, or constantly worrying about it; conflict between family members
- Potential liability

**Risk to problem dog**

- Physical injury – from other dog or person, or from owner trying to stop the behaviour
- Emotional injury – stress in encountering the stimuli; stress in anticipating the owner's reaction
- Relinquishment

---

**18.1** Risks inherent in owning a dog with a history of aggressive behaviour.

Factors that need to be considered when evaluating risk might include:

- Owner's willingness and ability to keep others safe
- Owner's willingness and ability to follow treatment recommendations
- Diagnosis
- Overall temperament and size of the dog
- Frequency, intensity, severity and predictability of aggressive incidents.

One major factor to consider is the owner's willingness and ability to follow the treatment plan. Are they adequately able to avoid the aggression-inducing encounters? Are children involved, either as household members or as targets of the aggression? These factors can increase the risk and influence the prognosis.

## Diagnosis

As with all aspects of veterinary medicine, it is important to have an accurate diagnosis to develop the appropriate prognosis and treatment plan. In the absence of a primary diagnosis, it is necessary to have at least a working list of differential diagnoses. By ruling out obviously incorrect diagnoses, better focus can be made on efforts along more specific paths of investigation.

### Medical conditions

Obvious, and not so obvious, medical conditions need to be ruled out, or at least taken into consideration when working up a case (see Chapter 1).

- Any disease process that causes pain, such as orthopaedic disease, can lower an animal's threshold to display aggression.
- An encounter with another dog that caused pain (as when bitten by a dog during a fight or when an electronic stimulation was delivered) can predispose the dog to display aggression in similar circumstances.
- Gastrointestinal disorders, while not contributing directly to the aggression, may also lower the threshold for aggressive displays by causing the dog to be irritable.
- Sensory deficits can lead a dog to 'over-react' and so show aggression in situations in which it is startled, such as when a person suddenly reaches a hand over its head.
- Neurological abnormalities should also be considered in some circumstances, such as when presented with a dog with potentially idiopathic aggression.

A complete physical examination is an essential prerequisite, with other diagnostic tests as appropriate.

### Differential diagnoses: types of aggression

Functional types of aggression toward unfamiliar people that may be diagnosed are listed in Figure 18.2 along with characteristics and treatment

| Diagnosis | Offensive or defensive posture? | Triggers | Victim characteristics | Location | Age of onset | Development | General treatment recommendations |
|---|---|---|---|---|---|---|---|
| Fear-related aggression | Usually defensive, but can appear offensive as a result of learning | Potentially any type of action by an unfamiliar person that could be perceived by the dog as a threat (e.g. direct approach or reaching towards or over the dog) | Individual characteristics may heighten the risk, as a result of either learned aversive associations or unfamiliarity, e.g. very large people; bearded men. Familiar person that has unfamiliar characteristics, or one that surprises the dog may induce same response | Any location, but increased risk in novel environment or when animal's personal space is invaded | Any age | Often related to not being adequately exposed to people during socialization period. Could be due to an experience that caused pain or fear at any age | Avoidance of fear-eliciting triggers Tools: headcollar; muzzle DSCC to triggers No direct punishment ± Anti-anxiety medications ± Pheromone therapy |
| Territorial aggression | Often offensive, but can be defensive | Individuals approaching the dog's property, such as its house, garden, car | Anyone approaching the dog's property | The dog's territory, some of which may not be immediately obvious, such as kennel guarding in the clinic | Usually around time of social maturity: 1–3 years | May be related to the familiarity of the area, and how comfortable the dog is there versus elsewhere (so limited range of experience outside the home may increase the risk). Confidence is often a function of experience (e.g. withdrawal of passers-by) | Avoid dog being alone in 'its' territory and having access to trigger points like windows, doors, etc. Tools: headcollar; muzzle DSCC to triggers No direct punishment ± Anti-anxiety medications ( only with caution) ± Pheromone therapy |
| Assertive aggression | Offensive. If ambivalent (which is not uncommon) this usually suggests a lack of confidence in the situation | A perceived (whether real or not) challenge, e.g. staring or movement towards a key resource | Usually familiar people, but can display toward unfamiliar people, especially when behaviour has been reinforced | Any location, but usually at home or familiar location | Usually around time of social maturity: 1–3 years | Not very common. Thought to be more of an underlying biological predisposition – confident risk taker. Dogs can appear offensive in their posture but be emotionally fearful | Avoid triggering the dog's behaviour Tools: headcollar; muzzle DSCC to triggers No direct punishment ± Anti-anxiety medications (with caution) ± Pheromone therapy |

**18.2**   Differential diagnoses, characteristics and summary treatment recommendations for aggression toward unfamiliar people. Co-morbidity with other diagnoses is possible. (DSCC, desensitization and counter-conditioning.)

recommendations. Specific terminology varies widely between behaviourists, possibly with more contextual labels added. For example, defence of the car and the home might be differentiated, but essentially they are both protection of property and so functionally the same and are labelled 'territorial aggression' here. Treatment for the different types of aggression is relatively similar, the primary variables being location and the triggers that behaviour modification will address.

**Offensive aggression, defensive aggression and appeasement**
One way to differentiate types of aggression is to determine the body language and apparent intent of the dog. Dogs can react aggressively to a stimulus in either an offensive or a defensive manner.

- The body postures commonly associated with an *offensive* threat (Figure 18.3) are:
  - Ears pointing forwards
  - Eyes focused on the stimulus
  - Lips retracted vertically
  - Tail elevated
  - Body stance more forward-leaning or moving.

- The body postures commonly associated with a *defensive* threat (Figure 18.4) are:
  - Ears drawn backwards
  - Eyes diverted from the stimulus
  - Lips retracted horizontally
  - Tail tucked or lowered
  - Body stance more retreating or lowered.

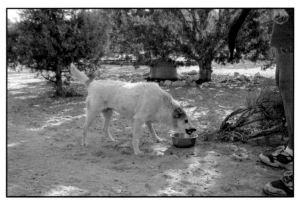

**18.3**   A dog that appears to be assertively aggressive. Note the vertical lip lift, elevated tail, forward body posture and piloerection.

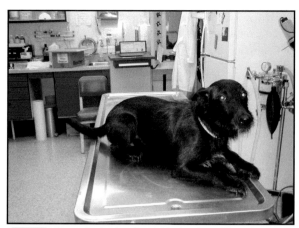

**18.4** Dog displaying fearful behaviour. Note the drawn-back ears, dilated pupils and stiff body posture.

Associated with either group of visual signals may be growling or barking at the stimulus, and perhaps physical contact with the teeth.

The relationship between posture and underlying emotion is not necessarily straightforward. It is perhaps simpler to determine the motivation of the dog that is clearly signalling one way or the other, but frequently dogs will display offensive, defensive and/or appeasement signals concurrently, indicating a mixed motivation or a state of conflict anxiety. When obtaining a history, it is important to determine not only the signalling that the dog currently delivers, but also signals that it displayed previously in other or similar situations.

A common presentation is of a dog that lunges toward approaching people with little provocation, teeth bared midway between vertical and horizontal lip retraction and tail elevated. Some are tempted to classify this dog as a confidently aggressive dog, but the history may say otherwise. Until a few months prior, the dog may have cowered and growled when approached by a person. Another piece of historical information often noted is that the dog once snapped at a person and, since then, it has displayed an offensive threat that is more effective at driving the person away than showing signs of fear while growling.

Understanding the underlying motivation is important when delivering the treatment plan and prognosis, since the prognosis might be different if the dog is fearful rather than completely confident, though in both situations the dog is responding to a perceived threat.

### Owner involvement
Owners and other people can play a significant role in their dogs' behaviour, for better or for worse.

It may seem obvious that a dog will become fearfully aggressive to people when harsh training techniques are used, such as 'alpha-rolling/pinning' or shaking the dog's scruff. Other types of harsh training may cause an association between pain and another stimulus, such as a dog given a harsh training ('choke') collar jerk or an electronic-collar stimulation ('shock') when the dog demonstrates interest or unruliness around an unfamiliar dog. This may lead to an association with unfamiliar dogs predicting something painful, leading to a fear of unfamiliar dogs and perhaps aggression to them as a result.

Human-handler miscommunication also occurs when a person becomes tense during certain situations. If the dog is somewhat unruly or aggressive toward unfamiliar dogs while on a walk, the owner may become concerned and tighten up on the lead, perhaps displaying their own tense body posture. This tension is conveyed to the dog, who also becomes anxious or protective in response (see Chapter 5).

A more common situation is when an owner differentially rewards or punishes a territorially aggressive dog, depending on who the visitor or 'intruder' is. Owners may state that they want a dog to protect their property from intruders, while being able to let other visitors enter their property. This is a very difficult situation in which to place a dog, requiring it to differentiate between 'good' and 'bad' people (see section on stimulus control in Chapter 5). It is the owner's job to identify true intruders, with the dog alerting them. Perhaps postal workers are most strongly defended against, since they intrude on to the territory without the owner escorting them; they make noise, rarely give the dog a treat or other reward, and retreat in apparent response to the dog barking – or at least this is how it may seem to the dog.

### Onset of aggression
Knowledge of when the aggressive behaviour began can help to indicate the correct motivation for the behaviour. This is difficult to determine if a dog is obtained as an adult.

When obtaining a history, it is important to determine not only when the problem began to be of concern to the owner, but also when the dog *first* displayed aggressive or other fearful behaviour. Earlier onset of aggression can be more disconcerting, especially when linked with a truly confident personality or when more advanced threats, such as biting, are more quickly employed. The dog that shows little aggression and has never growled or snapped at someone during its entire life and then, at age 10, bites someone when it is cornered and grabbed by its painful hips has a potentially better prognosis than the 1-year-old confident dog that displays severe offensive and largely unprovoked aggression the first time someone approaches it.

### Combinations of aggressive behaviours
It is important to keep in mind that any dog can have more than one behavioural problem, including multiple expressions of aggression. A dog could display offensive aggression, based on territoriality, toward people coming on to its property, but defensive aggression toward veterinary staff when examined.

The situation must be triaged to determine which of the different problems should be addressed first. If a dog is diagnosed with aggression of equal intensity and severity toward household members and toward unfamiliar people, the aggression toward familiar people should normally be addressed first. It is generally possible for owners to avoid unfamiliar people more easily than to avoid interacting with the dog in the household. However, the severity of the aggression shown to date must also be taken into consideration. If the dog has growled at the owners in a few predictable and avoidable situations, but has broken through the fence to attack a passing dog, then the latter should be addressed first. Even if the owner is unable to work fully on multiple problems concurrently, avoidance is almost always recommended in the interim until the problem can be fully addressed.

# Treatment

The aim of treatment is to manage the dog and change the underlying motivation sufficiently, so that the aggression is significantly decreased and the associated risk is reduced to an acceptable level (see Chapter 17). No assurance should be given that aggression will be 'cured', since it is a normal part of the behavioural repertoire of a dog. There can never be a guarantee that the dog will not display aggressive behaviour in the future and owners must be clear that it is not feasible to eliminate all signs of aggression completely. Medical factors contributing to irritability (e.g. chronic pain) should be recognized and treated as appropriate.

The overall goals are dependent on human- and dog-related factors. It may be helpful to owners to set up a step-wise goal-directed programme, so that all involved can more objectively see progress as well as problem areas. If owners are educated about the signs and triggers that the dog displays, they can more easily identify and avoid the triggers, as well as employ behaviour modification to decrease the dog's reaction to those triggers.

The goals of the owner must be taken into consideration. Without a full discussion and an understanding of their perceptions about the management and eventual outcomes of the treatment, there could be disappointment and frustration on the part of both the owner and veterinary surgeon. Is it the owner's goal to decrease the dog's chance of biting again? Do they want to be able to make their dog more comfortable in situations and lessen its anxiety, so that the aggression is less likely to be displayed? Or is the owner's goal to have a dog who never growls or even lifts its lip at a person, even in the most extreme circumstances?

It is important to determine how easy it is to avoid a specific situation while the owner helps the dog to respond more appropriately to the trigger. An example is an owner who wants to visit an off-lead exercise area (dog park) with their dog. Not only is it difficult to have complete control over a dog that is off-lead, but also it is difficult to predict whether all of the other dogs at the park will act in a socially appropriate manner. It is not feasible to guarantee that a dog will behave in a non-aggressive manner in these types of parks. With treatment, however, it is feasible that the owner's dog will be able to get aerobic exercise in other ways, walk calmly on-lead past other dogs, and even have off-lead exercise time with familiar dogs with known histories in a fenced area.

## Acute management strategies

Before moving to the heart of changing a dog's motivation, the owner must prevent the dog from performing the undesirable behaviour. Not only is this a safety recommendation, it also prevents the dog from being reinforced for performing the aggressive behaviour (see Chapter 5) and prevents the dog from practising and perfecting it.

### Avoidance

One method of helping to ensure safety is avoiding the situation in which the dog displays the behaviour. If a dog displays aggression toward visitors to the house, it should be placed in another room before the visitors arrive, or be kept away from windows, doors and fences, depending on the triggers of the aggression. The only exception is if the owner is actively working on behaviour modification with the dog and the visitor is being used as part of the treatment programme.

Some owners will state that avoiding does not solve the problem. While this is true, not letting the dog practise the behaviour is the foundation of the entire treatment plan and is a sound safety recommendation. If the dog will not tolerate confinement, then confinement training should also be part of the treatment plan.

### *Punishment, reassurance and reinforcement:*
Owners may have to change their own interactions with their dog, especially if they are using punishment-based techniques. Dogs that are physically corrected for unwanted behaviours (for example, acting fearfully or anxiously, growling, lunging, snapping and biting) may become more anxious and aggressive in association with the stimulus. Nor should the owner reassure the dog when it displays signs of aggression or other signs of anxiety, since this may lead the dog to believe that the behaviour is appropriate. Finally, owners must appreciate that the behaviour is further reinforced whenever the dog successfully threatens the stimulus and the stimulus retreats. The dog is choosing the behaviour because it feels it is appropriate for the situation and is unlikely to pick a different behaviour unless taught a new one; therefore the owner must control the situation if they cannot control the dog.

The dog should not be allowed off-lead in the presence, or potential presence, of the problem stimulus, whether it is another dog or a person. The lead should be leather or heavy nylon, with a sturdy metal buckle, and no more than 2 metres (6 feet) in length. Retractable leads should not be used, as they are thin and owners can have difficulty manipulating them to call the dog closer to them. Some dogs are actually less aggressive when they are allowed off the lead, perhaps due to their owners reacting in an anxious manner when the dog is on-lead (as described above), or an inability to get away if fearful when on-lead. However, most owners are unable to control their dog reliably when it is off-lead and so off-lead exercise cannot be recommended.

## Control and restraint aids

For the best control, the dog should wear a head-collar; this gives the owner control over the dog's forward movement, closes the mouth if necessary and redirects the dog's attention to the owner. It can also be worn with a long light lead or cord/drag line while loose in the house under supervision, so that the owner can safely grab the end of the line to control and redirect the dog. A useful 'side effect' of a head-collar is that, although it is not a muzzle, other people may think that it is and may not approach the dog so readily. If the dog or owner absolutely cannot tolerate the use of a headcollar, a front-attachment harness can be used for better control of forward movement. Tools that cause pain, such as prong/pinch, training/choke or electronic collars, should be avoided.

Muzzles can also be used. The caveat is that a muzzle should not be placed on the dog to let the dog 'fight it out' or otherwise become highly emotionally aroused. The recommended muzzle is one that allows the dog to pant, drink and safely vomit (if necessary), which usually means a basket muzzle. Nylon or cloth muzzles should be avoided for long-term use, as they need to be snug to be effective. However, they can be effective if needed for a short time, such as at a veterinary practice. Care must be exercised to avoid overheating when dogs are muzzled, and muzzles may be inappropriate in some climates.

The dog should be gradually acclimatized to wearing a headcollar or muzzle (see Chapter 17). A dog cannot be expected to tolerate a new tool that is just quickly placed upon its head without proper introduction. It is best to use food treats, attention and walks while the dog is wearing the headcollar or muzzle, rather than just putting it on to the dog when it encounters a potentially unpleasant person or dog.

## Long-term treatment strategies

### Owner control and consistent interactions

A key component of a behaviour modification programme is deference exercises. These are non-confrontational steps that will help the dog to learn to defer to people and their control in various situations and to become more responsive to the direction provided by others. Such a programme is sometimes referred to as 'Nothing in Life is Free' (Voith and Borchelt, 1982; see **client handout**) or 'Learn to Earn' (Campbell, 1999). These exercises require that the dog begins to earn all of its valued resources by responding to a command given by the owner. By doing this, the owner not only gains control but also interacts with the dog in a consistent manner. It helps to teach the dog to look to the owner for guidance when faced with a difficult situation. This alone may ameliorate the dog's uncertainty and aggression when meeting unknown individuals. It is very important that everyone who interacts with the dog follows the guidelines in the **client handout**.

*Eye contact:* Teaching a dog to make eye contact with its owner on command can be very useful. An eye-contact command can be used to get and keep the dog's attention in situations that may otherwise provoke fear or anxiety. It can also be a part of teaching the dog literally and figuratively to look to the owner for leadership. Separately, it also helps to desensitize and counter-condition a dog to being stared at.

*Down-stay:* Teaching a dog to 'down-stay' at increasing distances from the owner can help the dog to relax, as well as teach it that it is a good thing to be away from visitors and other such stimuli. The dog should be asked to 'down' and 'stay' at gradually farther distances from the owner, and for gradually longer times (see Chapter 5). This behaviour should be reinforced with a long-lasting food treat.

### Desensitization and counter-conditioning

In general, systematic desensitization and counter-conditioning (DSCC) are the main techniques that are utilized to change a dog's response to strangers (see Chapter 5). Specific characteristics of the stranger that can trigger aggression might include their gender, height, type of clothing, movement and so on, and should have been discovered during the history taking. The goal of these techniques is to replace unwanted behaviours (attempts at withdrawal and aggression) with a positive behaviour (remaining calm and focused on the owner).

- **Systematic desensitization** is the process of reintroducing the dog to the stimulus (e.g. unfamiliar people or dogs) through the use of a stimulus gradient, which should be established at the beginning of the treatment sessions.
- **Counter-conditioning** is the process of changing the emotional state in regard to the stimulus, usually from fear to a state of relaxation, in which the dog becomes classically conditioned to the stimulus (respondent counter-conditioning).
- **Counter-commanding** is the process of reinforcing a substitute behaviour that is incompatible with the unwanted behaviour (a sitting dog cannot lunge at the person) (operant counter-conditioning).

When these techniques are combined, the unwanted behaviour is replaced with a positive emotion and usually an incompatible behaviour through a gradual process of reintroducing the stimulus and rewarding the dog for the desired behaviour.

*Intensity and distance gradients:* The trigger or stimulus that was identified as causing the dog's fear and aggression should be reintroduced in a series of gradual steps or intensities. The common gradients that are used for DSCC are altering the intensity and changing the distance to the stimulus. The intensity can be changed by altering the location (in the house *versus* out on walks *versus* in the garden; Figure 18.5), speed of movement of the person, and different types of people (men, women, children). The DSCC should be started at the lowest intensity that results in no signs of anxiety or concern from the dog.

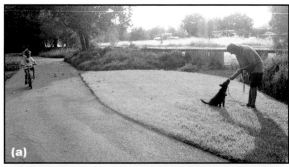

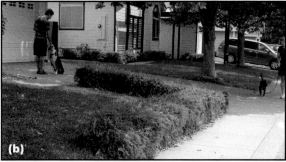

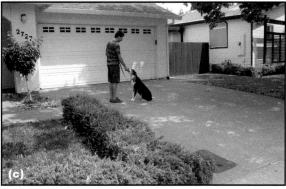

**18.5** Dogs being desensitized and counter-conditioned (DSCC) in a range of contexts.
**(a)** DSCC when away from home territory: position the dog off a pathway and give it a reinforcer (in this case a treat) when it is calm and focused on the owner while the stimulus (a child) goes by. **(b)** DSCC for territorial aggression: position the dog in a place where it responds less (in this case in the driveway instead of inside the house) and give it a reinforcer (in this case a treat) when it is calm and focused on the owner while the stimulus goes by. **(c)** Setting up for DSCC: have the owner and dog parallel to the area where the stimulus will pass by and have the dog in a sitting position; do not have either the owner's or the dog's back to the approaching stimulus, and have small treats in hand.

1. The stimulus (at the lowest intensity or furthest distance) is presented and the dog is given a reward for its new relaxed attitude and behaviours.
2. The stimulus is repeated over multiple sessions, while the dog is rewarded for the positive behaviour.
3. Once the dog is 'good' at a level of intensity and is anticipating the reward, the owner can move up to the next level by increasing the intensity of the stimulus or by decreasing the distance to the stimulus. They should not decrease the distance and increase the intensity at the same time, but only make one change at a time.

*Rewarding positive behaviour:* The owner will need things that the dog finds truly rewarding, such as very tasty treats, a highly rewarding toy, or attention from them (e.g. praise, petting, eye contact). This is not to be used as bribery, but instead given at the time when the dog is behaving calmly and non-aggressively, to counter-condition the dog to the trigger. It is important that *every* desired calm and relaxed behaviour be rewarded if possible (respondent counter-conditioning; see Chapter 5).

*Pace of training:* Owners need to understand that, just as the problem behaviour took time to develop, so they should expect incremental improvements rather than instant results. Common problems that can arise relate to progressing too quickly, especially by not controlling the stimulus intensity and not taking incremental steps. The owner should think through the steps needed before starting each DSCC session and it should constantly be borne in mind that the DSCC is to be performed at the dog's pace, not the owner's. If the steps are too large, or occur too quickly, the techniques will not be effective.

The owner needs to set up the dog to succeed. If they attempt DSCC when the dog is already anxious or highly aroused, they are likely to be ignored and the process will not proceed as planned. They should start in a quiet, neutral setting and only gradually build up to the situation where the problem occurs. The dog must first learn the task without distractions so that it can perform it reliably; and then distractions may be added into the training sessions.

The DSCC should be carried out in such small steps that the problem behaviour never occurs. If the dog reacts, either the intensity must decrease or the distance increase. A good understanding of the stimulus gradient and the response gradient will allow better control of training sessions and hopefully enhance the ability of the pet to learn and respond appropriately.

DSCC takes time and requires that the process be gradual. The owner should not progress faster than the dog can accept. Ideally each session should be kept short (3–5 minutes) and repeated frequently (several times daily or several times during a walk). Since progress is often slow, the owner should maintain a journal of the behaviour to track the dog's progress objectively. It is important to record the stimulus, intensity, distance, situation, and the dog's response.

*Body language:* It is vital that the owner understands and can evaluate the dog's body language for signs of general anxiety, aggression or disinterest (Figure 18.6). Should the dog display any early signs of anxiety or aggression during a session, the owner should move the dog away from the unfamiliar stimulus (person or dog), which ideally should not be moved except when they are in danger of being harmed. In this way the dog's behaviour does not dictate the behaviour of the stranger. However, the dog should only be moved to a distance at which anxiety or aggression is not displayed and should then be rewarded for its display of calm behaviour. At this point, the session should end. The owner should

| Anxiety |
|---|
| Lip licking |
| Lips drawn back |
| Yawning |
| Sniffing the ground |
| Scratching at a body part |
| Vocalizing; shifting eyes |
| Furrowed brow |
| Not accepting the reward or only accepting certain types of treats |
| Taking the treat in an altered manner (usually in a harsher manner) |
| Staring at the stimulus |
| Not obeying the owner's commands |

| Hostility |
|---|
| Stiffening |
| Raised lip(s) |
| Staring at the stimulus |
| Piloerection |
| Snarling, growling, barking, snapping, and/or biting |

**18.6**  Behavioural signs of anxiety and hostility.

always try to end the sessions on a good note by rewarding the display of the desired behaviour.

### Consequences of undesirable behaviour

Many people focus on how to punish inappropriate or unwanted behaviour, instead of on how to recognize and reward appropriate behaviour and how to change the underlying motivation and behaviours. The bulk of the treatment of aggression involves changing the motivation and rewarding the appropriate behaviour.

Despite someone's best efforts, aggressive incidents may occur. When talking with owners about what to do in these situations, these are the options available:

- Do nothing
- Redirect the dog to perform other commands, or to change its attitude
- Use negative punishment, such as a 'time-out' (see below)
- Use direct physical punishment (this is *not* recommended, as it can be extremely dangerous and often escalates the problem, as well as increasing fear and degrading the relationship with the owner).

***Doing nothing:*** If the owner cannot adequately, safely and quickly redirect the dog or take it to a time-out area, they should do nothing at that moment that would put the person or the dog in danger. This could mean walking out of the room and closing the door behind them if this can be done safely, or immediately going home if on a walk, or putting the dog into another part of the house. These actions should be taken without directly acknowledging the dog. Owners often are concerned about this type of reaction, believing that 'the dog won' and that it will become even more aggressive over time. However, if the owner cannot safely interact with their dog during the incident, there is nothing to be gained by forcing an interaction. This is not a battle and the fact that the dog reacted has more to do with poor control of the stimulus and/or the environment than with the dog wanting to 'win'. In

most cases the dog desires the end of the encounter and the removal of the stimulus, as the dog is usually fearful and defensive. A dog cannot learn when they are highly emotionally aroused and so training or changing its behaviour is not realistic once the dog is aggressively aroused.

***Counter-commanding and attitude changing:*** The owner can redirect the dog by either asking it to perform a command (counter-commanding) or changing the attitude by acting excited and happy.

Counter-commanding should work if the owner has a good relationship with the dog and if the dog already performs commands readily for the owner, even in high-arousal situations. This does not directly counter-condition the dog to the stimulus, but it can encourage the dog to focus on doing something else, such as performing a command or focusing on the owner, even if it remains somewhat anxious or aggressive, and it may allow the owner to remove the dog from the situation and thus prevent escalation of aggressive behaviour.

Similarly, trying to get the dog in a happier state by acting very happy in relation to it (Campbell, 1999) may produce little change in the dog's overall emotional state in the long run in relation to the stimulus, but it may get the dog out of that specific situation.

If the dog is very highly aroused or aggressive, neither of these techniques is likely to work. Owners do need to be careful of timing the 'jolly' routine or counter-commanding, as some dogs may perceive this as a reward for the aggressive behaviour. The owner has to be aware that, as with punishment, this is a small part of the entire treatment plan, and the dog should not be placed in situations that lead to aggressive arousal. As with doing nothing, there will be owners who will say that these techniques are rewarding to the dog and may cause an increase in the aggressive behaviour. However, when taken in the context of the overall treatment plan, the impact should be minimal, since these events should be a rarity. Each time one of these events occurs, it signals the need to re-evaluate management techniques that are allowing the dog to continue to perform the unwanted behaviours.

***Negative punishment: time-out area:*** Negative punishment is the removal of something the dog wants (see Chapter 5) and gives the owner another option in these circumstances. The main ways that it can be used are:

- Social isolation
- Removal of other things desired by the dog.

Since most dogs are social with people, being removed from the rest of the family or being taken away from a pleasurable place and subsequently placed in an undesirable location can be a very effective punishment. Social isolation should be in a restricted and unstimulating place, such as a bathroom or large closet where the dog normally does not spend time. There should be no toys, treats, food or specifically developed resting places in this room, and it should generally not be used by the dog for any other purpose (the twice-yearly bath does not count). The owners should not use the dog's crate or kennel for the time-out spot. It is imperative that the owner be prepared by having a long light drag-line attached to the dog's regular or headcollar, so that they can more safely grab the end of the line and lead the dog away. They should not grab the dog's collar to avoid getting bitten.

The other way in which this technique is used is to help to diffuse the situation and allow the dog and owner to calm down after an aggressive incident. When the dog is in a separate room, it allows everyone to relax; and by removing the dog from the room, the owner avoids having to use other forms of punishment on the dog.

The moment the dog shows any aggression directly toward a person (lip lifting, growling, baring its teeth, lunge, snapping, biting) the owner should bring it to the time-out area by taking the end of the attached drag-line in an unemotional and not angry manner. They should not verbally scold, physically punish or even look at the dog on the way to the time-out spot. The dog should be left in that area for just a few minutes, or as long as necessary for the dog and people involved to calm down. When releasing the dog, the owner should unemotionally open the door, allow the dog out under control and ignore it for a while. If the dog is whining, barking or scratching, the door should not be opened until the behaviour has stopped for a moment or so, since the behaviour must not be reinforced.

A 'bridging stimulus' will help the dog to learn to associate this period of social isolation with their mis-behaviour. This stimulus is a unique, often low-pitched tone (such as a kazoo or a phrase) that the dog hears only when it is being taken to social isolation. A low tone is preferred, because it is less arousing than a higher-pitched sound such as a whistle (McConnell, 1990). Each person in the household should know the tone and be prepared to use it appropriately. The moment the dog is aggressive, the tone should be used, the end of the drag-line picked up and the trip to social isolation should begin. With repetition the dog will learn to associate the sound of the bridging stimulus with a trip to social isolation. Once the dog has made this association, the bridging stimulus will help the owner to implement the punishment more effectively, even when they are farther away from the time-out area, such as when on a walk.

If the owner feels that they cannot safely remove their dog to its time-out area, they should not attempt to do so. Care must be exercised in using this technique if the behaviour does not begin to change, as it is likely that the dog is repeatedly being put in situations where it is uncomfortable and unable to learn appropriate responses. This probably means that the stimulus intensity is not controlled and the situation must be re-evaluated as a training situation.

### Medication

Although most dog aggression is based on some level of anxiety, it is usually not recommended to use medication as a first line of treatment. In most cases the concern is that owners will rely too heavily on the potential effects of the medication and not take the management or behaviour modification seriously, resulting in an unacceptable risk. A recommendation that this author generally follows is to see how adherent the owner is to the basic recommendations about implementation of safety measures and the relationship-building exercises within a predetermined follow-up period. If an owner is unwilling to implement these basic parts of the treatment plan, there is concern as to how seriously they are taking the aggression problem, as well as how compliant they will be even after the medication is prescribed. Certainly there are some dogs with such severe anxiety that there is little that can be done without some help from anti-anxiety medications, but these cases are much less common than the average dog diagnosed with aggression.

Another potential problem is that, by decreasing the anxiety level, medications may cause the dog to feel more comfortable approaching people and to display an elevated level of aggression, such as snapping or biting instead of growling. This is referred to as **disinhibition** and may be more likely when benzodiazepines are used. Disinhibition can occur if fear and anxiety are restraining the aggression; if these are lessened, the dog may be more likely to bite rather than less.

The medications used most often are in the selective serotonin reuptake inhibitor (SSRI) or tricyclic antidepressant (TCA)/anti-anxiety families (see Chapter 21). These medications can take up to 4–6 weeks before their full effects are seen.

There are no placebo-controlled double-blind studies in dogs that have demonstrated that medications are an effective part of a treatment plan for aggression, though they may be used in some cases (see Chapter 21).

Where owners are compliant with the treatment recommendations to the best of their ability but their dog is either not improving, or not improving quickly enough for the owner to be able to lead a reasonable life, or is suffering, anti-anxiety medications are a reasonable option to supplement the behaviour modification part of the treatment plan. Figure 18.7 gives dosages for some commonly used medications and Chapter 21 has more information on this topic.

| Drug type | Drug name | Dosage |
|---|---|---|
| SSRIs | Fluoxetine | 1–2 mg/kg q24h |
| | Paroxetine | 1–2 mg/kg q24h |
| | Sertraline | 1–3 mg/kg q24h |
| TCAs | Amitriptyline | 2–4 mg/kg q12h |
| | Clomipramine | 2–4 mg/kg q24h or divided twice daily |
| Benzodiazepines (rarely used) | Alprazolam | 0.05–0.1 mg/kg up to q8h |
| | Diazepam | 0.5–1.0 mg/kg up to q8h |

**18.7** Medications reported to be of use in helping treatment of canine aggression.

### Pheromone therapy

Pheromone products such as the dog appeasing pheromone DAP® may help to decrease a dog's anxiety (see Chapter 21). This product is available as a slow-release collar, or as a spray that can be sprayed in the environment or on to a cloth bandana that is tied around the dog's neck, or as a plug-in diffuser for inside the house. The product has been associated with helping to alleviate anxiety, but no studies have tested its effectiveness in treating canine aggression. Pheromone products are not absorbed systemically and do not interfere with psychotropic medications; therefore, they could be a safe and potentially effective supplemental help in treating aggression.

### Surgery

Castration of male dogs may have a slightly beneficial effect in decreasing aggression. A study by Neilson *et al.* (1997) concluded that <35% of dogs castrated specifically to decrease aggression toward unfamiliar dogs or toward unfamiliar people entering their territory had at least a 50% improvement in the aggression. The study also noted that there was no effect of age at castration, nor how long the dog had displayed the aggression, on the eventual outcome. While it is obviously not a cure-all, it may help to shift the balance in the owner's favour.

Some owners ask about removing a dog's canine teeth, or even all of its teeth, or filing them down so that the dog theoretically cannot do as much harm when it bites. This is sometimes called 'disarming'. It is not recommended, primarily due to the pain caused to the dog but also due to its ineffectiveness in reducing the motivation for the behaviour.

## Prognosis

Prognosis depends on the level of communication between veterinary surgeon and client (including diagnosis, follow-up and continued guidance), the owner's comprehension of the treatment plan, the make-up of their household, their belief in the treatment recommendations, their ability to follow those recommendations and their attachment to their dog, as well as the dog's relationship with its owner, its size, age and temperament, and the severity, frequency and intensity of its aggression (see Chapter 17).

Thus there are many factors that affect prognosis and blanket statements cannot be made. Some owners have a very low tolerance for aggression and they may not be able to give their dog the chance to improve, even when counselled about a relatively low severity of risk. Many of the prognostic factors discussed in Chapter 17 are just as relevant here.

## Follow-up

As in any aspect of veterinary medicine, it is important to have follow-up contact with the owner and their dog. It is unlikely that the owner can be given a full and complete treatment plan that requires no changes upon review, so it is suggested that they should be given small steps to work on between their follow-up visits. Breaking down the treatment plan into manageable segments helps the owner to achieve realistic goals and see successful outcomes more quickly, and not get so frustrated in having to complete all of the instructions after the first visit.

It is helpful to have the owner keep a journal, (recording with whom, where, when, how often and how severely the dog reacts) to evaluate the progress, or lack thereof, more objectively and see where the problems lie. If an owner has been diligent about keeping records and noted an improvement, they will be less likely to give up if the dog does display aggression at a later date. With objective observations, they can note that their dog actually had *not* displayed aggression for the past 4 weeks, say, when initially it had displayed aggression on a daily basis, or that improvement has been made in one specific context even if it has not yet improved overall.

## Prevention

Chapter 6 gives an excellent outline of the importance of socialization, as well as how to implement a successful plan specifically to help to prevent aggression.

Proper selection of the right dog for a particular household is important as well. The breed of the dog is important (some are known to be more likely to display aggression), but so is the specific genetics of an individual dog – there are individual differences between dogs. If an owner is selecting a dog from a breeder, they need to meet both parents to get the best idea of the dog's likely behaviour as an adult, though of course the puppy is not a clone of its parents. Additionally, they should find out exactly how that puppy has been raised since it was born, because this early experience can have a profound effect on the dog's behaviour later in its life. If an owner selects a dog from a shelter, there is obviously a lack of knowledge of its parents' behaviour. There is little research that shows validity in predicting future behaviour once the dog is adopted.

## Conclusion

Canine aggression is a common complaint from owners and can lead to a serious public health risk, as well as liability, when unfamiliar people and dogs are involved. It is imperative that veterinary surgeons talk with their clients regarding prevention of these problems as well as how to treat them when they arise. With proper humane behaviour modification and management techniques, as well as owner understanding and patience, the dog's aggression should improve over time.

## References and further reading

Appleby D, Bradshaw JWS and Casey RA (2002) Relationship between aggressive and avoidance behaviour by dogs and their experience in the first six months of life. *Veterinary Record* **150**, 434–438

Beaver BV (1994) Owner complaints about canine behavior. *Journal of the American Veterinary Medical Association* **204**, 1953–1955

Cakiroglu D, Meral Y, Sancak AA and Cifti G (2007) Relationship between the serum concentrations of serotonin and lipids and aggression in dogs. *Veterinary Record* **161**, 59–61

Campbell WE (1999) *The New Better Behavior in Dogs: A Guide to Solving All Your Dog Problems.* Alpine Publications, Crawford, Colorado

Christensen EL, Scarlett J, Campagna M and Houpt KA (2007) Aggressive behavior in adopted dogs that passed a temperament test. *Applied Animal Behaviour Science* **106**, 85–95

DeNapoli JS, Dodman NH, Shuster L *et al.* (2000) Effect of dietary protein content and tryptophan supplementation on dominance aggression, territorial aggression, and hyperactivity in dogs. *Journal of the American Veterinary Medical Association* **217**, 504–508

Hart BL and Miller MF (1985) Behavioral profiles of dog breeds. *Journal of the American Veterinary Medical Association* **186**, 1175–1180

Hsu Y and Serpell JA (2003) Development and validation of a questionnaire for measuring behavior and temperament traits in pet dogs. *Journal of the American Veterinary Medical Association* **223**, 1293–1300

Kroll TL, Houpt KA and Erb HN (2004) The use of novel stimuli as indicators of aggressive behavior in dogs. *Journal of the American Animal Hospital Association* **40**, 13–19

Landsberg GM (1991) The distribution of canine behavior cases at three behavior referral practices. *Veterinary Medicine* **86**, 1011–1018

McConnell PB (1990) Acoustic structure and receiver response in domestic dogs, *Canis familiaris*. *Animal Behaviour* **39**, 897–904

Neilson JC, Eckstein RA and Hart BL (1997) Effects of castration on problem behaviors in male dogs with reference to age and duration of behavior. *Journal of the American Veterinary Medical Association* **211**, 180–182

Patronek GJ and Dodman NH (1999) Attitudes, procedures, and delivery of behavior services by veterinarians in small animal practice. *Journal of the American Veterinary Medical Association* **215**, 1606–1611

Patronek GJ, Glickman LT, Beck AM *et al.* (1996) Risk factors for relinquishment of dogs to an animal shelter. *Journal of the American Veterinary Medical Association* **209**, 572–581

Reisner IR, Mann JJ, Stanley M *et al.* (1996) Comparison of cerebrospinal fluid monoamine metabolite levels in dominant-aggressive and non-aggressive dogs. *Brain Research* **714**, 57–64

Sacks JJ, Lockwood R, Hornreich J and Sattin RW (1996) Fatal dog attacks. *Pediatrics* **97**, 891–895

Segurson SA, Serpell JA and Hart BA (2005) Evaluation of a behavioral assessment questionnaire for use in the characterization of behavioral problems of dogs relinquished to animal shelters. *Journal of the American Veterinary Medical Association* **227**, 1755–1761

Virga V, Houpt KA and Scarlett JM (2001) Efficacy of amitriptyline as a pharmacological adjunct to behavioral modification in the management of aggressive behaviors in dogs. *Journal of the American Animal Hospital Association* **37**, 325–330

Voith VL and Borchelt PL (1982) Diagnosis and treatment of dominance aggression in dogs. *Veterinary Clinics of North America Small Animal Practice: Animal Behavior* **12**, 655–663

White MM, Neilson JC, Hart BL and Cliff KD (1999) Effects of clomipramine hydrochloride on dominance-related aggression in dogs. *Journal of the American Veterinary Medical Association* **215**, 1288–1291

## Client handouts (bsavalibrary.com/behaviour_leaflets)

- Adopting a rescue dog: the pros and cons
- Canine behaviour questionnaire
- Cognitive dysfunction syndrome
- Down–stay mat exercises
- Handling exercises for puppies and kittens
- Headcollar training
- How to find a good trainer
- Ladder of Aggression
- 'Leave it' exercises

- Muzzle training
- 'Nothing in Life is Free'
- Playing with your dog – toys
- Recall exercises
- Redirected aggression in dogs
- Request for information on problem behaviours
- Sit–stay exercises
- What your dog needs
- Your puppy's first year

# 19

# Aggression in cats

## Sarah Heath

## Introduction

Although aggression is more readily associated with dogs it is also a significant behavioural problem in a feline context. Owners most commonly approach the veterinary practice with concerns over aggressive behaviour toward family members or other cats in the same household, though sometimes aggression between cats in the neighbourhood or aggression toward people outside the family may result in an enquiry for help and advice.

### Incidence in referred population

In the UK, data from 2004 and 2005 relating to 249 cases of feline aggression seen by members of the Association of Pet Behaviour Counsellors (APBC) found that 41 cats (16.5%) were referred for aggression toward people. Of these, 26.8% were recorded as being aggressive during handling but only five (2%) were recorded as actually having bitten a person (usually their owner). The majority of cats (45.1%) referred for aggression toward people were single cats, whilst intra-specific aggression was most likely to be displayed by cats in homes with three or more cats (42%). Aggression toward other cats was recorded 73 times (29.3%). Of the 63 cats (25.3%) referred for aggression toward other cats in the home, 29 (46%) were living with one other cat in the home, 21 (33.3%) were living with two other cats in the home and 13 (20.7%) were living in a home with three or more other cats.

Those that were recorded as showing aggression toward other cats in the home were as likely to be an indoor cat (33.3%) as to have free or limited access outdoors. Thirty-one cats (49.2%) were obtained by the owners from a domestic environment and 23 (36.5%) were obtained from a rescue environment. Sixteen cats (25.4%) were obtained when they were between 9 and 12 weeks of age.

### Incidence in the feline population at large

The APBC figures above relate to cats that had been referred through their veterinary surgeon for behavioural treatment, but the prevalence of aggression in that population does not necessarily reflect the level of feline aggression in the population at large.

Clinical data collected from cats treated at Southampton University's referral clinic have been compared with data obtained from a general population survey carried out in the UK, and data from a published national diagnostic review from the United States (Bradshaw *et al.*, 2000; Casey, 2001). The results suggested that certain problems, particularly those of feline house soiling (both elimination and marking) and aggression (directed toward people or other household cats), were over-represented in the referral clinic population. In contrast, fearful and avoidance-related behaviour, whether toward unfamiliar people or other cats, was not as frequent as would be predicted from the incidence in the general population; and scratching behaviour was also under-represented in the referral population (Figures 19.1 and 19.2).

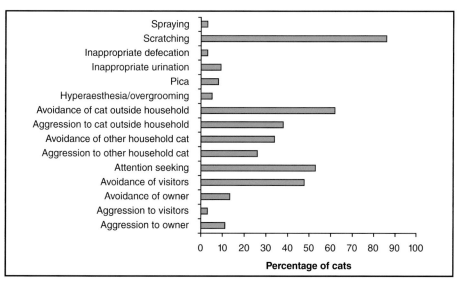

**19.1** Percentage of cats showing each category of 'undesirable behaviour' in the general population survey (*n* = 113). (Data from R. Casey.)

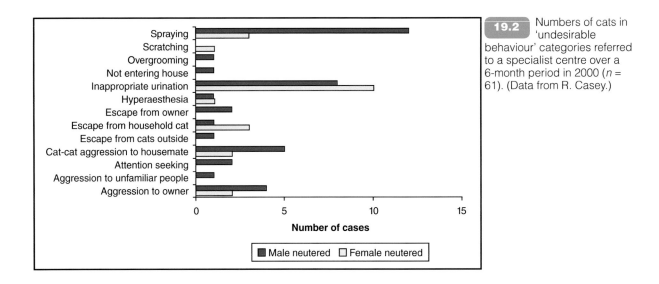

**19.2** Numbers of cats in 'undesirable behaviour' categories referred to a specialist centre over a 6-month period in 2000 (*n* = 61). (Data from R. Casey.)

Explanations for the discrepancies between the data from the referred population and from the two general cat populations are probably related to the potential impact of these different behaviours on the owners, and also to the level of knowledge amongst the general cat-owning population about behavioural therapy for cats. Problems of house soiling and inter-cat aggression can be difficult to live with and a high proportion of owners will be driven to seek help in order to resolve these issues. In contrast, cats that run and hide from fear-inducing situations may not pose a direct challenge to their owners and are often dismissed as being 'a bit nervous', so their owners will be less likely to seek help.

## Relevance of feline aggression to rehoming centres

Aggression is also a frequent reason given for the relinquishment of cats to rehoming centres and for cats being returned to these centres after adoption. In the UK, 14% of those cats that were relinquished to a shelter were as a direct result of specific behaviour problems: 2% because of house soiling, 3% because of aggression to people and 2.5% because of general problems of nervous or fearful behaviour. Five per cent of the cats were surrendered due to problems of intra-specific aggression, and this behaviour was cited as the most common behavioural reason for cats that had been re-homed being returned to the shelter (Casey *et al.*, in press). One study in the United States (New *et al.*, 1999) found that undesirable behaviours of relinquished cats played less of a role than in relinquished dogs. The study cited house soiling, destructive behaviour and a perception of the cat being overly active as the main behavioural reasons for feline relinquishment. In contrast to dogs the difference between relinquished and household cats was not statistically significantly different regarding the history of bites in the month before relinquishment. However, biting history was not known for 13.8% of relinquished cats, which potentially raises questions about the validity of this apparent lack of difference.

## Motivation for aggression

Aggressive behaviour is a sign and does not represent a diagnosis. It is an outward manifestation of the underlying emotional state of the cat and, whatever the target for the aggressive response (cat, human or other animal), the successful treatment of the problem will rely on an accurate assessment of the emotional basis for the behaviour. Obviously the threshold for the expression of an aggressive response can be lowered by internal or external stressors; and in clinical cases of aggressive feline behaviour, accurate history taking is essential to determine the factors that are involved in each case. In many situations the behaviour is multi-factorial in terms of the stimuli that elicit the emotional response and this highlights why 'recipe-book' approaches for the treatment of feline aggression are potentially dangerous. There can be no substitute for time taken to unravel the history in each individual case and prescribe treatment tailored for that individual cat and for that situation.

## Behavioural biology of feline aggression

The nature of aggressive responses in cats is related to their natural social and communication systems, which are just as relevant to cats living in a domestic situation as they are to cats in feral or wild environments. An understanding of natural feline behaviour is essential when managing behavioural signs that are problematic to owners of domestic cats.

Feline society is based on cooperative groups of females who are related to one another and live together in a mutually beneficial environment, which supports the successful rearing of kittens. Males are usually excluded from these social groupings and live their lives as solitary individuals who only venture into the main social context at times of breeding.

Within this social context it is important for fellow members of the group to recognize one another and affiliative behaviours (such as mutual grooming and mutual rubbing) are used to cement relationships and to exchange scent signals. The mixing of scents results in the formation of a group social odour, which reassures individuals that the social group is stable and enables them to relax in close proximity to one another.

Although levels of hostility within the related groups are low, intrusion by unrelated individuals is poorly tolerated since it poses a threat to resource availability and therefore a potential risk to offspring. As a result aggression to strangers can be intense. The relevance of this to the cat in a domestic setting is that additions to and removals from feline social groupings can be extremely stressful.

However, ultimate survival within feline society is an individual responsibility. Since physical aggression carries with it the risk of injury, it makes sense to avoid situations of potentially intense aggression that could result in a decreased ability to take care of oneself. Overt aggression is minimized by the use of elaborate distance-maintaining behaviours designed to diffuse tension, keep strangers at bay and discourage social interaction with individuals outside of the social group. These signals include postural and vocal communication, marking behaviours (such as urine spraying) and elaborate use of eye contact and facial communication, including ear positions. Fighting is usually the last resort in terms of behavioural defence strategies (Figure 19.3).

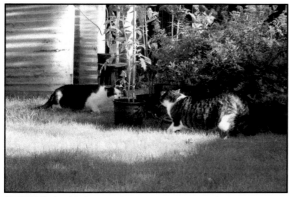

**19.3** In this interaction, two cats are using a combination of body language and vocalization to prevent escalation of the confrontation into physical violence. The ears are particularly expressive, indicating defensive motivation in both cats, and the weight distribution indicates that both individuals are preparing themselves to be able to swipe with their front paws in a defensive action. (Courtesy of A. Lummersheim.)

Although the traditional image of the cat as a solitary creature is not accurate, much of feline behaviour is based on individual survival and many of the fundamental behaviours, such as feeding, hunting, resting and eliminating, are performed in a solitary context and have no social significance.

## Feline aggression toward people

### Evaluation of presenting signs and history

It is important to remember that the term aggression is used to refer to a number of different behavioural responses, ranging from hissing and spitting to infliction of physical injury. History taking must include incident information, cat information, environmental information and human information.

### Health issues

The priority in all behaviour cases is to establish that the animal is in good physical health before investigating behavioural explanations for its responses.

In the case of feline aggression it is essential to consider any pain-inducing disease process (such as dental disease), central nervous system disease (such as brain tumours) or endocrine imbalance (such as hyperthyroidism or hypervitaminosis A) as possible differentials. In some cases of aggression associated with handling, the cats show signs of hyperaesthesia and may even display the classic signs of rippling skin and hypersensitivity to touch. A multi-disciplinary approach involving dermatology and behavioural medicine is to be encouraged in such cases. Aggressive responses may still remain after medical treatment for various reasons, including learning and poor environmental situations.

### Incident information

Provided that the animal is found to be in good physical health, the behavioural investigation can continue in order to identify the underlying emotional state. Relevant information about the specific incidents will include details about the cat, the person and the environment at the time of the aggression and owners should be encouraged to include as much detail as possible in their descriptions.

*Cat-related information:* An accurate description of the body language, facial expression and vocalization of the cat immediately prior to, during and after an aggressive encounter will be essential and for many owners it can be difficult to provide this with any degree of detail. If it is not possible for the veterinary surgeon to witness one of the events at first hand, it can be extremely beneficial to obtain video footage of the cat in action. Obviously this is not always practical and it is neither desirable nor ethical to set up aggressive encounters for the sake of the camera. It is also important to remember the potential legal implications of setting up situations that involve risk of injury to either the cat, its owners or other humans and to ensure that any advice that is given in cases of aggression is accompanied by suitable caveats regarding client safety. It can be helpful to have a series of photographs or illustrations of typical cat body language available when talking to clients and use these to enable them to describe their pet's behaviour (Figure 19.4).

*Environment-related information:* During the history-taking process it is important to ask questions about the circumstances surrounding the aggressive incident in terms of the physical context in which the behaviour occurred. For example, if the cat was in a restricted environment, such as a narrow passageway, it is more likely that the behaviour was defensively motivated than if it were in the middle of an open space. If the cat showed aggression to its owner when

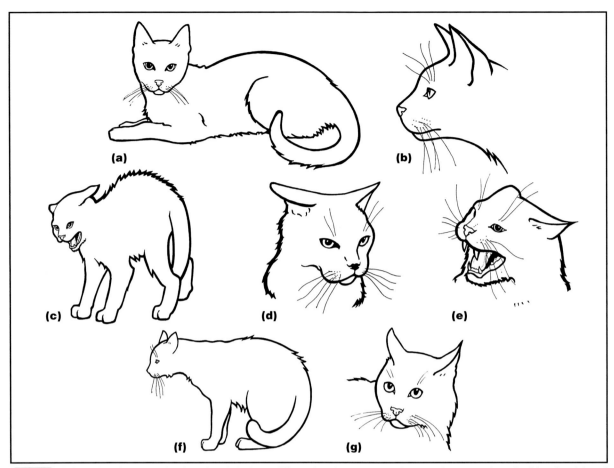

**19.4** Feline visual communication signals help to differentiate between an alert non-threatened cat **(a,b)**, a fearful and defensive cat **(c,d,e)**, and a confident aggressive cat **(f,g)**. Reproduced from *An Ethogram for Behavioural Studies of the Domestic Cat (Felis silvestris catus L.)* by the UK Cat Behaviour Working Group (1995); plates 3,4,5,6,7,16 and 17; by permission of Universities Federation for Animal Welfare (UFAW), Wheathampstead.

it was aroused by the sight of another cat outside the window, it is likely that the aggression was not primarily intended for the owner but was being redirected as a result of frustration.

Information about the environment (space available, routes of access and potential for escape) will be relevant since physical restriction is an important factor in terms of behavioural choice (see Chapter 4). Cats use physical conflict as a last resort in the wild and when aggression occurs readily within the domestic setting it is advisable to examine the environment from a feline perspective. Cats live in a three-dimensional world and make extensive use of vertical space in their environment (Bernstein and Strack, 1993). It is therefore important to consider this when investigating cases of aggression within a household with multiple cats, since lack of available vertical space may lead to a decrease in the cat's ability to regulate stress and a consequent increase in incidents of aggression.

## Client's attitudes, beliefs and behaviour

Although the lay interpretation of the word 'aggression' is a negative one and 'aggressive' behaviours are usually considered to be inappropriate, it is worth noting that aggressive responses form part of the normal behavioural repertoire of the cat. They are communicative methods used to change the outcome of a social interaction and it is the circumstances in which the responses are evoked that needs further investigation. Evaluating the emotional state of the cat and the trigger for that emotional reaction will be the basis of establishing a behaviour modification programme.

It is also worth noting that predation is functionally not a social behaviour but owners often misinterpret the natural predation sequence as a form of social interaction, especially when it is directed toward themselves. Predatory behaviours are learnt and perfected through play; as a consequence, owners may observe behaviour within the context of play which they are uncomfortable with and which they label as aggressive.

It is essential to understand that the natural response to social contact and the manner in which it is conducted varies significantly between cats and people. In general humans are low-frequency, high-intensity interactors for whom tactile contact is an important part of the greeting ritual, while cats are generally high-frequency, low-intensity interactors for whom fleeting greeting is often preferred to prolonged and restrictive social contact. Factors such as a lack of understanding of this discrepancy and kittens that are not adequately prepared for social interaction with humans are often implicated in the initiation of feline aggression directed toward people.

Human responses such as high-pitched screams, rapid movement and confrontational or punitive measures can all lead to an escalation in that tension and ultimately a more overtly aggressive response from the cat. This is especially true in aggression that is motivated by fear, or unwanted behaviour that is associated with predatory drives. It is common for the person to counter aggression with aggression in the mistaken belief that physical size is likely to win the day and their human stature puts them in a no-lose situation in competition with a cat. Because of the cat's innate behaviour and ability to cause harm, confrontation can be injurious and provocative and can lead to an increase in the incidence of conflict and in the intensity of the aggressive response.

Inappropriate responses on the part of the human may be responsible for initiating, rewarding and perpetuating aggressive behaviour.

## Risk assessment

The priority in cases of feline aggression toward people is to assess the risk of serious injury to those living with the cat or coming into contact with it. As a result of the limitations of natural feline behaviour, in terms of ability to diffuse conflict, it has to be accepted that the risk of injury is high once a cat has reached the point of engaging in physically aggressive behavioural responses. This fact serves to emphasize the importance of prevention in cases of feline aggression and this is dealt with at the end of this chapter.

Physical injury to people and zoonotic infections due to damage from claws and teeth are very real dangers. Children, the elderly and the immunocompromised could be considered to be at greater risk from feline aggression than others. Because of the possibility of cat scratch disease resulting from the introduction of bacteria from the teeth or claws, victims should be encouraged to seek medical attention if injured.

When carrying out a risk assessment it will be necessary to assess the owner's understanding of the behaviour and their willingness and ability to segregate the cat from vulnerable people while the behavioural treatment is in progress. The management of cats with aggressive behavioural signs is particularly challenging, since the option of muzzling is neither possible nor appropriate in the majority of cases. It is therefore essential to assess the ability of those dealing with the cat to avoid provocative situations and interactions and to implement the advice regarding prevention of arousal in the cat (see client handout).

## Diagnosis

The most common bases for aggression from cats to people include fear, anxiety, frustration and misdirection of predatory instinct. In some cases the victim may not be the primary target for the aggressive behaviour and a diagnosis of frustration aggression with redirection (often simply referred to as redirected aggression) may be made.

The majority of domestic cats are neutered and specific hormonal motivations for aggression by cats toward people are very rare. One example that is sometimes mentioned in the literature is aggression in lactating and nursing queens attributed to hormonally motivated defence of the litter, but the hormones merely serve to accentuate the likelihood of defensive behaviour in certain contexts. A queen that is overtly hostile to people is likely to have other problems relating to emotional factors such as fear or anxiety involved in her behavioural response, and prospective owners should resist the temptation to purchase kittens from such queens.

### Fear- and anxiety-related aggression toward people

A diagnosis of fear/anxiety-related aggression can be made when the aggression toward humans is associated with feline aggressive responses clearly triggered by a negative emotional reaction. It is important to look for any information that suggests the possibility of a previous traumatic experience involving people, or the use of inappropriate punishment for behaviour in the past. Kittens that have not received appropriate handling between 2 and 7 weeks of age may grow up to be wary of people and to have a predisposition to exhibit defensively aggressive behaviour as a result of feeling threatened by interactions that, from a human perspective, are seemingly insignificant or even sociable. The presence of inappropriate and unintentional reward of the present behaviour should also be considered.

Over time, fearful cats will learn that their aggressive responses are very effective at maintaining distance between themselves and any people of whom they are suspicious; before long the aggressive display may be used as a pre-emptive rather than a reactionary behaviour. In the early stages the cat will show noticeable signs of fear in terms of body language (e.g. crouching, dilated pupils, flattened ears) and vocalization (such as growling or hissing) and it is likely that there will be some attempt to use other defence strategies such as flight and hiding (Figure 19.5). In due course the cat will select aggressive responses more readily. By the time some of these cases come for treatment, the initial fearful motivation for the behaviour may be far from obvious and the cat may dispense with the preparatory body posturing and launch toward people in an overtly aggressive manner.

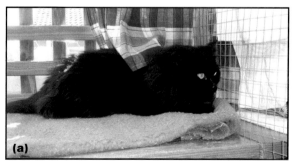

**19.5** Defensive strategies: **(a)** The crouched body posture, dilated pupils and fixated stare are signs of a negative state of emotion which is likely to make this cat defensive if approached rapidly. Slow cautious approach will be needed to avoid inducing an aggressive response. (continues) ▶

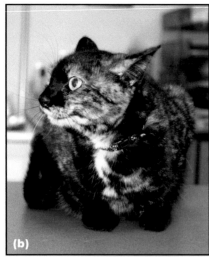

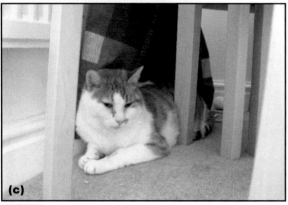

**19.5** Defensive strategies: **(b)** The dilated pupils, tense body posture and backward-rotated ears combined with the stiffened whiskers indicate the negative emotional state of arousal of this cat. (Courtesy of J. Hudson.) **(c)** The hunched and tense body posture, and selection of an inaccessible resting location, suggest that this cat is retreating from potential threat. The position of the ears indicates that the cat is scanning the environment for auditory information and the dilated pupils also illustrate the negative state of arousal of this individual.

Fear-related aggression may be triggered by very specific stimuli, such as restrictive handling. For example, it is possible for a cat to appear to be friendly to people while it has all four feet on the floor and has the option to use a flight response to defend itself, but to become overtly aggressive if picked up or an attempt is made to restrain it physically. The motivation for this aggression is fear and it is triggered by the removal of the cat's priority defence strategy of flight. The cat has not suddenly changed personality or become 'evil' but is responding to an underlying fear associated with the presence of perceived threat. People often misinterpret a cat's proximity for a willingness for interaction and physical contact.

### Frustration-related aggression toward people

In some situations of aggression toward people it is noted that the undesirable behaviour appears to be associated with circumstances in which the cat fails to receive an expected reward. Such behavioural responses are consistent with a state of frustration. In some of these cases there is a history of hand rearing

and there have been numerous anecdotal reports of such aggressive behaviour in hand-reared kittens. One study in the USA involving veterinary students hand rearing kittens and later testing them for aggressive behavioural responses failed to demonstrate a link between these factors (Cohn, 2005). However, it would be interesting to see the research repeated but with members of the public hand rearing the kittens, to see whether any differences of hand-rearing style occur and whether they are relevant to subsequent behavioural responses. Obviously hand rearing is not the only risk factor for developing aggression associated with frustration; cats that have been weaned normally by their mothers can go on to develop aggression of this sort, especially if they are continually rewarded for demanding behaviour during kittenhood and develop unrealistic expectations of human interaction.

Often aggression that is motivated by frustration is not an isolated behaviour and the cat also displays other frustration-related behaviours, such as excessive vocalization or indoor marking, in situations where it appears to be thwarted. Typical situations in which frustration-related aggression may occur include when the owner does not open a door or a can of food quickly enough, or tries to walk away from a cat during a period of interaction.

Frustration-related aggression may also develop in situations where behaviour that is not associated with human interaction has been thwarted. For example, a cat may show an aggressive reaction to people who walk close to it when it is watching another cat through a window and its intended interaction with the other cat cannot be completed. This is sometimes referred to as redirected aggression but a focus on frustration helps to emphasize what needs to be addressed in the treatment of the case.

### Misdirected predatory behaviour

One very common misconception amongst cat owners is that hunting is a behaviour that is performed only in order to satisfy hunger. In fact these two aspects of feline behaviour are independently controlled and while a hungry cat will be more highly motivated to hunt, even a well fed cat will respond to the stimuli of rapid movement and high pitched noise by displaying innate hunting responses (Biben, 1979). As a result a cat that is denied the opportunity to engage in hunting real prey or appropriate toys will often display predatory behaviour toward other rapidly moving objects, such as human ankles and hands. As the human reacts to the pain with a high shriek, this further stimulates the hunting response and the cat increases its response. Although such behaviour is often classified as a form of aggression, it is probably more appropriately considered as a form of predation (see Chapter 9), which is functionally and mechanistically different to negative emotional (affective) aggression.

The behavioural sequences involved in predation are practised and perfected through play and in some texts the term 'misdirected play aggression' may be used to describe a predatory form of behaviour that occurs in the absence of any normal potential prey.

While this may be an accurate description in some respects, it is important to remember that developing the skills necessary for predation underlies the behaviour (hence its consideration under this diagnostic category).

When taking the history it is important to ask questions about the cat's posture before and during the 'attacks' and also to determine the triggers that are leading to the behaviour. In many cases of inappropriate predatory behaviour, the behaviour is being inadvertently rewarded by the human response.

One feature of predatory behaviour is that the claws are usually protracted and the bite is not inhibited, unlike the behaviour in a social play context, and therefore cases of misdirected predatory responses toward humans run a high risk of causing appreciable injury. Elderly people and children are particularly at risk from this sort of behaviour.

During the history-taking process it is sensible to ask questions about the way in which the owner interacted with the cat when it was younger and especially about the ways in which they encouraged or stimulated its predatory responses. In many cases owners inadvertently encourage inappropriate responses by playing with kittens in a way that induces predatory attacks on human flesh. Examples include games that involve running fingers over the backs of sofas, or encouraging attacks on feet or hands under the duvet.

### Inappropriate social play behaviour

In some circumstances aggressive behaviours may be seen as part of interactive play. Although the behaviour is often associated with predatory sequences, one important difference is that the claws may be retracted and the bite inhibited. In cases of inappropriate play the cat often starts with acceptable playful interaction but becomes over enthusiastic and then inflicts actual damage. Lack of opportunity to act out the full predatory sequence during play can lead to frustration and it is not uncommon for such cases to be associated with other frustration-related behaviour patterns.

## Feline aggression toward other cats

Although people find it desirable to keep more than one cat in a household and to live in urban populations with a high density of cats in a relatively small area, it is not necessarily compatible with natural feline behaviour and problems can arise as a result. The motivation for the aggression in any particular case should be determined through a combination of observation and history taking, but the list of possible differentials is similar to that relating to aggression toward people. It includes aggression related to fear, anxiety and frustration, as well as inappropriate play.

It is important for owners to be able to interpret accurately the interactions between the cats. Accurate descriptions of body language, facial expression and vocalization before, during and after 'aggressive' incidents will help to achieve this (see Figure 19.4).

## Evaluation of presenting signs and history

In common with cases of aggression toward people, it is important to gather information about the cats involved in the confrontational behaviour as well as the environment in which the incidents take place. In addition to information about overt physical aggression, it is important to ask about passive signs of conflict such as visual threats, avoidance behaviour or restriction of movement through either the home or the neighbourhood (Figure 19.6) and the presence of other behavioural problems, such as urine marking, over-grooming, indoor toileting or obesity, that may be indicative of social stress.

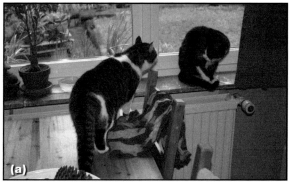

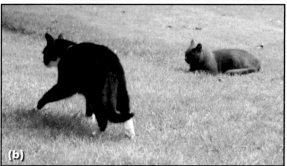

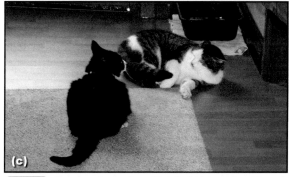

**19.6** Passive signs of conflict. **(a)** Using visual threat, the cat on the table intends to move the cat on the windowsill to a safe distance without the need for physical confrontation. **(b)** In this encounter between two strangers, the grey individual is displaying tense body posturing with mobile ears searching for information. It is avoiding eye contact with the other individual, who in turn takes a wide berth and moves slowly and deliberately so as to avoid inducing a chase response. **(c)** In this encounter between two cats in the same household, each cat is displaying tense body posturing and defensive ear positioning. The black and white cat is avoiding eye contact, while the tabby and white appears ready to launch a paw strike and if necessary roll over to release the other paws for defensive action. (Courtesy of A. Lummersheim.)

## Household cats

When aggression takes place between cats within the same household, it is important to establish how many social groupings are present. This is best achieved by observing tactile affiliative behaviour patterns such as allogrooming and allorubbing. These behaviours will be displayed between socially compatible cats (Bradshaw and Hall, 1999). By observing the cats closely over a period of 1–2 weeks, owners can build up a picture of the social relationships within the household.

The distribution of resources within the household will then need to be evaluated in the light of this information and an assessment made of the availability of core territory areas with appropriate resources for each of the social groups which exist within the household (see Chapter 4). In addition it will be important to assess the compatibility of the cats in terms of their requirements for social contact and in particular for social play.

Age differences between cats in the same household can sometimes be a significant factor in cases of inappropriate play and owners may misinterpret playful intent from younger cats as aggressive behaviour. When such play is directed toward older, or simply less sociable, individuals it can be misinterpreted by the recipient cat as well and lead to the onset of anxiety-related behavioural responses.

## Neighbourhood cats

In neighbourhoods it can be useful to evaluate the outdoor environment in terms of availability of visual vantage points and to monitor the distribution of cats within the territory in terms of space and time. Assessment of available passage tracks through the territory and the ability of cats to reach suitable latrine locations and resting places without running the gauntlet of other cats will help to evaluate the level of potential social stress within the feline community. It is important to be aware that cats who are not related to one another will prefer to use distancing behaviour to avoid unnecessary social contact and the neighbourhood should be assessed in terms of its ability to provide for this natural behaviour by offering visual cover and elevated resting sites.

## Risk assessment

It is obviously important to assess risk of physical injury in cases of intercat aggression but it should be remembered that increased risk of chronic stress, due to social incompatibility between cats in the same household or within the same neighbourhood, is probably more of a threat to the cat's welfare than physical confrontation.

With multi-cat households, honest assessment of space availability (in all three dimensions) and potential for appropriate resource distribution is a very important part of risk assessment. If it is not possible to create a safe and secure area within the home for all cats, it may be necessary to consider rehoming or permanent separation. In situations of neighbourhood tension the solution is more complicated: if people are unable to come to some agreement about a workable time-sharing system for their pets, it may be necessary to consider options such as enclosed outdoor runs or specialized garden fencing.

## Diagnosis

The most common causes of aggression between cats relate to:

- Social stress
- Fear and anxiety
- Frustration
- Inappropriate play.

### Aggression between cats in the same household

*Fear, anxiety, frustration and inappropriate play:* When aggression between cats in the household is motivated by fear, anxiety, frustration or inappropriate play in equivalent contexts to those described for human-directed aggression above, the approach to diagnosis will be similar to that described in relation to aggression toward people.

In some cases the other cat in the household is not the primary target of the aggression but happens to be more conveniently positioned than the intended victim and the aggression may be redirected as a result of frustration. This can then lead to social stress between individuals and a complex diagnostic picture as a result. When this is the case an understanding of all the emotional factors involved in the situation will be necessary in order to institute appropriate treatment.

*Social stress:* Cats are likely to show a specific anxiety-related aggression toward other cats when they perceive their vital survival resource (such as food, water, resting places and latrines) to be under threat. Consideration of natural feline social systems is crucial to understanding such behaviour and offering realistic means of controlling it.

Availability of suitable retreats where cats can hide is an issue in multi-cat households, since hiding is an important coping strategy in response to social challenge or change in the environment (see Chapter 4). Space is only one of the important resources within the home and availability of food, water and litter facilities should also be considered. Lack of access to these resources or competition over them may be a source of stress for feline inhabitants and lead to aggressive interactions.

Intercat aggression within the household is most likely to occur when a new cat is being introduced to the household and there is a high level of competition over resources (e.g. resting places, owner attention or food) or when one of the resident cats has been absent from the home, but it can also be precipitated following an incident of redirected aggression to a cat outside the social group. In a veterinary context the risk of aggression between cats in the same household when one resident returns home after a period of hospitalization, however brief, is something that is often overlooked and yet it is a relatively common occurrence. Poor socialization of one or more of the cats in the home and incompatibility between the social requirements of individuals within the household are also factors that need to be considered.

## Aggression to other cats in the general neighbourhood

Aggression to other cats in the neighbourhood is associated with social stress and is more likely in circumstances when the local population is destabilized by:

- The introduction of a newcomer
- When a feline despot (a cat that is proactively expanding its territory by displacement of other felines) is resident in the neighbourhood
- When there are one or more entire males in the local population
- The presence of queens in oestrus.

The defence of territory is linked to the defence of resources. When resources are provided in adequate supply, there is a reduction in territorial behaviour and aggression; but when populations increase in density, the risk of territorial aggression between cats is increased.

*Territories:* Feline territory is divided into three zones.

- The **core territory**, which is the area in which cats eat, sleep and play (and usually equates to the house, or part of it, for the domestic cat) needs to be safe and secure and free from potential intrusion by cats from other social groups.
- The **home range**, which usually includes latrine sites and observation platforms, is shared by cats in the immediate neighbourhood.
- The larger **hunting ranges** are shared by larger numbers of cats in the local vicinity.

Time-share systems are important in avoiding conflict within these territorial zones and in the majority of situations outright aggression is avoided. Conflict is most likely in the home range when cat densities are high. Invasion of core territories and threat to resources within homes can increase the risk of conflict.

Dawn and dusk are high risk times in terms of aggression and this may be due to the fact that prey is most active at these times, and there is increased competition for this important resource, or simply a consequence of the increased chance of feline encounters because more cats are out and about at these times.

*Feline despots:* Aggressive encounters between cats are significantly increased when a feline despot is present within a neighbourhood. These despotic cats not only show heightened territorial behaviour but also make repeated attempts to expand their territory. Entire males are most likely to be despotic but there is no exclusive association and other cats can behave in this way. In common with many territorially aggressive cats these individuals will display extreme aggression toward cats invading their home range but despotic individuals will also invade the core territory of other cats and attack them in their own homes. They are most active at dawn and dusk and their behaviour is often a source of deep tension between human neighbours in the vicinity.

*Entire males:* The majority of domestic cats are neutered and intercat aggression within neighbourhoods is consequently reduced but the risk of overt aggression is greatly increased in situations where two entire males live in close proximity. In such situations the aggression can be very serious. Neutering before 12 months of age has been shown to decrease fighting by as much as 88% (Hart and Cooper, 1984) and an earlier study (Hart and Barrett, 1973) suggested that postpubertal castration led to a similar level of reduction. This suggests that, in the case of male-to-male aggression, hormonal influences are more significant than learning.

Aggression between entire males and females is rare, although it may occur if the female is not ready to mate. It is important to consider the differential of normal mating behaviour when owners report that entire cats are acting in a hostile manner toward one another. The feline mating process is a very noisy event and it is not uncommon for inexperienced owners to misinterpret this as an episode of overt aggression.

## Principles of treatment

### Safety considerations

When an owner contacts the practice seeking advice about an aggressive cat, it is likely that there will be a time delay between that initial enquiry and the full behavioural consultation. In these circumstances it is *essential* to offer safety advice.

- **In all cases of feline aggression, owners must be advised to avoid situations that may induce or antagonize aggressive behaviour.**
- **They should also be advised to avoid confrontational measures at all times and to cease unintentional reinforcement of the behaviour by their own responses.**
- **The potentially serious nature of injury from cats must be emphasized and owners should be advised to seek medical attention if they have been badly bitten or scratched.**
- **Behavioural first aid in these situations should include:**
  - **Isolation of aggressively aroused cats**
  - **Separation of the cat and the potential victim (either feline or human)**
  - **Implementation of measures that will decrease the level of arousal, such as blocking visual access to potentially challenging situations (e.g. other cats in the garden).**

Following a full behavioural consultation, the aim of treatment is to deal with the specific cause of the aggression as well as to treat the learnt component of the present behaviour. Treatment may include a combination of approaches, including behavioural modification, environmental manipulation, conventional medication and pheromone therapy.

## Behavioural and environmental modification

### General measures

One of the most important considerations in the treatment of cases of feline aggression is establishing outlets for normal behaviour and ensuring that the cat's environment provides adequate opportunity to display natural coping strategies such as flight and hiding in situations of stress and social conflict (Figure 19.7). This is especially true in cases of cat-to-cat aggression but also applies to situations of conflict between cat and owner. Providing adequate environmental stimulation and opportunity for expression of predatory responses is the key to dealing with misdirected predatory behaviour and problems of inappropriate play.

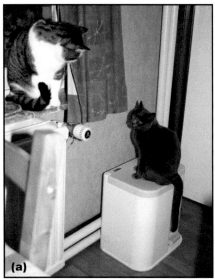

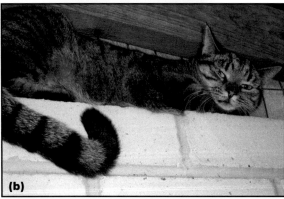

**19.7** Coping strategies. **(a)** In situations of social tension between cats, height can be used to provide more options for distancing from one another and avoiding outright confrontation. (Courtesy of A. Lummersheim.) **(b)** This shelter cat has retreated to an inaccessible and elevated location. Attempts to retrieve the cat will increase its perception of being threatened and increase the risk of defensive aggression in response.

Behavioural modification techniques that are designed to minimize the possibility of physical injury should be a priority and the use of barrier methods (such as restricted access, harnesses and house-lines) should be considered. In multi-cat households the practice of fitting a bell to the collar of the aggressive cat has been found to be beneficial in terms of giving other cats advance warning of its presence, allowing them time to take avoiding action. In cases involving despotic behaviour toward cats in the neighbourhood, time-share systems that allow the cats access to the home range at different times of the day can be very successful but rely on close cooperation between the respective owners, which is not always forthcoming. Increasing the attraction of remaining within their own core territory is another useful part of the treatment plan for despots and in extreme cases confinement in outdoor pens and enclosed gardens may be the only viable option for some of these cats.

Removal of confrontational interactions and unintentional reinforcement of inappropriate responses will also be an important part of the treatment plan. The perception on the cat's part that it is being restricted and threatened is a major factor in the onset of aggressive behaviour and, due to the cat's inability to diffuse conflict, it is important for owners to learn to recognize the very early signs of feline tension. This enables behavioural modification to be implemented as early as possible and to prevent escalation of the aggressive behaviour.

### Fear/anxiety-related aggression

Desensitization to fear-inducing stimuli, be they people or other cats, and counter-conditioning in order to establish acceptable behavioural responses (see Chapter 5) that are incompatible with aggression are the cornerstones of treatment in cases where fear and anxiety are the underlying motivations. In view of the cat's instinct to run from threatening situations, it may be necessary to use a controlled exposure technique in order to teach cats that stimuli are not threatening.

In controlled exposure the cat is not confronted with the fear-inducing stimulus in a confrontational manner and is always given a means of retreat from the perceived threat, albeit a controlled one. In other words, the cat may be restricted within an indoor pen, in order to prevent it from escaping from the room and never coming into the presence of the perceived threat, but the pen may be covered in the early stages of treatment to offer security and cardboard boxes may be provided in order to give temporary hideouts. It is very important that the cat is not faced with a full presentation of the fear-inducing stimulus without the option of avoidance, as would happen when using a flooding technique (in which the patient is exposed to a stimulus that evokes an undesired response and from which it is not allowed to escape until it learns to accept the situation).

### Anxiety at being handled

If aggression is triggered by human handling, it is advisable for the owner not to lift the cat off the ground during the early stages of treatment and only to have physical contact when the cat approaches them, rather than the other way around. Interactions should be limited to very short sessions and always terminated before agitation begins. The owner needs to learn how to read feline body language (see Figures 19.4 and 19.5) and predict when tension is rising. Tail twitching, flattened ears, stiffened shoulders and legs and dilated pupils should all be noted as signs of increasing arousal and risk of aggression.

If a cat begins to show aggression during handling, it is important not to touch the abdomen or other sensitive parts of the body. It is also important to resist the temptation to pull hands rapidly away from the cat, as this can cause it to tighten its grip and tear the skin. Instead the most appropriate reaction is to freeze and in order to make this response more appropriate it is advisable for owners to wear protective gloves and thick sleeves during treatment sessions.

The primary aim of treatment should be to work gradually to the situation where the cat is on the owner's lap unrestrained. Once this has been achieved it should be possible to condition the cat gradually to accept increased levels of restraint and handling and eventually to accept being lifted from the ground, but this may take some considerable time. It is important for owners to have realistic expectations of interaction with their cat and to appreciate that intense physical handling is not inherently rewarding for cats.

In order to increase the speed of acceptance of handling it is useful to use food rewards, though cats are not social feeders and are rarely motivated to work for their daily food ration. Treats that are used will therefore need to be of sufficient value as to be perceived as a reward by the cat. Limiting access to the chosen food to treatment sessions is recommended as this helps to increase the food's perceived value. In the early stages of treatment a positive association with the presence of a person is achieved by offering the food reward without any request for physical interaction; but as treatment progresses the cat should be rewarded for increasingly direct contact with the person (see **client handout**). It may help if the owner is given a listed sequence of behaviours that should be rewarded: only when the cat shows no signs of arousal or distress should the owner progress to the next stage in the sequence.

### General frustration

In cases of frustration-related aggression it is important to teach the cat to be more independent by encouraging independent play, through the use of items such as fishing-rod toys, and reward appropriate interactions with people while removing any unintentional reward for demanding interactions. The use of food-dispensing toys to provide the cat with some of their daily ration increases the control the pet has over its own circumstances while increasing foraging behaviour and can be quite useful (see Chapter 9).

### Social stress in the same house

In cases of aggression between cats in the same household the main element of the treatment plan is to respect the social groupings that exist and to implement resource distribution that allows the cats to coexist under the same roof and effectively avoid each other. Separate resting, feeding and toileting areas should be provided and adequate outlets for predatory behaviour should be established in order to decrease the likelihood of these behaviours being directed toward the other cat. Feeding is a solitary behaviour for cats and therefore it is not advisable to use food as a means of encouraging contact between cats. The aim is not to integrate the cats or to make them friends. In some cases, separation for some part of each 24-hour period may be necessary to allow some individuals to be calm and relaxed.

### Frustration resulting in redirection of aggression toward another cat in the household

A common scenario within multi-cat households, especially when the cats are restricted to indoors, is for aggression between housemates to be redirected as a result of a frustrated reaction to stimulation from outside the home. In such situations it is important to deal with the primary motivation for the aggression as well as work to restore the relationship between the two housemates. Measures such as keeping other cats out of the garden and blocking visual access to the cats outside will be an important part of the treatment plan.

### Predatory behaviour

Aggression associated with misdirected predatory behaviour is primarily treated by providing adequate opportunity to express these normal behavioural sequences (see Chapter 9). Since these behaviours are naturally rehearsed and perfected through play, it is important to provide cats with suitable toys. Often simple ones are best and ones that offer unpredictable, rapid movement and high-pitched sound are ideal. The piece of string and rolled-up piece of paper work very well, provided that an owner is on hand to move them in an unpredictable and exciting fashion, and it is easy to add to the value of this sort of play by rolling the paper down the stairs or along ledges and incorporating an element of agility into the game.

## Medication

In cases where systemic illness or pain is found to be an initiating factor for the behaviour, appropriate medical treatment should be instituted immediately. However, in many cases of feline aggression the behaviour is found to result from environmental and behavioural factors alone. Some may consider the use of medication in cases where the aggression is the result of normal feline responses to an inadequate environment, but medication must never be used to mask situations that compromise feline welfare. Its use cannot be justified in isolation from environmental manipulation and appropriate behavioural therapy techniques.

In cases of fear- or anxiety-based aggression, on the other hand, medical treatment may be a necessary part of the treatment regime. The drugs that are commonly used in these situations are not licensed for cats and the dose rates are based on individual experience and anecdotal evidence rather than controlled trials or published data. In cases where the cat is showing fearful behaviour toward specific identifiable stimuli, treatment with selegiline at 1.0 mg/kg once a day is recommended by the author. In cases where the cat is experiencing less specific anxiety which is fuelling an aggressive response, clomipramine at 0.25–0.5 mg/kg once a day or fluoxetine at 0.5 mg/kg once a day may be appropriate (see Chapter 21 for further details relating to the precautions necessary when considering the use of these medications).

## Pheromone therapy

There are currently two commercially available synthetic analogues of fractions from the so-called feline facial pheromone complex and both of these may be considered useful adjuncts to a behavioural therapy programme in cases of feline aggression.

Feline facial pheromone fraction F4 (Felifriend®) has been specifically marketed in Europe for situations involving aggression and has also been advocated as a means of preventing intra-specific aggression when introducing an unfamiliar feline to an existing resident (Pageat and Tessier, 1997a). However, there have been mixed reports over its efficacy in these situations. Some clinicians report an obvious panic reaction in cats when F4 has been used to treat aggression between cats in the same household and this reaction appears to be most pronounced when the aggression has been present for some time. One possible explanation is that the visual signal in such an encounter results in conflict between an aversive visual and appeasing odour signal. The conflicting signals then cause the cat to panic (Pageat, 1999). This reaction has also been reported in situations where F4 has been used to deal with aggression from cats to people, but other work has shown that the 'pheromone' can be very successful in decreasing hostility in the context of the veterinary consultation (Pageat and Tessier, 1997b).

Feline facial pheromone fraction F3 (Feliway®) is marketed as a familiarization odour and is indicated in cases of aggression that are related to social tension within the home or to anxiety-related behaviours. The aim is for F3 to make each cat feel more secure and relaxed within the home and thereby reduce conflict and make aggression less likely. It has been reported to be successful in cases where overt aggression is mild but there are obvious signs of social tension between the residents (Ogata and Takeuchi, 2001).

As with any product, correct application is necessary in order to achieve the best results and it would appear that many reported failures of F3 relate to inappropriate use rather than a lack of efficacy. Appropriate advice about leaving diffusers switched on for 24 hours a day and positioning them in undisputed areas of the house where social tension is at its lowest level is important. See Chapter 21 for further details on the use of pheromones.

## Prevention of feline aggression problems

### Prevention of aggression toward people

The cornerstone of prevention for aggression toward people is to teach humans to have realistic expectations of feline interaction and social behaviour and to teach cats how to accept human handling.

There has been a lot of research into the factors that affect a cat's friendly interaction with people (e.g. Moelk, 1979; Karsh, 1983; Turner *et al.*, 1986; Reisner *et al.*, 1994; McCune 1995) and these are important when considering the prevention of aggression problems. They include:

- The human handling that kittens receive in the period between 2 and 7 weeks of age in terms of frequency, duration and style
- The number of different handlers that a kitten experiences at this age and the characteristics of those handlers in terms of age and sex
- Factors relating to the boldness of the kitten's parents and their reaction to being handled by people.

One of the recognized factors predisposing to problems of perceived aggression toward humans is inappropriate play behaviour involving aggressive displays toward human hands and feet. The provision of toys that allow cats to complete the behavioural sequence by grabbing at the toy, and even opening it to reveal food items inside (see Chapter 9), can help to reduce the incidence of this sort of interaction with people.

### Prevention of aggression toward cats

The most important principles for preventing aggression between cats in the same household are:

- To select potential housemates after considering natural feline behaviour
- To restrict the number of cats within the household to socially compatible levels
- To pay careful attention to the introduction process if further cats are to be introduced (Levine *et al.*, 2005), always ensuring that all cats have free and immediate access to their essential resources without running the gauntlet of other cats (see **client handout**).

In order to reduce aggression problems between cats in the neighbourhood it is important to:

- Provide a secure demarcation between outdoor and indoor territory
- Make access to the outside world predictable.

Limiting visual intrusion into the home from cats outside is also beneficial and providing high-up resting places within the garden from which cats can observe their territory in safety should also be considered. In situations of severe overpopulation in the neighbourhood, the provision of accessible outdoor latrines may also be helpful.

## References and further reading

Association of Pet Behaviour Counsellors (2005) *Annual Review of Cases.* www.apbc.org.uk
Bernstein P and Strack M (1993) Home ranges, favoured spots, time sharing patterns and tail usage by fourteen cats in the home. *Animal Behavioural Consultants Newsletter* **10**(3), 1–3
Biben M (1979) Predation and predatory play behaviour of domestic cats. *Animal Behaviour* **27**, 81–94

Bradshaw JWS (1992) *The Behaviour of the Domestic Cat*. CAB International, Wallingford

Bradshaw JWS, Casey RA and MacDonald JM (2000) The occurrence of unwanted behaviour in the pet cat population. *Proceedings, Companion Animal Behaviour Therapy Study Group Study Day,* pp. 41–42

Bradshaw JWS and Hall SL (1999) Affiliative behaviour of related and unrelated pairs of cats in catteries: preliminary report. *Applied Animal Behaviour Science* **63**, 251–255

Bradshaw JWS and Lovett RE (2003) Do domestic cats form hierarchies? *BSAVA Congress Scientific Proceedings*, p. 104

Carlstead C, Brown J L and Strawn W (1993) Behavioural and physiological correlates of stress in laboratory cats. *Applied Animal Behaviour Science* **38**, 143–158

Casey RA (2001) A comparison of referred feline clinical behaviour cases with general population prevalence data. *BSAVA Congress Scientific Proceedings*, p. 529

Casey RA, Vandenbussche S, Bradshaw JWS and Roberts MA (in press) Reasons for relinquishment and return of domestic cats (*Felis silvestris catus*) to rescue shelters in the UK. *Anthrozöos*

Cohn E (2005) The effects of queen (*Felis sylvestris*) rearing versus hand-rearing on feline aggression and other problematic behaviours. *Current Issues and Research in Veterinary Behavioural Medicine*, ed. D Mills *et al.*, pp. 201–202. Purdue University Press, West Lafayette, Indiana

Hart BL and Barrett RE (1973) Effects of castration on fighting, roaming and urine spraying in adult male cats. *Journal of the American Veterinary Medical Association* **163**, 290–292

Hart BL and Cooper L (1984) Factors relating to urine spraying and fighting in prepubertally gonadectomized cats. *Journal of the American Veterinary Medical Association* **184**, 1255–1258

Karsh EB (1983) The effects of early handling on the development of social bonds between cats and people. In: *New Perspectives on Our Lives with Companion Animals*, ed. AH Katcher and AM Beck, pp. 22–28. Pennsylvania Press, Philadelphia

Levine E, Perry P, Scarlett J and Houpt KA (2005) Intercat aggression in households following the introduction of a new cat. *Applied Animal Behaviour Science* **90**, 325–336

Lindell EM, Erb HN and Houpt KA (1997) Intercat aggression: a retrospective study examining types of aggression, sexes of fighting pairs and effectiveness of treatment. *Applied Animal Behaviour Science* **55**, 153–162

McCune S (1992) *Temperament and the Welfare of Caged Cats*. PhD thesis, University of Cambridge

McCune S (1995) The impact of paternity and early socialisation on the development of cats' behaviour to people and novel objects. *Applied Animal Behaviour Science* **45**, 109–124

Moelk M (1979) The development of friendly approach behaviour in the cat: a study of kitten mother relations and the cognitive development of the kitten from birth to eight weeks. *Advances in the Study of Behaviour* **10**, 163–224

New JC, Salmon MD, Scarlett JM *et al.* (1999) Characteristics of dogs and cats and those relinquishing them to 12 US animal shelters. *Journal of Applied Animal Welfare Science* **2**, 83–96

Ogata N and Takeuchi Y (2001) Clinical trial of feline pheromone analogue for feline urine marking. *Journal of Veterinary Medical Science* **63**, 157–161

Pageat P (1999) Attachment pheromones in the dog. *Proceedings, 2nd International Conference on Veterinary Behavioural Medicine*, p.7

Pageat P and Tessier Y (1997a) Usefulness of the F4 synthetic pheromone for preventing intra-specific aggression in poorly socialised cats. *Proceedings of the First International Conference on Veterinary Behavioural Medicine*, ed. DS Mills *et al.*, pp. 64–72. Universities Federation for Animal Welfare, Potters Bar

Pageat P and Tessier Y (1997b) F4 synthetic pheromone: a means to enable handling of cats with a phobia of the veterinarian during consultation. *Proceedings, 1st International Conference on Veterinary Behavioural Medicine*, pp. 108–111

Reisner IR, Houpt KA, Hollis NE and Quimby FW (1994) Friendliness to humans and defensive aggression in cats: the influence of handling and paternity. *Physiology and Behaviour* **55**, 1119–1124

Rochlitz I, Podberseck AL and Broom DM (1998) The welfare of cats in a quarantine cattery. *Veterinary Record* **143**, 181–185

Turner DC, Feaver J, Mendl M and Bateson P (1986) Variations in domestic cat behaviour toward humans: a paternal effect. *Animal Behaviour* **34**, 1890–1901

## Client handouts (bsavalibrary.com/behaviour_leaflets)

- Avoiding aggression in cats
- Avoiding house soiling by cats
- Avoiding urine marking by cats
- Cognitive dysfunction syndrome
- Feline behaviour questionnaire
- Handling exercises for an aggressive cat
- Handling exercises for puppies and kittens

- Introducing a new cat into the household
- Request for information on problem behaviours
- Taking your cat in the car
- What your cat needs

# 20

# Repetitive and compulsive behaviour in dogs and cats

## Andrew U. Luescher

## Introduction

Repetitive or sustained, apparently abnormal behaviours performed out of context (but not linked to an identifiable pathology) have been described more commonly in various species of laboratory, farm and zoo animals than in small companion animals. These behaviours have variously been termed stereotypic behaviour, stereotypies, compulsive behaviours, or obsessive compulsive behaviours (for a review of these terms see Mason and Rushen, 2006). They can generally be linked to conditions of confinement and specific husbandry practices.

In companion animals, repetitive behaviour that was not caused by an identifiable medical disorder or lesion was historically attributed to a partial seizure disorder. Treatment with seizure-controlling medication was usually unsuccessful and patients were frequently euthanized. The concepts developed to explain repetitive behaviours in other species were for the first time applied to small animals by Luescher *et al.* (1991). Researchers at the National Institute of Health (NIH) reported that acral licking, a specific repetitive behaviour in dogs, was susceptible to treatment with a drug used for human obsessive compulsive disorder (OCD) (Goldberger and Rapoport, 1990). Thus, a theoretical framework had been developed that included ethological concepts and neurophysiological information. The first treatment success based on this shift in paradigm was published by Overall (1994).

Repetitive behaviour can have various causes, many of which are medical. However, even repetitive behaviours that are not based on an identifiable medical condition vary as to their aetiology: they may be a normal part of the species-typical repertoire, they may be conditioned, or they may be environmentally induced abnormal behaviours. Even the latter are not a homogeneous group of behaviours. They differ vastly in their appearance, their focus and the level of cognition that appears to be involved. Some are uniformly repeated motor patterns where the focus appears to be on performance of the motor pattern itself. These behaviours are correctly called **stereotypies** (Garner, 2006). Other behaviours result from fixation on a goal and may be labelled as **compulsive behaviours**. Some of these are relatively simple, such as staring at objects on the floor, but some are very complicated rituals that appear to involve a high level of cognition. For example, a German Shepherd Dog had a ball in the backyard.

Whenever let into the yard he would find a leaf, pick it up, deposit it on top of the ball, then lie down a few feet from the ball and stare at the leaf. When the wind blew the leaf away, he would go pick it up and place it back on the ball.

Some behaviours usually considered to be compulsive appear to involve 'hallucination'. One example of this was a Border Collie who, whenever he passed under a certain tree, stopped to stare into the canopy apparently frightened.

Theoretically, the classification of environmentally induced stereotypic behaviour has consequences for drug choice in treatment, with stereotypies supposed to be more amenable to treatment with dopaminergic drugs, and compulsive disorder (**CD**) to treatment with serotonergic drugs. This has never been documented in clinical trials (Hewson *et al.*, 1998b; Irimajiri *et al.*, 2009) and has not been reported even as anecdotal information. Also, in many cases of stereotypic behaviour it may be unclear what category it would fall into. For example, is a tail-chasing dog fixating on its tail or just repeating the same motor pattern? Is a 'fly snapping' dog (which appears to be snapping after imaginary flies) just repeating the snapping motion, or does it imagine that there are flies, i.e. it hallucinates? Dogs licking their carpus repeatedly and excessively have been considered to be a model for human OCD and responded to treatment with clomipramine, a drug used to treat OCD in humans. How is a dog to be classified that licks its carpus, but also licks other objects or performs licking as a vacuum activity?

Because of these difficulties and the fact that, so far, categorization of the behaviours into stereotypies and compulsive behaviours has yet to have clear and consistent clinical relevance, in the remainder of this chapter all these behaviours are grouped together under the label of compulsive behaviours (but not *obsessive* compulsive behaviour, since homology with this human disorder has not been proved and because some of these behaviours are likely to be stereotypies more akin to human tic disorders).

## Definition of compulsive behaviour

A working definition of compulsive behaviour has been proposed (Hewson and Luescher, 1996) as:

> ... *behaviours that are usually brought on by conflict, but that are subsequently shown outside of the original context. The behaviours*

*might share a similar pathophysiology (e.g. changes in serotonin, dopamine and beta-endorphin systems). Compulsive behaviours seem abnormal because they are displayed out of context and are often repetitive, exaggerated or sustained*

Overall and Dunham (2002) describe them as:

*'... repetitive, ritualistic behaviours, in excess of any required for normal function, the execution of which interferes with normal, daily activities and functioning'.*

## Causes and risk factors

### Environmental factors
In agreement with the theory for stereotypic behaviour in farm animals, compulsive behaviours are considered to be a consequence of stress (see Chapter 13), frustration or conflict (Luescher *et al.*, 1991; Cabib, 2006).

- **Frustration** refers to the situation in which an animal is motivated to perform a behaviour, but is prevented from doing so.
- **Conflict**, or 'motivational conflict', results from two opposing, similarly strong motivations (such as approach and withdrawal).

The label 'conflict behaviours' is defined as behaviours shown in situations of motivational conflict, but is also used for behaviour resulting from frustration or any other situation in which an animal does not have a contextually appropriate response for reducing arousal. Various forms of conflict behaviours have been studied in a great variety of species (Hinde, 1970).

Conflict behaviour often results from long-term housing in a restricted barren environment that does not contain the appropriate releasers for species-typical behaviour, and that the animal is not capable of acting upon with predictable outcome (lack of controllability). It can also result from motivational conflict (one of the motivations usually being fear) or frustration. Disease that increases stress or irritability may contribute to CD, as may other stressful conditions (e.g. a social conflict with another dog or cat, or separation anxiety).

Conflict behaviours that are elicited by prolonged and/or repeated exposure to the causal situation are particularly likely to develop into compulsive behaviour.

### Physical stimuli
In some cases, an animal may start to lick a lesion or sutures and then start also to lick other parts of the body, causing lick granulomas in sites unrelated to the lesion. This suggests that physical lesions or irritations, such as those caused by allergy, may trigger CD in some cases. It is assumed (but not proven) that the stress associated with a lesion or irritation can contribute to the development of CD in an already susceptible animal, and that the irritation can initially

direct the compulsive behaviour towards a particular body site. However, in any such case it would need to be ruled out if there is irritation or pain, or a lack of sensation in the target area, that may elicit licking, rubbing or scratching, or self-mutilation behaviour.

### Conditioning
Owner attention may reinforce existing compulsive behaviours or may condition normal conflict behaviours to the extent that they appear compulsive. Performance of the behaviour only in the owner's presence is suggestive of a conditioned behaviour.

### Genotype
A genetic predisposition is probably present in most cases of CD. Individuals may be genetically susceptible to develop a compulsive behaviour, or the genotype may determine which, if any, compulsive behaviour an animal will develop. Some breed predispositions for compulsive behaviours are listed in Figure 20.1 and have also been reported (Overall and Dunham, 2002).

| Breed or type | Common abnormal repetitive behaviour |
|---|---|
| Doberman Pinscher | Flank sucking |
| English Bull Terrier | Spinning in tight circles. Sticking head under or between objects and freezing |
| Staffordshire Bull Terrier | Spinning in tight circles |
| German Shepherd Dog | Tail chasing (Overall and Dunham, 2002) |
| Australian Cattle Dog | Tail chasing (Blackshaw *et al.*, 1994; Hartigan, 2000) |
| Miniature Schnauzer | Checking hind end |
| Border Collie | Visual fixations, e.g. shadow staring |
| Large-breed dogs | Persistent licking, causing granulomas |
| Siamese/Burmese cat | Wool sucking (Luescher *et al.*, 1991) (see Figure 20.2) |

**20.1** Abnormal repetitive behaviours typically seen in certain breeds of dog and cat.

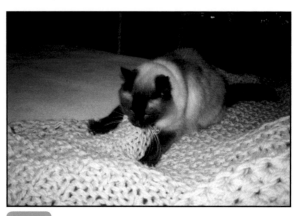

**20.2** A Himalayan cat sucking on a wool blanket.

## Temperament

Frequent co-morbidity with other anxiety disorders suggests that an anxious disposition may be a risk factor for CD. In a caseload analysis at the Purdue University animal behaviour clinic (unpublished data) where the response of dogs to various situations (handling and restraint by owner; strangers at home and away from home; children; other dogs at home and away from home; environmental stimuli such as loud noises) were examined, it was found that dogs with CD responded significantly more often with defensive aggression than dogs with other behavioural problems. This again supports the idea that temperament can be a risk factor for CD.

## Age

Overall and Dunham (2002) reported the mean age of onset of CD in dogs as just below 2 years and discuss the similarity with the onset of OCD in people during adolescence. In an analysis of the author's caseload, age of onset was 1.48 years, which was not significantly different from the mean age of onset of behaviour problems in general of 1.52 years and may thus not be meaningful. Furthermore, Moon-Fanelli *et al.* (2007) reported different ages of onset for flank-sucking and blanket-sucking Doberman Pinschers. In other species, such as horses, there are also clear differences in the average age of onset for different abnormal repetitive behaviours. Global statements on age of onset must therefore be interpreted with caution.

## Evaluation of the patient

### Clinical examination

The first essential step is a medical assessment, so that relevant medical causes for stereotyped behaviour can be identified and treated. A minimal medical database includes a physical examination with a basic neurological examination. The latter includes (Oliver and Lorenz, 1993):

- Observation of the animal (movement, balance)
- Symmetry of face and eye position
- Testing of the menace reflex, the eye blink reflex, vestibular eye movement and pupillary reflex
- Assessment of sensation on nose and lower jaw, and jaw tone
- Symmetry of larynx, pharynx and tongue
- Testing of the gag reflex
- Palpation of masseter, trapezius and brachiocephalicus muscles to assess atrophy
- Palpation of spine
- Testing of hopping and proprioceptive positioning
- Testing of hearing (by making a noise behind the animal and watching for a reaction).

The examination also includes a complete blood cell count, blood chemistry profile and possibly urinalysis. Additional tests such as a thyroid profile, dermatological tests, allergy testing, a complete neurological exam and imaging may be needed, depending on the specific case.

## Presenting signs and history

Once overt medical causes have been ruled out, a diagnosis of CD is primarily based on a detailed history. The history may be divided into three parts:

- Information about the animal's life history and management
- Assessment of the animal's disposition or temperament
- Focus on the compulsive behaviour itself.

### Life history and management

Information should be obtained about the original acquisition of the animal (source; age when acquired) and about its management, including exercise, confinement, training (including punishment techniques for the unwanted behaviour), feeding and interaction between the pet and the owner.

### Assessment of the animal's disposition

This may be achieved by giving the client a long list of situations and asking them to describe the animal's behaviour in each context (see behavioural profile questionnaire **client handout**). The behaviour is then scored as neutral, happy, submissive, fearful/anxious, hyperexcitable, or offensively or defensively aggressive. Temperament-related problems should be addressed before treatment of a specific behaviour problem is attempted.

### The compulsive behaviour

General information on the problem includes:

- A description of the situations in which the behaviour occurs (triggers of the behaviour)
- The behaviour of the animal and people just before the event
- The compulsive behaviour itself
- The body language of the animal
- The behaviour of the owner and behaviour of the animal immediately after the event
- The ease or difficulty with which the animal can be distracted.

These will allow the veterinary surgeon to understand the form of the behaviour, inciting situations and environmental factors sustaining the behaviour, which may need to be changed in the treatment phase of the consultation. Also recorded are:

- The frequency and duration of the compulsive behaviour (this allows assessment of treatment response by looking at a change in either or both)
- The age of the animal at the onset of the problem and any correlated changes
- Previous attempts by the owner to treat the problem (this information may help to determine whether attention seeking is a component of the behaviour).

Since a general description of the behaviour will be tainted by the owner's perception of the problem, it is useful to ask them to describe the three most recent incidents of the behaviour in detail (again: situation and trigger, behaviour including body language, behaviour of owner and of animal after the event). It is also useful to ask them to describe the earliest incidents, if possible, as a comparison between the most recent and the earliest incidents may shed some light on the development of the problem (identifying how it began may help to differentiate the problem from other disorders).

Owners should be encouraged to bring along a video recording showing the behaviour. From the recording it is often possible to evaluate more detailed properties of the behaviour of the animal (e.g. uniformity or variability), the reaction of the owner, conflict behaviours, how responsive the patient is to its environment while performing the behaviour, and its sense of balance.

## Client's attitudes, beliefs and behaviour

It is important to recognize and address the attitude and beliefs of the client, to ensure that their expectations remain realistic. The correction of inappropriate owner behaviour may be an essential component of the treatment strategy. Some important areas to consider include the following.

- The owner may have misapprehensions about the motivation for the behaviour. The animal is not doing it to 'annoy' the owner, nor is the problem a sign of poor temperament or a 'crazy' individual. However, attention-seeking behaviours must be differentiated and the role of inadvertent reinforcement identified and corrected.
- These problems often arise when there is a significant level of inconsistency and unpredictability in the animal's routine. The importance of predictability and control and owner consistency in the animal's life may need to be explained, emphasizing how animals view their interactions with the family members.
- Some cases may require medication and the client's attitude to this intervention needs to be assessed. Resistant owners may be persuaded about the importance of this type of intervention if they can understand that the problem has an important neurological basis.

## Risk evaluation

Compulsive behaviour can interfere with normal function, be associated with self-harm directly (e.g. acral lick) or indirectly (e.g. chronic musculoskeletal damage from repetition over time) and impact the human–animal bond (Moon-Fanelli and Dodman, 1998). These problems pose several risks to the patient's wellbeing, depending on the exact presenting complaint. Frequently, owners consider the impact on the dog–owner relationship to be minimal and this may explain why many of these cases are not presented as a problem requiring management, but the behaviours can be extreme (Moon-Fanelli *et al.*, 2007). For example, an English Bull Terrier responded with stereotyped pouncing towards any object on the floor. He was unable to eat from a dish and the food needed to be presented on paper. He was also unable to drink from a water bowl, and the owners had to provide the dog with water from a bottle to avoid dehydration.

## Diagnosis

Compulsive disorders can be expressed through a wide variety of specific behaviours, from visual fixations to tail spinning, coprophagia or polydipsia, and each has its own specific differentials which need to be evaluated. In the following section, a range of general differentials are considered, but it is important that careful evaluation is made of all differentials (specific and general). It may be necessary to begin treatment on the basis of a tentative diagnosis.

The diagnostic features of CD are as follows:

- The behaviours are often repetitive, exaggerated or sustained actions that interfere with normal functioning
- The behaviours are displayed out of context and are not purely conditioned responses
- The behaviours are usually brought on initially by conflict
- The behaviours may subsequently be shown outside the original context
- The behaviours are not due to some other physical lesion or pathological process.

## Differential diagnoses

### Seizures

Seizures need to be differentiated from compulsive disorder. Animals performing compulsive behaviours are obviously aware of their surroundings, can be distracted (though sometimes with difficulty) from performing the behaviour and do not show a post-ictal phase. In contrast to seizures, animals perform the compulsive behaviour usually when alert and interacting with their environment. Also, seizures do not follow the pathogenesis typical for CD.

### Central lesions

Neurological disorders such as forebrain and brainstem lesions may cause an animal to walk aimlessly in large circles. Circling in tighter circles with a head tilt indicates likely involvement of the vestibular system (Oliver and Lorenz, 1993). In these cases circling is related to a balance disorder. Circling has also been attributed to lumbosacral stenosis or cauda equina syndrome. Hydrocephalus has been suggested as a cause of circling in Bull Terriers (Dodman *et al.*, 1996); the same study reported that circling Bull Terriers had an abnormal electroencephalogram (EEG) indicative of seizure activity.

Tail-dock neuroma may draw a dog's attention to its hind end but the author is not aware of any case in which tail-dock neuroma was a proven cause for circling behaviour or aggression to the tail.

### Sensory neuropathies

Sensory neuropathies can induce chewing on the feet. Pain sensation in the distal extremities is reduced. The condition can be hereditary and is then usually apparent in young animals (Oliver and Lorenz, 1993). A trigeminal sensory dysfunction has been hypothesized to be responsible for the orofacial pain syndrome in cats that results in self-mutilation through repetitive chewing and clawing in the oral cavity (Rusbridge *et al.*, 2008).

### Dermatology

Any dermatological lesion or skin gland disease resulting in itching or pain can cause licking. Dermatological lesions may also increase stress and increase the likelihood of the animal developing CD. On the other hand, emotional stress can predispose an animal to develop dermatological disease (Virga, 2004). Dermatological lesions such as pre-existing wounds or pressure-point granulomas can also direct compulsive licking towards a particular area.

Dermatological conditions that need to be considered include parasitic infestation, staphylococcal furunculosis, dermatophytosis, endocrine dysfunction and allergy.

Licking or scratching can worsen many dermatological lesions, resulting in an itch–lick or itch–scratch cycle. Licking or scratching may persist long after the initiating dermatological cause has been removed (Reisner, 1991).

### Musculoskeletal

Tail-tip fractures, arthritic joints, etc. may draw the animal's attention to the painful region and may mimic or instigate compulsive behaviour towards that region.

### Acute conflict behaviour

Whenever an animal is in a situation of frustration or motivational conflict, it is normal for it to perform an acute conflict behaviour. In contrast to compulsive behaviour, acute conflict behaviour is shown only in conflict situations and not when an animal reaches a threshold of arousal for other reasons, such as anticipation of being fed, i.e. in contrast to compulsive behaviour, acute conflict behaviour is not shown in situations in which there is no outside stimulus inducing a conflict.

### Conditioned behaviour or play

Any behaviour, including conflict behaviour and play behaviour, can become conditioned by the owner (or possibly another social partner) paying attention to the patient. Such behaviour is only shown in the presence of the social partner. It is therefore always necessary to ask if the problem is also performed when the animal is alone (e.g. outside in the garden or in another room). Information about other attention-seeking and play behaviour exhibited by the animal may be helpful.

## Behavioural biology of the condition

Compulsive disorder arises as a result of a pathological process in the central nervous system. The pathophysiology of CD is not well understood and may vary between types of stereotypic behaviour. Stereotypies and compulsive behaviours, by definition, differ with regard to their pathophysiology. Furthermore, it has been suggested that oral and locomotor stereotypic behaviours may involve activation of different dopaminergic systems (Cabib, 1993).

Most evidence of pathophysiological mechanisms stems from pharmacological studies. Large doses of dopaminergic drugs such as amphetamine or apomorphine are effective in inducing stereotyped behaviour in animals, while the dopamine antagonist haloperidol results in suppression of spontaneously occurring stereotyped behaviour (Kennes et al., 1988). The relationship with clinical CD is unclear.

Beta-endorphin antagonists may be at least temporarily effective in suppressing compulsive behaviour (Dodman et al., 1988; White, 1990). Thus, beta-endorphins have been implicated in CD, at least in the initial stages of the development of the disorder.

As in human OCD, drugs inhibiting serotonin reuptake have sometimes been found to be effective in the treatment of CD in dogs (Wynchank and Berk, 1998; Goldberger and Rapoport, 1990; Hewson et al., 1998b; Irimajiri et al., 2009). The effectiveness of such drugs implies that serotonin is involved in animal CD. Direct evidence of serotonin involvement has also been presented (Vanderbroek et al., 1995), but the role of serotonin in CD is not well understood, in particular since it is difficult to separate its role as a neurotransmitter and as a neurohormone.

## Development of compulsive behaviour

The definition of CD provided in this chapter predicts that compulsive behaviours are first shown in a specific conflict situation (acute or normal conflict behaviour) and that, with prolonged or repeated conflict, they may generalize to other contexts in which the animal experiences a high level of arousal. As the number of eliciting contexts increases, the threshold of arousal needed to elicit the compulsive behaviour decreases. In extreme cases, this can result in an animal performing the compulsive behaviour incessantly unless it eats, drinks or sleeps; and in some cases it can even interfere with these behaviours.

In a clinical trial involving 51 dogs with CD it was found that this process was reversed during treatment. When the severity of CD was rated as improving, the number of contexts in which the behaviour was displayed also decreased (Hewson et al., 1998b).

## Treatment

Treatment consists of:

- Changing the animal's environment and social interactions to avoid triggers and provide more consistency
- Behaviour modification
- Pharmacological intervention (in most cases).

If the animal is self-harming, acute management may require preventing access to that region of the body, for example with bandages or a muzzle. All interactive punishment for the behaviour must be stopped, since it is likely to increase conflict and distress and possibly the performance of the compulsive behaviour. An increase in daily exercise, play and enrichment activities should be instituted as soon as possible.

In the following section, treatment is listed in order of implementation. The steps are summarized in Figure 20.3.

| Step | Details |
|------|---------|
| 1. Identify and remove cause of conflict, frustration and specific stressors that trigger the behaviour, or desensitize to these stimuli | |
| 2. Reduce general stress within environment | Avoid inconsistent interactions; all interactions should be in a command–response–reward format<br>Provide animal with opportunities to control aspects of its environment<br>Provide a consistent routine<br>Stop all forms of owner-administered punishment<br>Provide enough regular exercise off the property<br>Provide food twice daily |
| 3. Pharmacological intervention and possible dietary manipulation to increase systemic uptake of tryptophan | |
| 4. Response substitution | Prevent compulsive behaviour if possible unless animal is supervised<br>Distract animal when compulsive behaviour is anticipated or initiated; give command for an alternative (incompatible) behaviour; and reward animal for performing the alternative behaviour |

**20.3** Treatment recommendations for compulsive disorder (CD).

## Identifying and removing triggers

Since CD is stress related in most cases, an attempt should be made to identify (in the history) and remove the cause of stress. In some cases, particularly those of self-directed oral behaviour, an environmental cause may not be identifiable. In other cases, an inciting cause can be identified but cannot be removed. In such cases, it may be possible to desensitize the animal to the trigger or cause (see Chapter 5).

## Reducing general stress

Stressors may be additive: once a compulsive behaviour is established, other stress-inducing conditions (so-called modulating factors) may serve to perpetuate it. Therefore attempts should be made to reduce environmental stress as much as possible.

The most stressful situation for an animal is one over which it has no control, and in which it cannot predict what is going to happen. Lack of predictability and control over the environment may arise from:

- Inconsistent owner–animal interactions
- Lack of training to commands and thus inconsistent use of commands
- Inappropriate use of punishment
- An inconsistent routine
- Frustration of motivations such as those for social interaction or for exploration.

All of these factors should be addressed. Casual interaction should be avoided and replaced with highly structured interactions in a command–response–reward format. For dogs, formal obedience sessions allow for consistent interaction and also are likely to render the owner's behaviour towards the dog more consistent in the long term, because the owner develops a habit of using consistent commands. For cats, it is recommended that owners provide regular quality time at a time of day when it can be provided consistently. Owners are advised to play with their cat with toys or to clicker-train them to do tricks such as retrieving a ball.

Punishment is aversive, usually unpredictable and stressful, and should never be used in animals affected with CD. An acceptable alternative to punishment is **response substitution**: if the animal engages in an inappropriate behaviour it is distracted with a noise, a command is issued, and the animal is rewarded for obeying the command (see below).

A regular routine increases the predictability of the animal's environment. It is particularly important that feeding and exercise are provided on a consistent daily basis in the same place in the owner's routine. Sufficient exercise off the property should be provided to dogs for its physiological effect and to meet dogs' need for exploration and social interaction with other dogs by sniffing and leaving scent marks. In most cases, two daily walks of about 20 minutes each may be sufficient, but this will vary with breed and age (see Chapter 3).

A large variety of interesting toys, which can be provided on a rotational basis, may serve as a non-specific means of decreasing arousal. Particularly attractive toys such as those that dispense food can be given at times when the performance of the compulsive behaviour is likely. Food-dispensing toys such as balls with a hole filled with dry food may satisfy a cat's motivation to hunt.

## Pharmacotherapy

If the owner is opposed to the use of drugs it is sometimes possible to treat severe cases of CD with environmental and behaviour modification alone. In most cases, however, drug therapy may prove necessary or will at least facilitate treatment. An important reason not to delay pharmacological treatment is that the drugs used to treat CD become less effective the longer the behaviour has been going on (Hewson *et al.*, 1998b).

### Serotonin reuptake inhibitors

As is the case with human OCD, pharmacological intervention is most likely to be achieved with serotonin reuptake inhibitors (SRIs). Compounds that inhibit the synaptic reuptake of biogenic amines including serotonin, and thus their degradation by the pre-synaptic neuron, are believed to potentiate the actions of these molecules. However, their therapeutic effect is usually delayed by several weeks (Goldberger and Rapoport, 1990). This indicates that their effect is unlikely to be due to the accumulation of serotonin in the synapse alone which does not exceed three to five times the normal value (Fuller, 1994) but to be due to a cascade of events triggered by the accumulation of neurotransmitter (Baldessarini, 1996). For example, auto-receptors desensitize after chronic administration of an SRI, resulting in increased release of serotonin, while reuptake is still inhibited (Baldessarini, 1996). In addition, serotonin is not only released at synapses, but also from axonal swellings (varicosities) acting on many peripheral targets as a neuromodulator and neurohormone (Weiger, 1997).

- A double-blind randomized placebo-controlled study of **fluoxetine** on 62 dogs with acral lick lesions concluded that the drug was effective in controlling the condition over a 6-week period, and both licking behaviour and lesion scores continued to improve during a 2-month follow-up treatment period (Wynchank and Berk, 1998).
- A clinical trial involving 51 dogs with a variety of compulsive behaviours has been performed for the tricyclic antidepressant **clomipramine** (Hewson *et al.*, 1998b); it showed that clomipramine was effective in reducing the severity of oral and locomotory compulsive behaviours. A case series suggested effectiveness of clomipramine for tail chasing in terriers (Moon-Fanelli and Dodman, 1998).
- Clinical trials on cases of acral lick dermatitis have shown an ameliorating effect of clomipramine, fluoxetine and **sertraline** (Rapoport *et al.*, 1992).
- **Paroxetine** has also been used clinically, but its effect has not been evaluated scientifically.

Recommended drugs, dose rates, side effects and contraindications are listed in Figure 20.4. See Chapter 21 for further pharmacological information.

***Discontinuation of SRI drugs:*** The drug therapy is usually continued for at least a month after satisfactory clinical resolution of the problem has been achieved, and the animal is then weaned off gradually by giving a 75% dose for 2 weeks, a 50% dose for 2 weeks and a 25% dose for 2 weeks before the drug is discontinued completely. If the behaviour reappears during the weaning process, the dose is increased again and maintained at the effective level for some time (2–4 weeks perhaps) before resuming weaning.

It is extremely important to wean off reuptake blockers gradually. During treatment with these blockers, neurotransmitter accumulates in the synapse. Among other effects, this results in a down-regulation of receptors. Once the drug is discontinued, the amount of neurotransmitter in the synapse is suddenly much lower, but the receptors remain down-regulated for some time. This may result in a rebound effect, i.e. the compulsive behaviour may reappear worse than ever (Hewson C.J., personal communication, 1997).

### Tricyclic antidepressants and anxiolytics
Tricyclics other than clomipramine, or merely anxiolytic drugs, are highly unlikely to have sufficient effect on CD, because they have a much weaker effect on serotonin reuptake and because compulsive behaviour, once well established, can be performed even when the animal is not in a high state of anxiety.

### Buspirone
Buspirone is another drug acting on the serotonin system, but it is an agonist at 5-HT1A autoreceptors and so decreases the synthesis and release of serotonin. It also increases dopamine and noradrenaline (norepinephrine) turnover (Baldessarini, 1996) and is not considered effective for treatment of OCD or as an adjuvant in humans (Grady *et al.*, 1993; Baldessarini, 1996). Buspirone was likewise ineffective in the treatment of an apparently compulsively circling dog and may even have exacerbated the problem (Overall, 1995).

### Beta-endorphin antagonists
Beta-endorphin antagonists such as naloxone, nalmefene and naltrexone have been suggested for use in treatment. They have high first-pass metabolism and a short half-life, and most are only available as injectables. Only naltrexone is available as an oral formulation, because in humans its first metabolite, 6-beta naltrexol, is an active beta-endorphin antagonist. However, this metabolite is not formed in dogs (Garrett and el-Koussi, 1985) and clinical suppression of compulsive behaviour is short lasting (Dodman *et al.*, 1988). In spite of a report supporting its effectiveness at 2.2 mg/kg orally q12–24h (White, 1990), its value for the treatment of CD is questionable.

### Dopamine antagonists
Dopamine antagonists such as haloperidol appear to be a logical choice to treat stereotypic behaviour. However, effective doses of haloperidol for companion animals are not well established and its use is complicated by potentially serious side effects.

| Drug | Dose rate | Side effects | Contraindications |
|---|---|---|---|
| Clomipramine (Clomicalm, Novartis) | Dogs: 2–3 mg/kg q12h (may increase up to 6 mg/kg q12h) Cats: 0.5–1 mg/kg q24h | Sedation; urine retention; change in appetite; diarrhoea; vomiting. Also lowering of seizure threshold and arrhythmias | Liver disease; history of seizures; cardiovascular problems; hyperthyroidism or use of thyroid medication; glaucoma; diabetes mellitus |
| Fluoxetine (Reconcile, Lilly) | 1 mg/kg q12–24h | Sedation; increased anxiety; animal seems 'withdrawn'; loss of appetite; urine retention. Possible lowering of seizure threshold. With all serotonin active drugs there is rare possibility of development of serotonin syndrome. Giving drug with food should reduce likelihood of gastrointestinal upset. Tricyclic antidepressants can alter thyroid hormone levels | Simultaneous use of MAO inhibitors. Diabetes mellitus patients may be difficult to regulate because of fluctuation of blood glucose levels |
| Paroxetine | 1 mk/kg q12–24h | | |
| Sertraline | Dogs: 1–3 mg/kg q24h | | |

**20.4** Pharmacological treatment of compulsive disorder.

Landsberg *et al.* (1997) suggest 1–4 mg per dog orally q12h. This author has used it in only a few cases in dogs at 1–2 mg per dog, and invariably with adverse effects (the behaviour got worse and one dog became aggressive).

### L-Tryptophan

It may be possible to influence serotonin metabolism with the nutritive amino acid, L-tryptophan, a serotonin precursor (Fuller, 1994). Since L-tryptophan competes with other large neutral amino acids for uptake into the brain, careful dietary formulation is essential to maximize the effectiveness of supplementation (Clark and Mills, 1997).

## Specific behaviour therapy

In most cases the suggested environmental changes and drug therapy will not eliminate the problem completely. In these circumstances, a programme of response substitution can be implemented. Where the behaviour occurs with great frequency, it may be impractical to implement this behaviour modification procedure until environmental modification and drug treatment have reduced the frequency of occurrence of the behaviour.

Response substitution has to be implemented with great consistency in order to be effective. It is very important that the animal is not given a chance to perform the compulsive behaviour unless the owner is present and can respond appropriately.

### Dogs

The patient is initially trained with positive reinforcement to perform a desirable behaviour that is incompatible with the compulsive behaviour. A dog licking its carpus might be trained to lie with its head on the floor between its paws. Whenever the dog cannot be supervised, it is put into a situation where it cannot perform the compulsive behaviour. As often as the dog can be closely supervised (perhaps by the use of an 'umbilical cord' technique), it is put in the situation in which it is likely to perform the behaviour. Every time it shows any inclination to perform the compulsive behaviour it is distracted – if necessary by pulling on a lead connected to a head halter. The command for the alternative behaviour is then given. The dog either performs or is gently made to perform the alternative behaviour and is then rewarded. The reward can be progressively delayed, so that the dog has to stay in the chosen position for increasingly longer times before the reward is given.

The distraction is very important. If the dog is not distracted before a command (i.e. attention) is given, the treatment attempt could result in aggravation of the problem through inadvertent reinforcement of the behaviour.

### Cats

A similar programme is recommended for cats. The cat is continuously supervised or placed in a position in which it will not perform the behaviour. Every time the cat is about to perform the compulsive behaviour, it is distracted (startled), and then its attention is reorientated by throwing a toy. If a cat is trained to commands, the same method as for dogs can be used.

## Prognosis

At the behaviour clinic of the Ontario Veterinary College, the above treatment strategy resulted in approximately two-thirds of owners being satisfied with the outcome. The remaining one-third included owners with poor compliance, as well as owners who elected not to attempt treatment. A caseload analysis revealed that outcome was negatively affected by problem duration (Luescher, 1997). It is therefore important to treat CD as early as possible. Owners who used food treats contingent on the dog's behaviour had better treatment success than owners giving treats not dependent on the dog's behaviour (Luescher, 2004). It is likely, though not validated by research, that a return to a CD may be possible if the situations that trigger the behaviour return, such as unpredictable interactions, conflict situations, decreased exercise and lack of enrichment.

## Follow-up

It is suggested that cases be followed up by phone 1 week after the initial consultation and a scheduled revisit 4–6 weeks later. A five-point Likert scale to rate the severity of CD has been validated (Hewson *et al.*, 1998a) and applied clinically. It simply requires the clinician to ask the following question:

*I would like to get an overall idea of how bad is the licking behaviour that you see at present. By "bad" I mean how often he/she licks and how long he/she licks for. Taking everything together during the past 5 days, would you say that the licking you have seen has been:*

- *Extremely bad*
- *Very bad*
- *Quite bad*
- *Somewhat bad*
- *Not at all bad.*

The ratings obtained with this scale have been shown to correlate with the number of contexts in which the behaviour is shown and with the frequency and duration of the episodes. All three of these parameters will be reduced gradually during the course of successful treatment.

If there is no improvement at follow-up 4–6 weeks after the initial consultation, a history of the behaviour in the interim is taken and the differential diagnosis is reconsidered. If the diagnosis is considered to be correct, possible modulating factors and reinforcing stimuli are assessed. The management and behaviour modification techniques are reviewed and owner compliance is addressed. If it is concluded that the diagnosis was correct, factors that might maintain the behaviour have been eliminated as far as possible, and the owner has put all required measures into place, the dose of the drug is increased.

If there is still no improvement in another 4 weeks, the drug therapy may be changed again (dose increase, combination therapy or change of drug).

Response substitution will need to be emphasized and practical ways of improving its effectiveness need to be found.

## References and further reading

Baldessarini RJ (1996) Drugs and the treatment of psychiatric disorders, depression and mania. In: *Goodman & Gilman's The Pharmacological Basis of Therapeutics, 9th edn*, ed. JG Harman *et al.*, pp. 431–459. McGraw Hill, New York

Blackshaw J, Sutton RH, Boyhan MA (1994) Tail chasing or circling behaviour in dogs. *Canine Practice* **19**, 7–11

Cabib S (1993) Neurobiological basis of stereotypies. In: *Stereotypic Animal Behaviour: Fundamentals and Applications to Welfare*, ed. AB Lawrence and J Rushen, pp. 119–145. CAB International, Wallingford

Cabib S (2006) The neurobiology of stereotypy II: the role of stress. In: *Stereotypic Animal Behaviour: Fundamentals and Applications to Welfare, 2nd edn*, ed. G Mason and J Rushen, pp. 227–255. CAB International, Wallingford

Clark J and Mills DS (1997) Design consideration for the evaluation of tryptophan supplementation in the modification of equine behaviour. In: *Proceedings of the First International Meeting Veterinary Behavioural Medicine*, ed. DS Mills *et al.*, p. 220. Universities Federation for Animal Welfare, Potters Bar

Dodman NH, Knowles KE, Shuster L *et al.* (1996) Behavioral changes associated with suspected complex partial seizures in Bull Terriers. *Journal of the American Veterinary Medical Association* **208**, 688–691

Dodman NH, Shuster L, White SD *et al.* (1988) Use of narcotic antagonists to modify stereotypic self-licking, self-chewing and scratching behavior in dogs. *Journal of the American Veterinary Medical Association* **193**, 815–819

Fuller RW (1994) Mini-review: Uptake inhibitors increase extracellular serotonin concentration measured by brain microdialysis. *Life Sciences* **55**, 163–167

Garner JP (2006) Preservation and stereotypy – systems-level insights from clinical psychology. In: *Stereotypic Animal Behaviour: Fundamentals and Applications to Welfare, 2nd edn*, ed. G Mason and J Rushen, pp. 121–152. CAB International, Wallingford

Garrett ER and el-Koussi AEA (1985) Pharmacokinetics of morphine and its surrogates. V. Naltrexone and naltrexone conjugate pharmacokinetics in the dog as a function of dose. *Journal of Pharmaceutical Science* **74**, 50–56

Goldberger E and Rapoport JL (1990) Canine acral lick dermatitis: response to the antiobsessional drug clomipramine. *Journal of the American Animal Hospital Association* **27**, 179–182

Grady TA, Pigott TA, L'Heureux F *et al.* (1993) Double-blind study of adjuvant buspirone for fluoxetine treated patients with obsessive-compulsive disorder. *The American Journal of Psychiatry* **150**, 819–821

Hartigan PJ (2000) Compulsive tail chasing in the dog: a mini-review. *Irish Veterinary Journal* **53**, 261–264

Hewson CJ and Luescher UA (1996) Compulsive disorder in dogs. In: *Readings in Companion Animal Behavior*, ed. VL Voith and PL Borchelt, pp. 153–158. Veterinary Learning Systems, Trenton, New Jersey

Hewson CJ, Luescher UA and Ball RO (1998a) Measuring change in the behavioural severity of canine compulsive disorder: the construct validity of categories of change derived from two rating scales. *Applied Animal Behaviour Science* **60**, 55–68

Hewson CJ, Parent JM, Conlon PD *et al.* (1998b) Efficacy of clomipramine in the treatment of canine compulsive disorder: a randomized, placebo-controlled, double blind clinical trial. *Journal of the American Veterinary Medical Association* **213**, 1760–1766

Hinde RA (1970) *Animal Behaviour, 2nd edn*, pp. 396–421. McGraw Hill, New York

Irimajiri M, Luescher AU, Douglas G *et al.* (2009) Fluoxetine HCl treatment for compulsive disorder in dogs: a placebo-controlled clinical trial. *Journal of the American Veterinary Medical Association* [accepted for publication]

Kennes D, Odberg FO, Bouquet Y and DeRycke PH (1988) Changes in naloxone and haloperidol effects during the development of captivity induced jumping stereotypy in bank voles. *Journal of Pharmacology* **153**, 19–24

Landsberg G, Hunthausen W and Ackerman L (1997) *Handbook of Behaviour Problems of the Dog and Cat*. Butterworth-Heinemann, Oxford

Lawrence AB and Rushen J (eds) (1993) *Stereotypic Animal Behaviour: Fundamentals and Applications to Welfare*, CAB International, Wallingford

Luescher AU (1997) Factors affecting the outcome of behavioral treatment. *Meeting of the American Animal Hospital Association*, San Diego, California

Luescher AU (2004) Factors predicting the outcome of canine behavior cases. *ACVB scientific session, 141st American Veterinary Medical Association Annual Convention*, Philadelphia, Pennsylvania, July 24–28

Luescher UA, McKeown DB and Halip J (1991) Stereotypic and obsessive-compulsive disorders in dogs and cats. *Veterinary Clinics of North America: Small Animal Practice* **21**, 401–413

Mason G and Rushen J (eds) (2006) *Stereotypic Animal Behaviour: Fundamentals and Applications to Welfare, 2nd edn*. CAB International, Wallingford

Mills D and Luescher A (2006) Veterinary and pharmacological approaches to abnormal repetitive behaviour. In: *Stereotypic Animal Behaviour: Fundamentals and Applications to Welfare, 2nd edn*, ed. G Mason and J Rushen, pp. 286–324. CAB International, Wallingford

Moon-Fanelli AA and Dodman NH (1998) Description and development of compulsive tail chasing in terriers and response to clomipramine treatment. *Journal of the American Veterinary Medical Association* **212**, 1252–1257

Moon-Fanelli AA, Dodman NH and Cottam N (2007) Blanket and flank sucking in Doberman Pinschers. *Journal of the American Veterinary Medical Association* **231**, 907–912

Oliver JE and Lorenz MD (1993) *Handbook of Veterinary Neurology, 2nd edn*, pp. 9–10. WB Saunders, Philadelphia

Overall KL (1994) Use of clomipramine to treat ritualistic stereotypic motor behavior in three dogs. *Journal of the American Veterinary Medical Association* **205**, 1733–1741

Overall KL (1995) Animal behavior case of the month. *Journal of the American Veterinary Medical Association* **206**, 629–632

Overall KL and Dunham AE (2002) Clinical features and outcome in dogs and cats with obsessive-compulsive disorder: 126 cases (1989–2000). *Journal of the American Veterinary Medical Association* **221**, 1445–1452

Rapoport JL, Ryland DH and Kriete M (1992) Drug treatment of canine acral lick: an animal model of obsessive compulsive disorder. *Archives of General Psychiatry* **49**, 517–521

Reisner I (1991) The pathophysiological basis of behavior problems. *Veterinary Clinics of North America: Small Animal Practice* **21**, 207–224

Rusbridge C, Heath S, Gunn-Moore DA and Johnson N (2008) Causes, treatment, monitoring: feline orofacial pain syndrome. *Veterinary Times* **38**, 12–13

Vanderbroek I, Odberg FO and Caemaert J (1995) Microdialysis study of the caudate nucleus of stereotyping and non-stereotyping bank voles. *Proceedings of the International Society for Applied Ethology*, p. 245

Virga V (2004) Behavioral dermatology. *Clinical Techniques in Small Animal Practice* **19**, 240–249

Weiger WA (1997) Serotonergic modulation of behavior: a phylogenetic overview. *Biological Reviews of the Cambridge Philosophical Society* **72**, 61–95

White SD (1990) Naltrexone for treatment of acral lick dermatitis in dogs. *Journal of the American Veterinary Medical Association* **196**, 1073–1076

Wiepkema PR (1985) Abnormal behaviours in farm animals: ethological implications. *Netherlands Journal of Zoology* **35**, 279–299

Wynchank D and Berk M (1998) Behavioural changes in dogs with acral lick dermatitis during a 2 month extension phase of fluoxetine treatment. *Human Psychopharmacology – Clinical and Experimental* **13**, 435–437

---

## Client handouts (bsavalibrary.com/behaviour_leaflets)

- Canine behaviour profile
- Canine behaviour questionnaire
- Cognitive dysfunction syndrome
- Down–stay mat exercises
- Headcollar training
- How to find a good trainer
- 'Leave it' exercises

- Muzzle training
- 'Nothing in Life is Free'
- Playing with your dog – toys
- Request for information on problem behaviours
- Sit–stay exercises
- What your dog needs

# 21

# Pharmacology and pheromone therapy

## Sharon L. Crowell-Davies and Gary M. Landsberg

## Introduction

Psychoactive substances can alter an animal's motivation to engage in particular behaviours. Via this process, they can be a valuable adjunct to more traditional environmental management and behaviour modification programmes, but such interventions should never be used as the sole treatment modality. At best, it may entirely resolve the pet's behaviour while it is receiving treatment; however, unless necessary changes in the environment, owner education and retraining of the pet are achieved, the problem behaviours are likely to resume sooner or later after treatment is discontinued.

That said, research has shown that, at least for some behaviour problems, improvement in the pet's behaviour occurs more quickly, and is greater, if behaviour modification and environmental management are supplemented by appropriate medications or pheromones (e.g. King *et al.*, 2000; Gaultier *et al.*, 2005; Simpson *et al.*, 2007).

Before prescribing any psychoactive substance for a behaviour problem, it is necessary to determine the diagnosis, using the medical and behavioural history and any test results. Very few psychoactive substances are currently approved for the treatment of behaviour disorders in animals. Use of generic drugs, including generics developed for humans, is allowed in both the European Community and the United States under specific conditions.

New drugs for the treatment of psychiatric disorders in people regularly appear on the market but are typically prohibitively expensive for the average pet owner. In addition, there is usually a lack of data on animals, except for early research on the drug that involved laboratory animals. Generally, it is best for the general practitioner to use, firstly, drugs that are approved for use for a given problem in a given species and, secondly, generics that have been used for animals by specialists and experts in the treatment of behaviour problems, with resultant publication of information on the generic drug's efficacy and potential side effects in a given species. In the UK the choice of drug should follow the principles within the prescribing cascade. The older psychiatric drugs available as generics for human patients will be less expensive than newly released drugs and there will have been time for specialists in behaviour to pursue understanding of their efficacy in veterinary populations.

## Practical aspects of administering psychoactive drugs and special considerations

### Patient evaluation

All patients should receive a careful health check as part of the evaluation of problem behaviour (see Chapter 1) but this may need to be more extensive if psychopharmacology is being considered. For example, it is important to establish liver function when intending to use a drug that is to be administered over a relatively extended period of time and which is metabolized by the liver. Thus, it is recommended that a general blood profile is routinely evaluated before medication is prescribed, with further tests as necessary or indicated by the specific drug. Since many medications are not authorized for use in animals or perhaps for the indication for which they are being used, the implication of use of the drug in this context should be explained to the client and documented, such as through the use of a special release form (Figure 21.1).

### Oral administration

Psychoactive drugs used for the treatment of behaviour problems are typically given orally. With regards to administration, there are two major groups: those that must be given consistently, once or twice a day for extended periods of time; and those that are only given on an 'as needed' basis. In many cases the animal's behaviour problem (e.g. fear or aggression) may make administration of medication problematic, especially with the tricyclic antidepressants, which have a very bitter flavour.

Chewable meat-flavoured tablets have been developed for some approved drugs, which can facilitate the process. However, not all animals like these tablets and so extra efforts to get the medication into the pet must still be undertaken. It may be necessary to establish a routine of giving the pet treats before any attempt is made to add medication. This can be done with both cats and dogs by identifying a highly palatable food that is given as a small amount at approximately the same time every day. Once this ritual is established, attempts can be made to insert the medication into the treat. When a dog anticipates a highly palatable treat it will often gulp it without pausing to taste. In some cases the efficacy of this routine is improved by using several different treats and varying which one contains the medication,

## Consent for Special Therapy

I have been informed by _____
that (drug name) _____ is being recommended for the condition _____
_____ presented by my pet (pet's name) _____ . I understand
that this application of the medication represents a special investigational use of the drug (i.e. is outside its
licensed indication), but is in accordance with published guidelines. In addition to the potential benefits of this
special therapy, the risks of using medication in this way have been explained to me.

I hereby give my consent as owner or primary guardian of this animal for the above drug to be used on my
animal.

Signature of Client: _____
Date: _____

Signature of Clinician: _____

**21.1**   An example of a special therapy consent form.

thus hopefully preventing a consistent alteration in taste from discouraging the animal from taking the medicated food.

Cats can be somewhat more difficult, as they seldom gulp food the way dogs do. Nevertheless, if a routine is established in which the cat anticipates a small helping of a favourite food (e.g. tuna, sardines, tuna juice), voluntary consumption can sometimes be attained by slowly adding increasing amounts of the drug to the treat. The medication, which may need to be compounded because of the small doses required, can be suspended in a solution of a liquid flavour that the cat likes and that is compatible with the usual treat. Suddenly adding an entire dose may put the cat off, but the cat may readily accept a gradual change in flavour.

For both cats and dogs, it can also be beneficial to give a highly palatable medication-free treat immediately after they have voluntarily taken their medicine.

### Transdermal medication
Administering medications via transdermal routes is often easier than administering an oral medication, especially in cats, but transdermal systems have not been shown to be effective for these drugs. Blood levels achieved when a dose equivalent to the oral dose is administered via the transdermal route are substantially lower than blood levels achieved when the medication is administered via the oral route. Raising the concentration of medication in transdermal patches or gels to levels that lead to comparable blood levels is likely to result in dermatitis (Ciribassi *et al.*, 2003; Mealey *et al.*, 2004).

### Competition animals
Additional restrictions may apply to the use of psychoactive medications in animals that are used for competition in shows, racing, agility or other activities. Regulations regarding the use of specific drugs for animals used in specific competitions vary by breed,

species, country and type of competition. Although it is ultimately the responsibility of the owner to ensure that they comply with regulations before entering their animal in a given competition, the veterinary surgeon should be familiar with such regulations as they apply to competitions common in their country of practice.

Sometimes it is in the best interests of the animal to place it on medication for a period of time while the behaviour disorder is treated, even though this makes use of the animal in competition impossible during that time. The considerate owner should remove the animal from competition to allow optimal treatment of the disorder. In these cases, the veterinary surgeon should be aware of how long the animal will need to have been free from the medication before the drug has been entirely eliminated and the animal can be returned to competition.

### Pregnant and lactating females
When a pet has a major behaviour problem, use of psychoactive medications for a long period of time is often necessary. Since these medications typically pass through the placenta to the fetus and can also enter the milk of the bitch or queen, initiating or continuing their use in pregnant or lactating females should be avoided if at all possible.

### Serotonin syndrome (SS)
Serotonin syndrome is the term used for the potentially fatal toxicity that can result if multiple medications that facilitate the action of serotonin (5-hydroxytryptamine, or 5-HT) are combined, in excess. Foods containing large amounts of L-tryptophan (the precursor to serotonin) and drugs that increase presynaptic release of serotonin, inhibit the metabolism or the reuptake of serotonin back into the presynaptic neuron, or facilitate the action of serotonin at the postsynaptic neuron can all lead to SS. As many medications used to treat behavioural disorders affect serotonin in one of these ways, care should be taken in combining these drugs. Also, if the patient is placed

on any of the psychoactive medications that facilitate serotonin activity, other medications that the pet is on should be reviewed for their potential to induce toxic levels of serotonin activity. These include, but are not limited to, amitraz (for ectoparasite control) and tramadol (analgesic). Note should also be made of any herbal supplements used by the owner that may impact on serotonin (e.g. St John's wort). A useful reference on psychoactive herbs has been produced by Schwartz (2005).

## Commonly used classes of medication: actions and side effects

What follows is a summary of the types of medication, their actions, indications and side effects for the most commonly used classes of medication in the treatment of behavioural disorders in cats and dogs. The reader is referred to Crowell-Davis and Murray (2006) for more extensive information on this subject.

### Selective serotonin reuptake inhibitors (SSRIs)

#### Action
SSRIs inhibit the reuptake of serotonin, causing an increase in serotonergic neurotransmission by allowing serotonin molecules to act for extended periods of time. With prolonged use, there is also down-regulation of the postsynaptic serotonin receptors.

#### Indications
While the main use of SSRIs in humans is as antidepressants, it is for their other effects, i.e. anxiolytic, anti-compulsive and anti-aggressive effects, that they are primarily used in animals .

#### Clinical guidelines
Onset of effect is usually slow. While some improvement may be observed within the first 2 weeks, 6–8 weeks of daily medication may be required before the maximum efficacy of a given dose of a given medication is observed. SSRIs should always be given regularly, and never on an 'as needed' basis.

#### Contraindications, side effects and adverse events
Side effects include aggression, agitation, anorexia, anxiety, constipation, decreased appetite, diarrhoea, hyponatraemia, insomnia, irritability, sedation, seizures and tremor. Decreased libido, considered a side effect in humans, may be a beneficial effect in some pets, including neutered pets that exhibit excessive or inappropriate sexual behaviour.

SSRIs should never be given with monoamine oxidase inhibitors (MAOIs) such as selegiline. Overdose, and combination with tricyclic antidepressants (TCAs) and/or azapirones can lead to SS. Therefore, combination with TCAs, azapirones and other medications that facilitate serotonin activity, such as tramadol, must be done very cautiously.

#### Specific medications
Of the SSRIs listed in Figures 21.3 and 21.4, fluoxetine is the most commonly used in veterinary practice and has now been developed as a veterinary preparation. In combination with behaviour modification, fluoxetine has been shown to be effective in the treatment of separation anxiety in dogs (Simpson et al., 2007). It is effective in the treatment of urine spraying in cats (Pryor et al., 2001) and also in the treatment of acral lick dermatitis (ALD) in dogs, for which it is more effective than fenfluramine (Rapoport et al., 1992; Stein et al., 1992; Karel, 1994; Wynchank and Berk, 1998).

### Serotonin and noradrenaline reuptake inhibitors (SNRIs)

#### Action
SNRIs inhibit the reuptake of serotonin and noradrenaline (norepinephrine), causing an increase in activity of both of these molecules by allowing them to act for extended periods of time. With prolonged use, there is also down-regulation of the postsynaptic serotonin and noradrenaline receptors. In veterinary medicine, the most commonly used SNRIs are the TCAs. In addition to affecting the activity of serotonin and noradrenaline, the TCAs have antihistaminic and anticholinergic effects and are $\alpha$-1 adrenergic antagonists. There is wide variation in these five actions among the TCAs (Figure 21.2), resulting in substantial variation in their clinical effect.

| Drug | Receptors affected | | | | | |
|------|-----|------|------|------|------|-----------|
|      | NA | 5-HT | $\alpha$-1 | $\alpha$-2 | $H_1$ | Muscarinic |
| Amitriptyline | ± | ++ | +++ | ± | ++++ | ++++ |
| Clomipramine | + | +++ | ++ | 0 | + | ++ |
| Desipramine | +++ | 0 | + | 0 | 0 | + |
| Doxepin | ++ | + | ++ | 0 | +++ | ++ |
| Imipramine | + | + | ++ | 0 | + | ++ |
| Nortriptyline | ++ | ± | + | 0 | + | ++ |

**21.2** Biochemical activity of some tricyclic antidepressants used to treat dogs and cats (data from Crowell-Davis and Murray, 2006). All medications require several weeks of daily administration to reach full efficacy. Doses are given in Figures 21.3 and 21.4. $\alpha$-1, alpha-1 adrenergic; $\alpha$-2, alpha-2 adrenergic; $H_1$, histamine 1; 5-HT, serotonin; NA, noradrenaline (norepinephrine).

### Indications

TCAs are used for the same types of behaviour problems that SSRIs are used for (see above), specifically for their anxiolytic, anti-compulsive and anti-aggressive effects.

### Clinical guidelines

Like the SSRIs, TCAs must be given daily, or in some cases twice daily, for a period of several weeks before full efficacy is achieved.

### Contraindications, side effects and adverse events

Because of the substantial variation in biochemical activity of the various TCAs and the different ways in which various species metabolize them (see Figure 21.2), side effect profiles vary widely. In general, the more common side effects include appetite changes, ataxia, cardiac arrhythmias, changes in blood pressure, constipation, decreased tear production, diarrhoea, mydriasis, sedation, tachycardia and urinary retention.

TCAs should never be given with an MAOI and should be used cautiously and at low doses with other medications facilitating serotonin activity, including SSRIs and azapirones.

### Specific medications

The specific TCAs that are most commonly used in veterinary practice are listed in Figure 21.2. Of these, clomipramine is the most serotonin-specific and is available as a veterinary preparation. Combined with behaviour modification, clomipramine has been shown to be effective in the treatment of separation anxiety in dogs (King *et al.*, 2000). It has also been shown to be effective in the treatment of storm phobia when used in combination with behaviour modification and a benzodiazepine (alprazolam) (Crowell-Davis *et al.*, 2003). In cats it has been shown to help control urine spraying (King *et al.*, 2004) and may be useful in a wider range of anxiety-related behaviour problems in this species.

## Azapirones

### Action

Azapirones are serotonin 1-A agonists.

### Indications

Azapirones may be of benefit in anxiety disorders and phobias.

### Contraindications, side effects and adverse events

Sedation and increased anxiety have been reported in cats (Hart *et al.*, 1993). Cats also exhibit increased affiliative social behaviour, a side effect that is typically considered beneficial.

Azapirones should not be given with MAOIs and should be used cautiously and at low doses with SSRIs and TCAs.

### Clinical guidelines

Azapirones do not produce dependence or physical addiction, even after several months of treatment (Robinson, 1985). While desirable behaviour changes may be observed within the first week, several weeks of daily administration may be required for the maximum efficacy to be attained. Azapirones often need to be given multiple times daily for optimal effect, making them difficult for some pet owners to use.

### Specific medications

Buspirone is given to dogs at 0.5–2.0 mg/kg q8–24h and to cats at 0.5–1.0 mg/kg q12h.

## Benzodiazepines

### Action

Benzodiazepines facilitate the action of the inhibitory transmitter gamma-amino-butyric acid (GABA) in the central nervous system (CNS), thereby causing decreased neurotransmission throughout the CNS. Behavioural effects relate to their action within the hypothalamus and limbic system.

### Indications

Benzodiazepines are anxiolytic medications with a rapid onset of action. They are useful in a variety of anxiety disorders and phobias, especially when the delayed onset of action of the SNRIs or SSRIs is a problem.

### Clinical guidelines

Clinical efficacy ranges from about 3 hours for the shorter-acting benzodiazepines such as alprazolam to about 10 hours for the longer-acting benzodiazepines such as clorazepate. However, individual response is highly variable, as is the optimum dose for a given patient.

One of the great benefits of benzodiazepines is that they can be used in combination with a wide variety of other medications, including psychoactive medications, without adverse consequences.

*Test dosing:* When starting a patient on a benzodiazepine, it is useful for the owner to give a test dose when the fear-inducing situation or stimulus is not present, so they can observe the pet for side effects and adverse reactions. If the pet does not exhibit any side effects, it can then be tested under the circumstances in which fear occurs, e.g. when it is left alone or during a thunderstorm. In the former case, it is highly desirable to have a video camera positioned to tape the pet's response to the situation. Ideally, the benzodiazepine should be given 30–60 minutes prior to exposure to the fear-inducing stimulus, as this will allow time for it to be absorbed and become active in the CNS. If the pet has not been medicated when prolonged exposure to the fear-inducing situation is about to begin, the drug can still be given but will probably not be as effective.

*Potential addiction:* While benzodiazepines can be very beneficial for short-term or occasional use, daily dosing at higher doses for several weeks or months is likely to produce physical addiction. Occasionally this is necessary because use of a benzodiazepine is identified as being the only treatment modality that the patient responds to with improvement of clinical signs. In these cases, when the problem is finally resolved, discontinuation of medication must be done gradually, as a general rule by decreasing the dose by no more than 25–33% each week, taking at least a month before the patient is off all medication. In practice, an even slower withdrawal is often necessary.

***Tolerance and rebound:*** Two other phenomena that can occur with the use of a benzodiazepine are tolerance and rebound. Patients that develop tolerance require a steadily increasing dose of medication in order to maintain clinical efficacy. If repeated increases of dose are required over a period of weeks in order to maintain efficacy, the eventual development of addiction is likely. Rebound can occur when patients that have been on a benzodiazepine for several weeks, but have not become addicted, are suddenly taken off medication. In this case, the original behaviour problem returns abruptly and at a greater intensity and/or frequency than originally exhibited. Thus, even if physical addiction is not suspected, gradual withdrawal is necessary if a pet has been on a benzodiazepine several times a week for a period of weeks.

***Effect on aggression:*** The use of benzodiazepines in aggressive animals is controversial. Some of the early research indicated that benzodiazepines could cause a substantial decrease in aggressiveness, but subsequent research showed that aggression increased in some cases. This is because, while fear aggression may decrease as fear is decreased due to the anxiolytic effect of benzodiazepines, there is also the potential for a loss of inhibition, leading to increased aggression. Generally, benzodiazepines should not be the first drug of choice when treating aggressive animals, even fear aggressors. However, they may be of benefit to fear aggressors that do not respond adequately to other treatments (Crowell-Davis and Murray, 2006).

***Effect on learning:*** The effect of benzodiazepines on learning is variable, leading to their use in treatment of some behaviour problems likewise being controversial. Comprehensive review of the literature reveals that, while certain benzodiazepines at certain doses interfere with specific types of learning in specific species, other benzodiazepines, doses, types of learning and species may function quite normally. Thus, their use should not be entirely ruled out when treating a fearful animal in which various learning processes are being carried out as part of the behaviour modification programme (Crowell-Davis and Murray, 2006).

### Contraindications, side effects and adverse events

Side effects include anxiety, ataxia, hallucinations, increased appetite, increased friendliness, insomnia, muscle relaxation, muscle spasticity, paradoxical excitation and sedation. A number of cases of idiopathic hepatic necrosis have been reported in cats as a consequence of administering diazepam (Levy, 1994; Levy *et al.*, 1994; Center *et al.*, 1996; Hughes *et al.*, 1996).

### Specific medications

Alprazolam, a short-acting benzodiazepine, has been shown to be effective as part of a comprehensive treatment programme for storm phobia in the dog (Crowell-Davis *et al.*, 2003).

Diazepam has the advantage of being widely used in veterinary medicine for various purposes, including in relation to anaesthesia. Therefore, most practices have some form of the drug available and most practitioners are familiar with its use. It is available as tablets, suspensions, injectable solutions and rectal gels. The half-life of diazepam is 2.5–3.2 hours in the dog and 5.5 hours in the cat (Löscher and Frey, 1981). Its principal metabolite is nordiazepam, which has a half-life of 21.3 hours in the cat and 3.6–10 hours in the dog (Vree *et al.*, 1979; Löscher and Frey, 1981; Plumb, 2008). Oxazepam is another active metabolite predominant in the dog, with a half-life of 3.5–5.7 hours. The exact metabolism of diazepam, including which metabolites it is converted to in what proportions, varies substantially between species, resulting in sizeable variation in clinical effect and side effects.

## Monoamine oxidase inhibitors (MAOIs)

### Action

Monoamine oxidase (MAO) is found in the outer mitochondrial membrane of many types of tissue, including the heart, liver, kidneys, spleen, platelets, and the peripheral and central nervous systems. MAO-B is the primary catabolizer of the oxidative de-amination of multiple catecholamines, including β-phenylethylamine, dopamine, adrenaline (epinephrine), noradrenaline and serotonin in the CNS. MAO-A is the primary catabolizer of exogenous amines introduced via food or drugs in the intestinal tract and liver, including tyramine. MAO enzymes also de-aminate long-chain diamines.

MAOIs interfere with the action of MAO-A and MAO-B. They have multiple additional actions that are not covered in the name of the medication but are nevertheless often important to understanding their action in the body. Selegiline, the MAOI that is most used in animals, also inhibits the uptake of catecholamines, induces the release of catecholamines from their intraneuronal stores, inhibits activity of presynpatic catecholamine receptors, and stimulates action potential–transmitter release coupling. Thus, MAOIs are drugs that have complex actions on the body, a characteristic with potentially serious consequences when attempting to combine an MAOI with any of a broad spectrum of other medications.

An additional complication of using MAOIs in veterinary practice is the fact that different species have different ratios of MAO-A and MAO-B, both in specific organ systems and throughout the body. An MAOI that works a given way in one species may have a dramatically different effect and different sets of side effects in other species.

### Indications

MAO-B inhibitors have been shown to increase lifespan when given regularly to healthy mice and rats. Selegiline, which is primarily an irreversible inhibitor of MAO-B activity when administered at clinical doses, is authorized for use in dogs in many countries, although the licensed indications vary with geographical region. It is used in the treatment of canine cognitive dysfunction in geriatric dogs, and in Europe it is authorized for the treatment of emotional disorders. It has some anxiolytic effects but is generally not considered a first choice drug as other medications have anxiolytic effects that are as good or better, without severely limiting what other medications can be administered.

### Contraindications, side effects and adverse events
CNS toxicity, sometimes leading to death, can result from combining selegiline or any MAOI with a variety of other medications, including commonly used ones such as amitraz, amitriptyline, clomipramine, fluoxetine, paroxetine and tramadol. Side effects reported in dogs include restlessness, agitation, vomiting, disorientation, diarrhoea and diminished hearing.

### Specific medications
Selegiline (also known as L-deprenyl) is given to both dogs and cats (Landsberg, 2006) with cognitive decline associated with ageing at a dose of 0.5–1.0 mg/kg orally daily, in the morning. Medication should be given for at least a month before assessing whether or not it is beneficial to the patient.

## Antipsychotics

### Action
Antipsychotics block the action of dopamine. In addition they have a variety of other effects, including antihistaminic activity, antagonism of dopamine receptors, α-adrenergic blockade and muscarinic cholinergic blockade. One of the main uses of antipsychotics in animals is derived from its effect of ataraxia, i.e. decreased emotional arousal and indifference to various stimuli. Antipsychotics also cause decreased motor activity.

### Indications
Antipsychotics are often used, inappropriately, as a primary treatment modality for disorders of anxiety and fear. True anxiolytics alleviate fear while leaving the animal otherwise functioning at relatively normal levels, both emotionally and physically. Antipsychotics simply decrease motor activity and decrease all emotional responsiveness. Thus, they are not suitable as a stand-alone treatment for such disorders as storm phobia or separation anxiety.

Antipsychotics can be useful supplements to anxiolytics for cases in which the animal's behavioural response is so intense that there is a real risk it will harm itself. This includes animals that are prone to truly hysterical behaviour, jumping through glass or screens, or running without stopping even if that means running off a balcony or cliff. In such cases, modest use of antipsychotics early during treatment can ensure that the patient survives uninjured while real progress is made in the treatment of the primary disorder.

### Clinical guidelines
Most antipsychotic agents have an immediate effect and do not require regular dosing. Thus, they can be used 'as needed' for their behavioural quietening effect.

### Contraindications, side effects and adverse events
There is a wide variety of side effects, including extreme ataraxia, decreased social behaviour, difficulty initiating movement, motor restlessness, muscle spasm, stiffness due to increased muscle tone and tremors.

### Specific medications
The antipsychotic most commonly used for its sedative effect in small animals is acepromazine maleate (ACP), given orally to dogs at a dose of 0.5–2.0 mg/kg as needed and cats at a dose of 1.0–2.0 mg/kg as needed. Lower doses should be used when acepromazine is being given as a supplement to other psychoactive medications, such as a combination of fluoxetine and diazepam.

Haloperidol (at a dose of 20 mg/m²) is a butyrophenone antipsychotic, that is reported in the French literature (Pageat, 1998) together with a number of related neuroleptics, for the management of certain forms of aggression and repetitive behaviour problems in the dog. However, the reports relating to its clinical use in the English literature have been invariably unfavourable (Dodman, 1998; Luescher, 1998).

### Doses
Drug formularies for dogs and cats are provided in Figures 21.3 and 21.4, respectively.

| Drug | Dose for dogs | Use/Comments | References |
|---|---|---|---|
| **Benzodiazepines (BZs)** | | | |
| | | Drugs in this class may be combined with TCAs | |
| Alprazolam | 0.01–0.1 mg/kg q8–12h | Fearfulness, phobias, separation anxiety, noise sensitivities. Occasionally for aggression; beware of disinhibition | Landsberg *et al.* (1997); Overall (1997); Horwitz and Neilson (2007) |
| Chlordiazepoxide | 2.0–6.5 mg/kg orally q8h | Laboratory data available; no clinical uses documented | Crowell-Davis and Murray (2006) |
| Clonazepam | 0.1–0.5 mg/kg q8–12h | Noise sensitivities, anxiety | Crowell-Davis and Murray (2006) |

**21.3** Formulary of behavioural agents for dogs. All doses oral unless stated otherwise. (continues) ▶

| Drug | Dose for dogs | Use/Comments | References |
|------|---------------|--------------|------------|
| **Benzodiazepines (BZs) (continued)** | | | |
| Clorazepate | 0.55–2.2 mg/kg q4–24h | Fears and phobias, such as thunderstorm phobia | Forrester *et al.* (1990); Shull-Selcer and Stagg (1991) |
| Diazepam | 0.55–2.2 mg/kg q6–24h | Individual variation in dose and effect; start with low dose and increase to effect over days. If used in aggression, disinhibition is possible | Plumb (2008) |
| Flurazepam | 0.1–0.5 mg/kg q12h | Noise sensitivities, anxiety | Crowell-Davis and Murray (2006) |
| Lorazepam | 0.02–0.1 mg/kg q12–24h | Generalized anxiety | |
| | 0.02–0.5 mg/kg q8–12h | Noise sensitivities and some aggression | Crowell-Davis and Murray (2006) |
| Oxazepam | 0.04–0.5 mg/kg qh | Noise sensitivities, anxiety | Landsberg *et al.* (2003) |
| **Azapirones** | | | |
| Buspirone | 0.5–2.0 mg/kg q8–12h | Fearfulness, phobias | Hart *et al.* (1993); Papich (2007) |
| **Tricyclic antidepressants (TCAs)** | | | |
| | | May be combined with benzodiazepines or melatonin | |
| Amitriptyline | 1–3 mg/kg q12h or 2–6 mg/kg q24h | Reactivity, aggression, generalized anxiety, compulsive self-trauma, noise sensitivity | Reich *et al.* (2000); Papich (2007) |
| Clomipramine | 1–2 mg/kg q12h or 2–4 mg/kg q24h | Separation anxiety, noise sensitivity | Moon-Fanelli and Dodman (1998); King *et al.* (2000); Simpson (2000); Crowell-Davis *et al.* (2003) |
| | 1–3 mg/kg q12h | Canine compulsive disorders; higher dosages may be needed over time for better control | Hewson *et al.* (1998) |
| Desipramine | 1.5–3.5 mg/kg orally q24h | Very limited use, not much data available | Rapoport *et al.* (1992) |
| Doxepin | 3–5 mg/kg q12h | Self-trauma, acral lick dermatitis, compulsive behaviour | Landsberg *et al.* (2003) |
| Imipramine | 1–2 mg/kg q12h or 2–4 mg/kg q24h | Generalized anxiety, separation anxiety with urine elimination component, narcolepsy | Marder (1991); Landsberg *et al.* (1997); Overall (1997); Coleman (1999) |
| Nortryptiline | 1–2 mg/kg q12h | Especially useful for the treatment of cataplexy | Landsberg *et al.* (2003) |
| **Selective serotonin reuptake inhibitors (SSRIs)** | | | |
| | | May be combined with buspirone | |
| Citalopram | 0.5–1.0 mg/kg q24h | Aggression, compulsive disorders, urine marking | Landsberg *et al.* (2003) |
| Fluoxetine | 0.5–2 mg/kg q24h | Impulsive uninhibited aggression, separation anxiety, compulsive disorders, anxiety | Dodman *et al.* (1996); Melman (1995); Simpson *et al.* (2007) |
| | 1 mg/kg q12–24h | Compulsive disorders: divided doses may be needed | |
| Fluvoxamine | 1–2 mg/kg q24h | Compulsive disorders, aggression, anxiety | Landsberg *et al.* (2003) |
| Paroxetine | 0.5–2 mg/kg q24h | Generalized anxiety, aggression (some cases), compulsive disorders (some cases) | Reisner (2003) |
| Sertraline | 1–3 mg/kg q24h | Compulsive behaviours, including acral lick | Rapoport *et al.* (1992); Larson and Summers (2001) |
| **Atypical antidepressants** | | | |
| Trazadone | See Chapter 15 | | Gruen and Sherman (2008) |
| **Monoamine oxidase inhibitors (MAOIs)** | | | |
| Selegiline | 0.5 mg/kg q24h (UK) 0.5–1.0 mg/kg q24h (USA) | Give in the morning. Authorized for use in Europe for emotional disorders. Only licensed in USA for the treatment of cognitive dysfunction and Cushing's disease | Coleman (1999); Calves (2000); Landsberg *et al.* (2003) |
| **Anticonvulsants** | | | |
| Carbamazepine | 4–8 mg/kg q12h | Compulsive tail chasing, spinning | Holland (1988); Overall (1997) |
| Phenobarbital | 2–3 mg/kg q12h | May be combined with propranolol | Walker *et al.* (1997) |

**21.3** (continued) Formulary of behavioural agents for dogs. All doses oral unless stated otherwise. (continues) ▶

| Drug | Dose for dogs | Use/Comments | References |
|---|---|---|---|
| **Beta antagonists** | | | |
| Propranolol | 2–3 mg q12h | Combined with phenobarbital | Walker *et al.* (1997) |
| **Narcotic antagonists** | | | |
| Naloxone | 11–22 mg/kg i.v., i.m. or s.c. as required | Compulsive disorders | Brown *et al.* (1987); Dodman *et al.* (1988); Kenny (1994); Overall (1997) |
| Naltrexone | 1 mg/kg s.c. or 2.2 mg/kg orally q12–24h | Compulsive self-licking, self-chewing | Dodman *et al.* (1988); Overall (1997) |
| **Alpha-1 adrenergic blocking agents** | | | |
| Nicergoline | 0.25–0.5 mg/kg q24h | Negative age-related behavioural changes | Ogawa *et al.* (1993); Penaliggon (1997) |
| **Progestogen hormones** | | | |
| Delmadinone | 1.5–2.0 mg/kg (<10 kg); 1.0–1.5 mg/kg (10–20 kg); 1.0 mg/kg (>20 kg) s.c. or i.m. | By injection only | NOAH (2001–2002) |
| Megestrol acetate | 1 mg/kg q24h; if not improved, double dose after 14 days and possibly double again after another 7 days | Aggression, mounting, territorial marking, roaming, excitability and destructiveness. Undesirable side effects are more likely at higher doses; the lowest dose needed for effect is advised | NOAH (2001–2002) |
| **Dopamine agonists** | | | |
| Cabergoline | 5 mg/kg q24h for 5 days | Pseudopregnancy and its behavioural sequelae | Harvey *et al.* (1997) |
| **Xanthine derivatives** | | | |
| Propentofylline | 5 mg/kg q12h | Dullness, lethargy and dampened demeanour in older dogs | Sieffge and Katsuyoshi (1985) |
| **Supplements** | | | |
| alpha-Casozepine | 15 mg/kg q24h | Mild anxiety | |
| ʟ-Tryptophan | 10 mg/kg q12h | Supplementation may have an effect on certain types of aggressive behaviour | DeNapoli *et al.* (2000) |
| SAMe | 10–20 mg/kg q24h | Mood disorders, liver disease | |
| **Hormones** | | | |
| Melatonin | 0.1 mg/kg q24h | May be combined with tricyclics | Aronson (1999) |

**21.3** (continued) Formulary of behavioural agents for dogs. All doses oral unless stated otherwise.

| Drug | Dose for cats | Use/Comments | References |
|---|---|---|---|
| **Benzodiazepines (BZs)** | | | |
| Alprazolam | 0.125–0.25 mg/cat q8–12h | Urine spraying, fearfulness. Rapid onset of action | Marder (1991); Seibert (2003) |
| Clonazepam | 0.05–0.2 mg/kg q12–24h | Limited details available for usage recommendations | Virga (2002); Papich (2007) |
| Clorazepate | 0.02–0.4 mg/kg q12–24h | Urine spraying, generalized anxiety, fears and phobias | Overall (1997) |
| Diazepam | 0.2–0.4 mg/kg q12–24h | Urine spraying, generalized anxiety. Risk of hepatic necrosis (see text) | Cooper and Hart (1992); Overall (1997) |
| Flurazepam | | No reports of clinical studies of use in pets | |
| Lorazepam | 0.05 mg/kg q12–24h | Limited details available for usage recommendations | Papich (2007) |
| Oxazepam | 0.2–1.0 mg/kg q12–24h | | Landsberg *et al.* (1997) |
| **Azapirones** | | | |
| Buspirone | 0.5–1.0 mg/kg q12h | Urine spraying, anxiety states, intercat aggression, psychogenic alopecia | Houpt (1991); Hart *et al.* (1993); Overall (1994); Sawyer *et al.* (1999) |

**21.4** Formulary of behavioural agents for cats. All doses oral unless stated otherwise. (continues) ▶

| Drug | Dose for cats | Use/Comments | References |
|------|---------------|--------------|------------|
| **Tricyclic antidepressants (TCAs)** | | | |
| Amitriptyline | 0.5–1.0 mg/kg q12–24h | Urine spraying, generalized anxiety, aggression, nocturnal awakening, psychogenic alopecia | Houpt (1991); Overall (1997); Sawyer *et al.* (1999) |
| Clomipramine | 0.25–0.5 mg/kg q24h (The author [SCD] has used a total daily dose of 6 mg/kg in healthy young animals that have responded, but not sufficiently, to the highest label dose) | Urine spraying, anxiety states, psychogenic alopecia. Higher dosages may be needed for compulsive disorders; practitioners should use caution and increase the dose slowly over time | Dehasse (1997); Overall (1997); Sawyer *et al.* (1999) |
| Doxepin Imipramine Nortryptiline | 0.5–1.0 mg/kg q12–24h | Very limited information on usage in cats for behaviour problems | Papich (2007) |
| **Selective serotonin reuptake inhibitors (SSRIs)** | | | |
| Fluoxetine | 0.5–1.0 mg/kg q24h | Urine spraying, psychogenic alopecia, aggression | Hartmann (1995); Overall (1997, 1999); Pryor *et al.* (2001) |
| Fluvoxamine | 0.25–0.5 mg/kg q24h | The adverse effect profile of fluvoxamine in cats has not been well established | Landsberg (2004) |
| Paroxetine | 0.25–0.5 mg/kg q24h | Urine spraying, aggression. Monitor for constipation, urinary retention | Pryor (2003) |
| Sertraline | 0.5–1 mg/kg q24h | Situational sensitivities. Limited information available on dosage and use | Virga (2002); Seibert (2003) |
| **Monoamine oxidase inhibitors (MAOIs)** | | | |
| Selegiline | 1.0 mg/kg q24h (UK) 0.5–1.0 mg/kg q24h (USA) | Give in the morning | Coleman (1999); Calves (2000); Ramsey (2008) |
| **Anticonvulsants** | | | |
| Carbamazepine | 25 mg/cat q12h | Aggression | Schwartz (1994) |
| **Hormones** | | | |
| Medroxyprogesterone acetate | 10–20 mg/kg s.c. or i.m. | Injection only. Urine marking | Hart (1980) |
| Megestrol acetate | 5 mg/cat q24h for 1–10 days; then 5 mg q48h for 2 weeks; then 5 mg twice a week | Urine marking. Side effects include weight gain, mammary hyperplasia/neoplasia, blood dyscrasias. Undesirable side effects are more likely at higher doses. The lowest dose needed for effect is advised | Hart (1980) |
| **Beta antagonists** | | | |
| Propranolol | 0.2–1 mg/kg q8h or as required | Bradycardia is a possible side effect | Neilson *et al.* (1997) |
| **Serotonin antagonist antihistamines** | | | |
| Cyproheptadine | 0.5 mg/kg q24h | Urine spraying | Kroll and Houpt (2001) |
| **Supplements** | | | |
| alpha-Casozepine | 15 mg/kg | Mild anxiety | Beata *et al.* (2007) |
| SAMe | 100 mg/cat q24h | Mood disorders, liver support | Papich (2007) |

**21.4** (continued) Formulary of behavioural agents for cats. All doses oral unless stated otherwise.

## Pheromone therapy

Pheromones are a natural form of therapy based on the chemical signals used by animals in communication, and for which there are evidence-based data to document their efficacy in a variety of anxiety-based disorders in dogs and cats. Pheromones have the advantage that they do not require oral administration. For both dogs and cats they are formulated to be sprayed on to specific sites or diffused into the air in the pet's environment. Pheromones are generally species-specific and, since they are not taken internally (but largely trigger external receptors), they have no known contraindications. Adverse reactions appear rare and to relate to the presentation of mixed messages to the animal that may lead to confusion.

In cats, a number of pheromones are released during facial marking:

- The **F3 fraction** of the feline facial pheromone is deposited by the cat throughout its environment by facial rubbing to mark out boundaries and passageways. It is suggested that this pheromone provides emotional stability, perhaps by helping to distinguish known objects from unknown. The absence of the pheromone likely creates an increase in anxiety
- The **F4 fraction** of the feline facial pheromone is used for allomarking, which may be observed in cats that live together or between a cat and a dog or cat and human that are well socialized. By applying the F4 fraction to an unfamiliar animal or person, the probability of non-aggressive contact is increased (Pageat and Gaultier, 2003).

The **dog appeasing pheromone** is found in the sebaceous glands of the mammary chains of the lactating bitch. It is suggested that its function is to calm and reassure (or appease) the puppies (Pageat and Gaultier, 2003). Effects of the dog appeasing pheromone may be more subtle than those of the feline facial pheromones and so concurrent behaviour modification will generally be required to achieve a successful outcome and reduce relapse (Mills, 2005).

## Action

Pheromones are chemical substances used for communication between individuals within a species. They are perceived by the vomeronasal organ (VNO), which is part of the accessory olfactory tract. Pheromones bind to pheromone-binding proteins (PBP) that are specific for that pheromone. This allows activation of specific receptors that stimulate structures within the limbic system that alter the emotional state of the pet, or activate physiological effects such as the release of hormones. Since receptors are generally only found in the species that produces the pheromone, they are species-specific in their actions. In many species of animals, including cats, the *flehmen* (gape) response enhances the perception of sexual pheromones by opening the incisive ducts and aspirating the pheromones into the VNO. In dogs, tonguing (i.e. flicking of the tongue against the incisive papilla) probably aids in the perception of pheromones (Pageat and Gaultier, 2003).

Several classes of pheromone have been described:

- **Releasers** induce immediate modification to the physiology of the receiver, such as the release of a hormone. Sexual pheromones are releasers. With releasers, the results appear more or less immediately and additional behaviour therapy may not be necessary once the response has become established in the given context
- **Primers** induce modification of an emotional state. Primers such as feline facial pheromone and dog appeasing pheromone are used as an adjunct to other forms of behaviour therapy and environmental modification.

## General indications

Pheromones are useful for reducing a wide range of fear- and anxiety-induced behaviours in cats and dogs, and their trade names have become synonymous with their formulation.

- **Feliway**® (CEVA Sante Animale, Libourne, France) is a synthetic version of the F3 fraction of the feline facial pheromone, which may be effective in the control of stress, anxiety, urine marking and vertical scratching, as well as when introducing cats to situations that might evoke fear or anxiety such as a new home, veterinary hospital or car ride. It might be particularly useful in improving appetite, social interactions and play, when these have been inhibited by fear or anxiety. It may also be a useful adjunct for any disease process in which stress and anxiety might be a contributing factor, such as interstitial cystitis.
- **Felifriend**® (CEVA Sante Animale, Libourne, France), the F4 fraction of the feline facial pheromone, is currently available in parts of Europe. The indications for Felifriend® are to assist in developing a comfortable relationship between a resident cat and a newcomer, and toward unfamiliar people.
- **DAP**® (CEVA Sante Animale, Libourne, France), a synthetic version of the dog appeasing pheromone, may be useful in conjunction with behaviour therapy for separation anxiety, fear of fireworks and storms, and to facilitate introduction into novel or potentially fear-evoking environments such as new homes, shelters, veterinary clinics or car rides.

## Choice of delivery system

*Feline facial pheromone:* Feliway® (the F3 fraction) is available as a spray that can be used on specific spots where the cat might be marking (i.e. urine or scratching) or on blankets or into carriers or crates to reduce anxiety associated with crating, car travel or unfamiliar environments (e.g. veterinary clinics). For urine marking and scratching, each marked site as well as prominent objects that the cat might mark should be sprayed daily for at least 30 days. For multi-cat households the spray should be used twice daily for 45 days.

A plug-in diffuser is also available, which delivers the pheromone throughout the environment. The diffuser can be used for urine marking in multi-cat households and to help to reduce fear and anxiety associated with other pets, changes in the household or moving to a new home.

Felifriend® (the F4 fraction) is available as a spray that, when applied to the hands prior to handling a cat, may increase familiarization and decrease aggression to a new person. Although not specifically labelled for this use, it may also help to reduce fear and aggression toward other pets when applied to a cloth and then rubbed on the cat's head or flanks.

Anxiety reduction may be further complemented by the use of Feliway® in the environment. The success of both F3 and F4 pheromone treatment can be assessed by an increase in facial marking throughout the environment, including previously marked areas (in the case of F3), and in the marking of people or animals that are unfamiliar or with whom a cat has previously shown avoidance or aggression.

***Dog appeasing pheromone:*** DAP® is also available in a variety of delivery forms, including a spray that can be used to help the dog to adapt to specific sites or locations (e.g. cages, bedding, cars). The diffuser may be more practical for reducing anxiety, such as when first adopting the pet or when there are changes to the household or schedule. DAP® is available as a collar that is activated by the dog's body temperature and releases pheromone for about 28 days. This is especially useful for managing problems that occur outdoors, but the collar must not be allowed to get wet or else it will become less effective and/or its duration seriously curtailed.

***Efficacy of sprays and diffusers:*** When using the spray on a blanket or crate, it should be applied about 10–15 minutes in advance and repeated if needed up to every 1–2 hours. Diffusers deliver pheromones to 50–70 $m^2$ (about 650 square feet) for about 4 weeks. At least one diffuser should be used per floor or separate airspace, and efficacy may be compromised where air-conditioning is fitted.

While peak pheromone levels should be reached in the environment in about 24 hours, it may take up to 30 days or longer to assess the full effect of the pheromone and behaviour therapy combination.

### Contraindications, side effects and adverse events

Since the pheromone is a natural compound that targets only the specific species external chemical receptors for which it has been produced, there is no toxicity risk, nor contraindications and no effects on other species. They are safe for sick or aged pets and can be used safely in combination or with any drugs, including psychotropic agents. The collar loses efficacy when wet and the sprays should be tested on a small area before using on fabrics, walls or furniture, in case of a mark being left.

### Specific indications

***Feline facial fraction F3:*** The spray form of Feliway® has been shown to reduce urine marking in 74.7–96.7% of cases and resolve the problem in 33–96.7% of cases (Pageat and Tessier, 1997a; White and Mills, 1997; Frank *et al.*, 1999 ; Ogata and Takeuchi, 2001). In a 10-month follow-up study, 77% of cats remained under control, with 62% of owners ceasing the spray and 38% still using it intermittently (Mills and White, 2000). The pheromone diffuser was also found to be significantly more effective than the placebo at reducing urine marking (Mills and Mills, 2001).

Pheromone spray has also been shown to reduce anxiety-induced scratching (marking) (Pageat and Gaultier, 2003). Compared with the placebo, the feline pheromone spray significantly reduced marking when sprayed into vacation homes in advance of the cats'

arrival. With pheromones, the cats ate sooner and were less likely to wander away from the home (Pageat and Tessier, 1997a).

Spraying feline pheromone on a blanket or towel 30 minutes before placing cats into a veterinary hospital cage resulted in a significant increase in grooming and interest in food compared with the placebo (Griffith *et al.*, 2000). Over a 24-hour period, cats with the pheromone sprayed into their own cage had significantly greater food intake than cats in cages treated with the carrier substance of the pheromone spray alone (Griffith *et al.*, 2000).

In a study of the effects of feline pheromone spray on car-ride anxiety, somatic signs (vomiting, urination and defecation) as well as the owner's subjective score of the signs of anxiety (vocalization, agitation, salivation) were significantly improved in the pheromone group compared with the placebo (Gaultier *et al.*, 1998; Pageat and Gaultier, 2003).

In a small double-blinded crossover study of nine cats with idiopathic cystitis, there were no statistical differences between the groups but there was a trend towards fewer days with clinical signs and reduced episodes of cystitis when using the Feliway® diffuser (Gunn-Moore and Cameron, 2004). This and other medical indications in which stress is implicated deserve further investigation.

***Feline facial fraction F4:*** Felifriend® when applied to the hands has been shown to reduce fear and anxiety when introducing cats to new people, including veterinary examinations or during introduction to a shelter environment (Fillon, 1999; Kakuma and Bradshaw, 2001; Bonnafous *et al.*, 2005). Felifriend® may also be used as an aid in the prevention of intraspecific aggression when introducing new cats. Using a cloth, Felifriend® can be applied daily to the head and flanks of both the new cat and the existing cat, until allomarking is seen (Pageat and Tessier, 1997b).

***Dog appeasing pheromone:*** DAP® may be useful for reducing anxiety or in facilitating adaptation to new surroundings. In one study on separation anxiety (Gaultier *et al.*, 2005), the pheromone diffuser plus behaviour therapy resulted in no significant difference in improvement compared with that seen with clomipramine plus behaviour therapy, though the sample size was too small to suggest that the two substances are of equivalent efficacy. Improvement was seen in dogs that were fearful of fireworks, using a combination of sound-recording desensitization and a pheromone diffuser (Mills *et al.*, 2003; Levine *et al.*, 2007). The combination of a pheromone diffuser and sound desensitization has also been shown to decrease signs of storm phobia (Crowell-Davis and Imirijami, 2008).

Pheromones may be particularly useful in helping pets to adapt to new and potentially stressful environments. For example, the use of a pheromone diffuser was effective at relaxing dogs in a veterinary clinic, reducing barking in a shelter environment and reducing barking and stress-related signs when introducing puppies and shelter dogs into their new homes (Osella *et al.*, 2005; Tod *et al.*, 2005; Mills *et al.*, 2006; Taylor and Mills, 2007). In another double-blind study, the diffuser was found to reduce barking and arousal and increase appeasing behaviours in puppy classes (Graham *et al.*, 2007).

The pheromone spray may also help dogs to adapt to specific areas such as crates or bedding. In one study where DAP® was sprayed into the car about 10 minutes prior to travel, there was greater improvement in the DAP® group for physical signs such as car sickness, urination, salivation, vomiting and defecation in comparison with the placebo (Gaultier and Pageat, 2003).

Similarly the use of a DAP® collar led to improvement in car travel problems, with the greatest improvement in dogs with nausea, tenseness, excitable restlessness and running around (Estellès and Mills, 2006). The pheromone collar has also been shown to be effective in helping puppies adapt to new homes after adoption from a petshop by reducing initial signs of distress, and in reducing fear of owners and of unfamiliar people during the first 2 weeks following adoption (Gaultier *et al.*, 2008; Gaultier *et al.*, 2009).

Another application that may be particularly beneficial is the use of pheromone collars during puppy classes. Not only was there a significant improvement in fear and anxiety and more play between puppies wearing pheromone collars in class, compared with the placebo group, but also a 1-year follow-up found that the DAP® group puppies were more social and adapted faster to new situations and environments at all time points (Denenberg and Landsberg, 2008).

## References and further reading

Aronson L (1999) Animal behavior case of the month: extreme fear in a dog. *Journal of the American Veterinary Medical Association* **215**, 22–24

Beata C, Beaumont-Graff E, Coll V, Cordel J, Marion M, Massal N, Marlois N and Tauzin J (2007) Effect of alpha-casozepine (Zylkene) on anxiety in cats. *Journal of Veterinary Behaviour: Clinical Applications and Research* **2 (2)**, 40–46

Bonnafous L, Lafont C, Gaultier E *et al.* (2005) Interest in the use of a new galenic form of the feline allomarking pheromone (F4) analog Felifriend during medical examination. In: *Current Issues and Research in Veterinary Behavioral Medicine*, ed. D Mills *et al.*, pp. 119–122. Purdue University Press, West Lafayette, Indiana

Brown SA, Crowell-Davis S, Malcolm T and Edwards P (1987) Naloxone-responsive compulsive tail chasing in a dog. *Journal of the American Veterinary Medical Association* **190**, 884–886

Calves S (2000) Pharm profile: selegiline. *Compendium on Continuing Education for the Practicing Veterinarian* **22**, 204–205, 214

Center SA, Elston TH, Rowland PH *et al.* (1996) Fulminant hepatic failure associated with oral administration of diazepam in 11 cats. *Journal of the American Veterinary Medical Association* **209**, 618–625

Ciribassi J, Luescher A, Pasloske KS *et al.* (2003) Comparative bioavailability of fluoxetine after transdermal and oral administration to healthy cats. *American Journal of Veterinary Research* **64**, 994–998

Coleman ES (1999) Canine narcolepsy and the role of the nervous system. *Compendium on Continuing Education for the Practicing Veterinarian* **21**, 641–650

Cooper L and Hart BL (1992) Comparison of diazepam with progestin for effectiveness in suppression of urine spraying behavior in cats. *Journal of the American Veterinary Medical Association* **200**, 797–801

Crowell-Davis S and Imirijami M (2008) Pheromones: recent advances and clinical cases. *North American Veterinary Conference Proceedings*, p.141

Crowell-Davis SL and Murrray T (2006) *Veterinary Psychopharmacology.* Blackwell Publishing, Ames, Iowa

Crowell-Davis SL, Seibert LM, Sung W *et al.* (2003) Use of clomipramine, alprazolam and behavior modification for treatment of storm phobia in dogs. *Journal of the American Veterinary Medical Association* **222**, 744–748

Dehasse J (1997) Feline urine spraying. *Applied Animal Behavior Science* **52**, 365–371

DeNapoli JA, Dodman NH, Shuster L, Rand WM and Gross KL (2000) Effect of dietary protein and tryptophan supplementation on dominance aggression, territorial aggression, and hyperactivity in dogs. *Journal of the American Veterinary Medical Association* **217**, 504–508

Denenberg S and Landsberg GM (2008) Effects of dog-appeasing pheromones on anxiety and fear in puppies during training and on long-term socialization. *Journal of the American Veterinary Medical Association* **233**, 1874–1882

Dodman NH (1998) Pharmacologic treatment of aggression in veterinary patients. In: *Psychopharmacology of Animal Behavior Disorders*, ed. NH Dodman and L Shuster, pp.17–30. Blackwell Science, Malden, Massachusetts

Dodman NH, Donnelly R, Shuster L *et al.* (1996) Use of fluoxetine to treat dominance aggression in dogs. *Journal of the American Veterinary Medical Association* **209**, 1585–1587

Dodman NH, Shuster L, White SD *et al.* (1988) Use of narcotic antagonists to modify stereotypic self-licking, self-chewing, and scratching behavior in dogs. *Journal of the American Veterinary Medical Association* **193**, 815–819

Estellès MG and Mills DS (2006) Signs of travel-related problems in dogs and their response to treatment with dog-appeasing pheromone. *Veterinary Record* **159**, 140–148

Fillon F (1999) Efficacy of Felifriend® in improving the cat's tolerance to clinical examinations during a veterinary consultation. *Proceedings, 24th World Small Animal Veterinary Congress.* WSAVA, Lyon

Forrester SD, Brown SA, Lees GE and Hartsfield SM (1990) Disposition of clorazepate in dogs after single- and multiple-dose oral administration. *American Journal of Veterinary Research* **51**, 2001–2005

Frank D, Erb HN and Houpt KA (1999) Urine spraying in cats: presence of concurrent disease and effects of pheromone treatment. *Applied Animal Behaviour Science* **61**, 263–272

Gaultier E, Bonnafous L, Bougrat L *et al.* (2005) Comparison of the efficacy of a synthetic dog-appeasing pheromone with clomipramine for the treatment of separation-related disorders in dogs. *Veterinary Record* **156**, 533–538

Gaultier E, Bonnafous L, Vienet-Legue D *et al.* (2008) Efficacy of dog-appeasing pheromone in reducing stress associated with social isolation in newly adopted puppies. *Veterinary Record* **163**, 73–80

Gaultier E, Bonnafous L, Vienet-Legue D *et al.* (2009) Efficacy of dog-appeasing pheromone in reducing behaviours associated with fear of unfamiliar people and new surroundings in newly adopted puppies. *Veterinary Record* **164**, 708–714

Gaultier E, Pageat P and Tessier Y (1998) Effect of a feline appeasing pheromone analogue on manifestations of stress in cats during transport. In: *Proceedings of the 32nd Congress of the International Society for Applied Ethology*, Clermont-Ferrand, p. 198

Gaultier E and Pageat P (2003) Effects of a synthetic dog appeasing pheromone (DAP) on behaviour problems during transport. In: *Proceedings, 4th International Behavior Meeting*, Caloundra, Australia, pp. 33–35

Graham D, Mills DS and Bailey G (2007) Evaluation of the effectiveness of synthetic DAP (Dog Appeasing Pheromone) in reducing levels of arousal and improving learning in puppy classes. *Proceedings, CABTSG Study Day*

Griffith CA, Steigerwald ES and Buffington CA (2000) Effects of a synthetic facial pheromone on behavior of cats. *Journal of the American Veterinary Medical Association* **217**, 1154–1156

Gruen ME and Sherman BL (2008) Use of Trazodone as an adjunctive treatment for canine anxiety disorders: 56 cases. *Journal of the American Veterinary Medical Association* **223**, 1902–1907

Gunn-Moore DA and Cameron ME (2004) A pilot study using synthetic feline facial pheromone for the management of feline idiopathic cystitis. *Journal of Feline Medicine and Surgery* **6**, 133–138

Hart BL (1980) Objectionable urine spraying and urine marking in the cat: evaluation of progestin treatment in gonadectomized males and females. *Journal of the American Veterinary Medical Association* **177**, 529–533

Hart BL, Cliff KD, Tynes VV and Bergman L (2005) Control of urine marking by use of long-term treatment with fluoxetine or clomipramine in cats. *Journal of the American Veterinary Medical Association* **226**, 378–382

Hart BL, Eckstein RA, Powell KL and Dodman NH (1993) Effectiveness of buspirone on urine spraying and inappropriate urination in cats. *Journal of the American Veterinary Medical Association* **203**, 254–258

Hartmann L (1995) Cats as possible obsessive-compulsive disorder and medication models. *American Journal of Psychiatry* **152**, 8

Harvey MJA, Cauvin A, Dale M, Lindley S and Ballabio R (1997) Effect and mechanisms of the anti-prolactin drug cabergoline on pseudopregnancy in the bitch. *Journal of Small Animal Practice* **38**, 336–339

Hewson CJ, Luescher AU, Parent JM *et al.* (1998) Efficacy of clomipramine in the treatment of canine compulsive disorder: a randomized, placebo-controlled, double blind clinical trial. *Journal of the American*

*Veterinary Medical Association* **213**, 1760–1766

Holland CT (1988) Successful long term treatment of a dog with psychomotor seizures with carbamezepine. *Australian Veterinary Journal* **65**, 389–392

Horwitz DF and Neilson JC (2007) *Blackwell's Five Minute Veterinary Consult Clinical Companion: Canine and Feline Behavior*. Blackwell Publishing, Ames, Iowa

Houpt KA (1991) House soiling: treatment of a common feline problem. *Veterinary Medicine* **86**, 1000–1006

Hughes D, Moreau RE Overall KL *et al.* (1996) Acute hepatic necrosis and liver failure associated with benzodiazepine therapy in six cats, 1986–1995. *Journal of Veterinary Emergency and Critical Care* **6**, 13–20

Kakuma Y and Bradshaw JWS (2001) Effects of a feline facial pheromone analogue on stress in shelter cats. *Proceedings, 3rd International Congress on Veterinary Behavioral Medicine*, pp. 218–220

Karel R (1994) Fluoxetine use in dogs provides animal model for human mental disorders. *Psychiatric News* **29**, 12

Kenny DE (1994) Use of naltrexone for the treatment of psychogenically induced dermatoses in five zoo animals. *Journal of the American Veterinary Medical Association* **205**, 1021–1023

King JN, Simpson BS, Overall KL *et al.* (2000) Treatment of separation anxiety in dogs with clomipramine: results from a prospective, randomized, double-blind, placebo-controlled, parallel-group multicenter clinical trial. *Applied Animal Behaviour Science* **67**, 255–275

King JN, Steffan J, Heath SE *et al.* (2004) Determination of the dosage of clomipramine for the treatment of urine spraying in cats. *Journal of the American Veterinary Medical Association* **225**, 881–887

Kroll T and Houpt KA (2001) A comparison of cyproheptadine and clomipramine for the treatment of spraying cats. *Proceedings, 3rd International Congress on Veterinary Behavioural Medicine*, pp. 184–185

Landsberg G (2004) A behaviorist's approach to compulsive disorders. Proceedings, ACVIM Forum, Minneapolis

Landsberg G, Hunthausen W and Ackerman L (1997) *Handbook of Behaviour Problems of the Dog and Cat*. Butterworth Heinemann, Oxford

Landsberg G, Hunthausen W and Ackerman L (2003) *Handbook of Behaviour Problems of the Dog and Cat, 2nd edn*. Elsevier Saunders, Philadelphia

Landsberg G and Wilson AL (2005) Effects of clomipramine on cats presented for urine marking. *Journal of the American Animal Hospital Association* **41**, 3–11

Landsberg GL (2006) Therapeutic options for cognitive decline in senior pets. *Journal of the American Animal Hospital Association* **42**, 407–413

Larson ET and Summers CH (2001) Serotonin reverses dominant social status. *Behavioural Brain Research* **121**, 95–102

Levine ED, Ramos D and Mills DS (2007) A prospective study of two self-help CD based desensitization and counter-conditioning programmes with the use of Dog Appeasing Pheromone for the treatment of firework fears in dogs (*Canis familiaris*). *Applied Animal Behaviour Science* **105**, 311–319

Levy JK (1994) Letters to the editor: The author responds (original letter entitled Adverse reaction to diazepam in cats) *Journal of the American Veterinary Medical Association* **205**, 966

Levy JK, Cullen JM, Bunch SE *et al.* (1994) Adverse reaction to diazepam in cats. *Journal of the American Veterinary Medical Association* **205**, 156–157

Löscher W and Frey H-H (1981) Pharmacokinetics of diazepam in the dog. *Archives Internationales de Pharmacodynamie et de Therapie* **254**, 180–195

Luescher UA (1998) Pharmacologic treatment of compulsive disorder. In: *Psychopharmacology of Animal Behavior Disorders*, ed. NH Dodman and L Shuster, pp. 203–221. Blackwell Science, Malden, Massachusetts

Marder AR (1991) Psychotropic drugs and behavioral therapy. *Veterinary Clinics of North America: Small Animal Practice* **21**, 329–342

Mealey KL, Peck KE, Bennett BS *et al.* (2004) Systemic absorption of amitriptyline and buspirone after oral and transdermal administration to healthy cats. *Journal of Veterinary Internal Medicine* **18**, 43–46

Melman SA (1995) Use of Prozac in animals for selected dermatological and behavioural conditions. *Veterinary Forum* **12**, 19–27

Mills D (2005) Pheromonatherapy: theory and applications. *In Practice* **27**, 248–255

Mills DS, Estellès MG, Coleshaw PH and Shorthouse C (2003) Retrospective analysis of the treatment of firework fears in dogs. *Veterinary Record* **153**, 561–562

Mills DS and Mills CB (2001) Evaluation of a novel method for delivering a synthetic analogue of feline facial pheromone to control urine spraying by cats. *Veterinary Record* **149**, 197–199

Mills DS, Ramos D, Estellès MG and Hargrave C (2006) A triple blind placebo-controlled investigation into the assessment of the effect of Dog Appeasing Pheromone (DAP) on anxiety related behaviour of problem dogs in the veterinary clinic. *Applied Animal Behaviour Science* **98**, 114–126

Mills DS and White JC (2000) Long-term follow up of the effect of a pheromone therapy on feline spraying behaviour. *Veterinary Record* **147**, 746–747

Moon-Fanelli AA and Dodman NH (1998) Description and development of compulsive tail chasing in terriers and response to clomipramine treatment. *Journal of the American Veterinary Medical Association* **212**, 1252–1257

Neilson JC, Eckstein RA and Hart BL (1997) Effects of castration on problem behaviors in male dogs with reference to age and duration of behavior. *Journal of the American Veterinary Medical Association* **211**, 180–182

NOAH (2001–2002) *Compendium of Data Sheets for Veterinary Products 2001–2002*. National Office of Animal Health, Enfield

Ogata N and Takeuchi Y (2001) Clinical trial of a feline pheromone analogue for feline urine marking. *Journal of Veterinary Medical Science* **63**, 157–161

Ogawa N, Asanuma M, Hirnta H *et al.* (1993) Cholinergic deficits in aged rat brain are corrected with nicergoline. *Archives of Gerontology and Geriatrics* **16**, 103–110

Osella MC, Bergamasco L and Costa F (2005) Use of a synthetic analogue of a dog appeasing pheromone in sheltered dogs after adoption. In: *Current Issues and Research in Veterinary Behavioral Medicine*, ed. D Mills *et al.*, pp. 270–273. Purdue University Press, Purdue, Indiana

Overall KL (1994) Animal behavior case of the month: use of buspirone to treat spraying associated with intercat aggression. *Journal of the American Veterinary Medical Association* **205**, 694–696

Overall KL (1997) *Clinical Behavioral Medicine for Small Animals*. Mosby, St Louis, Missouri

Overall KL (1999) Intercat aggression: why can't they all just get along? *Veterinary Medicine* **94**, 688–693

Pageat P (1998) *Pathologie du Comportement du Chien, 2nd edn,* p183. Editions du Point Vétérinaire, Maisons-Alfort, Paris

Pageat P (1999) Experimental evaluation of the efficacy of a synthetic analogue of cat's facial pheromones (Feliway) in inhibiting urine marking of sexual origin in adult tom-cats. *Journal of Veterinary Pharmacology and Therapeutics* **20** (suppl. 1), 169

Pageat P and Gaultier E (2003) Current research in canine and feline pheromones. *Veterinary Clinics of North America: Small Animal Practice* **33**, 187–211

Pageat P and Tessier Y (1997a) Usefulness of the F3 synthetic pheromone Feliway* in preventing behaviour problems in cats during holidays. *Proceedings, 1st International Conference on Veterinary Behavioural Medicine*, p. 231

Pageat P and Tessier Y (1997b) Usefulness of the F4 synthetic pheromone for prevention of intraspecific aggression in poorly socialized cats. *Proceedings , 1st International Conference on Veterinary Behavioural Medicine*, pp. 64–72

Papich MG (2007) *Handbook of Veterinary Drugs, 2nd edn.* Elsevier Saunders, Philadelphia

Penaliggon J (1997) The use of nicergoline in the reversal of behaviour changes due to ageing in dogs: a multi-centre clinical field trial. *Proceedings, 1st International Conference on Veterinary Behavioural Medicine*, pp. 37–41

Plumb DC (2008) *Veterinary Drug Handbook, 6th edn.* Iowa State University Press, Ames, Iowa

Pryor P (2003) Animal behaviour case of the month. *Journal of the American Veterinary Medical Association* **223**, 1117–1119

Pryor PA, Hart BL, Cliff KD *et al.* (2001) Effects of a selective serotonin reuptake inhibitor on urine spraying behaviour in cats. *Journal of the American Veterinary Medical Association* **219**, 1557–1561

Ramsey I (2008) *BSAVA Small Animal Formulary, 6th edn.* BSAVA Publications, Gloucester

Rapoport JL, Ryland DH and Kriete M (1992) Drug treatment of canine acral lick: an animal model of obsessive-compulsive disorder. *Archives of General Psychiatry* **49**, 517–521

Reich MR, Ohad DG, Overall KL and Dunham AE (2000) Electrocardiographic assessment of antianxiety medication in dogs and correlation with serum drug concentration. *Journal of the American Veterinary Medical Association* **216**, 1571–1575

Reisner IR (2003) Diagnosis of canine generalized anxiety disorder and its management with behavioural modification and fluoxetine or paroxetine: a retrospective summary of clinical experience (2001–2003). *Journal of the American Animal Hospital Association* **39**, 512

Robinson DS (1985) Buspirone: long-term therapy. *Proceedings of anxiety disorders: an international update*, Düsseldorf, Germany, pp. 93–100. Bristol-Myers, New York

Sawyer LS, Moon-Fanelli AA and Dodman NH (1999) Psychogenic alopecia in cats: 11 cases (1993–1996). *Journal of the American Veterinary Medical Association* **214**, 71–74

Schwartz S (1994) Carbamazepine in the control of aggressive behavior in cats. *Journal of the American Animal Hospital Association* **30**, 515–519

Schwartz S (2005) *Psychoactive Herbs in Veterinary Behavior Medicine*. Blackwell, Ames, Iowa

Seibert L (2003) Antidepressants in behavioral medicine. *Western*

*Veterinary Conference*

Seibert L (2006) Antipsychotics. In: *Veterinary Psychopharmacology*, ed. SL Crowell-Davis and T Murray, pp. 148–165. Blackwell, Ames, Iowa

Shull-Selcer E and Stagg W (1991) Advances in the understanding and treatment of noise phobias. *Veterinary Clinics of North America: Small Animal Practice* **21**, 353–367

Sieffge D and Katsuyoshi N (1985) Effects of propentofylline on the micromechanical properties of red blood cells. *Drug Development Research* **5**, 147–155

Simpson BS (2000) Canine separation anxiety. *Compendium on Continuing Education for the Practicing Veterinarian* **22**, 328–339

Simpson BS, Landsberg GM, Reisner IR *et al.* (2007) Effects of Reconcile (Fluoxetine) chewable tablets plus behavior management for canine separation anxiety. *Veterinary Therapeutics* **8**, 18–31

Stein DJ, Shoulberg N, Helton K *et al.* (1992). The neuroethological approach to obsessive-compulsive disorder. *Comprehensive Psychiatry* **33**, 274–281

Taylor K and Mills DS (2007) A placebo controlled study to investigate the effect of Dog Appeasing Pheromone and other environmental and management factors on the reports of disturbance and house soiling during the night in recently adopted puppies (*Canis familiaris*). *Applied Animal Behaviour Science* **105**, 358–368

Tod E, Brander D and Wran N (2005) Efficacy of a dog appeasing pheromone in reducing stress and fear related behaviour in shelter dogs. *Applied Animal Behaviour Science* **93**, 295–308

Virga V (2002) Which drug and why: an update on psychopharmacology. *Proceedings: Atlantic Coast Veterinary Conference*

Vree TB, Baars AM Hekster YA *et al.* (1979) Simultaneous determination of diazepam and its metabolites N-desmethyldiazepam, oxydiazepam and oxazepam in plasma and urine of man and dog by means of high-performance liquid chromatography. *Journal of Chromatography* **162**, 605–614

Walker R, Fisher J and Neville P (1997) The treatment of phobias in the dog. *Applied Animal Behaviour Science* **52**, 275–289

White JC and Mills D (1997) Efficacy of synthetic feline facial pheromone (F3) analogue (Feliway) for the treatment of chronic non-sexual urine spraying by the domestic cat. *Proceedings, 1st International Conference on Veterinary Behavioural Medicine*, pp. 242

Wynchank D and Berk M (1998) Fluoxetine treatment of acral lick dermatitis in dogs: a placebo-controlled randomized double blind trial. *Depression and Anxiety* **8**, 21–23

## Client handouts (bsavalibrary.com/behaviour_leaflets)

- **Complementary therapies for behaviour problems**

# 22

# Complementary therapies

## Samantha Lindley

## Introduction

Cultural differences have a significant impact when it comes to prescribing behaviour-modifying drugs such as the tricyclic antidepressants and monoamine oxidase inhibitors. Owner resistance to such medication is thought to be greater in the UK than elsewhere and clients often seek an alternative. It is important that the consulting veterinary surgeon can give honest and informed advice to a client considering such an option for their pet.

Complementary therapies are now widely employed in veterinary practice to deal with a range of diseases (Figure 22.1). Almost as widely they are regarded with suspicion, partly as a result of a lack of understanding and partly because there is sometimes little or no experimental scientific evidence to support even a mechanistic hypothesis for treatment – with the exception of acupuncture, dietary manipulation and, to an extent, touch and massage. For this reason these three will be dealt with in detail and the remaining therapies discussed more briefly later in the chapter. This is not to suggest that acupuncture is superior to, for instance, homeopathy, but simply that there is a greater scientific understanding of the former and many different opinions about the latter.

| Therapy | Purported mode of action |
|---------|--------------------------|
| Diet | Control of satiety to manipulation of neurotransmitter levels |
| Acupuncture | Via nervous system, pain gate mechanisms, opiates, serotonin, noradrenaline (norepinephrine) and other neurotransmitters, RNA expression |
| Herbalism | Natural source of biologically active chemicals |
| Touch therapy | Via nervous system – modulation of neurotransmitter release |
| Homeopathy | Principle of similars – extreme dilutions of chemicals that can provoke certain signs will have therapeutic effects depending on the characteristics of the individual |
| Bach flowers | Small (almost homeopathic) amounts of flower essence used to treat personality rather than disease |
| Reiki and Shen | Channelling of 'energy' by therapist into patient |

**22.1** Complementary therapies commonly used in veterinary practice.

One of the reasons why there is so little evidence about the efficacy of such treatments in the management of behaviour problems is that very few animals need major psychiatric intervention (Scott and Mayhew, 2001), since behaviour therapy alone is often effective (Podberscek *et al.*, 1999). There is also enormous variability in treatment between individuals with similar conditions, which means that many centres need to be involved for a suitably homogeneous population to be identified for inclusion in any controlled study. There are insufficient numbers of practices employing these techniques to generate the numbers required for confident statistical analysis. In addition, many therapies are given alongside management changes and so their independent effects are difficult to measure. Also, since there is no need to demonstrate efficacy or comparability as a regulatory requirement, there is little incentive for organizations to invest in potentially expensive trials that will provide no obvious return. Non-commercial sources of funding are also much more limited than for conventional medicines. The available evidence is therefore quite limited.

The evidence that convinces most people is that 'it worked for my pet' or 'it worked for me'. Such beliefs, although important in arousing interest and ultimately shaping further research, are at the bottom of the hierarchy of evidence (Figure 22.2).

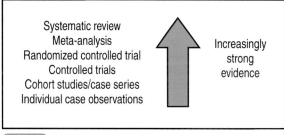

Systematic review
Meta-analysis
Randomized controlled trial
Controlled trials
Cohort studies/case series
Individual case observations

Increasingly strong evidence

**22.2** Hierarchy of evidence.

The assumption is that if A is treated with B, then B is responsible for C (where A = the problem, B = the intervention and C = the outcome or 'cure'). The intervention is assumed to be the cause of the cure, but B includes non-specific effects over and above any specific effects of the therapy. These include:

- Chance
- Natural history of the disease

- The therapeutic relationship (between owner, therapist and pet)
- The placebo effect (i.e. the real neurophysiological changes that may occur as a result of an interaction with a patient).

In any study of specific efficacy, B must represent only the specific effects of the therapy (e.g. the insertion of a needle through the skin in the case of acupuncture) and the study must therefore be designed to allow all the non-specific effects to be accounted for. This is only achieved at the level of randomized controlled trials, but even at this level there is room for controversy in terms of numbers and trial design.

## Assessment of the potential for complementary therapy

There are a number of important factors to consider when assessing a potential complementary therapy for a behavioural disorder.

Everything possible should have been done to establish the motivation underlying the behaviour; and a behaviour management programme should have been instituted and its effects assessed. If this has not been done, any subsequent success will inevitably be attributed to the medicine or therapy that is next employed, which will falsely elevate its success rate. Most behaviour problems respond successfully to behavioural management changes and a high proportion resolve spontaneously.

Any physical causes should have been ruled out as far as is reasonable to do so and all relevant blood work done. Complementary therapy is not an alternative to a conventional and thorough assessment of the patient. Missing any physical causes and components will delay recovery and compromise welfare (see Chapter 1).

If an assumption is being made that an animal's mental state is severely disrupted by neurotransmitter imbalance, the available evidence suggests that conventional psychotherapeutic agents will be effective more rapidly than will alternative therapy. The only evidence for an exception to this is in the treatment of acral lick dermatitis (see later) with acupuncture. It may be that the animal's physical state or reaction to these drugs, or the owner's refusal to countenance such treatment, means that alternatives must be sought but this does not alter the observation that a compromise is being made.

It follows that any treatment must be well tolerated by the animal, physically and emotionally. For example, traumatizing a cat by repeated car journeys to receive acupuncture is clearly not in its overall best interests unless a dramatically beneficial effect can be demonstrated.

**It is important to realize that therapies regarded as 'alternative' are not necessarily better or harmless.**

## Diet

It can be proposed that diet alters behaviour in two ways:

- Dietary manipulation supposedly alters neurotransmitter balances and affects mood
- Dietary intolerance or sensitivity may be the cause of behavioural problems.

### Dietary manipulation

At its most simple, dietary manipulation can be feeding a dog before it is left alone, to promote feelings of satiety, wellbeing and sleepiness. In other circumstances, it has been suggested that feeding practice may alter the animal's mood state; for example, the 'raw meaty bones' diet (raw meat, bones and yoghurt) is controversially claimed to improve mood because it gives increased fill and eliminates potentially problematic additives.

The theory behind specific dietary manipulation is that the feeding of certain substances at certain times in relation to other dietary components can increase levels of (particularly) serotonin, one of the neurotransmitters related to elevated mood and targeted in the treatment of affective disorders. The usual technique is to feed a carbohydrate-heavy food, such as pasta, between 30 minutes and 3 hours after the main protein meal. Research has shown that carbohydrate increases brain serotonin by stimulating insulin production (Fernstrom and Wurtman, 1972) and thereby facilitating L-tryptophan transfer across the blood–brain barrier. Tryptophan competes with large neutral amino acids for transportation across the blood–brain barrier. The tryptophan content of dietary proteins is often low and so the levels of other large neutral amino acids increase relative to plasma tryptophan after a high-protein meal. Thus, in the absence of insulin stimulation, this can lead to decreased tryptophan transport across the blood–brain barrier and reduced serotonin synthesis (Fernstrom 1977, 1986), even if a tryptophan supplement is provided. It is perhaps for this reason that a low-protein diet is recommended in some cases to elevate mood. However, what is important is not the protein level but rather the relative proportions of different amino acids and their uptake.

Although there is some evidence to show the effect of fatty and carbohydrate-rich foods, as well as specific foods on mood and cognitive function in humans (Brostoff and Gamlin, 1998), there is clearly a complex relationship between glucose, insulin and other hormones as well as consequent effects on the neurotransmitters. It is difficult to say whether such a feeding regime may normalize an imbalance or whether its effects may be entirely dependent on the background and baseline levels of the individual. Individual sensitivities to certain foodstuffs, absorption factors and metabolism will also play a role in any possible effects of the food on mood. Only a limited amount of work has been done on humans suffering from affective disorder (e.g. women with premenstrual depression (Brostoff and Gamlin, 1998)) and extrapolation between species should always be made with caution.

## Milk proteins

Interest in the tranquillizing effects of mother's milk on the young and the agents mediating these effects has been evident in the literature for many years (Laird and Drexel, 1934), but during more recent investigations it has been discovered that a tryptic hydrolysate alpha s1-casein and its decapeptide alpha casozepine displayed anti-anxiety effects in certain rat behaviours (Miclo *et al.*, 2001) and a reduction in blood pressure and cortisol levels in stressed human subjects (Messaoudi *et al.*, 2005). Further experimental studies in rats (Violle *et al.*, 2006) compared the effects of alpha s1-casein and diazepam in tests that demonstrate different aspects of anxiety-related behaviour in rats (conditioned defensive burying and the elevated plus-maze). Whilst the anxiolytic effects of both substances appeared similar in the tests, the milk protein did not produce the disinhibition state in the rats that was observed after diazepam administration. These observations and other studies have led to the production of alpha casozepine as a nutraceutical for use in cats and dogs. Trials into anti-anxiety effects in dogs and cats have shown some effects in favour of alpha casozepine, but the numbers included in the studies have been small and more work needs to be done to evaluate general efficacy (Beata *et al.*, 2007ab). The product appears to be safe, which is important when one is unsure of 'real' or 'placebo' effects, but, because it is safe, there may be a tendency to use the product prior to, or instead of, proper evaluation of the cause of the animal's anxiety, thereby delaying diagnosis. Since pain and anxiety are inextricably linked (and chronic pain causes the same physiological changes in the body as chronic stress), animals presenting as anxious may well be in pain; in addition, an inappropriate environment will not be cured by the administration of milk protein or any drug.

## Docosahexaenoic acid (DHA)

DHA is known to be an important component of the nervous system and is vital for the normal development of the brain and the retina in particular. DHA is transferred across the placenta and can be synthesized in the liver, but it has been suggested that the rate of synthesis in young mammals may not be optimal. DHA can be supplied from external sources such as fish, eggs and some meat and is now available as an addition to puppy food or included in puppy food to produce 'more trainable' puppies.

The hypothesis is that a depletion of DHA from the developing retina and brain (and the resultant abnormalities in electroretinogram and learned behaviours (Innis, 2003)) causes changes in cognitive performance, behaviour and the transmission of visual and auditory information. Studies in infant humans fed a normal milk preparation or breast milk compared with a DHA-enhanced diet showed that babies with the enhanced DHA diet had improved psychomotor tests at 4 months of age. The animal studies in rats, mice and puppies appear to focus on differences between enhanced DHA diets and deficient DHA diets, showing a significant improvement in certain cognitive and learning behaviours in favour of the DHA-enhanced

diets. What appears to be lacking from the animal evidence is a comparison with enhanced DHA and 'normal' DHA diets. One study on beagle puppies in particular looked at puppies who were in effect 'doubly' deficient in DHA, since their mothers had also been fed a DHA-deficient diet during gestation. It is not clear from these studies whether 'normal' puppy diets are considered to be DHA deficient and how puppies would perform if 'normally' fed and enhanced-DHA fed puppies were compared (Gamoah *et al.*, 1999; Birch *et al.*, 2000; Hoffman *et al.*, 2005).

## Antioxidants

Antioxidants are now widely available as supplements for pets, especially for the treatment of cognitive dysfunction in older animals. Their function is chiefly to counteract damaging free radicals, but different products contain a variety of other preparations that have been shown to be beneficial in influencing the effects of brain ageing. Their use in the aged animal is covered in Chapter 12 and so will not be covered further here.

## Effectiveness of dietary manipulations

In a clinical context, these dietary manipulations tend to be incorporated along with other behaviour management techniques, which are arguably effective alone. It is difficult to conceive that the effect of such a manipulation on a fundamental imbalance could be potent enough to correct an affective disorder. Other changes in management associated with the new dietary regime are likely to have a mild but normalizing effect on mood, because most of them are based on providing consistency, control and predictability for the animal – all important factors in reducing stress and decreasing anxiety.

Where dramatic changes have been noted, it may well be that, rather than causing a change in neurotransmitter balance per se, the dietary manipulation has removed from the animal's diet a foodstuff responsible for a dietary intolerance.

# Dietary intolerance or sensitivity

A dietary intolerance or sensitivity is defined as an 'abnormal response to an ingested substance'. It is important to note that this is a clinical condition that may be the cause of behavioural problems and not a therapy. Without a change of food, the behaviour problem will be difficult (if not impossible) to modify and thus consideration of the diet is imperative.

The term sensitivity is often favoured for this condition since it includes both allergic-type responses and intolerances that do not affect the immune system. Both 'sensitivity' and 'intolerance' are used in the literature, and the term allergy is often erroneously applied by the public or lay press.

The condition in companion animals was probably first extrapolated from anecdotal changes observed in horses fed different diets. Reducing the protein content of a dog's diet became the trend as a treatment for so-called hyperactivity problems and aggression (DeNapoli *et al.*, 2000). Since most of these animals would not have been suffering from an intolerance to their food, many were not 'cured' by this approach.

In human medicine there is still division about the effects of food on general wellbeing, as well as behaviour. However, Egger *et al.* (1989) reported an increasing interest in the effects of food on epilepsy in children and in dogs, and described clinical sign crossover in patients suffering from migraine, seizure and hyperkinetic syndrome. An unpublished case series of nine dogs from Glasgow University Veterinary School describes seven cases of apparently diet-responsive epilepsy, several of which were associated with behaviour problems that also resolved on cessation of seizures, and there are a number of studies noting an apparent link between coeliac disease (gluten sensitivity), cerebral calcifications and epilepsy (Cuvellier *et al.*, 1996).

Dietary sensitivity can cause a wide range of behaviour problems, including aggression, anxiety and compulsive disorders. Because the behaviour is often not predictable, seems out of context and does not respond to conventional management, owners are often bewildered and confused as to why their pet is behaving in this way, especially when they have apparently managed it correctly. Even if a diagnosis is reached and confirmed, in the case of severe aggression some of these animals must be euthanized because it is too dangerous to live with the possibility of them obtaining the wrong food.

**History taking**
The history might include:

- Chronic gastrointestinal signs (mild to severe), including: vomiting; diarrhoea; pica; coprophagia; excessive consumption of plants (including grass); flatulence; borborygmi; erratic eating habits; excessive frequency or volume of faeces for digestibility of diet; excessive yawning; excessive stretching ('praying' type)
- Chronic skin disease, including: aural and anal sac problems (not of seasonal occurrence, no specific diagnosis reached); poor dry, scurfy or fluffy coat
- Previous sensitivities
- Irrational unpredictable behaviour (as determined by the clinician rather than the owner)
- Sudden change of character
- Change of food recently
- Poor toilet training, or breakdown in toilet training
- Poor learning or concentration
- Hyperactivity (as determined by the clinician rather than the owner)
- Lethargy
- Refractory seizures.

These points should be covered in detail: many owners fail to appreciate the potential significance of coprophagia, pica and diarrhoea; many owners have animals that vomit frequently but are not presented to the veterinary surgeon for this problem. All the points are suggestive factors only; the more evidence that there is, the more likely it is that sensitivity is present. Note that, although the animal may have a sensitivity affecting the skin or gut, it may not be affecting its behaviour.

Absence of signs is not sufficient to discount a diagnosis of sensitivity. Questions to ask in assessing for sensitivity include the following:

- Did the animal show any dietary intolerances as a puppy or kitten?
- Have the owners noticed any change in behaviour, skin or gastrointestinal function after previous dietary changes? (Note that absence of behavioural change after previous dietary manipulation does not exclude diagnosis of sensitivity)
- Was the diet changed prior to the behaviour change? (Note that animals may develop sensitivities to a food that they have always been fed; absence of change is not an exclusion criterion for diagnosis.)

A positive answer to any of the following history questions increases the likelihood of clinical disease rather than dietary sensitivity specifically:

- Is the behaviour unpredictable?
- Does the animal show mood swings?
- Does the animal behave differently from day to day or in similar situations?
- Has there been a sudden change in established character?
- Is the behaviour bizarre, extreme or completely out of character?

As well as these specific questions, a complete history should always be taken. It is not uncommon for animals to be, say, competitive but also suffering from mood swings due to a sensitivity. The first problem may be relatively easy to resolve in normal circumstances by the application of behavioural modification, but erratic behaviours will remain if food sensitivity is part of the problem.

Behaviour problems caused by sensitivity to diet can include any presentation and can be very specific (e.g. dog-to-dog aggression) or generalized (e.g. a non-specific anxiety). One hypothesis is that the effects of sensitivity alter thresholds: either the threshold to a particular behaviour occurring is lowered, or the animal is in a heightened state of arousal and therefore much closer to that threshold. A particular set of stimuli may then trigger a full and apparently irrational behaviour that seems to be disproportionate to the evoking stimulus.

**Diagnosis**
Diagnosis is based on one or more of the following:

- Irrational, unpredictable behaviour
- History of gastrointestinal or skin disorders, which are undiagnosed and unresolved
- Behavioural management has not affected any change or has only given partial relief of clinical signs
- Behaviour so bizarre, extreme or contradictory that it does not lend itself to any obvious management change.

Causes may include a primary gastrointestinal disorder in which the gut becomes more permeable, allowing larger molecules to be absorbed. These molecules are not adequately metabolized to an inactive form and have a direct or indirect effect on brain or neurotransmitters (Brostoff and Gamlin, 1998). Since diet and certain forms of epilepsy have been linked, it is possible that some of the behaviours are manifestations of seizure-like activity (e.g. complex partial seizures). It has also been suggested that the death of bacteria in the gut as a result of bacterial overgrowth secondary to bowel irritation facilitates the release of toxins into the blood, with direct or indirect effects on the brain (Mugford, 1987). Certainly, gut discomfort alone is not enough to explain some of the more extreme behaviours seen.

Anecdotal observations of a small number of cases suggest that neutering an animal may change the way it deals with the food, such that sensitivities may manifest or worsen after neutering.

*Diagnostic tests:* All patients should have routine haematological and biochemical screening. Some screening procedures are claimed to identify culprit foods (Jeffers *et al.*, 1991; Halliwell, 1993) but these have only been used for dermatological and gastrointestinal problems. In the author's experience, the most reliable test still appears to be the exclusion diet – partly, one suspects, because the intolerance does not always involve an immune response.

Unpublished case reports (Mugford and Lindley, 1993–1997; Scott, 1997–2001) note a small but significant number of referred behaviour cases (1–2%) having confirmed congenital portosystemic shunts or other disturbances of liver vascularization resulting in encephalopathic signs. These dogs do not present as stunted, seizuring animals, with head pressing and classically postprandial behaviour changes; instead they present with a range of intermittent behavioural abnormalities, including anxiety and aggression. There are potential pitfalls with feeding these undiagnosed patients a highly digestible moderate-protein diet: (i) that such a diet may improve signs but leave the condition undiagnosed; and (ii) that the provision of a diet in which the protein content is moderate, but highly available to the animal, may result in severe exacerbation of the signs along with gastrointestinal disturbances. Worsening of signs on two different exclusion diets should therefore alert the clinician to the possibility of encephalopathy.

Ideally, each patient should be screened by a dynamic bile-acid test. These findings also add further weight to the need for routine blood testing before prescribing potentially hepatotoxic medication such as barbiturates and tricyclic antidepressants.

The only reliable way of identifying either immune-based or non-allergic sensitivity is by feeding an exclusion diet. If possible, this should be done in isolation with no other management changes. If positive changes are observed on such a diet, the animal should then be challenged with the original food.

If more than one condition is suspected (for example, a dog is consistent about protecting resources and placing limits on how the owner behaves, but also displays unpredictable, inconsistent aggression over non-valuable items), the first step would be to put in place a relevant behaviour modification plan, together with a note of caution regarding the need for further workup relating to diet. If the dog continues to behave unpredictably despite implementation of the behaviour modification measures, clinical causes should be reassessed. If signs of a dietary sensitivity are present, and if liver shunts, hypothyroidism, other hormonal problems and pain (as far as possible) have been ruled out (see Chapter 1), a dietary trial should begin.

### Treatment

The treatment of dietary sensitivity can produce dramatic and rewarding changes and should always be considered in refractory cases, preferably before embarking on psychopharmacy. However, some animals are too dangerous and any change could elicit sustained and unprovoked attacks; hence, even though a diagnosis may be reached, the prognosis may have to be guarded.

Treatment (and confirmation of diagnosis) is by feeding an exclusion diet. The type of diet that has been shown to be the most successful test for most individuals is home prepared and with two components: one protein source and one carbohydrate source, each preferably from foods that have not been eaten previously by the dog, or at least do not form part of its normal ration (e.g. fish and potato), fed at a ratio of 1 part protein to 3 parts carbohydrate. The diet is usually fed to appetite but, as a guide, 0.5–0.75 kg carbohydrate should be fed twice a day for a 20 kg dog. A proprietary diet is not a sufficient test in this first stage, though the aim is to wean the animal on to such a diet.

### Possible difficulties in treatment

*Individual sensitivity:* Each individual has its individual sensitivity. Some animals are sensitive to a large number of ingredients; some are unable to tolerate large quantities of a single ingredient (but are normal when permitted only a rationed amount); others might react quickly and explosively to a small amount of certain 'normal' foods. No one food is more of a culprit than another; rice, for example, may be implicated as much as beef. Intolerances are more likely to develop to what is frequently encountered than to specific foodstuffs of a particular type (Brostoff and Gamlin, 1998).

*Repeated intolerance:* In a few patients, intolerances appear to develop to whatever they are fed. There may be a dramatic improvement on the exclusion diet, then a deterioration; a new diet results in another improvement, but this again only lasts a short time, and so on. This may indicate an underlying primary gut problem such as inflammatory bowel disease.

Repeated intolerance can be difficult to manage but cycling the exclusion diets can be helpful. For example, the animal may tolerate 3 weeks of fish and potato, alternated with 3 weeks of chicken and rice, but not the same diet continually. This phenomenon is recognized in humans (Brostoff and Gamlin, 1998) and as a sign of irritable bowel syndrome, but may also be the result of somatovisceral effects of myofascial trigger points (Simons *et al.*, 1999), though this has yet to be investigated in the dog.

***Exacerbation:*** It is possible that the patient may become worse on the test diet. This is of particular concern in aggressive animals and owners should be warned of this in advance. Physical signs may also worsen and these may be an early warning signal. In humans this is perceived as 'getting worse before getting better'. In dogs, it is preferable to change the protein at this point and then, if there is still no change, change the carbohydrate. An exacerbation of signs is regarded as a positive result (i.e. the test is confirmed) and another protein/carbohydrate selection usually resolves both the exacerbation and the original signs.

***Increased urination:*** Uncontrollable increased urination may occur, especially with dogs used to a dry diet. In this case cooking all food in a microwave with minimal water, or substituting rice for the potato, can help.

***Insatiable hunger:*** In this case, the quantities fed should be increased and the carbohydrate changed from potato to rice (which is more calorie dense). If the test is positive, fat in the form of oil may be added (with care).

### Weaning
Ideally, the animal is gradually weaned on to the closest proprietary food. Sometimes the patient will deteriorate even on this and needs to be fed a balanced home-cooked diet for life. More care needs to be taken with the transition for an aggressive animal: one home-cooked ingredient is substituted at a time (e.g. potato for rice, fish for chicken, home-cooked for proprietary).

It should be remembered that the constitution of proprietary foods may alter. Thus changes in behaviour on apparently the same food may indicate not a new intolerance but the re-emergence of the original problem.

### Trial time
A behaviour change is usually seen within the first 2 weeks of feeding an exclusion diet, though some individuals may take longer. Any positive trends at 2 weeks would indicate the need to extend the trial time.

It is sometimes the case that future unrelated gastrointestinal disturbances temporarily appear to trigger the same behavioural disturbance although the food has not been changed. This should settle after the condition has been treated or has resolved, but unremitting behavioural alterations indicate a need to change the diet again.

### Vitamin supplements
At the initial stage of testing it is best to avoid the specific addition of vitamin supplements, since these are often wheat based or contain substances such as

fish oils. Once the cause has been established, the closest proprietary food is selected and tested. If the animal needs to be maintained on home-cooked food, vitamin supplements may be introduced with caution (as are all new foods).

### Dietary intolerance or sensitivity in cats
Applying the same criteria for judging unpredictable behaviour and some gastrointestinal signs can be problematic in cats. However, many of the same judgements *can* be applied and home-cooked exclusion diets may be fed with the same expected results.

## Acupuncture

### Mechanism of action
Acupuncture is defined as 'the insertion of a solid needle into the body with the intention of alleviating pain and disease and for the maintenance of health'. The technique is incorporated into traditional Chinese medicine, which is a system working through a variety of theories involving the flow of 'vital energy' around the body along lines or channels (meridians). Arguably, the action of piercing the skin can be seen as simply a way of stimulating the nervous system to respond in a wide variety of ways.

From extensive research (Filshie and White, 1998) it is known that acupuncture:

- Needs an intact nervous system to work
- Is blocked by naloxone and six other opiate antagonists
- Stimulates A-delta (rapid) pain fibres, which in turn inhibit C (slow) pain fibres via interneurons in the substantia gelatinosa of the spinal cord and stimulate areas of the brain via spinothalamic tracts to produce serotonin and noradrenaline (norepinephrine)
- Produces cerebrospinal fluid (CSF) and humoral changes (from cross-circulation studies)
- Up-regulates mRNA expression for proencephalin.

### Possible mechanism in behavioural problems
If a clinical condition is exacerbating or causing an animal's behavioural disturbance, acupuncture may alleviate some of the clinical signs (e.g. chronic pain, gastrointestinal disturbance) and relieve the behavioural signs, though it does not treat a behavioural problem *per se.*

However, it is known that serotonin, noradrenaline and endogenous opiates are released after acupuncture stimulation. It has also been suggested that acupuncture may result in the release of oxytocin, a hormone important in bonding and nurturing relationships (Uvnas-Moberg *et al.*, 1993). This is likely to have an effect on other mood-related neurotransmitters and hormones such as glutamate, dopamine and prolactin, since none has its effects in isolation. There is still a question as to whether or not the changes in concentration of these neurotransmitters are sufficiently high and maintained for long enough after stimulation by acupuncture to produce the kinds of changes in secondary messenger systems that are responsible for the clinical effects. Alternatively, acupuncture could operate by a different mechanism not yet elucidated.

## Human studies

### Addictions

The general trend of evidence in human studies is that acupuncture can be helpful in the treatment of withdrawal symptoms, rather than the actual addiction itself. A recent study comparing acupuncture and a placebo in treatments to give up smoking indicated that acupuncture was no better than the placebo. The placebo response, having a neurophysiological effect of its own, was substantial (White *et al.*, 2000).

### Depression

Electroacupuncture stimulation has been found to influence the brain. A study comparing amitryptiline treatment with electroacupuncture treatment for human patients with depression in a controlled multi-centre trial (Luo *et al.*, 1998) showed that electroacupuncture had a better therapeutic effect for anxiety somatization and cognitive disturbance of depressed patients and fewer side effects than amitryptiline. However, patients needed to be treated daily on an in-patient basis, which limits its practicality for veterinary use. It remains to be established whether sufficient changes in endogenous neurotransmitter levels occur after acupuncture therapy to change secondary messenger systems, up-regulate RNA and maintain the antidepressive effect.

### Anxiety

A review of a variety of acupuncture trials looking at treatment of anxiety with acupuncture was inconclusive, partly because the trials were of variable quality (Pilkington *et al.*, 2007).

## Animal evidence

Clinical observations only are available at present about the following conditions.

### Anxiety states

A small number of the author's patients have responded either negatively or equivocally to weekly electroacupuncture treatment for 6 weeks. Based on the medical evidence above, it would be preferable to try daily or at least twice-weekly treatment, alongside behaviour management changes.

### Compulsive conditions

Field data (Scott, 2000) suggest that acral lick dermatitis responds dramatically to acupuncture therapy, with once-weekly treatments usually required for only 3–4 weeks. Relapse rate is low and the compulsion to lick appears to be abolished rapidly, allowing the lesion to heal.

A randomized controlled double-blind trial is currently being conducted into the use of acupuncture to treat so-called idiopathic cases (i.e. assumed to be behavioural, all other causes, including local/referred pain, hypothyroidism, atopy and food sensitivity,

having been excluded) at Glasgow University Veterinary School. While this condition has been shown to respond well to serotonergic drugs such as clomipramine (Goldberger and Rapaport, 1991), the apparent response to acupuncture is much faster than one would expect for a similar serotonergic mechanism of action. Preliminary results are inconclusive partly because of logistical difficulties and the emerging trends give more information about the nature of acral lick dermatitis than the use of acupuncture, particularly that so-called 'idiopathic' acral lick dermatitis (this is generally considered to be behavioural in origin) is apparently not as common as originally thought. Many patients have musculoskeletal pain and underlying skin disorders; few have much evidence of environmental stress or conflict that may be expected to contribute to a compulsive disorder.

Generalized compulsive licking in cats and dogs, over-grooming in cats or compulsive licking of isolated areas are good candidates for acupuncture. Locomotor stereotypic behaviours such as spinning or tail chasing may theoretically respond but currently no data are available. In the author's experience, many cats that attack their tails or run about in a frenzied manner (so-called feline hyperaesthesia syndrome) have undiagnosed spinal pain.

## Contraindications, response, reactions and cautions

The only real contraindications to acupuncture treatment are refusal by the owner or active resentment by the animal. There are no known contraindications to its use in pregnancy, except from a medico-legal standpoint. Most animals tolerate acupuncture treatment well and become progressively more relaxed with subsequent treatments. Usually, there is a brief improvement after the first treatment, perhaps lasting several days, with the condition returning to normal intensity after this time. Subsequent treatment responses are expected to be greater and more enduring.

Since there is a possibility of a condition worsening after acupuncture treatment, the owner should be warned of the theoretical possibility of adverse behaviour changes, which would be only temporary. This is seen as a positive response to needling; treatment would continue but stimulation of needles and duration of needling would be decreased. Cathartic reactions to treatment have been reported by human patients but not in animals.

Except for the treatment of acral lick dermatitis (above), a maximum of six treatments should be anticipated before seeing a response with behaviour problems, and the prognosis remains guarded until further data are available.

## Transcutaneous spinal electroanalgesia (TSE)

TSE is the reported effect of stimulating the dorsal spinal cord via surface electrodes (MacDonald and Coates, 1995). Although mechanisms of action have been postulated (Towell *et al.*, 1997), none has been convincingly demonstrated to explain its effect. TSE was first used to treat chronic pain in humans. Observations on human mood alterations suggested that there was a positive mood elevation in subjects without pain (Towell *et al.*, 1997).

In animal patients, observations suggest that the majority become relaxed during treatment. In a small field study (Lindley, 1998), six patients suffering from affective disorder which would otherwise have been treated with anxiolytic medication were instead treated daily at home with TSE for 20 minutes. Four showed a level of response compatible with that expected from psychopharmacy.

## Touch therapy

Touch triggers a range of changes in the nervous system, from local chemical responses to the release of endogenous opioids. Massage, which involves the skin, fascia and muscles, is a more intense stimulation and may have a more potent effect in terms of relaxation. However, those animals that need it most – the frightened and anxious ones – might find such an interaction threatening and intimidating.

Stroking along the ventral surface of rats releases small amounts of oxytocin; the hormone is associated with bonding, sedation, mild anxiolysis and mild analgesia. Stroking pet dogs releases significantly more mood-elevating neurotransmitters than a control activity (Odendaal, 2002) and physiological relaxation of the heart (McGreevy *et al.*, 2005).

TTouch therapy was developed in 1978 from the Feldenkrais method, which was developed to help people to focus on their bodies (Fogle, 1999a,b). The TTouch technique involves stimulating the skin only, with tiny rhythmic circular movements. This has an indirect effect on the rest of the body, including the central nervous system, and also releases oxytocin (amongst other hormones), which is important in bonding and nurturing. Thus the act of touching and stroking a pet may increase the affiliative tendencies of the animal; alternatively, owners using this technique are spending more time touching their pet in a formally structured action, which may in itself bring about an adjustment in their relationship.

Animals should not need to be restrained for touch therapy. It is a positive action that owners can perform at home to help anxious animals but one should be wary about advocating its use for aggressive animals, particularly if status is an issue or if the motivation is uncertain.

## Homeopathy

### Proposed mechanism

Homeopathy works on the principle of 'like treating like'. A submolecular amount of a substance that has the potential at higher concentrations to cause the signs seen is used to counter the signs of disease. A true homeopathic consultation treats the patient holistically, which is essential for the management of any behavioural case, and advice on nutrition and lifestyle are often given in conjunction with sugar tablets or with tinctures deemed appropriate for the particular condition.

Some practitioners claim that, as a system, it is impossible to test homeopathy in the way other treatments are tested (e.g. randomized controlled trials). However, similar difficulties exist when trying to test other treatments for a particular kind of behaviour problem: each animal is an individual, and its individual environment plays a part. Nonetheless generic treatments are available and double-blind placebo-controlled studies are beginning to be undertaken in relation to behaviour problems.

### Evidence

Case studies report success (Day, 1992) but the potential for other treatments and owner placebo effects (potentially very important in treating any behaviour condition) should be recognized. Simply receiving a full and thorough consultation and understanding of the problem can have significant effects on the perception and progress of the problem by the owner and consequent effects on the animal. Cracknell and Mills (2007) undertook a double-blind placebo-controlled study to evaluate the response of dogs with firework fears to a homeopathic intervention; they found a significant response in both treatment and placebo groups, but no difference between the two.

### Choosing treatments

Certain treatments are said to be useful for certain behavioural signs but the nature of homeopathy relies on an assessment of the individual ('constitutional remedy') rather than on a set of signs indicating a particular disease that can be treated with a particular remedy. It is therefore inappropriate to list remedies as though they can be prescribed for specific behaviour problems; instead, the reader is referred to Day (1992) and Macleod (1989) for further information.

## Herbal remedies

Herbalism involves using parts of a plant known to have pharmaceutical properties, rather than a single active ingredient isolated from it. Traditionally, the practice is accompanied by a thorough assessment of the animal's temperament, environment, diet and other aspects of its life, and this alone may be valuable, as in the case of homeopathy. Some commercially available supplements combine herbal extracts with specific nutritional supplements (e.g. Senilife™ consists of a range of antioxidants and *Ginkgo biloba* extract, which also has antioxidant properties)

Therapeutic dosages should be used, but then the major drawback is potential toxicity. Most owners perceive herbs to be safer than drugs but many are potentially toxic or react adversely with other medication. The concentration of active ingredients varies with the specific species or subspecies of herb used, time of harvest, region of growth, part used, and methods of preparation and preservation; therefore responses may be more variable between doses or prescriptions, depending on the source.

Some preparations are prepared specifically for animals and have been used for years with no apparent reported ill effects. By not claiming medicinal properties, but rather an effect as an aid in the management of various conditions, many herbal preparations are available over the counter, rather than on prescription through the veterinary profession. For example, Skullcap and Valerian (Dorwest Herbs Ltd) is available as a licensed medicine on the 'General Sales List' in the UK for the 'symptomatic relief of anxiety, nervousness, excitability and travel sickness'.

There is a temptation for owners to extrapolate from human conditions and treat their pets with substances untested for animals. A scientifically evaluated guide to herbal and related remedies is now available (Ernst, 2006), as well as a specific guide to psychoactive herbs for veterinary use (Schwartz, 2005) to which the reader is referred for further information.

Awareness of veterinary herbalism is of particular importance because of the potential for interaction with psychoactive medication. In humans there have been cases of serotonin syndrome reported following the concomitant use of serotonin reuptake inhibitors with St John's wort (Stevinson and Ernst,1999) and so owners should routinely be asked if they are currently, have previously or intend in future to use any of these supplements.

## Aromatherapy

Given that dogs and cats respond so strongly to smell, it may be assumed that the use of specific aromas to stimulate a sense of wellbeing and relaxation or to inhibit unwanted behaviours may be useful. In fact, the potency of such a therapy may be its drawback. Because pet animals are so sensitive to smell, one dominating odour may cause disruption since it may effectively obliterate the ability to detect important signals and messages from the physical environment and from conspecifics. Some dogs and cats appear to attempt actively to mask odours on their coats by rubbing or finding another, stronger odour in which to roll.

The theory is that odours act via the hypothalamus to influence mood and therefore other body systems, since mood and organic function are intimately linked. To be effective, the smell must trigger a particular association since it is purported that the scent from the aromatherapy oil triggers the limbic system, which governs emotional responses and is involved with the formation and retrieval of learned memories. It would be difficult to anticipate which of a vast array of smells may have the desired effect on an individual.

A controlled trial looked at the use of lavender to calm travel-induced excitement in dogs and showed a reduction in movement and vocalization in the dogs exposed to lavender compared with dogs exposed only to the ambient odours (Wells, 2006). However, this study does not prove a specific effect of lavender; other strong odours may have a similar effect and the effect may be via distraction rather than a real 'aromatherapy' effect. Also the study covered only 3 days of exposure; it is not known whether or not this effect is maintained.

Pheromone therapy (the use of conspecific social odours or pheromones to treat a wide range of animal behaviour problems) has a good evidence base and has now become part of mainstream behavioural practice (see Chapter 21).

## Bach's flower remedies

Dr Bach hypothesized that disease could be treated not by tackling the pathology itself but by alleviating the negative emotional state of the patient (Bach, 1933). Thus a variety of diseases may be treated by the same remedy if the patients all have similar 'personalities'. For example, people whose negative emotional state is a tendency to show an excessive need for companionship may suffer from gallstones, headaches or gastric upsets, but for each condition the treatment would be the same: heather. Dogs suffering from hyperattachment with frequent diarrhoea and cystitis would also be treated with heather.

The preparations are infusions of plant and flower parts preserved in brandy and diluted in spring water. Therapeutic concentrations of plants are undetectable, but it is claimed (as in homeopathy) that molecular changes occur in the carrier as a result of the preparation.

### 'Rescue remedy'

'Rescue remedy' is a combination of various Bach flower remedies used by owners to calm emotional animals, with reported good effect. According to current evidence these remedies are not associated with specific therapeutic effects (Ernst, 2006). Two randomized controlled trials in humans for treatment of anxiety with 'Rescue remedy' concluded that they were an effective placebo in this context (Armstrong and Ernst, 1999; Walach et al., 2000).

## Reiki and Shen

*Shen* is a Chinese term for the spiritual element of an individual's psyche; *reiki* is a Japanese word meaning 'universal life energy'. This form of therapy is based on the principle that the practitioner channels and directs energy to the patient. It is reputed to have powerful effects on mind and body.

Touch is not usually applied but the patient often feels a sensation of extreme warmth in certain body areas. The act of lying peacefully in a non-threatening environment may itself have beneficial effects and the techniques may be extremely effective ways of triggering the 'placebo' response, a potent neurophysiological response that can be directed, conditioned and now, potentially, augmented by certain agents (Benedetti, 2006).

A systematic review of 23 placebo-controlled randomized trials in humans suggested a positive result in half the studies, but because of methodological difficulties no firm conclusions could be drawn (Astin et al., 2000). Owners report positive effects in behaviourally disturbed animals and such an approach is unlikely to do harm, although Ernst

(2006) cited psychiatric illness as a contraindication to treatment – presumably since this would delay effective treatment.

## Conclusion

It is not been the intention to belittle or to dismiss any form of healing either described or omitted here. Healing remains partly art, simply because we do not understand enough about our interactions with each other and our environment even to start to formulate concepts of how such systems might work. Most of the systems described will at least do no harm in themselves and that should be the first maxim of any treatment. Owner confidence and perception play a significant part in pet behaviour problems and the relationship between counsellor, pet and owner is no less important. Time taken during a consultation and the impression of empathy with owner and pet are therapeutic tools not to be underestimated in behavioural therapy and are usually found in a 'complementary' or integrated consultation.

Despite these positive considerations, it is important to bear the following in mind:

- The temptation to stop current medication to the detriment of the animal without thorough discussion and evaluation of correct dosage reduction regime should be discouraged
- Behaviour therapy should be continued alongside any other intervention
- Any additive that is effective will inevitably have side effects, since no additive can be completely specific
- Animals should be monitored and reassessed for the manifestation of any relevant or unconnected clinical condition
- Thorough communication and trust need to be established between the therapist and the veterinary surgeon responsible for the wellbeing of the patient
- A **client handout** explaining the pros and cons of such therapies may be helpful in dealing with enquiries.

Only if these considerations are followed may it be possible to safeguard the interests of the owner for their animal's welfare and to evaluate each of these and other therapies objectively and rationally.

## References and further reading

Armstrong NC and Ernst E (1999) A randomised, double blind, placebo controlled trial of Bach Flower Remedy. *Perfusion* **11**, 440–446

Astin J, Harkness E and Ernst E (2000) The efficacy of spiritual healing: a systematic review of randomised trials. *Annals of Internal Medicine* **132**, 903–910

Bach E (1933) *The Twelve Healers and Other Remedies*. CW Daniel & Co., Saffron Walden

Beata C, Beaumont-Graff E, Coll V *et al.* (2007a) Effect of alpha-casozepine (Zylkene) on anxiety in cats. *Journal of Veterinary Behavior* **2**, 40–46

Beata C, Beaumont-Graff E, Diaz C *et al.* (2007b) Effects of alpha-casozepine (Zylkene) versus selegiline hydrochloride (Selgian, Anipryl) on anxiety disorders in dogs. *Journal of Veterinary Behavior* **2**,175–183

Benedetti F (2006) Placebo analgesia. *Neurological Science* **27** (suppl. 2), S100–S102

Birch EE, Garfield S, Hoffman DR *et al.* (2000) A randomized controlled trial of early dietary supply of long-chain polyunsaturated fatty acids and mental development in term infants. *Developmental Medicine and Child Neurology* **42**, 174–181

Blakemore JC (1994) Gastrointestinal allergy. *Veterinary Clinics of North America: Small Animal Practice* **24**, 655–695

Brostoff J and Gamlin L (1998) *The Complete Guide to Food Allergy and Intolerance, 3rd edn*, pp. 243–260. Bloomsbury Press, London

Cracknell NR and Mills DS (2007) A double-blind placebo-controlled study into the efficacy of a homeopathic remedy for fear of firework noises in the dog (*Canis familiaris*). *The Veterinary Journal* **177**, 80–88

Cuvellier JC, Valle L and Nuyts JP (1996) Celiac disease, cerebral calcifications and epilepsy syndrome. *Archive of Pediatrics and Adolescent Medicine* **3**, 1013–1019

Day C (1992) *The Homeopathic Treatment of Small Animals*. CW Daniel & Co., Saffron Walden

DeNapoli SS, Dodman NH, Shuster L *et al.* (2000) Effect of dietary protein content and tryptophan supplementation on dominance aggression, territorial aggression and hyperactivity in dogs. *Journal of the American Veterinary Medical Association* **217**, 504–508

Egger J, Carter CM, Soothill JF and Wilson J (1989) Oligoantigenic diet treatment of children with epilepsy and migraine. *Journal of Pediatrics* **114**, 51–58

Ernst E (2006) *The Desktop Guide to Complementary and Alternative Medicine – An Evidence-based Approach, 2nd edn*. Churchill Livingstone, London

Fernstrom JD (1977) Effects of the diet on brain neurotransmitters. *Metabolism* **26**, 207–223

Fernstrom JD (1986) Acute and chronic effects of protein and carbohydrate ingestion on brain tryptophan levels and serotonin synthesis. *Nutritional Review* **44**, 25–36

Fernstrom JD and Wurtman RJ (1972) Elevation of plasma tryptophan by insulin in rats. *Metabolism* **21**, 337–342

Filshie J and White A (1998) *Medical Acupuncture – A Western Scientific Approach*. Churchill Livingstone, London

Fogle B (1999a) *Natural Cat Care*. Dorling Kindersley, London

Fogle B (1999b) *Natural Dog Care*. Dorling Kindersley, London

Gamoah S, Hashimoto M, Sugioka K *et al.* (1999) Chronic administration of docosahexaenoic acid improves reference memory-related learning ability in young rats. *Neuroscience* **34**, S33–S37

Goldberger E and Rapaport JL (1991) Canine acral lick dermatitis: response to the antiobsessional drug clomipramine. *Journal of the American Animal Hospital Association* **27**, 179–182

Halliwell REW (1993) The serological diagnosis of IgE mediated allergic disease in the domestic animal. *Journal of Clinical Immunoassay* **16**, 103–108

Hoffman L, Kelley R and Waltz D (2005) *For Smarter, More Trainable Puppies: effect of docosahexaenoicacid on puppy trainability*. Eukunaba Symposium, Seville

Innis SM (2003) Perinatal biochemistry and physiology of long-chain polyunsaturated fatty acids. *Journal of Pediatrics* **143** (Suppl. 4), S1–S8

Jeffers JG, Shanley KJ and Mege EK (1991) Diagnostic testing of dogs for food hypersensitivity. *Journal of the American Veterinary Medical Association* **198**, 245–250

Laird DA and Drexel H (1934) Experimenting with food and sleep. I. Effects of varying types of foods in offsetting sleep disturbances caused by hunger pangs and gastric distress – children and adults. *Journal of the American Diet Association* **10**, 89–94

Lindley S (1998) The use of transcutaneous spinal electroanalgesia in canine anxiety disorders. *BSAVA Congress 1998 Scientific Proceedings: Clinical Research Abstracts*

Luo H, Meng F, Jia Y and Zhao X (1998) Clinical research on the therapeutic effect of the electro-acupuncture treatment in patients with depression. *Psychiatry and Clinical Neuroscience* **52** (Suppl.), S338–S340

MacDonald AJR and Coates TW (1995) The discovery of transcutaneous spinal electroanalgesia and its relief of chronic pain. *Physiotherapy* **81**, 653–661

Macleod G (1989) *Dogs: Homeopathic Remedies*. CW Daniel & Co., Saffron Walden

McGreevy PD, Righetti J and Thomson PC (2005) The reinforcing value of physical contact and the effect on canine heart rate of grooming in different anatomical areas. *Anthrozoos* **18**, 236–244

Messaoudi M, Lefranc-Millot C, Desot D *et al.* (2005) Effects of a tryptic hydrolysate from bovine milk alpha s1 casein on hemodynamic responses in healthy human volunteers facing successive mental and physical stress situations. *European Journal of Nutrition* **44**, 128–132

Miclo L, Perrin E, Driou A *et al.* (2001) Characterisation of alpha-casozepine, a tryptic peptide from bovine alpha(s1)-casein with benzodiazepine-like activity. *FASEB express article* **15**, 1780–1782

Mugford RA (1987) The influence of nutrition on canine behaviour. *Journal of Small Animal Practice* **28**, 1046–1055

Odendaal J (2002) *Pets and Our Mental Health: The Why, the What, and the How*. Vantage Press, New York

Pilkington K, Kirkwood G, Rampes H *et al.* (2007) Acupuncture for anxiety and anxiety disorders – a systematic literature review. *Acupuncture in Medicine* **25**, 1–10

Podberscek AL, Hsu Y and Serpell JA (1999) Evaluation of clomipramine as an adjunct to behavioural therapy in the treatment of separation-related problems in dogs. *Veterinary Record* **145**, 365–369

Schrader E (2000) Equivalence of St John's Wort extract (Ze 117) and fluoextine: a randomised controlled study in mild-moderate depression. *International Clinical Psychopharmacology* **15**, 61–68

Schwartz S (2005) *Psychoactive Herbs in Veterinary Behavior Medicine.* Churchill Livingstone, New York

Scott S (2000) The use of acupuncture as a treatment for canine acral lick dermatitis. *Research in Veterinary Science* **68** (Suppl. A), 36

Scott S and Mayhew IG (2001) Guest editorial: Pharmacological treatment in behavioural medicine. *The Veterinary Journal* **162**, 5–6

Simons DG, Travell JG and Simons PT (1999) *Travell & Simons' Myofascial Pain & Dysfunction. The Trigger Point Manual. Vol. 1: Upper Half of Body.* Williams & Wilkins, Baltimore

Stevinson C and Ernst E (1999) Safety of Hypericum in patients with depression. *CNS Drugs* **11**, 125–132

Towell AD, Williams D and Boyd SG (1997) High frequency non-invasive stimulation over the spine: effects on mood and mechanical pain tolerance in normal subjects. *Behavioural Neurology* **10**, 61–65

Uvnas-Moberg K, Bruzelius G, Alster P and Lundeberg T (1993) The antinociceptive effect of non-noxious sensory stimulation is mediated partly through oxytocinergic mechanisms. *Acta Physiologica Scandinavia* **149**, 199–204

Violle N, Messaoudi M, Lefranc-Millot C *et al.* (2006) Ethological comparison of the effects of a bovine alpha s1 casein tryptic hydrolysate and diazepam on the behaviour of rats in two models of anxiety. *Pharmacology, Biochemistry and Behaviour* **84**, 517–523

Walach H, Rilling C and Engelke U (2000) Bach Flower Remedies are ineffective for test anxiety: results of a blinded, placebo controlled randomised trial. *Forschung für Komplementarmedizin Klass Naturheilkund* **7**, 55

Wells DL (2006) Aromatherapy for travel induced excitement in dogs. *Journal of the American Veterinary Medical Association* **229**, 964–967

White AR, Rampes H and Ernst E (2000) Acupuncture for smoking cessation. *Cochrane Database Systematic Review* **2**, CD000009

## Client handouts (bsavalibrary.com/behaviour_leaflets)

- **Complementary therapies in behaviour problems**
- **Your puppy's first year**

# 23

# Managing and rehoming the rescue dog and cat

## Sheila Segurson

## Introduction

Over the past several decades, as more and more people have chosen to include pets as members of their households, pet owners have become more responsible regarding their care and more aware of welfare issues that affect dogs and cats. Despite this development, some people remain unaware about responsible pet ownership and opt to relinquish their pet to a shelter. Others may have housing or financial difficulties that make it difficult to keep their pet; or they may care deeply about their pet but it has a medical or behaviour problem and they have exhausted their resources for management and treatment. Many people who relinquish pets feel that they are acting in their pet's best interest, because someone else will be able to provide it with a better home. They may not understand that, with regard to behaviour, the reason they feel they can no longer keep their pet may prevent it from being chosen for adoption.

Landlord and housing issues are usually the most commonly cited reasons for relinquishment to shelters, but, when the underlying causes are evaluated, behaviour problems are the most common causes of relinquishment of dogs and the second most common cause of relinquishment of cats. Common problems leading to relinquishment of dogs are: lack of housetraining; destructive behaviour; high energy level; and aggression. Behaviour problems that lead to relinquishment of cats include: house soiling; problems with other pets in the household; aggression; and destructive behaviour (Salman *et al.*, 2000). Australian data reveal that escaping from the yard, boisterousness and barking are the most common behavioural reasons for dog relinquishment (Marston *et al.*, 2004).

Because behaviour problems are such a frequent reason for relinquishment and because of the importance of behaviour in successfully rehoming dogs and cats, many shelters are developing comprehensive behaviour plans. These often include:

- Behavioural evaluation and assessment
- Methods to reduce stress and enrich shelter pets' lives
- Training and behaviour modification programmes
- Pre-adoption screening and counselling
- Post-adoption follow-up to prevent and/or treat potential problems in the home.

The task of rehoming and saving animal lives involves a coordinated effort among animal shelters, foster homes and breed rescue groups. Highly successful rehoming programmes are very unlikely to exist without a comprehensive plan for interplay between different animal groups. Breed and other rescue groups are often better able to counsel potential adopters regarding the behavioural and medical care needed for a particular breed, and are often able to care for and rehabilitate pets with behaviour problems that the shelter is unable to handle. Because of the seasonal nature of the canine and feline reproductive cycles, foster homes are also crucial to a shelter's success. They are able to house kittens, puppies and adults temporarily during times of high shelter occupancy and can also provide the shelter with valuable data regarding the pet's behaviour in a home environment.

According to one study, 67% of dogs and 53% of cats relinquished to a shelter visited a veterinary surgeon at least once in the year preceding relinquishment (Salman *et al.*, 1998). Private veterinary practices may be the only professionals providing advice to the pet owner after adoption, and therefore play a critical role in prevention of relinquishment to shelters and successful rehoming of recently adopted pets. This chapter includes information to help to familiarize the veterinary surgeon with behavioural evaluation in shelters, techniques to match pets to new owners, and methods to increase the likelihood that the pet will remain in its new home. For owners considering a new pet, the **client handout** gives helpful advice about the advantages and disadvantages of adopting a dog from a rescue group or shelter.

## Shelter behaviour plan

The goals of a shelter behaviour plan are to:

- Increase the likelihood that a pet will be adopted and stay in its new home
- Decrease the likelihood that a pet who is a public safety risk will be placed in a home
- Increase the quality of life for pets in the shelter's care
- Decrease the likelihood that pets will be surrendered to the shelter in the first place.

Shelters should attempt to create a welcoming environment for the public (Figure 23.1), which encourages visitors to spend time there and potentially choose to adopt a pet or volunteer at the shelter. The shelter behaviour plan ensures that there is a solid foundation of programmes to serve the public and manage the shelter population.

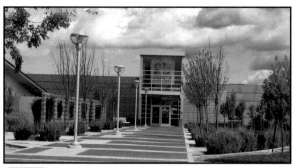

**23.1** Shelters attempt to create a welcoming environment for potential adopters, in an effort to increase the likelihood that people will visit the shelter and choose to adopt a pet.

Key components of a shelter behaviour plan are included in the chart below (Figure 23.2). A solid plan for evaluation, basic care, treatment, counseling and rehabilitation is crucial to the success of an adoption program. This plan should be devised by a behaviour advisory committee comprised of: a shelter manager and/or director, veterinary surgeon, shelter behaviour

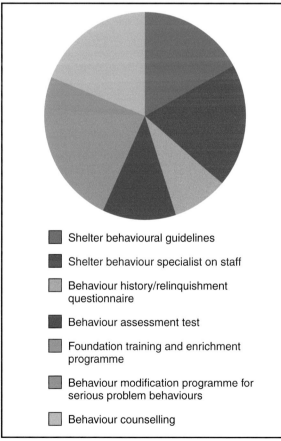

- Shelter behavioural guidelines
- Shelter behaviour specialist on staff
- Behaviour history/relinquishment questionnaire
- Behaviour assessment test
- Foundation training and enrichment programme
- Behaviour modification programme for serious problem behaviours
- Behaviour counselling

**23.2** Key components of a shelter behaviour programme and their estimated relative resource requirement.

specialist, and, in the case of dogs, a local dog trainer. It is valuable for a veterinary surgeon to be included on this committee, as a veterinary surgeon is able to provide input regarding the interplay of medical and behaviour problems (see Chapter 1), as well as the impact of behaviour programmes on infectious diseases. The plan should include a manual with detailed descriptions of all of the items in the Key Components chart. Similar to shelter infectious disease protocols, this plan serves as a guideline to aid the shelter in managing and minimizing behaviour problems.

### Shelter behaviour specialist

Shelters maximize the success of their behaviour programmes by hiring an employee whose primary responsibility is to manage the behavioural needs of the shelter population and to train staff/volunteers to execute the plan. The behaviour specialist must be someone who, in addition to understanding canine and feline behaviour, also understands shelter population dynamics and can utilize their behavioural skill and training to maximize adoptions from the shelter. Ideally the specialist should have successfully completed an academic and practical training programme regarding pet behaviour that leads to certification.

## Behaviour assessment in shelters

The ultimate goal of an animal shelter or rescue centre is to find suitable homes for as many dogs and cats as possible. Behaviour is evaluated through intake interviews and questionnaires with relinquishing owners, behaviour assessment tests performed in the shelter, and observations and results of training the pet in the shelter environment. The goal of the evaluation is to identify behaviour problems or concerns, and to match the pet to a suitable family.

The term temperament is often used by animal shelters when attempting to assess pet behaviour. While this term was historically used to describe personality, and the words character, temperament and personality are often used interchangeably in the non-scientific literature, it is useful to distinguish between them when discussing behavioural assessment in shelters.

- **Character** may be considered a product of the environment in which a pet lives, and the pet's experiences in that environment. It refers to the habits and manner of responding to its environment that a pet has developed secondary to its experiences.
- **Temperament** may be used to describe a pet's natural or innate manner of responding to its environment, particularly its emotional responses. Temperament is based on a pet's genetic constitution and early experiences.
- **Personality** represents a combination of character and temperament. it refers to an overall way of responding to the environment, based on past experience and genetic tendencies.

While a pet's character can be influenced by modifying its environment, its temperament is a stable characteristic. Temperament forms the foundation of personality; character influences that foundation but cannot fundamentally change it. Because personality is the manifestation of genetic background, experiences and method of responding to the environment in *multiple* different circumstances, an accurate prediction of a pet's personality is unlikely to be possible in the shelter environment.

## Common problems

Although many shelters undertake behavioural evaluations, there is no generally accepted technique for assessing canine and feline behavioural traits, no standardized terminology for describing these, and no test or questionnaire being used in shelters that has been validated, via peer-reviewed research, to be highly predictive of the pet's behaviour in its new home. Common problems with many test evaluations include:

- Time available to assess personality
- Effect of stress on behaviour
- Standardization.

### Time available to assess personality

A one-time meeting or experience is unlikely to provide an accurate assessment of the pet's personality. A pet's behaviour may be different in different circumstances, and these differences constitute their uniqueness. In addition, it is difficult to assess a pet's potential for house soiling or destructiveness when the assessment is not performed in a home environment. Thus, it is virtually impossible to assess personality by means of a single test. Personality is something that is learnt about a dog or cat by observing their reactions over a broad range of environments and experiences. Most shelters do not have the time or the resources to do this, and thus they are assessing behaviour at only a specific or limited point in time, rather than true personality.

### Effect of stress on behaviour

Although many shelters attempt to provide a comfortable and enriched home for pets, shelters are a stressful place for many animals (Figure 23.3) and stress often changes their behaviour. Some pets will behave more aggressively when stressed, some will tend to hide, some perform repetitive or destructive behaviours, and some will be quieter and more inhibited (see Chapter 13). The behaviour of a highly stressed animal may very well not represent its true personality.

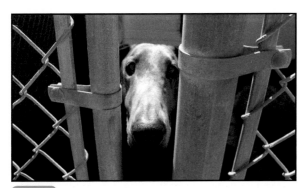

**23.3** Shelters can be a stressful environment for pets.

### Standardization

In order to serve as a valid diagnostic tool, the behaviour assessment test must be standardized. It must be performed using the same techniques and in the same manner with every dog or cat. Because part of performing an assessment includes observing body language, it is very common that when the pet shows signs of fear or anxiety, with or without aggression, the evaluator starts to behave in a more careful and guarded manner. While this is a normal and appropriate response by the evaluator, their behaviour is not consistent between tests and may further exacerbate the pet's stress and anxiety. Given that behaviour evaluators are observing unique individuals, it may be impossible to truly standardize a test in a real-life setting, where the evaluator must protect themselves from injury, and especially when more than one evaluator is used.

## Public safety and adoptability

Shelters must often make difficult decisions regarding which pets are suitable to be placed for adoption. They evaluate canine and feline behaviour in an effort to determine whether a pet is a significant public safety (bite) risk, whether the pet is adoptable from the shelter and, lastly, what steps they can take to improve that pet's adoption potential.

### Public safety risk

Shelters are entrusted with protecting the public from dangerous or vicious animals. Behavioural evaluation may help to identify animals that pose a serious risk.

### Adoptability

Due to the number of pets entering the shelter and limited resources, some shelters are unable to house animals humanely for the long term. Many make decisions regarding placement for adoption based upon a pet's likelihood of being adopted from that shelter. Factors that affect adoptability include the pet's age, sex, breed (or mix), size, colour, underlying stress level and behaviour. A pet that has a poor chance of being adopted at a particular shelter might be euthanized (if local laws or societal policy allow) or transferred to a rescue programme where it is more likely to be adopted (Figure 23.4).

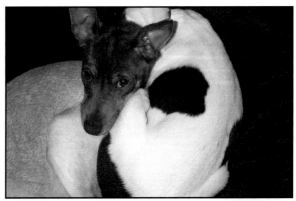

**23.4** Although this terrier was of a highly adoptable size, age and breed for most shelters, it was extremely fearful in the shelter environment. Its behaviour improved once it had been placed in a foster programme and eventually it was placed successfully in a home.

Pets that are housed in shelters long term (e.g. where there is a no-kill policy) often develop stress-related behaviour problems, which can manifest as withdrawal from social interaction, repetitive behaviours or other undesirable behaviours. The pet's chances for adoption decrease the longer it stays in the shelter and so, as well as being a welfare concern, it is in the shelter's best interest to find more suitable options for rehoming of less adoptable pets.

### Improving adoption potential

Behaviour is one of the few factors affecting adoptability that can be changed. Shelters that easily find homes for highly adoptable pets have often developed behaviour and training programmes to resolve or manage behaviour problems.

## Personality assessment

The Ancient Greeks, most notably Hippocrates and Galen, first described the four humours (or temperaments) as ideas regarding personality and health in humans. These personality types were defined as phlegmatic, choleric, sanguine or melancholic. It is from this model that many models of human (and animal) personality were later developed. During Ivan Pavlov's well known experiments, he evaluated the behaviour of his dogs and argued that different personality types responded differently to his experiments. He classified the dogs into the same four personality types, describing them as:

- Sanguine (easily excited/emotionally aroused but calms quickly/good inhibition)
- Phlegmatic (not easily excited and calms quickly if aroused)
- Choleric (easily excited with poor ability to calm/inhibit itself)
- Melancholic (not easily aroused and with poor inhibition).

These personality types were further developed by Hans Eysenck, who provided major contributions to the field of human personality assessment – a field that has made great progress. In contrast, validation of canine personality assessment techniques has lagged behind. Since Pavlov, research regarding canine personality and behaviour has primarily focused on the temperaments of guide dogs and working dogs, though studies of shelter dog behaviour are increasing in frequency. Research regarding feline behaviour assessment is sparse.

## Intake interviews and questionnaires

Obtaining historical information about the pet is a primary method of diagnosing behaviour problems in owned dogs and cats but is not the primary method of behaviour assessment used in some shelters. Behavioural questionnaires for pets entering a shelter are typically designed to obtain information regarding the pet's environment (relinquishing owner's lifestyle, housing, pet's exposure to other animals), behaviour problems and training. Many shelters suspect that information from relinquishing owners may not provide an accurate representation of the pet's personality and studies in shelters lend support to this concept (Segurson et al., 2005; Stephen and Ledger, 2007). A validated standardized questionnaire (Serpell and Hsu, 2001), such as the University of Pennsylvania's C-BARQ© (Canine Behavioural Assessment and Research Questionnaire), may be considered as an ancillary tool to guide adoption and placement decisions.

### Behaviour assessment tests

Because of concerns regarding the reliability of information provided by relinquishing owners and the potential influence of the previous owner's lifestyle and management of the pet on its behaviour problems, many shelters rely primarily upon a wide range of behavioural assessment tests to help adopters select a dog or cat, and to guide decisions on euthanasia, placement and treatment. Most of the assessments fall into two categories:

- Tests that evaluate the pet's response to interactions commonly performed by a pet owner on a regular basis
- Tests that are provocative and attempt to determine a pet's response to extremely challenging circumstances.

Because provocative tests place the evaluator at risk of injury, many shelters use an artificial hand or dummy to evaluate portions of the test that are most likely to result in aggression. This practice is of questionable validity, as dogs demonstrate the ability to discriminate between artificial and real hands (Tempany and Mills, 2008).

The lack of validation of assessment tests is a serious cause for concern as it may not only condemn animals unnecessarily, but also provide false assurances (Taylor and Mills, 2006; Christensen et al., 2007; Braem et al., 2008). However, lack of validation does not mean that the tests do not have value, only that confidence in their results is more limited. Until validated tests are developed and published, it is crucial that shelters adhere to standards that maximize the value of their assessment protocol (Diederich and Giffroy, 2006). These include, at minimum:

- Utilization of a standardized test
- Training of staff regarding how to evaluate canine and feline body language, as well as how to perform and evaluate the test
- Assessment of reliability of the test for the circumstances under which it is performed (assessing reliability involves assessing whether the same tester, or multiple different testers, will perform the test consistently each time)
- Use of standardized criteria and terminology for evaluating the results of the test
- Obtaining follow-up information on the pets regarding outcome: euthanasia, transfer to a different facility, adoption, and problems in the new home (if rehomed).

While it is becoming standard practice for shelters to perform canine assessments, feline assessments are performed less frequently, and some shelters do not perform them.

## Testing

The shelter advisory committee should create a behavioural assessment manual that clearly defines the test itself, provides definitions for behaviour and terminology, and lays down criteria for outcome decisions. Staff who perform behavioural evaluations should undergo extensive training about interpretation of pet body language and how to perform the test in a standardized and unbiased manner. They should also receive periodic reviews in an effort to assess inter- and intra-rater reliability. This is best accomplished by video-recording assessments and then meeting to discuss modification of techniques in order to improve reliability, as well as provide further education regarding body language interpretation.

Evaluators should work in teams in order to ensure safety and to avoid missing subtle body language signals. While this is the ideal method, unfortunately many shelters do not have enough physical or human resources and an evaluator will assess the pet alone. The test is typically performed in a room designated for behaviour evaluations, which is free of potentially stressful distractions such as loud noises and other animals. If housed in indoor kennels, dogs should be walked outside to eliminate before testing (a housetrained dog may otherwise 'fail' the test because it needs to eliminate and is not interested in interact- ing with people).

Every dog, cat, kitten and puppy that is admitted to the shelter should be tested. Some shelters post- pone testing for pets with medical problems, but this practice is not recommended. While the disease probably influences the pet's behaviour, it is impor- tant to evaluate its behaviour early in its tenure at the shelter. For ill animals, the assessment may serve to guide handling recommendations or behaviour modification plans.

Most shelters perform their test 3–5 days after admission, since a study in one shelter reported that it takes 3 days for stress levels to start decreasing (Hennessy *et al.*, 1997). Pets entering the shelter are quite stressed and providing them with an adjustment period may allow the shelter to evaluate behaviour more accurately. However, if the shelter does not provide animals with appropriate levels of physical environmental enrichment and social interaction, they may get more stressed the longer they are in the shelter. In this case, it is more appropriate to perform the test soon after admission.

### Components of the assessment

Shelters usually assess categories of behaviour that may influence the likelihood that the adopter will be satisfied with the pet. Examples of elements of an assessment include:

- Sociability
- Handleability
- Playfulness
- Food bowl and possessive aggression (dogs only)
- Reaction to life-sized toddler doll (dogs only)
- Reaction to dogs and cats.

### Sociability

An assessment of sociability attempts to determine whether the pet enjoys interacting with people. This is usually evaluated by initially standing or sitting in an evaluation room and observing whether the pet chooses to interact with people versus its environment.

### Handleability

This part of the assessment attempts to determine whether the pet accepts handling such as petting or hugging, lifting into the arms, gently grabbing the skin or lifting a paw, and if so whether it tolerates rough handling. Evaluators may simulate rough handling by gently pinching the pet's skin or holding a paw despite clear body language signals that the pet is mildly uncomfortable (see Ladder of Aggression in Chapter 2). This may be utilized in an effort to determine what type of home to place the pet in (young children *versus* older children *versus* adults only).

### Playfulness

The evaluator attempts to engage the dog in games of tug-of-war and retrieving, or the cat in play with a wand-type toy. During this part of the evaluation, the shelter is attempting to determine whether the pet likes to play; and if the pet does play, the evaluator observes whether or not it calms down appropriately after playing. A dog that retrieves and plays interactive games with people may be much easier to exercise and manage in a home environment. A dog that has difficulty disengaging from an emotionally excited or aroused state may be more difficult to train and man- age. During feline evaluations, the evaluator pets or lifts the cat after playing with it in an effort to determine whether play induces overexcitement or aggression.

### Food bowl and possessive aggression

The evaluator provides the dog with a bowl of food and then a valuable chew toy. An assistant restrains the dog and the evaluator uses an artificial hand to determine whether the dog behaves aggressively with regard to these items (Figure 23.5). A dog that growls, snaps or bites during this part of the assessment should be placed in a behaviour modification programme. While many shelters successfully treat this problem, some do not have the resources to do so and opt for euthanasia.

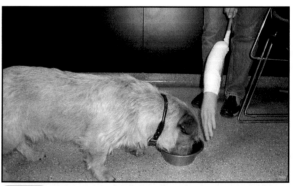

**23.5** Using a synthetic hand and arm to assess for food bowl aggression. To protect the evaluator from injury, the dog is restrained on a lead.

### Reaction to life-sized toddler doll

This part of the assessment evaluates the dog's response to a doll, which is usually held in the evaluator's arms or moved on the ground. One study of this revealed that it was not able to reliably and significantly predict a dog's aggressive response (or lack thereof) to children (Kroll *et al.*, 2004). While some shelters use this procedure, it is not recommended as a predictive tool for aggressive behaviour toward children.

### Reaction to dogs and cats

Some shelters evaluate the pet's response to other animals (conspecifics and other species) but many are not able to assess these characteristics. Because a positive (or negative) response to one dog or cat does not necessarily mean a positive (or negative) response to *all* dogs or cats, potential adopters should always attempt to bring their own existing pet to the shelter to meet the new dog or cat before deciding on whether or not to take the shelter pet home. Ideally, adopters should temporarily care for a friend's pet in order to assess the disruption that a new pet provides to the home environment, before deciding to adopt a new pet.

## Evaluation of test results

There is no standardized system for scoring and evaluating the test results. While some shelters use ethograms, most use a 'pass', 'questionable' or 'fail' score, a numerical scoring system, or a graded score (A, B, C…) to evaluate the pet. These techniques are often quicker and simpler, but without extensive training they are more likely to result in inconsistency. Utilization of these graded or scored techniques can be a functional method of evaluation if the scores are based upon clearly defined behavioural descriptions.

## Using test results to guide decisions

Shelters should have a written scoring or assessment system that will help to guide classification and outcome decisions. The Asilomar Accords (www.asilomaraccords.org) were created by a coalition of humane organizations in the United States in an effort to end the euthanasia of healthy and treatable pets in animal shelters. The Accords provide shelters with definitions as a standard for categorizing animals, as well as guidelines for data collection and reporting. Data collection allows the shelter to determine where they can improve their behaviour programmes, as well as track progress. From these guidelines, pets are classified (with emphasis on behaviour for this discussion) as follows (where 'treatable' refers to treatment by a reasonable and caring pet owner in the community):

- Healthy (no sign of behaviour or medical problems)
- Treatable / Rehabilitatable (behaviour problem present, but can become 'healthy' after treatment)
- Treatable / Manageable (behaviour problem present, but unlikely to be completely resolved; pet likely to have a satisfactory quality of life with treatment and does not pose a significant public health risk)
- Unhealthy / Untreatable (behaviour problem present that poses a health or safety risk and pet is unlikely to become 'healthy' or 'treatable' with treatment).

Shelters that follow the Asilomar Accords guidelines form a behaviour advisory panel in order to draft guidelines regarding which problems fit into each category. The panel should comprise staff members of different shelters in the community and people who are knowledgeable about the standard of care for pets in the community, such as veterinary surgeons, dog trainers, behaviourists and kennel owners. The shelter then utilizes the assessment test and the classification system to make decisions about pets in their care.

Keeping track of outcome over time (adoption success, adoption counselling needed, adoption return, euthanasia) will help the shelter to modify and improve the behaviour programme. Development of criteria for classification is made on a community-wide basis, and often varies from community to community, depending on that community's characteristics. The shelter classifies problems according to what a reasonable and caring pet owner would do, and not according to the resources within the shelter. Classification will guide but does not mandate outcome.

A shelter may not currently have the resources to rehabilitate a behaviour problem, such as food bowl aggression, but as the shelter and community develop the behaviour plan, treating that problem may become an achievable goal.

Classification of behaviour problems helps to prioritize treatment. Because of the nature of behaviour problems, a problem might be interchangeable between categories for an individual animal, depending on behavioural changes over time and response to treatment. A pet in the manageable category who does not respond to treatment poses a significant public health risk, and one whose quality of life is significantly adversely affected could be reclassified as untreatable and unhealthy. Because many potentially rehabilitatable behaviour problems will require continued maintenance and preventive techniques in the new home, they are classified as manageable.

A word of caution: while behaviour assessment is a useful tool for evaluating pet behaviour in shelters, it has not yet been determined to be an accurate diagnostic tool as a predictor of pet behaviour and personality. Because behaviour assessment tests affect life-and-death decisions, it is critical that more behaviour studies are performed and published in order to determine which pet personality characteristics can be reliably predicted in shelters.

## Foundation training and enrichment programmes

The most common behaviour problems among shelter pets are relatively simple ones such as pulling on the lead or jumping up on people. The behaviours may be caused by a lack of basic training or by a lack of environmental enrichment that results in hyper-excitability or attention-seeking behaviour. They often significantly impact on adoptability, as people looking for a dog tend not to choose one that displays unruly behaviour.

## Foundation training

Because these problems are less time consuming to resolve than more complicated ones, every shelter should have a foundation training programme in place before considering treatment for more serious problems. The shelter behaviour specialist (or a trained assistant) should evaluate the pet at the outset of the training process to ensure that the standard treatment protocol is appropriate for that pet. The added benefit of training programmes is that they teach staff and volunteers the principles of behaviour and training, which then serve as a foundation for more complicated problems, if the shelter chooses to address them.

### Cats

Stressed cats often inhibit their behaviour, thus attention-seeking problems similar to those seen in dogs are much less common. It is important to recognize that the quiet non-interactive cat in the shelter should be considered as serious a problem as an attention-seeking dog. Many cats withdraw and reduce interactivity with their environment and visitors the longer they stay in the shelter. This behaviour hinders their adoptability (whereas in dogs overly interactive behaviours deter adopters). Most adopters want their new cat to interact with them and do not understand that many shelter cats are withdrawn due to stress, and that the withdrawn behaviour may not be a normal part of their behavioural repertoire. The foundation training programme for cats should emphasize handling, grooming and environmental enrichment (Figure 23.6). The foundation programme for cats aims to reduce stress and quickly identify problems.

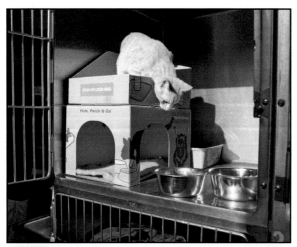

**23.6** Environmental enrichment for a shelter cat. This 'Hide, Perch & Go' box (devised by the British Columbia SPCA) serves as a method of stress reduction by offering a hiding place and perch. The box transforms into a carrier when the cat is adopted.

## Enrichment

Shelters should attempt to provide pets in their care with humane housing and enriched environments. Enrichment improves the lives of shelter animals, as well as the morale of staff and volunteers. Many studies document the effects of kennelling on animal stress as well as the positive effects of environmental enrichment in reducing stress.

Enrichment in the form of human interaction (play, petting, training), exercise, provision of toys, increasing the complexity of the enclosure, provision of a hiding place/sleeping area, group housing (for pets that enjoy interacting with other pets), bedding and sensory enrichment (olfactory, auditory and visual) can all reduce stress and result in calmer pets. Reducing stress reduces the likelihood of development of new behaviour problems, as stress can lead to aggressive and other fearful responses in a pet that has not behaved in such a way in the past.

The enrichment provided depends upon the populations of dogs and cats in the shelter, staffing (including volunteers) available to provide enrichment, level and types of disease present, and education of staff and volunteers about infectious disease control. An enrichment programme can greatly improve the welfare of pets during their stay in the shelter (see client handouts).

## Behavioural modification programme

Behaviour modification programmes in shelters must be embarked upon with caution. First and foremost, the shelter must meet the physical and mental enrichment needs of the pets in the shelter. Once these needs are met, more complicated problems might be treated. In considering treatment of serious problems such as human-directed aggression in cats and dogs, the shelter must consider whether it has the resources available to treat the problem adequately, and must also consider liability issues. A pet with a history of aggression might place staff and volunteers at risk of personal injury. Even if well managed, a behaviour problem must be disclosed to adopters, which will reduce the number of people interested in adopting the pet. In many situations, the shelter may be held liable for a pet with a documented history of aggression that then bites or injures someone in its new home.

Because of these concerns, behaviour modification plans in shelters should perhaps be focused on problems with less liability risk, such as fears and anxieties without a history of aggression. A pet being treated for a problem in the shelter environment must have a detailed treatment plan, people dedicated to follow the plan, a treatment/training log and scheduled re-evaluations. Pets receiving behaviour modification should be re-evaluated by the behaviour specialist every week, and by the shelter manager and behaviour specialist once a month. An example of a generalized anxiety behaviour modification plan for a shelter with a well developed behaviour programme is included in Figure 23.7. This plan contains a template for a treatment plan; a more detailed plan is necessary for individual animals.

| Definition |
| --- |
| Generalized anxiety is persistent and profound fear of objects, people, animals, or any unexpected movement/stimulus in the environment, with poor recovery after exposure. Over time, anxious behaviour becomes independent of any stimulus and is manifested as hypervigilance, severe avoidance, escape behaviour and/or anxiety. In order to be considered for treatment, the dog must not have shown any signs of aggression. |

| Treatment |
| --- |
| 1. Create consistent, routine and structured environment. The dog should be fed, walked and interacted with at the same times each day. |
| 2. Reduce kennel stress (provide hiding place in kennel; reduce access to things that increase the dog's stress; environmental enrichment). If no response, consider foster home. |
| 3. Initially only people that the dog is comfortable with are allowed to interact with it. The dog must work (sit, eye contact, or touch hand) to earn anything it wants (e.g. food, attention, access to outdoors). |
| 4. Teach 'coping skills' to increase the dog's feeling of control over its environment. |
| 5. Clicker training. |
| 6. 'Check it' cue to teach the dog to approach fear-inducing items in order to earn a reward. |
| 7. Medications: consult with veterinary surgeon regarding all dogs with generalized anxiety. Anti-anxiety medication is often necessary. The dog must not be categorized as unhealthy or untreatable until medications have been provided for a minimum of 8 weeks. |
| 8. Trainers must keep a daily log of treatment and behaviour modification. |

| Re-evaluation |
| --- |
| The training log and treatment plan must be reassessed and, if necessary, modified once weekly. Dogs that are not making significant progress after 1 month *must* be started on anti-anxiety medications (if not already on them). All dogs in treatment must be reviewed by behaviour review committee once monthly. |

| Outcome |
| --- |
| • Dogs that respond to treatment (significant reduction or elimination of anxiety) can be put up for adoption and their status (including recommendations for rehoming) identified to adoption staff. |
| • Dogs that show progress after 8 weeks but are not ready for maintenance will receive continued treatment pending behavioural review. |
| • Dogs that do not respond (display significant anxiety which drastically impacts their quality of life) after 8 weeks of behavioural modification and drug therapy will be considered for transfer to a specialty facility or euthanasia. |

**23.7** Template for behaviour modification plan for generalized anxiety.

## Behaviour counselling

Many behaviour problems are 'manageable' rather than 'rehabilitatable' when one considers rehoming the pet. Even relatively simple problems such as pulling on the lead may recur if management of the problem is not maintained in the new home. Behaviour counselling in shelters includes pre-adoption screening, counselling at the time of adoption and post-adoption follow-up. It serves several important functions:

- Providing services matching pets and people, thereby matching personality and lifestyle of the adopter to that of their new pet
- Providing full disclosure about behaviour problems to potential new owners, which helps to guide the adopter's decision
- Educating pet owners regarding the pet's basic behavioural needs and care
- Educating shelter staff, volunteers and the public about safe and humane treatment of behaviour problems
- Serving as a post-adoption resource for new owners to ensure continued treatment and management of the problem
- Providing post-adoption follow-up in an effort to identify and treat problems as soon as they occur.

### Pre-adoption screening programmes

Pre-adoption screening programmes have been developed in an effort to increase the likelihood that adopters will be satisfied with their new pet, and reduce the likelihood that the pet will be rejected by the new owner. Matching pets to an appropriate adopter is the next step in the shelter's behaviour plan. Currently, most shelters categorize or rate pets according to family lifestyle and the skill levels of pet owners.

Because small children often scare under-socialized dogs and cats and because families with children are more likely to surrender their pet to a shelter, most shelters only allow the most stable dogs and cats to be adopted into homes with small children. Some pets may be classified as being allowed into homes with older children (i.e. over 12 years) only and others are restricted for placement in adult-only homes. Some shelters do not allow small dogs to be adopted into homes that already have a larger dog; and some shelters do not allow cats to be adopted to homes that contain dogs.

While shelters have the pets' best interests as their primary consideration, stringent adoption criteria are now sometimes preventing suitable pet owners from adopting the pet that they want from a shelter, as criteria based on the family (children in the home) do not take into consideration the pet owner's competence and interest in animal behaviour.

A standardized pet–owner matching programme, ASPCA Meet Your Match™ Feline-ality™ and Canine-ality™ (Weiss 2007ab), is being evaluated and utilized in shelters in the United States. This programme assesses both pet behaviour (through an assessment test) and adopter lifestyle/preferences (through a survey). Based upon the adopter's evaluation, pet owners are provided with a colour coded 'guest pass' that suggests that a certain category (purple, orange or green) of cat or dog would be most suitable for them. The pets are assigned a colour and one of nine descriptions (Figure 23.8) based on their behaviour assessment test.

With regard to cats, these categories fit in a grid composed of two primary components: 'valance' and 'independence–gregariousness'.

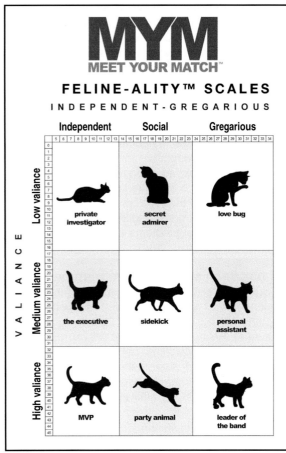

FELINE-ALITY™ SCALES
INDEPENDENT-GREGARIOUS

**23.8**  ASPCA Meet Your Match™ Feline-ality™ scales (reproduced with permission).

- **Valiance** refers to cat's reaction to novel stimuli and stimulating environments. A low-valiant cat has a tendency to hide or avoid interaction when novel stimuli (e.g. strangers in the house) are present.
- **Independence–gregariousness** refers to the cat's interest in interacting with people, acceptance of handling and attention-seeking behaviour.

For example, a cat with the highest degree of independence (low tolerance for interaction and handling) and lowest degree of valiance (low tolerance for stimulating environments) would be assigned a purple colour and called a 'private investigator'.

When an adopter selects a particular cat, an adoption counsellor educates the potential owner about why the cat may be suitable for them and any potential problems they may face if they adopt that cat.

There are several advantages to the Meet your Match™ programme. First and foremost, it is a standardized matching programme and data indicate that it increases adoptions, reduces euthanasia and reduces shelter returns. In addition, all categories of pet are provided with flattering descriptions; thus, even the cats and dogs that are more challenging to place are identified with a description that increases the likelihood that they will find a suitable home.

### Adoption screening for pets with treated and managed problems

Pets with a history of *any* treated behaviour problem should have a behaviour record in the adoption screening/counselling area of the shelter. Maintenance requirements for the problem must be explicitly defined for adoption staff and potential adopters. When an adopter is interested in a pet, the record allows the shelter to identify the shelter's treatment plan and educate the owner orally and in writing regarding how they will need to manage the problem on an ongoing basis, if necessary. All pets with treatable and manageable problems must be the subject of behavioural counselling before and after adoption. A shelter behavioural modification and training programme is of limited usefulness without proper behavioural counselling for the adopter.

## Behaviour counselling at the time of rehoming

At the time of rehoming, adopters should be educated about the following topics:

- Normal pet behaviour and body language
- Management of the environment, to prevent problems (crate training, litterbox management, exercise, enrichment)
- Common problems (scratching furniture, stealing food off worktops) and prevention/treatment
- Behavioural resources in their community
- Recommended reading about pet behaviour.

Teaching adopters preventive measures regarding problems increases the likelihood that the pet will remain in the home, but most adopters are so excited about their new pet that they do not absorb much of what the adoption counsellor is trying to teach them, and forget about written informational materials once they get home. Education at the time of adoption should therefore be focused on the most important items:

- How they should expect their pet to behave when it gets home
- Management to prevent house soiling and destruction (Figure 23.9)

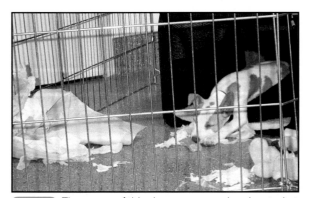

**23.9**  The owner of this dog was properly educated at the time of adoption regarding how to manage their new pet's environment. While the pet did destroy something, it was not anything of significant value to the owner and was therefore an acceptable outlet for the behaviour while the dog was being trained.

- Telephone number for the shelter's behaviour helpline
- Treatment of any pre-existing problems.

A range of useful **client handouts** are provided.

## Post-adoption follow-up

Ensuring successful adoption is the final portion of the shelter's behaviour plan. Because behaviour problems are common in the general pet population, they are also common in pets adopted from a shelter and include fearfulness, house soiling, aggression and unruly behaviour. Estimations vary from shelter to shelter but up to 25% of adopted dogs are returned to the shelter. Given the prevalence of behaviour problems and the aforementioned data, it is clear that post-adoption follow-up is an essential aspect of the adoption process for shelters.

A follow-up programme ensures guidance for ongoing or new problems, and assesses the accuracy of the behavioural assessment test and plan. Detailed education about pet behaviour, as described in the previous section, should be offered by means of lectures, training classes, behaviour helplines and recommended reading.

Most owners think that their new pet will immediately be content in their new home, but many pets are significantly stressed as they adjust to their new environment. Shelters and veterinary surgeons must teach owners that changes of environment and routine can be quite disruptive and that it is not uncommon to see lethargy and anorexia for a day or two after the pet gets to its new home. It is also important to emphasize the effect of stress on the pet's behaviour. Stress may lead to aggressive fearful behaviour in a pet who does not normally behave in that manner. More commonly, stressed pets are quieter and more inhibited than normal.

Owners should be made aware of the 'honeymoon period' after adoption. The calm and quiet behaviour that they see initially is unlikely to continue, and most pets start to relax and behave normally in their new home approximately 2–4 weeks after adoption. Unfortunately 'normally' is not necessarily what most owners prefer, as once the honeymoon period is over many pets start to become destructive or over-exuberant, or display other excitable yet undesirable behaviours (Figure 23.10) if not properly managed initially. If owners expect this to happen, the worst effects can be pre-empted and any change is a lot less distressing when it occurs.

Shelters should provide telephone follow-up for all adopted pets at 3 days, 3 weeks, 3 months and 1 year post adoption. Pets with managed pre-existing problems should receive a follow-up telephone call at 1 and 3 days and a follow-up visit with a behaviour counsellor at 1 week, 1 month and 3 months (or whenever is needed). While this is ideal, most shelters do not have enough employees to manage the large volume of calls that this protocol would necessitate. Phone calls for behaviourally healthy pets can be conducted by trained volunteers, who are also educated about treatment of basic problems and refer clients with pets with problems to the behaviour staff.

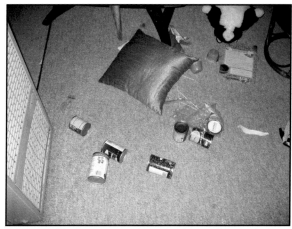

**23.10** The honeymoon is over – the newly adopted dog started to pull cans out of cupboards and chew on household items one month after adoption.

Volunteers can also staff the behaviour helpline. Follow-up calls and visits for pets with problems must be made by behaviour staff or highly trained and experienced volunteers.

## Conclusion

Rescue pets can make great companions, especially if obtained from a reputable shelter. Veterinary surgeons in practice have a responsibility not only to help and guide potential owners to appropriate sources, but also to support shelters and sanctuaries to ensure that they maintain standards that protect the welfare of the animals in their care and so fulfil their goals with regard to the successful rehoming of animals.

## References and further reading

Armstrong M, Avanzino R, Burns P *et al.* (2004) *The Asilomar Accords.* Available online at www.asilomaraccords.org

Braem M, Doherr MG, Lehmann D *et al.* (2008) Evaluating aggressive behavior in dogs: a comparison of 3 tests. *Journal of Veterinary Behavior: Clinical Applications and Research* **3**, 143–151

Christensen EL, Scarlett J, Campagna M and Houpt KA (2007) Aggressive behavior in adopted dogs that passed a temperament test. *Applied Animal Behaviour Science* **106**, 85–95

Diederich C and Giffroy J (2006) Behavioural testing in dogs: a review of methodology in search for standardisation. *Applied Animal Behaviour Science* **97**, 51–72

Diesel G, Pfeiffer DU and Brodbelt D (2008) Factors affecting the success of rehoming dogs in the UK during 2005. *Preventive Veterinary Medicine* **84**, 228–241

Diesel G, Smith H and Pfeiffer DU (2007) Factors affecting time to adoption of dogs re-homed by a charity in the UK. *Animal Welfare* **16**, 353–360

Gourkow N and Fraser D (2006) The effect of housing and handling practices on the welfare, behaviour and selection of domestic cats (*Felis sylvestris catus*) by adopters in an animal shelter. *Animal Welfare* **15**, 371–377

Hennessy MB, Davis HN, Williams MT *et al.* (1997) Plasma cortisol levels of dogs at a county animal shelter. *Physiology & Behavior* **62**, 485–490

Hiby EF, Rooney NJ and Bradshaw JWS (2006) Behavioural and physiological responses of dogs entering re-homing kennels. *Physiology & Behavior* **89**, 385–391

Kroll TL, Houpt KA and Erb HN (2004) The use of novel stimuli as indicators of aggressive behavior in dogs. *Journal of the American Animal Hospital Association* **1**, 13–19

Marston LC and Bennett PC (2003) Reforging the bond – towards successful canine adoption. *Applied Animal Behaviour Science* **83**, 227–245

Marston LC, Bennett PC and Coleman GJ (2004) What happens to shelter dogs? An analysis of data for 1 year from three Australian shelters. *Journal of Applied Animal Welfare Science* **7**, 27–47

McCobb EC, Patronek GJ, Marder A *et al.* (2005) Assessment of stress levels among cats in four animal shelters. *Journal of the American Veterinary Medical Association* **226**, 548–555

Salman MD, Hutchison J, Gallie-Ruch R *et al.* (2000) Behavioral reasons for relinquishment of dogs and cats to 12 shelters. *Journal of Applied Animal Welfare Science* **3**, 93–106

Salman MD, New JG Jr, Scarlett JM *et al.* (1998) Human and animal factors related to the relinquishment of dogs and cats in 12 selected animal shelters in the United States. *Journal of Applied Animal Welfare Science* **1**, 207–226

Segurson SA, Serpell JA and Hart BL (2005) Evaluation of a behavioral assessment questionnaire for use in the characterization of behavioral problems of dogs relinquished to animal shelters. *Journal of the American Veterinary Medical Association* **227**, 1755–1761

Serpell JA and Hsu Y (2001) Development and validation of a novel method for evaluating behavior and temperament in guide dogs. *Applied Animal Behaviour Science* **7**, 347–364

Stephen J and Ledger R (2007) Relinquishing dog owners' ability to predict behavioural problems in shelter dogs post adoption. *Applied Animal Behaviour Science* **107**, 88–89

Taylor KD and Mills DS (2006) The development and assessment of temperament tests for adult companion dogs. *Journal of Veterinary Behavior* **1**, 94–108

Taylor KD and Mills DS (2007) The effect of the kennel environment on canine welfare: a critical review of experimental studies. *Animal Welfare* **16**, 435–447

Tempany C and Mills DS (2008) Are dogs dummies when it comes to their perception of people? In: *Proceedings of the CABTSG Study Day 2008*, pp. 29–32

Weiss E (2007a) *Meet your match Canine-ality and Puppy-ality manual and training guide.* ASPCA, New York

Weiss, E (2007b) *Meet your match Feline-ality manual and training guide.* ASPCA, New York

Wells DL (2004) A review of environmental enrichment for kennelled dogs, *Canis familiaris. Applied Animal Behaviour Science* **85**, 307–317

## Client handouts (bsavalibrary.com/behaviour_leaflets)

- Adopting a rescue dog: the pros and cons
- Avoiding house soiling by cats
- Avoiding house soiling by dogs
- Avoiding urine marking by cats
- Canine behaviour questionnaire
- Cognitive dysfunction syndrome
- Down–stay mat exercises
- Environmental enrichment for cats in animal shelters
- Environmental enrichment for dogs in animal shelters
- Feline behaviour questionnaire
- Handling exercises for an aggressive cat
- Handling exercises for puppies and kittens
- Headcollar training
- How to find a good trainer
- Introducing a new cat into the household
- Ladder of Aggression
- 'Leave it' exercises
- Litterbox training
- Muzzle training
- Noise fear score sheet
- 'Nothing in Life is Free'
- Pet selection questionnaire
- Playing with your dog – toys
- Playing with your kitten
- Puppy socialization: getting used to new people
- Questionnaire to assess separation anxiety
- Recall exercises
- Redirected aggression in dogs
- Request for information on problem behaviours
- Sit–stay exercises
- Teaching your dog to go to a place on command
- The newly adopted rescue dog: preventing problems
- Treating a fear of car journeys using desensitization and counter-conditioning
- Treating a fear of the veterinary clinic using desensitization and counter-conditioning
- Treating separation anxiety in dogs
- What your cat needs
- What your cat needs: multi-cat households
- What your dog needs
- Your puppy's first year

# A glossary of behavioural terms

**Activity feeders**
Devices designed to make an animal work for its food ration. For example, the animal may have to push an object around for it to dispense food.

**Affective aggression**
Aggressive behaviour involving a marked mood change. This means it is associated with an assessment of the personal significance of any threat posed by the trigger or the response, e.g. competitive aggression. Predatory behaviour and play are not forms of affective aggression.

**Age-Related Cognitive and Affective Disorders (ARCAD) score**
A scoring system for the evaluation of age-related cognitive and affective disorders.

**Aggression**
A general term for all elements of attack, defence and threat behaviour.

**Agonistic behaviour**
All behaviours associated with fighting, including aggression, flight and appeasement behaviour.

**Allogrooming**
The act of grooming another individual.

**Allorubbing**
The act of rubbing against another individual.

**Anxiety**
The anticipation of danger or harm and associated emotional response.

**Appeasement behaviour**
Behaviour aimed at averting or diffusing aggression.

**Appetitive reinforcement**
Using the presentation or acquisition of something, such as food, to strengthen a behavioural response.

**ARCAD score**
See Age-Related Cognitive and Affective Disorders (ARCAD) score.

**Associative learning**
A form of learning in which the subject is required to make an association between two features or events.

**Avoiders**
Animals that associate with another individual colony member less than would be expected by chance.

**Basket-type muzzle**
A muzzle that encircles the mouth of a dog in a cage-like structure, preventing the dog from delivering a bite.

**Cat colonies**
Feline social groups formed whenever sufficient resources allow.

**Choke chain**
A chain link collar used in training to control a dog. Pulling the chain tightens the collar around the dog's neck. If the collar is properly applied it pulls and easily slides loose when tension is released (sometimes called a check chain); if applied improperly the collar remains tight and does not easily loosen.

**Classical (Pavlovian) conditioning**
Any procedure whereby a neutral stimulus comes to elicit a reflex response by being paired with a stimulus that regularly elicits that response.

**Classical (respondent) counter-conditioning**
Using an unconditional response, such as eating a treat, as a desired alternative to a problem behaviour, with the goal of creating a different emotional response to the target stimulus (strangers, animals, etc.)

**Cognitive dysfunction**
An age-related neurodegenerative disorder in dogs resulting in a decline in higher brain functions, including those involved in memory and learning. It is believed to resemble Alzheimer-type dementia in humans in both its symptomatology and pathophysiology.

**Conditional response**
A response to the association of an unconditional stimulus with a conditional stimulus.

**Conditional stimulus**
A stimulus that prior to any learning does not elicit a response, but following association with a stimulus that elicits an innate response becomes capable of eliciting a similar response.

**Conflict**
The product of two or more behaviours with a similar level of motivation competing for expression at the same time.

**Contiguity**
The relationship between two events in both time and/or place. Two events that occur in the same place and at the same time are said to be highly contiguous.

**Contingency**
The predictability of two events occurring together.

**Continuous reinforcement**
The provision of reinforcement every time a behaviour is performed.

# A glossary of behavioural terms

**Coprophagia**
Eating faeces.

**Core area**
The area within an animal's territory in which most recuperative, self-maintenance and social behaviours occur.

**Counter-conditioning**
The process whereby an animal learns a new response to a targeted stimulus (i.e. strangers, noise or other animals). This new response is different from, and incompatible with, the previously learned undesirable response.

**Critical periods**
Fixed short developmental stages involving irreversible learning. This term is inappropriately applied to dogs and cats, where the term sensitive phase is more appropriate.

**Dementia**
A general mental deterioration due to organic or psychological factors. In dogs it is often referred to as 'cognitive dysfunction'.

**Desensitization**
*See* Systematic desensitization.

**Differential reinforcement**
Reinforcement is only given for behaviours that meet a predetermined limit of frequency or duration.

**Differential schedule**
A method of reinforcement where the decision to reinforce a specific response is determined by some aspect of the behaviour. This can result in behavioural shaping or successive approximation to a final goal.

**Disorientation**
A delay in the recognition of people, places and objects, or total loss of such recognition.

**Dominance**
The relationship between two individuals that results in consistent precedence for resources, through one party giving way to the other. It is determined by observers from the outcome of repeated agonistic encounters.

**Dominance aggression**
A commonly used term for aggression occurring in differing circumstances; for example, in response to social provocation, aggression to owners in the context of competition, in response to dominant-appearing postures and interactions by the owner. The term is unreliable as a descriptive label and inappropriate as a diagnostic descriptor in favour of more descriptive and accurate terminology. It is unclear whether animals actually use an increase in social status as a motivating factor or whether they are responding to perceived threats.

Recent research suggests that social interactions between dogs over resources can be explained most easily by referring to their previous learning rather than any intrinsic social motivation (i.e. they are context- and subject-specific). Similarly, confusing terms include status-related aggression, dominance-related aggression and social conflict aggression.

**Dyad**
Two individuals or groups that interact with each other.

**Epigenesis**
The process involving the interaction between the environment and the individual's genotype to produce a given phenotype.

**Extinction**
The process resulting ultimately in the diminishing of a behaviour when no reinforcement is given after a response that is normally reinforced.

**Extinction burst**
The intensification of a behaviour as a result of frustration prior to its decline when reinforcement is withdrawn.

**Fear**
An emotion that induces an adaptive response that enables an animal to avoid situations and activities that could be dangerous.

**Flooding**
A psychotherapeutic technique whereby the patient is exposed to an arousing and possibly fearful stimulus without the opportunity of escape. Exposure continues until the animal shows no reaction to the stimulus. The goal of the technique is to desensitize the animal to non-harmful stimuli.

**Frustration**
The product of thwarting the expression of a motivated behaviour.

**Geriatric (senior) dog or cat**
The working definition is a dog or cat over 8 years old; however, the rate of ageing varies with breed, size, nutrition and lifestyle.

**Habituation**
Non-associative learning involving the reduction of a response through repeated exposure to the stimulus for the response and not the association of two events.

**Harness**
A restraint device embracing an animal's lower neck and chest.

**Headcollar**
A restraint device that encircles an animal's neck and muzzle (similar to a halter on a horse), to which a lead can be attached.

**House soiling**
The deposition of urine or faeces in an indoor location which the owner finds unacceptable.

**Housetraining**
The process of training an animal to eliminate in a desired location.

**Hyperkinesis/hyperactivity**
A rare clinical syndrome characterized by overactivity, attention deficits, impulsivity, high resting basal physiological parameters and a paradoxical calming response to amphetamines.

**Inappropriate elimination**
Elimination of urine or faeces that is not in the expected location.

**Instrumental (operant) counter-conditioning**
*See* Response substitution.

### Instrumental aggression
Aggression that has been learned through reinforcement of the behaviour (usually unintentional). For example, a dog that is aggressive towards people and is called off by offering it a treat.

### Intermittent reinforcement
The occasional provision of reinforcement in association with a particular behaviour.

### Irritable aggression
Aggressive behaviour associated with either underlying pain or emotional agitation, which alters the threshold of expression of aggression. It is a non-specific term and may include several ethologically different forms of aggression.

### Ladder of Aggression
A continuum of context-specific threat-averting gestures by dogs, with the least overt signals on the lowest rungs and progressing to overt aggression at the top.

### Latent learning
The acquisition of information that might affect behaviour at a later date without an apparent immediate change in behaviour.

### Marking
The deposition of urine (and less commonly faeces) to leave an olfactory message; unrelated to normal physiological emptying of the bladder or bowel.

### Meta-communication
The process whereby a communicative signal qualifies the behaviour that follows it. For example, a play bow which precedes a growl indicates that the growl is not indicative of an agonistic behaviour.

### Middening
The deposition of faeces in a prominent location, suggestive of marking behaviour.

### Negative punishment
The removal or withholding of a pleasurable event in response to a given behaviour, which decreases the probability of a behaviour recurring in similar circumstances in the future.

### Negative reinforcement
The removal or withholding of an unpleasant or aversive stimulus in response to a given behaviour, which increases the probability of a behaviour recurring in similar circumstances in the future.

### Neoteny
The slowing or delaying of adult developmental changes, leading to the retention of juvenile characteristics into adulthood. Neoteny is one of the processes that can lead to paedomorphosis.

### Noise phobia
An excessive fear response related to an auditory stimulus that is out of proportion to any actual or potential threat and is maladaptive for the individual.

### Nose-touch
Gentle nose to nose contact thought to be a greeting behaviour in cats.

### Observational learning (social learning)
Learning what to do in a given situation from observing the behaviour of another individual in that situation.

### Operant conditioning
Any procedure that makes a response more or less likely to occur as a result of its consequences.

### Overactivity
Term used to describe a condition when an animal is more active than might be expected. The condition is often a reaction to lack of stimulation at other times. Not to be confused with hyperkinesis.

### Paedomorphosis
The retention of juvenile morphological or behavioural characteristics into adulthood.

### Perichezia
Defecating around the home in unwanted locations.

### Periuria
Urinating around the home in unwanted locations.

### Pheromone therapy (pheromonatherapy)
The use in a clinical context of chemicals that are analogous to those naturally produced by animals for the purposes of intraspecific communication.

### Phobia
An excessive fear response that is out of proportion to any actual or potential threat and is maladaptive for the individual.

### Pica
An appetite for non-nutritive items such as stones, plastic or wool.

### Play aggression
Harm, or an apparent threat of harm, produced in the context of play. This is not a form of affective aggression.

### Positive punishment
The addition of an unpleasant or aversive stimulus in response to a given behaviour, which decreases the probability of a behaviour recurring in similar circumstances in the future.

### Positive reinforcement
The addition of a pleasant stimulus in response to a given behaviour, which increases the probability of a behaviour recurring in similar circumstances in the future.

### Preparedness
A biological predisposition allowing the more rapid formation of particular types of association. For example, certain breeds of dog may be more or less predisposed to develop noise fears, gun dog breeds being less at risk and some breeds of terrier being at greater risk.

### Prong collar (pinch collar; spike collar)
A chain link collar with blunt metal projections that protrude inwards. These are articulated such that when a dog pulls the projections stick into the neck. Pressure from the prongs is only relieved when tension is reduced.

### Puzzle feeder
A type of activity feeder where the animal is required to solve a puzzle to gain its food ration.

# A glossary of behavioural terms

**Rage**
A term which has been used in a variety of contexts to describe an extreme form of aggression but diagnostic criteria are inconsistent and not clear, and so the term is not of diagnostic value, though still widely used in the popular press.

**Redirected aggression**
Aggression that is directed to an individual but which arises as a result of the frustration of high arousal toward another. For example, redirected aggression by a dog can occur if an owner tries to intervene whilst the dog is barking at someone at the door. If the owner tries to pull the dog back, then the dog may momentarily turn and snap at the owner in an act of redirected aggression. Redirected aggression in cats may occur in a multi-cat household if one cat sees another posturing through a glass window. As the threat exchange escalates, the movement of a household cat nearby might provoke direction of the aggression toward the housemate. In both cases, the victim is not the same as the trigger of the aggressive behaviour.

**Reinforcement**
An event that increases or decreases the probability of an associated behaviour occurring again in similar circumstances. Often used in a narrow sense to mean a reward, i.e. something that increases behaviour.

**Resource-holding potential**
An index of competitive ability which allows the prediction of the outcome of interactions between competitors. It is determined by both physical attributes such as size, weight, age and the outcomes of previous encounters between familiar individuals.

**Respondent behaviour**
Behaviours that appear to be biologically linked to certain stimuli through an inherent predisposition, e.g. salivation in response to food.

**Response substitution**
The imposition of one behavioural reaction to a stimulus over another to the same stimulus. For example, a dog may be trained to go to bed instead of to bark when the doorbell rings.

**Sensitive phases**
Developmental stages when an animal is especially sensitive to learning a particular association that is relatively stable and enduring.

**Separation anxiety**
A group of separation-related problems characterized by a high level of anxiety in anticipation of the departure of a member of the household and subsequent behavioural reactions in the figure's absence, including vocalization, elimination, destructiveness and excessive salivation.

**Skinnerian (instrumental) conditioning**
This is also known as trial and error learning. *See* Operant conditioning.

**Social learning**
*See* Observational learning.

**Socialization period**
Stage of development during which young animals form primary social relationships beyond their immediate family and social behaviour emerges.

**Spraying**
The deposition of urine on vertical surfaces while a cat is in a standing posture.

**Status-related aggression**
*See* Dominance aggression.

**Stress response**
The body's physiological, psychological and behavioural responses to a challenge to its homeostatic state.

**Stressor**
A stimulus that elicits a stress response.

**Subordinance hierarchy**
A relationship based on alertness to deferent signals within individual relationships for determining relative rank.

**Systematic desensitization**
A psychotherapeutic technique in which the threshold at which an animal responds to a given situation is raised by exposing the animal to non-arousing levels of the component stimuli.

**Tail wrapping**
An affiliative signal consisting of intertwining of the tails of two cats, or laying of the tail of one cat over the back of another cat, other animal or human.

**Therapeutic bond**
The effective, social and professional relationship that binds the client and the veterinary surgeon and facilitates compliance with the treatment.

**Training discs**
A training aid consisting of a collection of sonorous discs, which are used to signal negative punishment, i.e. the discs are sounded and then food or some other reward removed.

**Umbilical cording**
Leashing a pet to its owner or a nearby piece of furniture whenever the owner is home and awake.

**Unconditional response**
An unlearned response.

**Unconditional stimulus**
The stimulus that evokes an unlearned response.

# Appendix

## Client handouts

This Appendix contains selected examples of the 37 handouts that accompany this Manual. To access the handouts, got to bsavalibrary.com/behaviour_handouts or scan the QR code on this page. Each document is provided as a PDF file with a text box in the top right-hand corner where practice details may be included prior to printing out. Readers may wish to print out a full set of handouts for their reference.

These handouts are the copyright of BSAVA. Readers may print out, copy and distribute these forms to their clients only as part of their consultation. Other than adding practice information, these handouts may not be altered in any way or used for any other purpose without prior written permission of the copyright holder, and may not be sold.

## Client questionnaires

The questionnaires have been designed for use by owners of dogs or cats with behavioural problems. The owner can be asked to fill in the form prior to, or during, the first behavioural consultation with the veterinary surgeon/counsellor.

These questionnaires are the copyright of BSAVA. Readers may print out and copy these forms for use with their clients only. They may not be altered in any way or used for any other purpose without prior written permission of the copyright holder, and may not be sold.

## Referral form

A referral form designed for use by general practitioners when referring cases for behavioural consultations is included. This referral form is approved by The British Veterinary Behaviour Association (BVBA) and was produced after consultation with the Royal College of Veterinary Surgeons.

The form is the copyright of the BVBA but readers may print out and copy it for their own use. It should not be used for any other purpose, and may not be sold.

# Canine behaviour questionnaire

Date _____

## Owner details

(Mr/Mrs/Miss/Ms) Surname/Family name _____ First name or Initials _____

Address _____
_____ Postcode _____

Phone (day) _____ (evening) _____
(mobile) _____ Fax _____
Email _____

**Please include as much information as possible. The more detail available, the more accurate our assessment of the case can be. Please use additional sheets where necessary.**

Have you owned a dog before?                         [   ] Yes        [   ] No
Have you owned this breed of dog before?      [   ] Yes        [   ] No
Have you owned other pets previously?          [   ] Yes        [   ] No

Please list other current household pets

| Type and breed | Name | Age | Spayed/neutered? | Relationship with dog (e.g. avoids, plays, fights) |
|---|---|---|---|---|
|  |  |  |  |  |
|  |  |  |  |  |
|  |  |  |  |  |
|  |  |  |  |  |
|  |  |  |  |  |

Please list the names, ages and occupations of other family members who live at home

| Name | Age | Occupation |
|---|---|---|
|  |  |  |
|  |  |  |
|  |  |  |
|  |  |  |
|  |  |  |

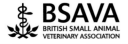

**BSAVA**
BRITISH SMALL ANIMAL
VETERINARY ASSOCIATION

# BSAVA CLIENT QUESTIONNAIRES: BEHAVIOUR SERIES

## Patient details

Name _____ Breed _____

Sex    [  ] Male    [  ] Female    [  ] Male neutered    [  ] Female spayed

Date of birth_____ Age when obtained (if known) _____

Date first acquired _____ Source _____

Reason(s) for obtaining this dog
_____
_____
_____

Has the dog ever been used for breeding?    [  ] Yes    [  ] No
If yes, at what age?  _____

How would you describe your dog's personality?
_____

Do you consider your dog to be:

[  ] Aggressive? (growling, snarling, snapping, nipping or biting in any circumstances)
[  ] Destructive?    [  ] Hyperactive/restless?    [  ] Disobedient?              [  ] Housetrained?
[  ] Nervous?        [  ] Excitable?               [  ] Noisy/excessive vocalization?
[  ] Depressed?      [  ] Demanding attention?     [  ] Playful?

## A    Medical history

1.    Please give a brief medical history, especially recurrent problems and treatment.
      Use an extra sheet if necessary
      _____
      _____
      _____

2.    Vaccination status    _____

3.    Date last wormed    _____

4.    Is your dog currently on any regular medications (such as allergy medication, heartworm treatment, herbal or homeopathic remedies)?

| Drug/remedy | Dose |
|---|---|
|  |  |
|  |  |
|  |  |

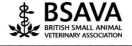
BRITISH SMALL ANIMAL
VETERINARY ASSOCIATION

Canine behaviour questionnaire
© BSAVA 2009
BSAVA Manual of Canine and Feline Behavioural Medicine, 2nd edition

# BSAVA CLIENT QUESTIONNAIRES: BEHAVIOUR SERIES

5.  Has your dog been on medication for his/her behaviour in the past?
    If yes, please list name and dosage (include herbals and homeopathics)

| Drug/remedy | Dose |
|---|---|
| | |
| | |
| | |

6.  Is your dog on any medication for his/her behaviour now?
    If yes, please list name and dosage (include herbals and homeopathics)

| Drug/remedy | Dose |
|---|---|
| | |
| | |
| | |

## B  Early history

1.  Please give details of the dog's early life, if known, including litter size, age of weaning, age when obtained, whether raised outside or indoors, if orphan or stray, whether hand-reared, etc.

    _____
    _____
    _____

2.  How much interaction did the puppy have with people in the first year of his/her life? _____
    _____

3.  What method of housetraining was used? _____

4.  How did you react to any mistakes during housetraining? _____

5.  Did your puppy attend puppy 'parties' or classes? If so, please give details_____
    _____

## C  Training and obedience

1.  Has your dog ever attended training classes?     [   ] Yes     [   ] No

2.  If Yes, please give details (when, where, age of dog, who took it to the class)_____
    _____

3.  What types of training techniques were used in the class? _____
    _____

4.  What training methods have you used? _____
    _____

5.  How well did your dog do in the class?     [   ] Very well        [   ] Average
                                                [   ] Poor            [   ] Was asked to leave
    If asked to leave, please say why _____

## BSAVA CLIENT QUESTIONNAIRES: BEHAVIOUR SERIES

6.    Do you think your dog is Good, Average or Poor at learning?  [ ] Good  [ ] Average  [ ] Poor

7.    What tasks will the dog reliably perform for you on command?
    [ ] Sit    [ ] Stay    [ ] Down    [ ] Fetch    [ ] Other _____

8.    Does your dog do 'tricks' (such as shake, rollover)? _____

9.    Does your dog pull when on the lead?    [ ] Yes    [ ] No

10.    Is your dog more obedient in some places than in others?    [ ] Yes    [ ] No
    If Yes, please give details: _____
    _____

11.    Is your dog more obedient with some people than with others?    [ ] Yes    [ ] No
    If Yes, please give details: _____
    _____

12.    How do you correct your dog when he/she misbehaves? _____
    _____

### D    Diet and feeding

1.    What types of food (and brands) do you give your dog? _____
    _____

2.    How much does he/she eat a day? _____

3.    When and where is the dog fed? (how often and at what time) _____

4.    If there is more than one dog in the home, how many food bowls are provided? _____
    Where are the food bowls situated? _____

5.    Who feeds the dog? _____

6.    Is the dog protective (stiffening, growling, snapping or biting) around the food?  [ ] Yes  [ ] No
    Details _____

7.    Is his/her appetite Good or Poor?  [ ] Good  [ ] Poor

8.    Does your dog eat Quickly or Slowly?  [ ] Quickly  [ ] Slowly

9.    What are his/her favourite foods? _____

10.    Do you have to be present for him/her to eat?  [ ] Yes  [ ] No

11.    How much does your dog drink each day (in pints or litres)? _____

12.    Do you add supplements or titbits to the diet?  [ ] Yes  [ ] No
    If yes, what and why? _____

13.    Is he/she given bones or chews? _____
    Is he/she possessive with these? _____

14.    Do you consider your dog to be at the correct weight?  [ ] Yes  [ ] No
    Please fill in your dog's weight _____

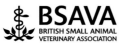

---

# BSAVA CLIENT QUESTIONNAIRES: BEHAVIOUR SERIES

## E    Daily activities

### Sleeping and waking
1.    Where does your dog sleep? _____

2.    If your dog sleeps on the bed, who invites him/her up? _____

3.    When does the dog get up in the morning? _____

4.    Does your dog ever wake you at night?    [   ] Yes    [   ] No
      If yes, how often and why? _____

### Going outside
5.    When does your dog go outside and for how long? _____

6.    How does your dog ask to go outside? _____

7.    Does he/she roam free in a garden or yard? _____

8.    What type of fencing is used to restrain the dog? _____

9.    Is your dog keen to explore when on its own? _____

### Toileting
10.    Where does your dog tend to go to the toilet? _____

11.    Does your dog spot mark with small amounts of urine?    [   ] Yes    [   ] No
       If so, where? _____

12.    How often does he/she empty his/her bladder in a day? _____

13.    How frequently does he/she empty his/her bowels? _____

### Exercise
14.    What sort of exercise (e.g. walking on/off lead, running off lead, agility training) does your dog
       receive and how much?

| Type | Purpose | Amount | Frequency |
|------|---------|--------|-----------|
|      |         |        |           |
|      |         |        |           |
|      |         |        |           |
|      |         |        |           |
|      |         |        |           |

15.    Who takes the dog for exercise?

### Play/training
16.    Is there any specific time devoted to play and/or training on a daily basis?    [   ] Yes    [   ] No

17.    Does your dog play games with you or other family members?    [   ] Yes    [   ] No
       Details_____

18     Who initiates play: people or the pet? _____

19     What types of toys does your dog play with? _____

**BSAVA**
BRITISH SMALL ANIMAL
VETERINARY ASSOCIATION

Canine behaviour questionnaire
© BSAVA 2009
BSAVA Manual of Canine and Feline Behavioural Medicine, 2nd edition

# BSAVA CLIENT QUESTIONNAIRES: BEHAVIOUR SERIES

### 'Home alone'

20.   Is your dog left home alone in the house? _____

21.   Where does the dog stay during the day when no one is home? _____

22.   What does he/she do as you prepare to depart? _____

23.   Does your dog ever bark or whine when you leave?    [  ] Yes    [  ] No

24.   Does your dog ever [   ] vocalize, [   ] toilet, or [   ] engage in destructive behaviour while you are gone?

25.   Typically, how long is your dog alone without people on any given day? _____

26.   What arrangements are made for your dog when you go on holiday? _____

### Family routine

27.   What does he/she do during family meals? _____

28.   Has there been a change in your household routine (e.g. new work hours, new baby, moving, new roommate or visitors, boarding, diet change)?    [  ] Yes    [  ] No
      Details_____

### Favourite things

Please list 5 things your dog enjoys most; these may be foods, toys or activities

_____   _____   _____   _____   _____

## F    Interaction with family members

### The home environment

1.   What type of home do you have (e.g. flat/apartment, house) _____

2.   What areas of the house does your dog have access to? _____

3.   Where does your dog sleep at night? _____

4.   Does he/she have their own bed? _____

### Reaction to handling by family members

5.   Is there aggression in the following circumstances? This can include growling, snarling (showing teeth), lunging, nipping, snapping or biting. Please fill in the chart: (Y=Yes, N=No, N/A=doesn't apply). If biting has occurred in any of these circumstances, please describe the wound (tear, puncture, bruising)

|                        | Adult owner (female) | Adult owner (male) | Children | Any specific individual |
|------------------------|----------------------|--------------------|----------|-------------------------|
| Handling/grooming      |                      |                    |          |                         |
| Petting or hugging     |                      |                    |          |                         |
| Disturbed when resting |                      |                    |          |                         |
| Discipling             |                      |                    |          |                         |
| Walking on the lead    |                      |                    |          |                         |
| Taking food away       |                      |                    |          |                         |
| Taking other objects   |                      |                    |          |                         |

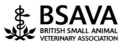

Canine behaviour questionnaire
© BSAVA 2009
BSAVA Manual of Canine and Feline Behavioural Medicine, 2nd edition

# BSAVA CLIENT QUESTIONNAIRES: BEHAVIOUR SERIES

## G    Interaction with others

### Reaction to visitors

1.    How does your dog behave when visitors come to the house (e.g. barking, door charging)?

_____

2.    Is the behaviour different toward familiar and unfamiliar people?    [  ] Yes    [  ] No
      If yes, describe _____

3.    Is the behaviour different toward people outside the house and people inside the house?
                                                              [  ] Yes    [  ] No
      If yes, describe _____

4.    Does your dog display aggression (growling, snarling, snapping or biting) to visitors to your home?
                                                              [  ] Yes    [  ] No
      If yes, describe _____

5.    Has your dog ever bitten or attacked anyone?    [  ] Yes    [  ] No

6.    Please fill in details of any regular visitors to the home

| Name (if known) | Purpose | Time & Days | Dog's reaction |
|---|---|---|---|
|  |  |  |  |
|  |  |  |  |
|  |  |  |  |
|  |  |  |  |

7.    What is the dog's response to other visitors?

| Frequent visitors | Occasional visitors | Rare visitors |
|---|---|---|
|  |  |  |

### Reactions to other people

8.    Please describe your dog's reaction to each of the following:

|  | In the home | Out of the home |
|---|---|---|
| Familiar men |  |  |
| Familiar women |  |  |
| Familiar children |  |  |
| Unknown men |  |  |
| Unknown women |  |  |
| Unknown children |  |  |
| Familiar dogs |  |  |
| Unknown dogs |  |  |
| Other animals |  |  |
| Crowds/busy areas |  |  |

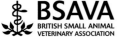
**BSAVA** BRITISH SMALL ANIMAL VETERINARY ASSOCIATION

Canine behaviour questionnaire
© BSAVA 2009
BSAVA Manual of Canine and Feline Behavioural Medicine, 2nd edition

## BSAVA CLIENT QUESTIONNAIRES: BEHAVIOUR SERIES

**Reactions to other animals**

9.  What is the reaction to other dogs when out at exercise?
    On a lead _____
    Free exercise _____

10. What is the reaction to other animals, e.g. squirrels, unfamiliar cats? _____
    _____

### H    Other behaviours

1.  Does your dog ever show inappropriate mounting or other sexual activity?   [   ] Yes   [   ] No
    If so, to whom or what?_____

2.  Is your dog ever protective over parts of his/her body (especially ears and feet)?   [   ] Yes   [   ] No
    If yes, which regions? _____

3.  Does your dog lick or chew on themselves more than you would expect?   [   ] Yes   [   ] No

### I    The current problem

1.  What is the current problem(s) you are having with your dog? Please describe it briefly_____
    _____
    _____

2.  When did it begin? _____

3.  How long has it been present? _____

4.  How old was the dog when it began? _____

5.  Where does the problem occur?_____

6.  With whom? _____

7.  How often? _____

8.  Other details _____
    _____
    _____

### J    Aggression

Please answer the questions below if the problem is aggression:

1.  Describe the most recent incident and the setting it occurred in (try to be very precise, as if you were drawing a picture):

    a)  Where was the dog? _____
    b)  Where was everyone in relation to the dog? _____
    c)  What was everyone doing before the incident? _____
    d)  What did the dog do?_____
    e)  What was the dog's body posture? Describe the position of ears, tail, face, hair on back, or draw a picture if necessary _____
        _____
        _____

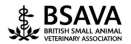

**BSAVA**
BRITISH SMALL ANIMAL
VETERINARY ASSOCIATION

Canine behaviour questionnaire
© BSAVA 2009
BSAVA Manual of Canine and Feline Behavioural Medicine, 2nd edition

## BSAVA CLIENT QUESTIONNAIRES: BEHAVIOUR SERIES

2. What was your reaction to the behaviour? _____

3. How did the dog react to your reaction? _____

4. Was there any punishment? _____

5. If there was a bite wound was it a puncture wound or a tear? _____

6. Going back in time, describe the 3 most recent incidents of the behaviour. Please use additional pages for this _____

7. How frequently does the problem occur?  [  ] Times per day      [  ] Times per week
    [  ] Times per month      [  ] Times per year

8. When does the problem occur?
    When left alone?      [  ] Always      [  ] Usually
    [  ] Rarely      [  ] Never
    When family members are present?      [  ] Always      [  ] Usually
    [  ] Rarely      [  ] Never

9. What has been done to correct the problem? _____

10. Is the problem getting:    [  ] Better    [  ] Worse    [  ] No change?

11. Do you suspect any cause? _____

### K    House soiling

If the problem is house soiling, does it take place:
When you are not present?      [  ] Yes    [  ] No
When someone is home?      [  ] Yes    [  ] No

### L    Destruction

If the problem is destruction, does it take place:
When you are not present?      [  ] Yes    [  ] No
When you are home?      [  ] Yes    [  ] No

### M    Other problems
What other behaviours does your dog engage in that are objectionable to you? _____
_____
_____

Does his/her behaviour cause arguments at home? _____
_____
_____

### N    You and your dog

1. How would you describe your relationship with this dog?
    Adult owners (female) _____
    Adult owners (male) _____
    Children _____

**BSAVA**
BRITISH SMALL ANIMAL
VETERINARY ASSOCIATION

Canine behaviour questionnaire
© BSAVA 2009
BSAVA Manual of Canine and Feline Behavioural Medicine, 2nd edition

## BSAVA CLIENT QUESTIONNAIRES: BEHAVIOUR SERIES

2.  What are your feelings about the dog's present behaviour?
    Adult owners (female) _____
    Adult owners (male) _____
    Children _____

3.  How would you ideally like your dog to be? _____

4.  Under what circumstances would you consider euthanasia? _____
    _____

5.  What is your expectation for change? _____

6.  Is there anything else you would like to add about your dog and its behaviour?
    Please give any other information you think is relevant to the case _____
    _____
    _____
    _____
    _____
    _____
    _____
    _____
    _____
    _____
    _____
    _____
    _____
    _____
    _____

Questionnaire completed by (print) _____

Signature _____ Date _____

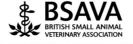

## BSAVA CLIENT QUESTIONNAIRES: BEHAVIOUR SERIES

# Feline behaviour questionnaire

Date _____

## Owner details

(Mr/Mrs/Miss/Ms) Surname/Family name _____  First name or Initials _____

Address _____
_____  Postcode _____

Phone (day) _____  (evening) _____
(mobile) _____  Fax _____
Email _____

**Please include as much information as possible. The more detail available, the more accurate our assessment of the case can be. Please use additional sheets where necessary.**

Have you owned a cat before?               [  ] Yes     [  ] No
Have you owned this breed of cat before?   [  ] Yes     [  ] No
Have you owned other pets previously?      [  ] Yes     [  ] No

Please list other current household pets

| Type and breed | Name | Age | Spayed/neutered? | Relationship with cat (e.g. avoids, plays, fights) |
|---|---|---|---|---|
|  |  |  |  |  |
|  |  |  |  |  |
|  |  |  |  |  |
|  |  |  |  |  |
|  |  |  |  |  |

Please list the names, ages and occupations of other family members who live at home

| Name | Age | Occupation |
|---|---|---|
|  |  |  |
|  |  |  |
|  |  |  |
|  |  |  |
|  |  |  |

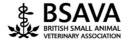
**BSAVA**
BRITISH SMALL ANIMAL
VETERINARY ASSOCIATION

Feline behaviour questionnaire
© BSAVA 2009
BSAVA Manual of Canine and Feline Behavioural Medicine, 2nd edition

## BSAVA CLIENT QUESTIONNAIRES: BEHAVIOUR SERIES

### Patient details

Name _____  Breed _____

Sex  [  ] Male   [  ] Female   [  ] Male neutered   [  ] Female spayed

Date of birth_____  Age when obtained (if known) _____

Date first acquired _____  Source _____

Reason(s) for obtaining this cat:

_____

_____

_____

Has the cat ever been used for breeding?     [  ] Yes     [  ] No
If yes, at what age?  _____

How would you describe your cat's personality?

_____

Do you consider your cat to be:

[  ] Aggressive? (growling, hissing, scratching, nipping or biting in any circumstances)
[  ] Destructive?   [  ] Hyperactive/restless?   [  ] Disobedient?
[  ] Nervous?       [  ] Excitable?              [  ] Noisy/excessive vocalization?
[  ] Depressed?     [  ] Demanding attention?    [  ] Playful?

### A    Medical history

1.    Please give a brief medical history, especially recurrent problems (such as fur balls and fight injuries) and treatment. Use an extra sheet if necessary

_____

_____

_____

2.    Vaccination status    _____

3.    Date last wormed    _____

4.    Is your cat currently on any regular medications (such as allergy medication, herbal or homeopathic remedies)?

| Drug/remedy | Dose |
|---|---|
|  |  |
|  |  |
|  |  |

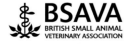

## BSAVA CLIENT QUESTIONNAIRES: BEHAVIOUR SERIES

5.  Has your cat been on medication for his/her behaviour in the past?
    If yes, please list name and dosage (include herbals and homeopathics)

| Drug/remedy | Dose |
|---|---|
|  |  |
|  |  |
|  |  |

6.  Is your cat on any medication for his/her behaviour now?
    If yes, please list name and dosage (include herbals and homeopathics)

| Drug/remedy | Dose |
|---|---|
|  |  |
|  |  |
|  |  |

### B    Early history

1.  Please give details of the cat's early life, if known, including litter size, age of weaning, age when obtained, whether raised outside or indoors, if orphan or stray, whether hand-reared, etc.

2.  How much interaction did the kitten have with people (frequency, numbers of people) in the first year of his/her life? _____

3.  What method of litter training was used? _____

4.  How did you react to any mistakes during litter training? _____

5.  Did your kitten attend kitten 'parties' or classes? If so, please give details _____

### C    Diet and feeding

1.  What types of food (and brands) do you give your cat? _____

2.  How much does he/she eat a day? Please state actual weight if known _____

3.  When and where is the cat fed? _____

4.  Who feeds the cat? _____

5.  How many food bowls are provided? _____

6.  Where are the food bowls placed? _____

7.  Is his/her appetite Good or Poor?    [ ] Good    [ ] Poor

**BSAVA**
BRITISH SMALL ANIMAL
VETERINARY ASSOCIATION

Feline behaviour questionnaire
© BSAVA 2009
BSAVA Manual of Canine and Feline Behavioural Medicine, 2nd edition

## BSAVA CLIENT QUESTIONNAIRES: BEHAVIOUR SERIES

8. Does your cat eat Quickly or Slowly?     [  ] Quickly     [  ] Slowly

9. What are his/her favourite foods? _____

10. How much water does your cat drink each day (in pints or litres)?_____

11. How much milk does your cat drink each day (in pints or litres)?_____

12. Do you add supplements or titbits to the diet?     [  ] Yes     [  ] No
    If yes, what and why? _____

## D     Daily activities

**Sleeping and waking and resting**

1. Where does your cat sleep at night? _____

2. Where does he/she sleep during the day? _____

3. Is your cat very active at night?     [  ] Yes     [  ] No

4. When does he/she get up in the morning?_____

5. Does your cat tend to seek out high places to rest?     [  ] Yes     [  ] No

6. Where can the cat normally be found during the day? _____

**Toileting**

7. Do you provide a litterbox?     [  ] Yes     [  ] No
    If Yes, how many are there? _____

8. Where is/are the box/boxes located? _____

9. Does the cat use a litterbox on a regular basis?     [  ] Yes     [  ] No

10. How often is/are the box/boxes cleared of waste material (scooped out)?_____

11. Does your cat ever eliminate outside the litterbox inside the house?     [  ] Yes     [  ] No
    If yes, please complete section I below.

**Going outside**

12. Does your cat have access to a garden or yard?     [  ] Yes     [  ] No

13. Is access controlled or free through a cat door?_____

14. How often do you see other cats in your garden?     [  ] Daily          [  ] Several times a week
                                                        [  ] Once a week     [  ] Rarely

15. How much time is spent outdoors by your cat each day?     In Summer _____
                                                             In Winter_____

**Roaming**

16. What area is available to the cat to roam? _____

17. How far does he/she roam on average?     [  ] Stays in the garden     [  ] May go to next door or two
                                             [  ] Further ranging

18. Does your cat stay away from home for several days at a time?     [  ] Yes     [  ] No

**BSAVA**
BRITISH SMALL ANIMAL
VETERINARY ASSOCIATION

Feline behaviour questionnaire
© BSAVA 2009
BSAVA Manual of Canine and Feline Behavioural Medicine, 2nd edition

# BSAVA CLIENT QUESTIONNAIRES: BEHAVIOUR SERIES

**Territory**

19.   Does the cat defend territory against other cats?      [  ] Yes      [  ] No
      If yes, describe his/her reaction _____

**Hunting**

20.   Does your cat catch prey and bring it into the house?      [  ] Occasionally      [  ] Regularly

21.   What type of prey does he/she catch? _____
      _____

**'Home alone'**

22.   How long is your cat alone without people on any given day? _____

23.   What arrangements are made for the cat if you are away from home for a while, e.g. on holiday?
      _____

**Play**

24.   Is your cat playful?      [  ] Yes      [  ] No

25.   Is there any specific time devoted to play on a daily basis?      [  ] Yes      [  ] No
      If so, how much? _____

26.   Who initiates play: people or the cat?      [  ] People      [  ] Cat

27.   What types of toys does your cat play with? _____

28.   Does your cat come when called or do any 'tricks'?      [  ] Yes      [  ] No

**Scratching**

29.   Do you have a scratching post?      [  ] Yes      [  ] No
      If yes, please describe it _____
      How many are available in the home? _____
      Where are they placed? _____

30.   Does your cat use the scratching post?      [  ] Yes      [  ] Sometimes      [  ] Never

**Family routine**

31.   Has there been a change in your household routine (e.g. new work hours, new baby, moving, new
      roommate or visitors, boarding, diet change)?      [  ] Yes      [  ] No
      Details_____
      _____

## E      The home environment

1.    What type of home do you have (e.g. flat/apartment – ground floor/upper floor, house)?
      _____

2.    How would you describe your home?      [  ] Quiet      [  ] Lively      [  ] Chaotic

3.    What areas of the house does your cat have access to? _____

4.    Please draw on a separate sheet of paper a map of the layout of your home with the cat's key
      areas (e.g. feeding, litterbox, favourite rest areas) indicated. Please indicate any windows through
      which the cat can see the outside

5.    Is your cat keen to explore?      [  ] Yes      [  ] No

**BSAVA**
BRITISH SMALL ANIMAL
VETERINARY ASSOCIATION

Feline behaviour questionnaire
© BSAVA 2009
BSAVA Manual of Canine and Feline Behavioural Medicine, 2nd edition

## BSAVA CLIENT QUESTIONNAIRES: BEHAVIOUR SERIES

6.    If you have more than one cat, when do you see them all in the same room? _____

7.    Do some cats spend most of their time in only certain locations?    [  ] Yes    [  ] No
      If yes, which cats and where do they stay? _____

### F    Interaction with others

1.    How does your cat behave when visitors come to the house? (e.g. hides, acts interested, interacts with them)? _____

2.    Is the behaviour different toward familiar and unfamiliar people?    [  ] Yes    [  ] No
      If yes, describe _____

3.    Is your cat quick to approach new people?    [  ] Yes    [  ] No

4.    Has your cat ever bitten anyone?    [  ] Yes    [  ] No
      If yes and this is NOT the primary complaint please give brief details of circumstances

      _____

      If yes and this IS the primary complaint, please complete section **J**

5.    Please fill in details of any regular visitors to the home

| Name (if known) | Purpose | Time & Days | Cat's reaction |
|---|---|---|---|
|  |  |  |  |
|  |  |  |  |
|  |  |  |  |
|  |  |  |  |

6.    What is your cat's response to other visitors?

| Frequent visitors | Occasional visitors | Rare visitors |
|---|---|---|
|  |  |  |

7.    Please describe your cat's reaction to each of the following:

|  | In the home | Out of the home |
|---|---|---|
| Familiar men |  |  |
| Familiar women |  |  |
| Familiar children |  |  |
| Unknown men |  |  |
| Unknown women |  |  |
| Unknown children |  |  |
| Familiar dogs |  |  |
| Unknown dogs |  |  |
| Familiar cats |  |  |
| Unknown cats |  |  |

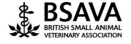

**BSAVA** BRITISH SMALL ANIMAL VETERINARY ASSOCIATION

Feline behaviour questionnaire
© BSAVA 2009
BSAVA Manual of Canine and Feline Behavioural Medicine, 2nd edition

# BSAVA CLIENT QUESTIONNAIRES: BEHAVIOUR SERIES

## G    Other behaviours

1.    When does your cat miaow?_____

2.    When does he/she growl?  _____

3.    When does he/she purr?  _____

4.    Is your cat aggressive when denied something it wants?    [  ] Yes    [  ] No

5.    Does your cat ever show inappropriate mounting or other sexual activity?    [  ] Yes    [  ] No
      If so, to whom or what?_____

6.    Does your cat Tolerate, Enjoy or Resist:
      Handling     [  ] Tolerate    [  ] Enjoy    [  ] Resist
      Grooming    [  ] Tolerate    [  ] Enjoy    [  ] Resist

7.    Does your cat lick or chew on itself more than you would expect?    [  ] Yes    [  ] No
      If yes, where on the body? _____

8.    How do you correct your cat when he/she misbehaves? _____

## H    The current problem
*Please also refer to specific sections below*

1.    What is the current problem you are having with your cat? Please describe it briefly _____
      _____
      _____

2.    When did it begin? _____

3.    How long has it been present? _____

4.    How old was the cat when it began?  _____

5.    Did the onset of the problem coincide with any event, or action, you can identify? _____
      _____

6.    Where does the problem occur?_____

7.    With whom? _____

8.    How often? _____

9.    Other details _____
      _____
      _____

10.   What has been tried to correct or change the problem?_____

11.   Is the problem getting:    [  ] Better    [  ] Worse    [  ] No change?

12.   Do you suspect any cause? _____

13.   Describe the 3 most recent incidents of the behaviour. Use separate pages as required
      _____
      _____
      _____
      _____

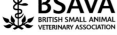

# BSAVA CLIENT QUESTIONNAIRES: BEHAVIOUR SERIES

**I    Elimination and marking problems (house soiling)**
*Please answer the questions below if the problem is elimination or marking (house soiling)*

**Elimination behaviour**

1.    Does the cat use a litterbox?    [  ] Yes    [  ] No    How often? _____

2.    Does the cat use the litterbox for:    [  ] Urine only    [  ] Faeces only    [  ] Neither

3.    Does the cat bury its urine?    [  ] Yes    [  ] No

4.    Does your cat bury its faeces?    [  ] Always    [  ] Usually    [  ] Occasionally
                                        [  ] Rarely    [  ] Never    [  ] Don't know

5.    Is there much digging and scratching in and around the litterbox?    [  ] Yes    [  ] No

6.    Does your cat ever eliminate outside the litterbox inside the house?    [  ] Yes    [  ] No

**Litterbox**

7.    How many litterboxes are there? _____

8.    What type (e.g. covered, uncovered)? _____

9.    What shape and size? _____

10.    Where is/are it/they located? _____

**Litter**

11.    What type of litter material do you use? _____

12.    Do you always use the same brand?    [  ] Yes    [  ] No

13.    Are there odour control granules added?    [  ] Yes    [  ] No

**Litterbox cleaning**

14.    How often is the litterbox cleared of waste material (scooped out)?_____

15.    How often is it completely cleared out and washed? _____

16.    What do you use to clean the litterbox? _____

17.    Have you recently changed the litter material or cleaning solution used?    [  ] Yes    [  ] No

18.    How often do you provide a completely new box? _____

**Problem details**

19.    Is the cat leaving faeces, urine or both outside the litterbox?    [  ] Faeces    [  ] Urine    [  ] Both

20.    How often does this occur?    [  ] Once a week    [  ] Once a month
                                        [  ] Once a day    [  ] Always

21.    What time of day do you usually find the urine or faeces outside the litterbox?
        (a.m., p.m., before work, overnight, etc.) _____

22.    How big is the spot of urine? _____

23.    How many times a day does your cat defecate? _____

24.    Do you recall the first time you found urine or faeces outside of the litterbox?    [  ] Yes    [  ] No
        If yes, please provide the details surrounding the incident_____
        _____

**BSAVA**
**BRITISH SMALL ANIMAL**
**VETERINARY ASSOCIATION**

Feline behaviour questionnaire
© BSAVA 2009
BSAVA Manual of Canine and Feline Behavioural Medicine, 2nd edition

# BSAVA CLIENT QUESTIONNAIRES: BEHAVIOUR SERIES

25. Where is the cat depositing urine/faeces outside the litterbox? Please list the room/rooms and all the locations in the room/rooms. Also specify if the deposits are found near windows, doors, plants, furniture, etc. How many spots/deposits are there in a given room?

| Room | Locations | Number of spots/deposits |
|------|-----------|--------------------------|
|      |           |                          |
|      |           |                          |
|      |           |                          |
|      |           |                          |
|      |           |                          |
|      |           |                          |

26. Please draw a floor plan of the house, noting litterbox location and sites of urination and/or defecation outside the litterbox. Please also include resting places in cases of conflict between cats and indicate any specific locations of such conflict

27. Has there been a change in litterbox location?　　[ ] Yes　　[ ] No
If yes, how recent was this? _____
From where to where? _____

28. Has there been a change in litter type?　　[ ] Yes　　[ ] No
If yes, how recent was this? _____
From what to what? _____

29. Has there been a change in litterbox cleaning routine?　　[ ] Yes　　　　[ ] No
Is the box cleaned less or more often?　　　　　　　　　[ ] Less often　　[ ] More often

30. When the problem first began, can you recall any unusual incident or anything that might have upset the cat? (For example, moving house, new roommates, unusual noises, new work hours, addition of another pet, a new baby, food changes) _____
_____

31. Have there been any recent changes in your personal routine?_____

32. Have there been any recent changes in living arrangements?_____

33. Have you ever caught the cat depositing urine or faeces outside the litterbox?　　[ ] Yes　　[ ] No
What was your response? _____
What was the cat's response? _____

34. What posture does the cat assume when urinating or spraying outside the box?
[ ] Standing　　[ ] Squatting

35. Where is the urine located?　　[ ] On the floor
　　　　　　　　　　　　　　　　　[ ] On the walls about 6 to 8 inches up from the floor?

36. Is this spraying or urination?　　[ ] Spraying　　[ ] Urination

37. Are there many cats outdoors in the immediate vicinity of your cat?　　[ ] Yes　　[ ] No

38. Is your cat agitated by the presence of other cats?　　[ ] Yes　　[ ] No

39. Are you the cat's first owner?　　[ ] Yes　　[ ] No
If no, were there similar problems in a previous home?　　[ ] Yes　　[ ] No

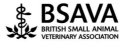

Feline behaviour questionnaire
© BSAVA 2009
BSAVA Manual of Canine and Feline Behavioural Medicine, 2nd edition

# BSAVA CLIENT QUESTIONNAIRES: BEHAVIOUR SERIES

40. If you have more than one cat, are there additional litterboxes?    [  ] Yes    [  ] No
How many? _____
Where are they? _____

41. Does this cat interact with the other cats in the home?    [  ] Yes    [  ] No

42. Does this cat fight with or avoid any of the other cats in the home?    [  ] Yes    [  ] No
If yes, which cat does it fight with or avoid? _____
Which cats does this cat associate with? _____

43. Does this cat have a previous history of urinary tract infections?    [  ] Yes    [  ] No

44. When was the last time a urine sample was examined? _____

45. What have you done in the past to try and change the behaviour? _____
_____

## J    Aggression
*Please answer the questions below if the problem is aggression:*

1. Describe the most recent incident and the setting it occurred in (try to be very precise, as if you were drawing a picture):

   a)  Where was the cat? _____
   b)  Where was everyone in relation to the cat? _____
       _____
   c)  What was everyone doing before the incident? _____
       _____
   d)  What did the cat do? _____
       _____
   e)  What was the cat's body posture? Describe the position of ears, tail, face, hair on back, or draw a picture if necessary _____
       _____
       _____

2. What was your reaction to the behaviour? _____

3. How did the cat react to your reaction? _____

4. Was there any punishment? _____

5. If there was a bite wound was it a puncture wound or a tear? _____

6. How frequently does the problem occur?    [  ] Times per day    [  ] Times per week
                                              [  ] Times per month   [  ] Times per year

7. When does the problem occur?
   When left alone?                  [  ] Always    [  ] Usually    [  ] Rarely    [  ] Never
   When family members are present?  [  ] Always    [  ] Usually    [  ] Rarely    [  ] Never

## K    Other problems

Does your cat have any other behavioural problems (e.g. scratching, excessive miaowing, plant eating)?
_____
_____
_____

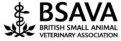

Feline behaviour questionnaire
© BSAVA 2009
BSAVA Manual of Canine and Feline Behavioural Medicine, 2nd edition

# BSAVA CLIENT QUESTIONNAIRES: BEHAVIOUR SERIES

## L    You and your cat

1.   How would you describe your relationship with this cat?
     Adult owners (female) _____
     Adult owners (male) _____
     Children _____

2.   What are your feelings about the cat's present behaviour?
     Adult owners (female) _____
     Adult owners (male) _____
     Children _____

3.   How would you ideally like your cat to be? _____

4.   Under what circumstances would you consider euthanasia? _____

5.   What is your expectation for change? _____

6.   Is there anything else you would like to add about your cat and its behaviour? _____
     Please give any other information you think is relevant to the case _____

     _____
     _____
     _____
     _____
     _____
     _____
     _____
     _____
     _____
     _____
     _____
     _____
     _____
     _____

Questionnaire completed by (print) _____

Signature _____ Date _____

**BSAVA**
BRITISH SMALL ANIMAL
VETERINARY ASSOCIATION

Feline behaviour questionnaire
© BSAVA 2009
BSAVA Manual of Canine and Feline Behavioural Medicine, 2nd edition

## BSAVA CLIENT HANDOUTS: BEHAVIOUR SERIES

# Adopting a rescue dog: the pros and cons
*Sheila Segurson*

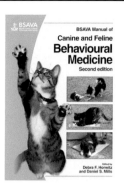

## Adopting a rescue dog: the pros and cons

**Many people choose dogs from rescue organizations or animal shelters; others avoid rescue dogs, due to worries about the dog's health or behaviour. Here are some of the advantages and disadvantages of adopting a dog from a reputable animal shelter or rescue group.**

## Breeds

⊕ By adopting a mixed-breed dog from a shelter, you might be reducing the risk of medical problems which are associated with purebreds.

⊖ Purebred dogs are also often available at shelters, but popular breeds may be difficult to acquire.

⊖ You may have less background information available than if you purchased a purebred from a reputable breeder, where you can obtain information about the dog's parents and ancestors, as well as research common behavioural characteristics and medical problems for the breed.

## Puppies

⊕ If you prefer a puppy, they are occasionally available at rescue centres.

⊖ While it is possible to adopt a puppy from a shelter, they may be much more difficult to find, and with unknown parentage their final form may be difficult to judge.

## Medical health

⊕ Most rescue dogs have had a veterinary exam, vaccinations, testing for and prevention of parasites, and are spayed or neutered. This thorough evaluation and treatment increases the likelihood that your new dog will be healthy.

⊖ Some dogs adopted from animal shelters or rescue groups may have diseases that they acquired while in the rehoming facility. Reduce this risk by asking your veterinary surgeon about reputable rescue centres with low risk of disease.

*continues* ▶

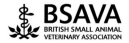
**BSAVA** BRITISH SMALL ANIMAL VETERINARY ASSOCIATION

# Adopting a rescue dog: the pros and cons

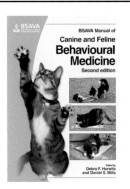

*continued*

## Behavioural health

⊕ Most rescue dogs have had a behaviour evaluation performed, in an attempt to determine their safety in a home and to match them to an appropriate home.

⊖ Many dogs at rescue organizations will have been surrendered because of behaviour problems. Find out as much as you can from the shelter about the dog's behavioural history, and the shelter's treatment of any problems, or post-adoption support policy. Ensuring a healthy relationship from the start is key.

## Training

⊕ Adopting an adult dog from a rescue centre may mean that you are acquiring an already obedient and housetrained dog.

⊖ Some dogs will have been surrendered because their owner did not have time to train them. If the shelter has not performed remedial training, you may be acquiring a dog that requires a significant investment in training. But if you are consistent, many training problems with previous owners will quickly disappear.

## Support

⊕ By adopting a rescue dog, you are supporting an organization whose primary goal is to save animals' lives and improve their welfare.

⊖ Ensure the shelter is reputable, with the animal's welfare considered foremost, or else you may not be supporting good welfare as much as you think you are.

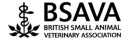

**BSAVA CLIENT HANDOUTS: BEHAVIOUR SERIES**

# Sit–stay exercises
*Ellen Lindell*

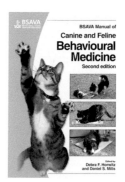

## Sit–stay exercises

Sit and stay exercises are designed to teach your dog to focus attention on you for direction, in order to receive behavioural cues.

## Principles

- Tiny food treats are used for positive reinforcement.
- In some cases the use of a headcollar and lead may be useful.
- Begin practising in a familiar area with minimal distractions. As your dog learns the task at hand, vary the location. Finally, add distractions.
- Initially, plan several short sessions over the course of the day. As you progress, sessions may vary from 5 to 15 minutes.

## Stage 1: Reward attention

1. Stand directly in front of your dog.
2. Show the treat to the dog, ask the dog to 'sit', give him/her the treat.*
3. Show the treat to the dog, say 'sit and stay', count to 2, reward with the treat.*
4. Repeat, randomly varying the count from 1 to 10 during each session.*

\* Reward your dog if he/she sits quietly and looks directly at you. During initial lessons, you may use the treat to lure attention to you.

- Throughout the lesson, encourage your dog to relax by repeating the word 'relax'.
- Your dog should remain in the 'sit' position until you calmly but clearly release him/her with a word such as 'OK'.

*continues* ▶

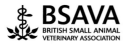
**BSAVA**
BRITISH SMALL ANIMAL
VETERINARY ASSOCIATION

**BSAVA CLIENT HANDOUTS: BEHAVIOUR SERIES**

## Sit–stay exercises

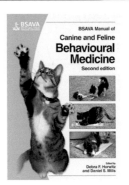

*continued*

---

### Stage 2: Reward relaxed attention

During initial sessions, your dog may be excited about earning treats. He/she may bark, or offer you other behaviours he/she has learned.

- Try to ignore any barking or pawing. Wait quietly; withhold the reward until he/she offers you the 'sit' as instructed.
- With repetition, the dog will begin to understand that the only way to earn a treat is to sit calmly and watch you. You may notice subtle relaxation of your dog's body posture. Reward these postures.

### Stage 3: Add distance and distractions

Once your dog can consistently sit–stay and quietly watch you for 10 seconds, you are ready to ask him/her to stay as you move away.

1. Stand directly in front of your dog.
2. Ask your dog to 'sit and stay' while you take a step away and return. Give a treat.*
3. Repeat the sequence, randomly varying the distance. Return to the dog and reward with the treat.*
4. As you progress, add some distractions such as clapping your hands, knocking on the floor or bouncing a ball.
5. Finally, walk to the door, and then knock on the door. After each event, return to the dog and give the treat.*
6. Alternate randomly between challenging tasks and simple ones.
7. Always end your lesson on a positive note. Pick an easy task such as a series of 1-second 'sits'.

* Reward your dog if he/she sits quietly and looks directly at you.

### Stage 4: Add challenging distractions

Sit–stay exercises can be used to manage many problem behaviours, including jumping up on guests and running after bicycles. The dog's reaction to these triggers can be reduced, but the process must be gradual.

*continues* ▶

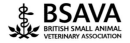
BRITISH SMALL ANIMAL
VETERINARY ASSOCIATION

## BSAVA CLIENT HANDOUTS: BEHAVIOUR SERIES

## Sit–stay exercises

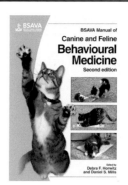

*continued*

Begin a lesson far enough away from the trigger that the dog is able to sit and stay. A lead and/or headcollar should be used for control, but this should not be a struggle. Use very delicious treats.

***Example:*** Sit–stay to control jumping up on guests (this exercise should not be attempted until the dog has mastered the sit–stay while a family member walks to the door, opens and closes door, and returns to the dog).

1. When the guest enters the house, the dog should be restrained by lead (and headcollar) several feet from the door, out of the path of the visitor.
2. The dog should sit and stay to earn high-value treats.
3. Keep the dog's attention, rewarding quiet behaviour, while guests settle.
4. Maintain the sit–stay for several minutes. Do not release the stay until the dog has relaxed and is not attempting to look toward the guests.
5. Once the dog is calm, he/she may be released to greet the visitors.
6. Guests should pet the dog only if he/she sits quietly.

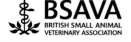

**BSAVA**
BRITISH SMALL ANIMAL
VETERINARY ASSOCIATION

## BSAVA CLIENT HANDOUTS: BEHAVIOUR SERIES

# Treating a fear of the veterinary clinic using desensitization and counter-conditioning
*Clara Palestrini*

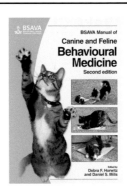

## Treating a fear of the veterinary clinic using desensitization and counter-conditioning

Fear of a specific place, such as the veterinary clinic, can be treated using a desensitization and counter-conditioning (DSCC) programme. In simple terms, your pet must be exposed to the fearful stimulus in such a way that he/she sees there is nothing to fear, and settles down. If the association with the stimulus can be turned into one that is positive, your pet may actually develop a positive attitude to the occurrence.

### 1 Preparation

- This programme generally involves multiple and controlled visits to the clinic, starting with visits involving no direct manipulation and only positive reinforcement of calm behaviours, followed by simulations of visits when the fear response is no longer present. It is therefore important that owners and the veterinary surgeon work together on this problem and agree on times for training.
- Prevent the pet from experiencing the triggers except during training sessions.
- Avoid taking your pet to the clinic unless it is part of the structured training programme or, of course, a medical necessity. Setbacks may occur if the pet is suddenly in need of medical attention, but its welfare must **not** be compromised by delaying such a need.
- Encourage calm and relaxed behaviours in the absence of the fear-inducing stimuli.

### 2 Expose your pet to the place of which it is afraid, starting at a very low level of exposure

- **Gradual desensitization** is the key. It is important to establish a *gradient* of the stimuli to be presented. During gradual exposure to these stimuli, it is important that they are only presented below the threshold at which the fearful behaviour is triggered.
- Take your pet on trips to the clinic but only expose him/her to a point where he/she remains calm and comfortable.
- For example, you may need to stay in front of the clinic door, or even in the car on the first few trips.

*continues* ▶

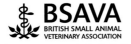

BRITISH SMALL ANIMAL
VETERINARY ASSOCIATION

**BSAVA CLIENT HANDOUTS: BEHAVIOUR SERIES**

# Treating a fear of the veterinary clinic using desensitization and counter-conditioning

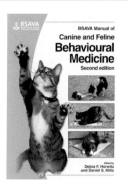

*continued*

---

### 3 Try to change your pet's perception by associating the place with something positive

- Make sure you know what your pet's most favoured rewards are and save these for the training sessions. For some pets, food is the strongest reinforcer, while others may be more responsive to a favoured play toy or social contact.
- The reward should be presented to your pet for non-fearful responses, such as a relaxed 'sit', along each step of the training gradient.

### 4 Strengthen the resilience of your pet

- As your pet's response improves, encourage him/her to accept more intense situations, such as staying in the waiting room.
- It is important to reward calm responses, such as a relaxed 'sit', along each step of the training gradient.
- **Advance along the gradient very slowly. If the pet shows even the slightest fear response he/she should be removed from the situation and the intensity of the next exposure must be reduced to one that remains below the fear threshold.**
- Gradually you should be able to enter the examination room with your pet remaining calm.

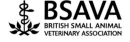

**BSAVA**
BRITISH SMALL ANIMAL
VETERINARY ASSOCIATION

**BSAVA CLIENT HANDOUTS: BEHAVIOUR SERIES**

What your cat needs

*Irene Rochlitz*

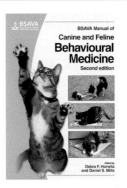

## What your cat needs

**The inside of your home is the heart of your cat's territory, where your cat should feel safe and comfortable. Here is a list of the important things to consider when arranging your house to meet your cat's needs.**

### Space

- There should be enough space for your cat, at least two rooms.
- More important than the amount of space is its quality. This means making sure your cat can make use of the space, especially the vertical dimension.
- Cats like to climb and spent a lot of time off the floor, on raised surfaces such as shelves placed at different heights, window sills, cat activity centres or even on the tops of wardrobes and cupboards if they can be reached easily.

### Food and water

- Your cat should receive a balanced diet that is correct for its lifestage (kitten, adult, senior).
- It is better to feed your cat several small meals during the day, rather than two larger meals.
- If your cat is overweight or easily bored, try stimulating 'hunting' behaviour by hiding pieces of dry food for your cat to discover, or using a puzzle feeder.
- Offer clean water next to the food bowl and also in a place away from the feeding area.

*continues* ▶

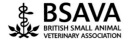

**BSAVA CLIENT HANDOUTS: BEHAVIOUR SERIES**

# What your cat needs

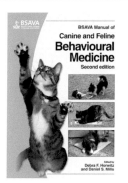

*continued*

## Litter tray (box)

- If your cats are kept indoors, there should be one litter tray per cat, plus one extra one. These should be in multiple locations to allow all cats easy access to them.
- Make sure the trays are kept clean and free of smells, by scooping out soiled litter once or twice a day.
- Clean the trays and replace litter as often as is necessary to keep them clean and odour-free.
- Place the trays in quiet but easily accessible areas; avoid busy areas or very remote locations.
- In multi-level houses, make sure there is a litter tray on each floor.
- Make sure the litter trays are big enough: at least 1.5 times the length of the cat, and that the cat can get in and out easily.
- Most cats prefer uncovered boxes and unscented, clumping fine-grained litter.
- Size of tray, placement and cleaning frequency may be different for kittens and senior cats.

## Resting and sleeping areas

- Cats spend a lot of their time resting and sleeping, so there should be plenty of comfortable areas for them throughout the home.
- Some of these areas should be raised off the floor on higher surfaces such as chairs, beds and shelves.

## Hiding places

- Being able to hide helps cats cope with challenges, changes and stress in their environment.
- Hiding places can be boxes, crates, baskets, wardrobes or cupboards with the door left open.
- A comfortable hiding place can also serve as a rest or sleep area, especially if it is raised off the floor and is a good look-out (vantage) point.

*continues* ▶

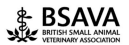
**BSAVA**
BRITISH SMALL ANIMAL
VETERINARY ASSOCIATION

© BSAVA 2009
BSAVA Manual of Canine and Feline Behavioural Medicine, 2nd edition

## BSAVA CLIENT HANDOUTS: BEHAVIOUR SERIES

# What your cat needs

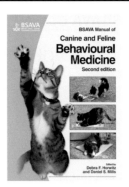

*continued*

## Claw scratching

- Claw scratching is a normal behaviour that cats do to stretch their muscles, keep their claws in good condition and also to leave scent that marks their territory.
- Good surfaces for scratching include scratch posts, sisal rope, hessian, rush matting, cardboard and pieces of carpet and wood.
- Scratching surfaces should be put at places of entry and exit into the home where new smells are brought in (for example, by the front door or the door to the garden/yard).
- Scratching surfaces should also be placed next to resting or sleeping areas, as cats often stretch and sharpen their claws after waking.
- Prominent surfaces such as corners of furniture are often used, so these can be covered with a suitable material for scratching, or scratch posts placed next to them.
- Cats often like vertical scratching surfaces that are high enough for them to stretch fully and with a vertical thread to pull the claws through, though horizontal scratching surfaces may also be used.

## Human contact

- Most cats enjoy having contact with their owner, so owners should spend time every day with their cats, preferably for at least 10 to 15 minutes a session, several times a day.
- Some cats will enjoy being petted and groomed and handled, while others will like to play.
- Try to identify the kind of toy your cat prefers to play with.
- Toys that mimic small prey are often best, if they flutter or squeak when touched, move rapidly or suddenly, or have feathers or are covered in soft fur so much the better.
- Other toys include 'fishing' rods, ping-pong balls, bouncy or self-propelling toys.
- Cats will get bored with playing with the same toys so there should be a variety and they should be replaced frequently.

*continues* ▶

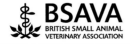
**BSAVA** BRITISH SMALL ANIMAL VETERINARY ASSOCIATION

**BSAVA CLIENT HANDOUTS: BEHAVIOUR SERIES**

# What your cat needs

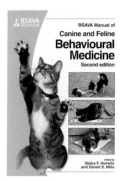

*continued*

## Activity and exploration

- It is important for cats to be active, as this helps prevent obesity and boredom, especially if your cat is kept indoors all the time.
- Offer your cat things to explore, such as large boxes, large paper bags and other structures.
- Access to the outdoors will provide your cat with a wide range of stimuli and opportunities for exercise but may be associated with certain dangers.
- If your cat is unable to go out freely, consider making a secure pen or other type of enclosure outdoors, or training your cat to go out on a harness and lead.
- Using techniques to stimulate feeding behaviour will also encourage activity.

## Stimulation of the senses

- Even if your cat is confined indoors, he/she can enjoy outdoor stimuli (sounds, sights and smells) by using window sills, viewing platforms near windows, or using secure balconies or other enclosures.
- Audiovisual products are available for cats, which contain images and sounds of nature that may be of interest to them.
- Catnip is a well-known stimulant that some cats enjoy.
- Some cats like to chew certain types of grass that can be grown in containers or pots.
- Surfaces that cats have used for scent marking (such as corners of tables and doors that cats have rubbed against) should not be cleaned too often.
- Many cats do not like household sprays containing citrus scents.

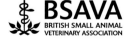

# Index

# Index

# Index

# Index